...n and Management
of Early Psychosis

A Preventive Approach

Second Edition

The Recognition and Management of Early Psychosis

A Preventive Approach

Second Edition

Edited by

Henry J. Jackson

and

Patrick D. McGorry

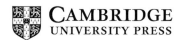

CAMBRIDGE
UNIVERSITY PRESS

CAMBRIDGE UNIVERSITY PRESS

Cambridge, New York, Melbourne, Madrid, Cape Town, Singapore, São Paulo, Delhi, Dubai, Tokyo, Mexico City

Cambridge University Press
The Edinburgh Building, Cambridge CB2 8RU, UK

Published in the United States of America by Cambridge University Press, New York

www.cambridge.org
Information on this title: www.cambridge.org/9780521617314

First published 2009
Reprinted with corrections 2010

Printed in the United Kingdom at the University Press, Cambridge

A catalogue record for this publication is available from the British Library

Library of Congress Cataloguing in Publication data
The recognition and management of early psychosis : a preventive approach / edited by Henry J. Jackson and Patrick D. McGorry. – 2nd ed.
    p.   ;   cm.
Includes bibliographical references and index.
ISBN 978-0-521-61731-4 (pbk.)
1. Psychoses.   I. Jackson, Henry J.   II. McGorry, Patrick D.   III. Title.
[DNLM: 1. Psychotic Disorders – diagnosis.   2. Psychotic Disorders – therapy.   WM 200 311 2009]
RC512.R43   2009
616.89–dc22
2008040778

ISBN 978-0-521-61731-4 Paperback

HENRY: The book is dedicated to my deceased parents Henry George and Elizabeth Jackson, who gave me love, support and encouragement, a sense of curiosity and imparted the importance of generosity and a commitment to helping others, and to my son Carl, for his love, support and independent perspectives.

PATRICK: The book is also dedicated to my deceased parents, Desmond and Margaret, who created unique opportunities for me to contribute, and my sons Liam, Niall and Fionn, who have quite different ones.

Contents

List of contributors   *page* xi
Foreword
Jan Olav Johannessen   xvii
Acknowledgements   xix

Section 1   Introduction   1

1   Rationale for and overview of the second
    edition of *The Recognition and
    Management of Early Psychosis*
    Henry J. Jackson, Patrick D. McGorry
    and Kelly Allott   3

2   Diagnosis and the staging model of
    psychosis
    Patrick D. McGorry, Kelly Allott and Henry
    J. Jackson   17

Section 2   Risk and vulnerability   29

3   Genetic vulnerability
    Daniel Weinberger and Gregor Berger   31

4   Environmental vulnerability and genetic–
    environmental interactions
    Jim van Os and Richie Poulton   47

5   Neurobiological endophenotypes of
    psychosis and schizophrenia: are there
    biological markers of illness onset?
    Christos Pantelis, Murat Yücel, Stephen
    J. Wood, Warrick J. Brewer, Alex Fornito,
    Gregor Berger, Tyrone Cannon and Dennis
    Velakoulis   61

Section 3   At-risk mental state   81

6   At-risk mental state and prediction
    Alison R. Yung, Joachim Klosterkötter,
    Barbara Cornblatt and Frauke Schultze-Lutter   83

7   At-risk mental state: management
    Lisa J. Phillips, Jean Addington and Anthony
    P. Morrison   107

**Section 4   Access and reducing delay
to treatment: reducing the duration
of untreated psychosis**   123

8   Duration of untreated psychosis:
    definition, measurement and
    association with outcome
    Max Marshall, Susy Harrigan and Shon Lewis   125

9   Improving the community's mental
    health literacy as a means of facilitating
    early intervention
    Anthony F. Jorm and Annemarie Wright   147

10   Pathways to care and reducing
    treatment delay in early psychosis
    Ross M. G. Norman and Ashok K. Malla   161

Section 5   The first episode   175

11   Initial assessment and initial
    pharmacological treatment in the acute
    phase
    Martin Lambert   177

12   Complete and incomplete recovery
    from first-episode psychosis
    Jean Addington, Tim Lambert and Peter
    Burnett   201

13   Preventive strategies in bipolar
    disorders: identifying targets for early
    intervention
    Philippe Conus, Michael Berk, Nellie Lucas,
    José Luis Vázquez-Barquero and Craig
    Macneil   223

**Section 6   The critical period: other
psychopathology and comorbidity**   241

14   Substance misuse in first-episode
    psychosis
    Darryl Wade, Leanne Hides, Amanda Baker
    and Dan Lubman   243

15   Suicide prevention in first-episode
    psychosis
    Paddy Power and Jo Robinson   257

16   Emotional and personality dysfunctions
    in early psychosis
    Max Birchwood, John Gleeson, Andrew
    Chanen, Louise K. McCutcheon, Shona M.
    Francey and Maria Michail   283

**Section 7   The critical period:
specific interventions**   303

17   Family intervention in early psychosis
    Catharine McNab and Don Linszen   305

18   Enhancing work functioning in early
    psychosis
    Eóin Killackey, Henry J. Jackson, David
    Fowler and Keith H. Nuechterlein   331

19   Relapse prevention in early psychosis
    John Gleeson, Don Linszen and Durk
    Wiersma   349

20   Treatment resistance in first-episode
      psychosis
      Christian G. Huber and Martin Lambert   365

Section 8   Service models   383

21   Using research and evaluation to inform
      the development of
      early-psychosis service models:
      international examples
      Meredith Harris, Thomas Craig, Robert B.
      Zipursky, Donald Addington, Merete
      Nordentoft and Paddy Power   385

Index   405

Contributors

Donald Addington
Professor and Chair, Department of Psychiatry,
University of Calgary Head, Regional Clinical Department
of Psychiatry, Foothills Hospital, Calgary, Canada

Jean Addington
Professor of Psychiatry, University of Toronto,
Director, Prime Clinic, First Episode Psychosis
Program, Centre for Addiction and Mental Health,
Toronto, Canada

Kelly Allott
Research Fellow and Clinical Neuropsychologist,
ORYGEN Research Centre and Department of
Psychiatry, University of Melbourne, Parkville, Australia

Amanda Baker
Associate Professor and Senior Clinical Psychologist,
Centre for Brain and Mental Health Research,
University of Newcastle, Callaghan, Australia

Gregor Berger
University Hospital Basel, Department of Psychiatry,
Basel, Switzerland and Deputy Chief Psychiatrist,
The Schlössli Clinic, Zürich, Switzerland, and
Senior Lecturer, University of Melbourne, Parkville,
Australia

Michael Berk
Professor of Psychiatry, Barwon Health and the Geelong
Clinic, ORYGEN Research Centre and Mental Health
Research Institute, University of Melbourne, Geelong,
Australia

Max Birchwood
Professor of Clinical Psychology, School of Psychology, University of Birmingham and Director, Birmingham Early Intervention Service, Birmingham, UK

Warrick J. Brewer
Associate Professor of Neuropsychology, ORYGEN Research Centre and Early Psychosis Prevention and Intervention Centre, Department of Psychiatry, University of Melbourne, Parkville, Australia

Peter Burnett
Medical Director, ORYGEN Youth Health, Clinical Associate Professor, Department of Psychiatry, University of Melbourne, Parkville, Australia

Tyrone Cannon
Staglin Family Professor, Departments of Psychology and Psychiatry and Biobehavioral Sciences, University of California at Los Angeles, California, USA

Andrew Chanen
Senior Lecturer, ORYGEN Research Centre, Department of Psychiatry, University of Melbourne and Consultant Psychiatrist and Associate Medical Director, ORYGEN Youth Health, Parkville, Australia

Philippe Conus
Maître d'Enseignement et de Recherche, Université de Lausanne, Médecin Associé, Département de Psychiatrie CHUV, Treatment and Intervention in Early Psychosis Program, Clinique de Cery, Switzerland

Barbara Cornblatt
Professor of Psychiatry, Albert Einstein College of Medicine Director, Recognition and Prevention Program, Zucker Hillside Hospital, Division of Psychiatry Research, Glen Oaks, New York, USA

Thomas Craig
Professor of Social Psychiatry, King's College London, Institute of Psychiatry Health Services and Population Research Department, Denmark Hill and Honorary Consultant Psychiatrist, South London and Maudsley NHS Foundation Trust, London, UK

Alex Fornito
Melbourne Neuropsychiatry Centre, Department of Psychiatry, University of Melbourne, Royal Melbourne Hospital, Sunshine Hospital and National Neuroscience Facility, Melbourne, Australia

David Fowler
Professor of Social Psychiatry, School of Medicine, Health Policy and Practice, University of East Anglia, Norwich, UK

Shona M. Francey
Coordinator, Early Psychosis Prevention and Intervention Centre, ORYGEN Youth Health, Parkville, Australia

John Gleeson
Acting Senior Advisor, Clinical Psychology, North Western Mental Health Program, Associate Professor of Psychology, Department of Psychology, University of Melbourne, Parkville, Australia

Susy Harrigan
Research Fellow, ORYGEN Research Centre, Department of Psychiatry, University of Melbourne, Parkville, Australia

Meredith Harris
Senior Research Officer, School of Population Health, University of Queensland, Queensland Centre for Mental Health Research, The Park – Centre for Mental Health, Richlands, Australia

Leanne Hides
Clinical Research Coordinator and Research Fellow, Substance Use Research and Recovery Focused Program, ORYGEN Research Centre, Department of Psychiatry, University of Melbourne, Parkville, Australia

Christian G. Huber
Clinical Fellow, Psychosis Early Detection and Intervention Centre, Department of Psychiatry and Psychotherapy, Centre for Psychosocial Medicine, University Medical Centre, Hamburg-Eppendorf, Hamburg, Germany

Henry J. Jackson
Professor of Psychology, School of Behavioural Science, Department of Psychology, University of Melbourne, Parkville, Australia

Anthony F. Jorm
Professorial Fellow, ORYGEN Research Centre and Department of Psychiatry, University of Melbourne, Parkville, Australia

Eóin Killackey
Senior Research Fellow and Clinical Psychologist, ORYGEN Research Centre and Department of Psychology, University of Melbourne, Parkville, Australia

Joachim Klosterkötter
Professor and Head of Department, Department of Psychiatry and Psychotherapy, University of Cologne, Cologne, Germany

Martin Lambert
Associate Professor, Consultant Psychiatrist, Psychosis Early Detection and Intervention Centre, Department of Psychiatry and Psychotherapy, Centre for Psychosocial Medicine, University Medical Centre Hamburg-Eppendorf, Hamburg, Germany

Tim Lambert
Professor and Chair, Psychological Medicine, University of Sydney Concord Medical School Head, Schizophrenia Treatments and Outcomes Research, Brain and Mind Research Institute, University of Sydney Director, First Episode Psychosis, Sydney, Australia

Shon Lewis
Professor of Adult Psychiatry, University of Manchester, Wythenshawe Hospital, Manchester, UK

Don Linszen
Professor of Psychiatry, Adolescent Clinic, Academical Medical Centre of the University of Amsterdam, Amsterdam, the Netherlands

Dan Lubman
Associate Professor, Substance Use Research and Recovery Focused Program, ORYGEN Research Centre, Department of Psychiatry, University of Melbourne, Parkville, Australia

Nellie Lucas
Research Fellow and Clinical Psychologist, ORYGEN Research Centre, Parkville, Australia

Craig Macneil
Senior Clinical Psychologist, Early Psychosis Prevention and Intervention Centre, ORYGEN Youth Health, Parkville, Australia

Ashok K. Malla
Professor and Canada Research Chair in Early Psychosis, Department of Psychiatry, McGill University Director, Clinical Research Division and Prevention and Early Intervention Program for Psychoses, Douglas Mental Health University Institute, Montréal, Canada

Max Marshall
Professor of Community Psychiatry, Division of Psychiatry, University of Manchester and Medical Director of Lancashire Care NHS Trust, The Lantern Centre, Preston, UK

Louise K. McCutcheon
Senior Project Manager, HYPE Training, ORYGEN Research Centre and Coordinator, HYPE Clinic, ORYGEN Youth Health, Parkville, Australia

Patrick D. McGorry
Professor of Youth Mental Health, University of Melbourne, Executive Director, ORYGEN Research Centre and Director of Clinical Services, ORYGEN Youth Health, Parkville, Australia

Catharine McNab
Psychologist, ORYGEN Youth Health, Parkville, Australia

Maria Michail
Trial Manager, COMMAND Trial, School of Psychology, University of Birmingham, Birmingham, UK

Anthony P. Morrison
Professor of Clinical Psychology, School of
Psychological Sciences, University of Manchester,
Manchester, UK

Merete Nordentoft
Professor and Chief Physician, Copenhagen University
Hospital, Psychiatric University Centre, Copenhagen,
Denmark

Ross M. G. Norman
Professor, Departments of Psychiatry and
Epidemiology and Biostatistics, University of Western
Ontario, Prevention and Early Intervention Program for
Psychoses, London, Canada

Keith H. Nuechterlein
Director, Center for Neurocognition and Emotion in
Schizophrenia, Professor, Departments of Psychiatry
and Psychology, Semel Institute for Neuroscience and
Human Behaviour, University of California at Los
Angeles, California, USA

Christos Pantelis
Professor of Neuropsychiatry and Scientific Director,
Melbourne Neuropsychiatry Centre, University of
Melbourne and Melbourne Health, Parkville, Australia

Lisa J. Phillips
Senior Lecturer, Department of Psychology, University
of Melbourne, Parkville, Australia

Richie Poulton
Professor and Director, Dunedin Multidisciplinary
Health and Development Research Unit, Department
of Preventive and Social Medicine, Dunedin School of
Medicine, University of Otago, Dunedin, New Zealand

Paddy Power
Lead Consultant Psychiatrist, Lambeth Early Onset
service, South London and Maudsley NHS Foundation
Trust and Honorary Senior Lecturer, Departments of
Psychological Medicine and Psychiatry and Health
Service and Population Research, Institute of
Psychiatry, King's College London, London, UK

Jo Robinson
Research Fellow, ORYGEN Research Centre and
Department of Psychiatry, University of Melbourne,
Parkville, Australia

Frauke Schultze-Lutter
Scientific-Psychological Head of Early Recognition and
Intervention Centre for Mental Crises, Department of
Psychiatry and Psychotherapy, University of Cologne,
Cologne, Germany

Jim van Os
Professor and Head, Department of Psychiatry and
Neuropsychology, South Limburg Mental Health
Research and Teaching Network, EURON, Maastricht
University, Maastricht, the Netherlands and Division of
Psychological Medicine, Institute of Psychiatry,
London, UK

José Luis Vázquez-Barquero
Head Professor, Department of Psychiatry
Director, Psychiatric Research Unit of Cantabria
(WHO Collaborating Centre), University
Hospital 'Marqués de Valdecilla', Servicio de
Psiquiatria, University of Cantabria, Santander,
Spain

Dennis Velakoulis
Clinical Director, Melbourne Neuropsychiatry
Centre, University of Melbourne and Melbourne
Health Director, Neuropsychiatry Unit, Royal
Melbourne Hospital, Melbourne, Australia

Darryl Wade
Clinical Psychologist and Honorary Senior Fellow,
Department of Psychiatry, University of Melbourne,
Parkville, Australia

Daniel Weinberger
Director, Genes, Cognition and Psychosis
Program, National Institute of Mental Health,
National Institutes of Health, Bethesda,
Maryland, USA

Durk Wiersma
Professor of Clinical Epidemiology of Psychiatric
Disorders, University Centre Psychiatry, Director,
Rob Giel Research Centre, University Medical Centre,
University of Groningen, Groningen, the Netherlands

Stephen J. Wood
Senior Research Fellow, Melbourne Neuropsychiatry
Centre, National Neuroscience Facility, Carlton South,
Australia

Annemarie Wright
Research Officer and Honorary Fellow, Department of
Psychiatry, University of Melbourne and ORYGEN
Research Centre, Parkville, Australia

Murat Yücel
ORYGEN Research Centre and Melbourne
Neuropsychiatry Centre, Department of Psychiatry,
University of Melbourne, Melbourne, Australia

Alison R. Yung
Professor, Department of Psychiatry, University of
Melbourne and ORYGEN Research Centre, Parkville,
Australia

Robert B. Zipursky
Professor and Chair, Department of Psychiatry and
Behavioural Neurosciences, Michael G. DeGroote
School of Medicine, McMaster University Vice
President, Mental Health and Addiction Services,
St. Joseph's Healthcare Hamilton and Hamilton Health
Sciences, Hamilton, Canada

Foreword

The concept of early intervention in psychiatric disorders is not a new one, but thanks to a number of researchers, including the editors of and contributors to this book, the area of early intervention has gained great prominence over the last two decades. When it comes to dealing with the serious psychiatric disorders, such as psychosis in general and schizophrenia in particular, I am of the opinion that the research, clinical and service developments that have originated from this work represents the most important step forward since the introduction of antipsychotic drugs in the mid 1950s.

Until recently, research carried out on patients with psychosis, including schizophrenia, has focused on heterogeneous samples. Studies reported on mixtures of old and young people; new and chronic cases; males and females; and people with very different symptoms (including various kinds of hallucination and delusion), long and short durations of illness, and long and short durations of untreated psychosis (DUP). All have been collapsed into the same groups and studied as if they required the same treatments and carried similar prognoses.

A major advancement introduced by the early-intervention paradigm, and resultant strategies, is that we study more 'refined' and better-defined diagnostic subgroups in our current research endeavours: that is, young people with first-episode psychosis (FEP), as opposed to older patients with longer durations of illness. We are able to study the impact of psychosis itself by studying such factors as DUP and duration of untreated illness. Furthermore, we can now focus on young people deemed to be at risk for developing a psychotic disorder, and as such, pursue the possibility of preventive strategies in this previously pessimistic field.

Although DUP is not a perfect measure and in itself relates to positive symptoms, currently, it is the best single measure for assessing delay in treatment. We need to develop and improve on this and other concepts. We need to gain better insight into the mechanisms underpinning the different responses to treatment experienced by various people. The ideas that psychosis is neurotoxic itself and that psychosis could be *socially* toxic both need to be further explored.

It is a paradox that the acceptance of the early-intervention paradigm as the 'correct' strategy should have to be 'proven' through extensive research. If we ask the question, 'Is it ethical to allow a young person suffering from psychosis to go undiagnosed and untreated and, if so, for how long?', the answer would be evident to most people. For some obscure reason, until just a few years ago, there was substantial resistance to the idea of early intervention. Researchers and clinicians advocating early-intervention strategies had to prove their case. This seems strange. One would imagine that efforts to bring young people to treatment earlier in the illness course would be welcomed by all – at least when considered from the purely humanistic position of shortening another person's severe mental suffering.

Luckily, there has been a shift in the tide, brought about by the important and impressive results from early-intervention services around the globe. There are strong indications that early intervention with FEP patients leads to a better prognosis, as measured by fewer negative symptoms, less suicidal ideation, fewer suicidal plans and attempts, and probably a reduction in suicides. Importantly, the provision of special adapted treatment programmes for FEP patients produces results superior to treatment as usual. Early-intervention research and clinical practice has also resulted in the adoption of more careful and adapted medical treatment strategies, with lower dosages of antipsychotic drugs now being the standard practice.

Several projects investigating the so-called 'prodromal' phase and the possibility of preventing 'at-risk' individuals from progressing into manifest psychosis

are so promising that we are now looking for the best way to develop and adapt clinical service systems for these patients. Linked to this are efforts to model a user-friendly service system to achieve early intervention. What is the best way to do this? And when is early *early*? The field has developed and introduced a variety of service models, and the last word has not been written in this connection. However, it has been demonstrated that two elements are necessary if one wishes to establish a system for early intervention: (1) low threshold for care/easy access to care, and (2) information about available help and early signs of serious psychiatric disorders. There also seems to be a consensus that some early-intervention active outreach strategies, such as the employment of detection teams, is a prerequisite to achieve early intervention; it is still somewhat dubious whether these themes should also have treatment tasks. Probably that is a question that should be further explored. Still, one should not confuse 'early-intervention services', which intervene *early*, with 'FEP services', which intervene without focusing on achieving earlier intervention.

In addition to its obvious clinical advantages, early recognition of psychosis opens new windows of opportunity for early-psychosis treatment and service research. For me personally, the possibility of developing better, more effective and adapted psychological treatments is the most challenging and rewarding task. There is, however, ample space and opportunity for other aspects of treatment research as well, for example for family treatments, such as multifamily group therapy.

This book takes the field a major step forward and sets a new standard for research, service development and clinical practice. It represents optimism in psychiatry and mental health, integrating treatment development with prevention strategies. It is practical, but theoretically well founded. There is no longer any excuse for not doing early intervention!

Jan Olav Johannessen, M.D. Ph.D.
Chief Psychiatrist, Stavanger University Hospital,
Stavanger, Norway

Acknowledgements

We both express our deepest gratitude to Dr Kelly Allott in assisting us with the editing of this book. The completion of this book is due in large part to her assiduity, attention to detail, warmth and charm.

Henry wishes to thank members of his family – Elissa, Chris, Tom and Sue – for their constant love and support, Dr Christine Simons for her warmth, helpful insights and wisdom, and Effie and Bill Patrikakos of Strathmos for supplying nourishment and an atmosphere of conviviality during the course of this project.

Patrick wishes to thank all of his family for their love and support, and their patience with and support for this long-term project, which has consumed so much life and energy over the past 20 years.

We thank all of our colleagues at EPPIC and its diaspora, as well as all our friends and colleagues from all parts of the globe who have been so committed to helping people with early psychosis, to understanding the nature of these illnesses, to establishing relevant youth-friendly mental health services in their countries, and to furthering development of the early psychosis paradigm. This has been a remarkable story of international cooperation and goodwill, which will one day be fully documented.

Finally, and most importantly, we would like to express our gratitude and admiration to all those who experience early psychosis. You have been our essential guides and teachers in our quest to improve understanding, detection and care.

SECTION 1

Introduction

Rationale for and overview of the second edition of *The Recognition and Management of Early Psychosis*

Henry J. Jackson, Patrick D. McGorry and Kelly Allott

Introduction and rationale

This is the second edition of our book entitled *The Recognition and Management of Early Psychosis* first published in 1999 (McGorry & Jackson, 1999). Although this book is a second edition, every single chapter is completely new. In fact, we have an almost completely different set of authors for this second edition. The chief reason for this resides in the explosion of literature on early psychosis over the last decade. Different areas of interest have emerged along with another generation of researchers, clinicians and colleagues from a diversity of countries around the globe. Represented in this book are authors from Australia, New Zealand, Canada, the UK, the USA, Spain, the Netherlands, Germany, Denmark and Switzerland.

Using the search terms, 'early psychosis', 'first onset psychosis', 'first episode psychosis', 'first episode schizophrenia', 'at risk for psychosis', 'ultra high risk for psychosis' and 'prodrom* psychosis', we conducted electronic database searches (PsycINFO, MEDLINE, and Web of Science) to locate relevant articles and book chapters from 1988 to 1997. We then did the same for 1998 to 2007. We chose these two 10-year periods because the first edition of our book, although published in 1999, was completed a year before that (1998). The results are shown in Table 1.1, which provides a breakdown according to search term, electronic database and decade.

From Table 1.1, it can be seen that the three databases identify widely different total numbers of papers and different numbers of papers within the seven specific search term categories. Of the three databases,

MEDLINE identifies the lowest number of total papers (4263 compared with the other two databases with 7750 and 9828, respectively). But it can be seen that irrespective of the database, there has truly been an explosion in the literature, with MEDLINE identifying a four-fold increase in publications for the 1998–2007 decade compared with the 1988–1997 decade, PsycINFO a 48-fold increase and Web of Science a 6.5-fold increase. Notably, the 'ultra high risk' and 'prodrome' categories have the lowest absolute numbers of publications uncovered in the 1998–2007 period, but very few articles were uncovered for the 1988–1997 decade, so there has been some increase in numbers over time for these two categories. This striking increase in the salience of the 'early psychosis' field reflects the growth of a major new paradigm in the mental health field.

Book overview

The book is organized into eight sections. The first introductory section, comprising this chapter and Ch. 2, provides an overview of the book's content and a staging-model approach to the prevention and intervention of early psychosis. In Ch. 2, McGorry, Allott and Jackson set the scene for a preventatively oriented approach to the recognition and management of early psychosis, and put forward a model for achieving this. The continuum of preventive intervention, namely, universal, selective and indicated prevention, developed by Mrazek and Haggerty (1994), is briefly reviewed. The authors then introduce a clinical staging model – a heuristic framework – which builds upon the

The Recognition and Management of Early Psychosis: A Preventive Approach, ed. Henry J. Jackson and Patrick D. McGorry.
Published by Cambridge University Press. © Cambridge University Press 2009.

Table 1.1. Number of citations pertaining to early psychosis in the decades prior to, and following, the first edition of *The Recognition and Management of Early Psychosis*

Search term	PsycINFO		MEDLINE		Web of Science	
	1988–1997	1998–2007	1988–1997	1998–2007	1988–1997	1998–2007
'early psychosis'	17	1071	388	1333	336	1838
'first onset psychosis'	5	133	174	509	144	767
'first episode psychosis'	42	2558	148	907	171	1834
'first episode schizophrenia'	89	3795	275	1210	361	2458
'at risk for psychosis'	6	85	3	2	473	2380
'ultra high risk for psychosis'	0	63	0	50	0	122
'prodrom* psychosis'	1	45	39	252	35	429
Cumulative total[a]	160	7750	1027	4263	1520	9828

[a] Note that there may be duplication of articles across search terms.

preventive intervention model by viewing psychosis as a stage-based illness, whereby each stage requires different treatment strategies and implies different prognoses. The rationale for a clinical staging approach to psychosis is, in part, related to the issues surrounding the validity of the diagnosis of psychotic disorder, particularly when prevention and early intervention is the focus. Issues impacting upon the validity of the diagnosis of psychosis include the fact that symptoms and syndromes are not necessarily concrete and stable across phases of disorder, especially at the earliest stages; the presence of 'non-specific' symptoms in the prodromal and first-episode phases of disorder that do not fall within the psychosis diagnostic category, but clearly require treatment; the phenotypic heterogeneity and continuum of patient presentations, which require clinical judgement as to their level of 'abnormality' or 'psychopathology'; and the relative non-specificity of neurobiological markers of illness. The authors, therefore, argue for a phase-of-disorder and treatment-oriented approach to diagnosis.

The remainder of the chapter is devoted to describing the early stages of the four-stage clinical staging model of diagnosis and intervention in psychosis, which guides the clinician in selecting the safest and most effective treatments that are most appropriate to the specific stage of illness. The clinical staging model

implies that early successful treatment may improve prognosis and prevent progression to more severe stages of disorder. In line with the theme of the book, the early stages of psychosis are unpacked in detail in relation to the staging model: stage 0, increased risk for psychosis; stage 1a, mild non-specific symptoms, mild/moderate fall in functioning; stage 1b, ultra-high risk (UHR) or prodromal phase; stage 2, first-episode psychosis (FEP); stage 3a, incomplete recovery or treatment resistance; and stage 4, sustained disability and treatment resistance. Over time, and with further research, the eventual aim is to move toward a 'clinicopathological' staging model as in other disorders, which incorporates clinical phenomena, functioning and neurobiological variables.

In Section 2 (Chs. 3 to 5), the broad and critical area of risk and vulnerability for psychosis is explored, with a specific focus on the role of genetic, neurobiological and environmental risk factors and their interactions in the expression of psychotic illness. Chapter 3 (Weinberger and Berger) provides a comprehensive overview of current knowledge regarding the complex area of psychosis genetics. The authors point out that despite family, twin and adoption studies revealing a high genetic liability, with a point estimation of 81%, single major-effect genes have not been detected and the precise molecular aetiology of psychosis currently remains unknown. The authors argue that the low effect size of individual marker loci and the heterogeneous phenotype of schizophrenia make replication of genome-wide linkage studies difficult. Nevertheless, linkage and allelic association studies have identified several candidate genes for susceptibility to psychotic disorder, including the genes for dysbindin (*DTNBP1*), neuregulin (*NRG1*), D-amino acid oxidase activator (*DAOA*; G72), regulator of G-protein signalling-4 (*RGS4*), catechol-*O*-methyltransferase (*COMT*), the 'disrupted in schizophrenia' genes (*DISC1* and *DISC2*) and the gene for brain-derived neurotrophic factor (*BDNF*). The authors also briefly describe the fields of intermediate phenotype (i.e. endophenotype) and epigenetic research, as adjuncts to traditional genetic approaches. It is argued that, to date, the evidence points towards either the involvement of multiple genes, with small effects across diverse populations or a heterogeneous aetio-pathology – or a combination of both. It is suggested that complex inheritance patterns of detrimental and protective genes may define the threshold for expression of psychosis, but only in the presence of certain environmental impacts (e.g. obstetric complications, substance use, stressful life events) and during critical developmental periods (e.g. prenatal, adolescence). The authors argue that, although the research base is still immature, genome-wide linkage studies and the identification of (new) genes in addition to intermediate phenotypes (e.g. cognitive dysfunction, abnormal brain function) is likely to improve the validity of diagnosis and provide inroads into formulating the staging model for psychosis and improving prevention and early intervention of the illness.

In Ch. 4, van Os and Poulton review the environmental risk factors for psychosis and their interaction with genetics. This approach differs from the linear gene–phenotype approach in that environmental risk factors are seen to play a *causal* role in the expression of psychosis and genes are believed to play an *indirect* role by moderating environmental impacts. Gene–environment relationships may reflect either gene–environment interaction ($G \times E$), which depicts how genetics moderate *sensitivity* to environmental factors to determine outcomes or gene–environment correlation (*rGE*), whereby differences in an individual's genotype may moderate

exposure to differential environments. In studies aimed at detecting $G \times E$, *rGE* may operate as a confounding factor and needs to be ruled out. The authors review the evidence for $G \times E$ in psychosis based on first- and second-generation studies. Most of the evidence for $G \times E$ in psychotic disorder comes from first-generation studies using non-specific or indirect (proxy) measures of genes and environment, including epidemiological studies; twin, adoption and family studies; studies examining psychosis liability using psychometric measures; and studies of environmental impact upon DNA sequence and DNA methylation. Newer second-generation studies have directly tested for interactions between particular measured genes and environments. Specifically, the interaction between *COMT* genotype and cannabis use has received the most research attention. The results of these studies have shown strong evidence for an increased risk for psychosis in individuals who carry the COMT allele encoding valine (Val) at position 158 and use cannabis during adolescence. Van Os and Poulton highlight some of the methodological challenges associated with $G \times E$ research and suggest future research directions. The authors make the case that, through increasing our understanding of the combination of genetic risk factors (i.e. genetic polymorphisms, endophenotypes) with environmental exposures, it will be possible to make more robust predictions regarding transition to psychosis, thus improving early identification and intervention.

Pantelis and colleagues tackle the exploding field of neurobiology and early psychosis in Ch. 5. They review the relevant research for at-risk-for psychosis populations and first-episode psychotic patients under headings of neuropsychology, psychophysiology, functional imaging and structural imaging. Key neuropsychological findings suggest that prior to psychosis onset there are relatively subtle impairments in self-ordered working memory tasks, certain types of memory requiring rapid and complex organization of material, and in olfactory identification ability.

Regarding psychophysiological markers, there are mixed findings: the authors conclude that mismatched negativity may be a marker of progression rather than an endophenotype in the traditional sense. Similarly, it is not entirely clear that P300 is a stable trait marker of illness as there is no clear evidence of progressive abnormality as with mismatched negativity, although this may suggest that the P300 may index poorer prognosis. In terms of P50, the authors conclude that this may be a more stable marker for the early recovery phase, although such deficits may be developmentally dependent. After exploring the available functional imaging studies conducted prior to and during the transition to psychosis, the authors review potential genes coding for brain maturation that may prove useful.

Finally, a number of brain structural abnormalities are identified as potential endophenotypes of schizophrenia and psychosis; however, a review of the studies in pre-psychotic individuals at high risk for transition to illness has not provided compelling evidence to support these abnormalities as illness-related markers (although some may prove promising). Rather, it would seem that many of the findings represent state-related abnormalities or changes that occur dynamically over the course of the illness.

The authors conclude that the dynamic brain changes occurring in adolescence and early adulthood may provide a context for interpreting some of the more important findings, where the most promising markers, such as certain executive functions (e.g. measured with self-ordered working memory tasks) and more direct measures of frontal lobe integrity (derived both from psychophysiology and functional and structural imaging), relate to frontal and perhaps temporal cortices; these are the brain regions that are changing dynamically during adolescence and early adulthood.

Nevertheless, Pantelis *et al.* sound a number of salutary warnings. They conclude that (1) the results reviewed by them do not support findings from studies of patients with more chronic psychosis; (2) the variables of interest may represent markers of illness progression and may not represent true endophenotypes; (3) other neurobiological factors may emerge with illness progression, or chronicity, or the same neurobiological factors may worsen; and (4) researchers have failed to take account of maturation as regards abilities and brain structures – the authors argue that brain structures are still developing around the time of the

key ages of onset for both males and females. Abnormalities in patients with FEP or UHR for psychosis may represent failure to mature.

In keeping with the book's focus on prevention and early intervention, Section 3 deals with the identification and treatment of individuals with an 'at risk mental state' (ARMS) and the prediction of their transition to FEP. Researchers from Australia, Germany and the USA, namely, Yung, Klosterkötter, Cornblatt and Schultze-Lutter, author Ch. 6, which focuses on defining the putative prodromal or UHR population and identifying the factors that predict transition to psychotic disorder in UHR individuals. Retrospective reports show that FEP is generally associated with a prodromal phase. The psychosis prodrome has been reported to include non-specific signs and symptoms (such as depressed mood, anxiety, sleep disturbance and deterioration in role functioning), subtle self-experienced cognitive and affective disturbances known as 'basic symptoms' (such as thought interference, disturbance of receptive language and visual perception disturbances), attenuated or subthreshold psychotic symptoms, neurocognitive deficits, and neurobiological changes measured via magnetic resonance imaging (MRI). Increasing improvements in the methods used to identify those truly at high risk for psychotic disorder has paved the way for early intervention strategies in this population and increased the possibility of minimizing distress and disability and delaying or even preventing the onset of full-blown psychotic disorder.

Yung and colleagues describe three strands of research that have focused on the identification of 'prodromal' or UHR individuals: (1) early intervention studies conducted at the Personal Assessment and Crisis Evaluation (PACE) clinic in Melbourne, Australia, using 'close-in' UHR criteria developed by their research group; (2) schizophrenia 'basic symptoms' research and intervention conducted at the Early Recognition and Intervention Centre for Mental Crisis (FETZ) in Cologne, Bonn, Düsseldorf and Munich, Germany, using early and late initial prodromal state criteria; and (3) genetic high-risk studies investigating the causes of schizophrenia undertaken at the Hillside Recognition and Prevention (RAP) programme in New York, USA. These methods of identification of people at risk of psychosis or schizophrenia have honed the identification from the general population rate of 1% to a rate of approximately 30%. However, some criticisms of this approach are highlighted, particularly the high false-positive rate that occurs in these selective samples. The second half of the chapter is mainly devoted to describing the predictive validity of a range of psychopathological (i.e. schizotypal features, positive psychotic phenomena, negative symptoms, basic symptoms, depression, anxiety and distress), clinical (i.e. poor functioning, substance use, stress), neurocognitive (i.e. working memory, olfactory identification, sensory gating) and neurobiological variables (i.e. hypothalamic–pituitary–adrenal axis function, brain structure and morphology) in predicting transition to psychosis. The goals of future work in this field are to improve the accuracy of predictive tools and further develop the most appropriate phase-specific interventions, while minimizing false positives and unnecessary iatrogenic harm.

In Ch. 7, Phillips, Addington and Morrison comprehensively review specific interventions for managing the broad range of symptoms and functional difficulties of individuals identified as having ARMS. Ethical considerations associated with the treatment of young people meeting ARMS criteria are flagged by the authors, including possible stigma associated with being labelled as having an ARMS, unnecessary treatment of 'false positives', how to discuss ARMS with individuals and their families, and how long treatment should be provided for. The bulk of the chapter is dedicated to outlining the case for and against specific interventions. Antipsychotic medication is reviewed first. Based on a limited number of studies with small samples, low-dose atypical antipsychotic drugs appear to at least delay, if not prevent, the conversion to fully fledged psychosis and enhance symptomatic and functional recovery, particularly in individuals in the late pre-onset period. However, there are potential risks and disadvantages associated with the use of antipsychotics in individuals with ARMS. These include the potential (serious) side effects associated with all antipsychotic medications (e.g. extrapyramidal side effects, weight gain, diabetes, sexual dysfunction), the possibility of 'feeding into' the commonly held belief that they are

going 'mad', the potentially greater prominence of non-psychotic phenomena that may be best treated via other methods, the alleviation of psychotic symptoms that may be rightly or wrongly experienced by the individual as pleasurable or functional, and reduced acceptability of antipsychotic medication (as indicated by poor adherence and higher dropout rates in medication arms of intervention studies with this population).

Only one published study has specifically examined the efficacy of psychological interventions in ARMS individuals, but the results were very positive, with individuals who received cognitive therapy being less likely to progress to psychosis or be prescribed antipsychotic drugs than individuals who were simply monitored. The authors argue that psychological interventions may be most effective and more acceptable to patients during the earlier stages of the putative prodrome, when presenting symptoms are less severe and less specific. Some of the disadvantages associated with providing psychological treatment include the fear and stigma that may be associated with being labelled as having an ARMS and being in 'therapy' and the possible development of a sense of helplessness, although these disadvantages may be addressed by the psychological intervention. Phillips and colleagues briefly review other potential approaches, including social interventions, monitoring and no intervention, of which the last is believed to be the most common, but least optimal scenario. Research into the type and length of intervention that is most effective in ARMS individuals is still in its early stages; however, a number of services worldwide are dedicated to treatment and ongoing research with this population. The authors describe four examples of this; namely, the Prevention Risk Identification, Management and Education (PRIME) clinic in Toronto, Canada; the Personal Assessment and Crisis Evaluation (PACE) clinic in Melbourne, Australia; the Early Detection and Intervention Team (EDIT) in Salford, UK; and the FETZ in Cologne, Germany. The chapter concludes with a case study and general recommendations.

Chapters 8 to 10 discuss the improvement of identification of psychosis and access to services and the relationship between duration of untreated psychosis

(DUP) and outcome. The definition, measurement and associated outcomes of DUP are first tackled by Marshall, Harrigan and Lewis in Ch. 8. Prior to conducting a systematic evaluation of the evidence for the strength and specificity of the relationship between DUP and outcome, the authors thoroughly review the difficulties in defining and measuring DUP, believed to account for the large variability in estimates of DUP across studies. They report the most likely sources of measurement error to be (1) difficulties and inconsistency in defining the onset and offset of DUP; (2) reduced reliability associated with retrospective assessment and illness status of the individual when they are recalling illness onset; (3) discrepancies between the reports of patients and carers (e.g. reporting of subjective and objective phenomena); (4) sample bias (e.g. including only patients who are hospitalized or have non-affective psychosis); and (5) failure to use standardized assessment instruments. Bearing these methodological issues in mind, Marshall and colleagues systematically review follow-up studies of patients with FEP that have examined the association between DUP and outcome and they attempt to determine the degree to which premorbid adjustment may confound any observed association. Primary outcome variables that were included were measures of symptoms, overall functioning and symptom remission. Secondary outcome variables were quality of life, social functioning and measures of relapse. Twenty-six cohorts, with a mean DUP of 124 weeks (103 weeks with exclusion of one outlier), were included in the meta-analysis. Results showed that by 6–12 months following first presentation there was a significant positive correlation between DUP and a range of primary and secondary outcomes (i.e. the longer the DUP, the worse the outcome). Sixteen multiple regression analyses (from nine studies) examined the relationship between DUP and outcome while controlling for premorbid adjustment. After controlling for premorbid adjustment, the association between DUP and outcome remained significant in 12/16 analyses; this association was particularly robust between DUP and positive symptoms. These data provide a clear rationale for reducing DUP through early detection and intervention.

In Ch. 9, Jorm and Wright examine the role of community mental health literacy as a means of facilitating early intervention in psychosis. Their rationale is to reduce DUP by facilitating better and earlier recognition of psychotic (and prodromal) symptoms and help-seeking from appropriate professionals by the person who is affected and/or those close to them. Jorm and Wright review public knowledge about psychotic disorders, specifically focusing on the recognition of psychosis, mental health 'first aid' skills and beliefs about mental health professionals and treatments. One approach to assessing public mental health literacy is to present people with a case vignette of a person with schizophrenia or psychosis and ask the respondent what they believe is wrong with this person. Research shows that although many people recognize a mental health problem of some kind only a minority correctly label it as psychosis. Another approach is to assess the public's beliefs about the helpfulness of particular professionals and also the helpfulness of treatments. Interestingly, as regards the latter, the public tend to favour psychological treatments and be negative about medication and admission to hospital. The authors also examined studies comparing the beliefs of the public and professionals and found some consensus, but also some discrepancies; they also found some improvements over time in the public's mental health literacy for psychotic disorders.

Jorm and Wright then review interventions to improve mental health literacy for psychotic disorders, including four community campaigns conducted in four different countries, school-based programmes, and individual training programmes. They conclude that community campaigns can enhance awareness in the community and with referral sources can increase help-seeking and reduce DUP, particularly where the median DUP is long to start with. School-based programmes and individual training programmes are described as promising but are still in their infancy. The need for more research into the nature, specificity and strength of the relationship between mental health literacy and DUP is highlighted by the authors.

In Ch. 10, Norman and Malla explore pathways and barriers to receiving care and methods of reducing delay into treatment for early psychosis. Their rationale for reducing DUP through early intervention is to improve outcomes, reduce unnecessary suffering and limit disruptions to social and role functioning commonly associated with psychotic illness. The authors first review what is known about the nature and determinants of help-seeking in early psychosis. Eight key observations regarding help-seeking are discussed: (1) help is often sought *before* the explicit onset of psychosis; (2) help-seeking is often initiated for reasons other than psychotic symptoms (e.g. dysphoria, anxiety, somatic concerns, deterioration in functioning); (3) help-seeking is often prompted by the actions of the sufferer's family or social network; (4) primary healthcare providers (e.g. primary care physicians) are often the first points of contact in accessing 'professional' treatment; (5) some barriers to help-seeking are potentially modifiable (e.g. knowledge of early warning signs and effectiveness of treatment); (6) once help is sought, there is wide variability in how readily it is provided (i.e. multiple contacts with helping professionals is common prior to the commencement of appropriate treatment); (7) there is considerable variation in who facilitates the final referral to appropriate services; and (8) accessing the appropriate service and receiving the correct diagnosis does not automatically denote prompt treatment.

In the next section, Norman and Malla explore the factors that predict treatment delay. There have been mixed findings regarding demographic and personal predictors of DUP; however, having fewer social contacts around the time of illness onset appears to be one factor that is relatively consistently associated with longer treatment delay. Some aspects of illness onset are more robust predictors of longer treatment delay, specifically poorer premorbid functioning, more gradual onset of illness and the presence of specific negative symptoms (i.e. apathy, social anhedonia). The authors conclude the chapter by describing approaches for reducing treatment delay for psychosis, including public education, training and education (i.e. 'up-skilling') of primary healthcare and social service providers, and the implementation of specific early detection programmes.

In Section 5, the chapters take on a practical clinical focus and are concerned with providing thorough and comprehensive assessment and treatment of the client experiencing a FEP or mania. In Ch. 11, Martin Lambert takes the reader through the various components of initial assessment and commencement of treatment – mostly pharmacotherapeutic in nature – of patients presenting with FEP. Key principles that underscore successful acute treatment (e.g. within the first 3 months) and provide a stable foundation for later treatment and maximum recovery are outlined first, including: (1) engagement and development of therapeutic alliance; (2) recognition of psychosis and understanding its personal context; (3) prompt non-traumatizing treatment of behavioural disturbances (e.g. agitation, pathological excitement, suicidal ideation); (4) achievement of symptomatic remission, functional recovery and quality of life; and (5) formulation of an individualized integrated treatment plan. Lambert then reviews the major elements of a comprehensive psychobiological assessment. These include detailed assessment of the individual's current and past psychiatric and personal history (with collateral information obtained from significant others); serial mental status examinations (MSEs); assessment of current and past comorbid axis I and II disorders and medical conditions, serial risk assessment, full biomedical evaluation, neuropsychological assessment and longitudinally based diagnostic evaluation. The remainder of the chapter is devoted to outlining best practice guidelines for pharmacological intervention in FEP, both non-affective and affective, including the management of psychiatric emergencies and the management of adverse events or side effects associated with pharmacological treatment (e.g. extrapyramidal motor symptoms, weight gain, metabolic syndrome, endocrine and sexual side effects). These guidelines are underpinned by a number of important principles: (1) the reduction of treatment delay improves antipsychotic response; (2) integrated treatment is a prerequisite for antipsychotic response (e.g. adjunctive psychosocial intervention); (3) separate approaches to initial pharmacotherapy are applied to non-affective and affective psychoses; (4) patients and relatives should be involved in treatment planning; (5) initial low-dose atypical antipsychotic treatment is recommended; (6) medication side effects should be avoided or treated early to promote response and future adherence; (7) comorbid psychiatric disorder(s) can reduce treatment response and, therefore, should also be treated early; (8) medication adherence should be regularly monitored; (9) pharmacotherapy should be adapted according to diagnostic shift; (10) early identification of patients with an unfavourable outcome is crucial; and (11) some patients require a longer period (e.g. over 8 weeks) to achieve treatment response and remission.

The initial assessment and treatment phase is commonly termed the 'early recovery phase', which may be characterized by either complete or, unfortunately in some cases (ranging from 9% to 30% in the first 1–2 years), incomplete recovery. Chapter 12 by Canadian and Australian researchers and clinicians, Jean Addington, Tim Lambert and Peter Burnett, is concerned with exploring potential reasons for incomplete recovery and providing guidelines for pharmacological, psychological and social treatments during the early recovery phase and beyond. The authors differentiate 'remission' from 'recovery'; in addition to *symptomatic* (*positive and negative symptoms*) *remission*, recovery represents the ability to effectively *function* in social, vocational and community domains. Achievement of complete recovery, therefore, generally represents a longer-term process. The first part of the chapter focuses on the initial 3 months of treatment (i.e. early recovery phase). Reasons and recommendations regarding an inadequate response to initial pharmacological treatment are addressed, including poor efficacy, poor tolerability and medication non-adherence. A major focus is devoted to the rationale for and provision of psychosocial treatments during the early recovery phase, particularly in relation to addressing functional recovery and adaptation to psychosis. Several psychosocial interventions are described, including psychoeducation, individual cognitive – behaviour therapy (CBT), phase-specific group treatment, vocational rehabilitation and family work.

The second part of Ch. 12 centres on incomplete recovery following the initial 3 months of treatment. It is imperative that incomplete recovery is identified as early as possible. Incomplete recovery may be characterized by ongoing positive symptoms; the presence of negative symptoms, depression and anxiety; deficits in

social and vocational functioning; poor quality of life; and/or cognitive deficits. When incomplete recovery is identified, the authors recommend a three-stage assessment and treatment approach. In stage 1, unmodifiable (e.g. long DUP, insidious illness onset, intellectual disability, neuropathology) and modifiable (e.g. comorbidity, inadequate psychosocial intervention, poor psychological adjustment, medication adherence) confounders of recovery must be identified. When there is a clear issue with medication adherence, stage 2 involves dealing with this via some form of adherence therapy or depot medication. In the situation where adherence has been effectively dealt with, but recovery remains incomplete, the clinician proceeds to stage 3, which involves determining whether incomplete recovery is a result of treatment resistance (estimated to affect at least 10% of patients with FEP). If treatment resistance is identified, the first line of treatment is clozapine. The authors conclude the chapter by describing treatment approaches for incomplete recovery, including medication strategies and individual, group-based and service-wide psychosocial treatments.

Although we ourselves remain skeptical around clarity of diagnosis in patients with first-episode bipolar disorder, we also acknowledge the burgeoning interest in this area. In Ch. 13, Conus and colleagues argue that Kraepelin's view of outcome for bipolar disorder was excessively optimistic. They conclude that, despite symptom remission, especially in the manic phase, assessment at follow-up shows poor functional or social recovery and high levels of comorbidity, including substance misuse. In line with principles of early intervention in psychosis, the authors make a case for early detection and early intervention in bipolar disorder, describing various factors responsible for the delay in diagnosing bipolar disorders and the unfavourable consequences associated with delayed diagnosis and treatment. The authors review extant treatment guidelines for bipolar disorders, concluding they are invariably based on patients with chronic disorders. They make the case for better definition of the disorder from vulnerability to initial onset to full-blown disorder, and the difficulties, but also the benefits, of doing so. They argue for treatments tailored to patients in the early phase of bipolar disorder and emphasize, in addition to pharmacotherapy, the imperative of providing psychological treatments to such patients, providing some guidelines to best practice in this regard. It is clear from this chapter that much more research is needed into the early identification and treatment of first-episode bipolar disorder and several suggestions as to future research directions are offered by the authors.

The 'critical period' is tackled by the next two sections of the book. First, specific topics pertaining to embedded, comorbid and/or secondary psychopathology in early psychosis are dealt with in Section 6. Substance use or misuse (i.e. abuse or dependence) is ubiquitous, is a problem in itself, is frequently comorbid with psychosis, and is a risk factor for other disorders and for relapse or retarded recovery from a psychotic break. In Ch. 14, Wade and colleagues report that individuals with psychotic disorders are at an increased risk for substance misuse and regular tobacco use compared with individuals with other mental disorders or the general population. In FEP, the lifetime rate of substance misuse is at least 40%, with the most frequently misused substances being cannabis and alcohol. For most individuals, the onset of substance misuse precedes the onset of positive psychotic symptoms, and many continue misusing substances despite involvement with treatment services. Wade and others outline the correlates and consequences of substance misuse in FEP, highlighting the poorer outcomes associated with ongoing substance misuse following entry into treatment. The authors describe three hypotheses that have been proposed to explain the high rate of substance use among individuals with psychosis: (1) that psychosis increases the risk of substance misuse (i.e. self-medication hypothesis); (2) that substance misuse increases the risk for psychosis; and (3) that there are common risk factors for both psychosis and substance misuse. To date, the second hypothesis has received the most empirical research support.

Wade and colleagues then review the evidence for the efficacy of psychological interventions targeting substance misuse in psychosis. Of the relatively few randomized controlled trials conducted to date, findings are mixed, but they do provide some support for psychoeducation, motivational interviewing, CBT and nicotine-replacement therapy in reducing substance misuse and improving secondary outcomes such as mood, other psychopathology and antipsychotic medication dosage. The authors conclude the chapter by providing guidelines for the implementation of interventions for substance misuse with individuals with FEP. These interventions need to be administered within the one treatment setting, via an integrated and comprehensive approach, and in a 'stepped-care' fashion. They include engagement, initial and ongoing assessment and formulation, assessment of motivation to address substance misuse, the provision of assessment feedback and psychoeducation, harm-minimization strategies, motivational interviewing and CBT.

Chapter 15, by Power and Robinson, focuses on the serious issue of suicide prevention and early intervention in FEP. Suicide is a perennial problem and has an elevated risk in psychosis, affecting up to 15% of individuals with psychotic disorders and representing the leading cause of unnatural death during the first 10 years of illness. Power and Robinson provide the legal definition of death by suicide and describe the process and manifestation of suicide during non-psychotic compared with psychotic phases, highlighting the diverse range of mental states and their potential effects on suicidal ideation and behaviour. The authors identify the first years after diagnosis of psychosis as critical, as suicide is more likely to occur during this stage of the illness, particularly during the early recovery phase (e.g. the months following discharge from hospital) – a period that may be characterized by the emergence of insight and feelings of hopelessness, depression and loss. Suicide risk assessment and formulation is, therefore, vital in early psychosis. The authors provide guidelines as to how to conduct comprehensive clinical suicide risk assessments and when hospitalization may be indicated. They emphasize the importance of a collaborative approach (involving the patient, carers and other services) to the initial risk formulation and risk management plan and careful documentation of the same. Power and Robinson provide a comprehensive review of the factors to consider when conducting suicide risk assessments. These include (1) biological risk factors, such as genetics/family history, neurochemical alterations, chronic illness (e.g. diabetes), medications and substance misuse; (2) psychological risk factors, such as stressful life events, poor coping style and personality traits (e.g. impulsivity); (3) wider family, social and cultural or religious risk factors; (4) service and treatment risk factors; and (5) protective factors.

Suicide risk management is described next, according to the continuum of preventive interventions described above: (1) selective interventions (i.e. screening and monitoring); (2) indicated interventions; and (3) universal interventions. Selective suicide interventions primarily encompass regular routine risk monitoring – the authors describe two specific examples of standardized service-wide suicide risk monitoring implemented in early psychosis services in London and Melbourne. Indicated suicide interventions are employed when a patient is assessed to be a suicide risk. Indicated interventions include acute suicide risk containment (e.g. increased contact with the service, removal of potential suicide means, hospitalization), pharmacological and physical treatments (e.g. atypical antipsychotic drugs, antidepressants, mood stabilizers, electroconvulsive therapy), individual and group-based psychological interventions, psychosocial interventions, and self-help. Finally, universal strategies target the whole clinic population by aiming to prevent suicide risk. Universal strategies include raising staff, carer and patient awareness; devising protocols and providing training in suicide prevention; regular debriefing and service reviews; implementation of early intervention models of mental health service provision; and adequate social services and social policies.

Complicating and debilitating emotional and personality dysfunction in early psychosis is covered in Ch. 16 by Birchwood and colleagues. The authors argue that emotional dysfunction is an endemic feature of early psychosis and is often inappropriately conceptualized as 'comorbidity'. They cite evidence for emotional dysfunction being present prior to onset, during the prodromal phase, and during the acute phase of early psychosis. Specifically, high levels of social anxiety, withdrawal, isolation, irritability and depression are the most prominent signs of emotional disturbance during these early phases of illness. Postpsychotic depression is also commonly experienced by patients

following remission of symptoms of FEP. The nature of the link between emotional disturbance and psychosis is explored in terms of three types of interaction: (1) the direct influence of emotional dysfunction in the development and/or maintenance of delusions and hallucinations; (2) emotional dysfunction and psychotic symptoms sharing a common developmental pathway (i.e. common risk factors); and (3) emotional dysfunction as a psychological reaction to psychosis. The implications and applications of CBT in the treatment of psychosis are briefly appraised. The authors argue that, given that the roots of CBT lie traditionally and theoretically in the treatment of 'affective' disorders, further research into CBT for psychosis needs primarily to involve theory-driven studies focusing on reducing the emotional and behavioural dysfunction of the illness, thereby being complementary to neuroleptic drugs in their treatment of psychotic symptoms. A number of research foci are suggested in line with this.

The remainder of Chapter 16 is dedicated to the neglected area of personality dysfunction, specifically borderline personality disorder (BPD) in FEP. Based on minimal research, the conceptualization and comorbidity of BPD and FEP are briefly reviewed, but the authors argue that further conceptual clarity is needed. Significant diagnostic and treatment conundrums are commonly faced by clinicians when presented with a young person displaying features of BPD and symptoms of psychosis, and treatment guidelines are lacking. The authors argue that this 'subgroup' of patients deserves a specialized treatment approach, which takes into consideration the complex interactions between the psychotic symptoms, which may be 'episodic', and the pervasive interpersonal difficulties, affect dysregulation and impulsivity associated with BPD, which may complicate recovery from FEP. Cognitive analytic therapy is a candidate intervention for this subgroup of patients because it has developed an integrated theoretical account of both BPD and psychosis. The theory, application and research of cognitive analytic therapy in patients with co-occurring BPD and psychosis are described in detail.

Section 7 also covers the critical period but is concerned with specific therapeutic interventions that move beyond the individual and their FEP symptoms.

Family interventions remain an important area, and in Ch. 17, McNab and Linszen summarize research on family factors in FEP research, including the experiences of families of individuals with FEP, particularly in relation to distress and grief. The authors dismiss earlier theories that identified families as 'causing' psychotic disorders. They examine the 'expressed emotion' construct in FEP and UHR clients and propose putative mechanisms for the link between expressed emotion and relapses. Reasons are advanced for the weaker link between expressed emotion and relapse in these two client populations compared with populations with chronic mental illness (e.g. schizophrenia).

The experiences of family members or caregivers of people with psychotic disorder are frequently overlooked. The authors attempt to rectify this and conclude that, despite the few and inconsistent findings, levels of distress and feelings of grief and loss of caregivers of people with recent-onset psychotic disorder are at least comparable to those experienced by carers of people with more chronic psychiatric difficulties. A second major strand of work is concerned with intervention. Findings linking expressed emotion and outcome in chronic schizophrenia have been used to justify the development of intervention programmes aimed at reducing expressed emotion rates in FEP. It is concluded that since expressed emotion is generally less entrenched in the FEP population interventions may prevent potential entrenchment by targeting loss and psychological morbidity and providing families with resources to stay involved with patients and maximize their caregiving capacity. A stage-based model of working with families is then introduced with sequential foci on the family experience, the teaching of skills and knowledge, building family support and resilience, and longer-term care. A Canadian and Australian comparison is made. Key principles underlying family work in the FEP population are highlighted, including patient consent and collaboration, tailored supportive interventions, the importance of ongoing psychoeducation, and strengthening or teaching effective coping strategies.

Moving away from individual interventions focused on reducing symptomatology (e.g. antipsychotic medication, CBT for positive symptoms), Ch. 18 focuses on interventions that aim to enhance vocational functioning in the early-psychosis population. Despite the achievement of symptom recovery for many individuals with FEP, Killackey and colleagues emphasize the barriers to employment and associated high unemployment rates among young people with FEP (~40%) relative to the general population (~5%). They also outline the huge economic and psychosocial costs associated with ongoing unemployment in this population and provide a clear rationale for early intervention in FEP specifically targeting vocational rehabilitation. Specific employment interventions that have been implemented for people with mental illnesses over the past several decades are critiqued, namely (1) industrial or work therapy; (2) social firms; (3) the clubhouse model (transitional employment, train and place); and (4) supported employment, best characterised by the individual placement and support (IPS) model. The latter two employment interventions have received the most systematic research and although there is some research support for the clubhouse model for individuals with mental illnesses in general, the authors argue, for various reasons, that this model may not be appropriate for young people with FEP. To date, supported employment, specifically IPS, has received the most empirical support (i.e. from randomized controlled trials) in individuals with established mental illness. Only one published study has focused on supported employment in the early-psychosis population, but found that it was effective. Killackey and colleagues go on to describe current research and the successful application of vocational intervention within specialized FEP services or with FEP populations around the world, specifically, in Australia, the USA and the UK. Some of the key principles that underlie successful delivery of IPS in FEP populations are outlined in the chapter. These principles include integration of the vocational intervention with the mental health treatment team; provision of the intervention in the community (as opposed to office based); an individualized approach to intervention; job search guided by consumer preference; focus on education and training as needed (because of the developmental stage/age of most individuals with FEP); ongoing support provided beyond the point that employment is obtained; and combining the vocational intervention with specific supplementary psychosocial interventions. Preliminary research findings are impressive and further research is ongoing.

In Ch. 19, Gleeson, Linszen and Wiersma examine the recovery phase in FEP, with a major focus on the prediction and prevention of relapse. The authors initially examine the concept and definitions of relapse. Allowing for the lack of consensus over definitions, the authors report relapse rates of 40–50% at 2 years, with rates increasing to 85% by 15-year follow-up. Factors associated with the risk for relapse are then reviewed. These include medication non-adherence, expressed emotion, substance (particularly cannabis) abuse, stress and life events, early warning signs, personality difficulties, poorer premorbid adjustment, cognitive deficits and possibly DUP. The prevention of relapse following FEP is then reviewed, with the important role of maintenance antipsychotic medication and psychosocial intervention (i.e. individual psychotherapy and family intervention) in preventing relapse being highlighted. The authors conclude the chapter with general treatment recommendations regarding relapse prevention and outline gaps in the knowledge base that require future research.

In Ch. 20, Huber and Lambert focus on early identification and intervention of treatment resistance in early-psychosis patients. Although research and standardized clinical practice in samples of those with FEP and treatment resistance is less developed than in samples of those with chronic schizophrenia, the authors outline the most appropriate pharmacotherapeutic approaches to treatment resistance in early schizophrenia, schizoaffective disorder, bipolar disorder and major depressive disorder. One of the barriers to effective early intervention in patients with treatment resistance is that definitions of such resistance for affective and non-affective psychoses do not exist, are not updated or remain controversial. Nevertheless, Huber and Lambert clarify that contemporary definitions of treatment resistance necessarily incorporate persistent positive, negative, affective and cognitive symptoms, poor social and vocational functioning, and poor quality of life. All of these facets of the illness need to be addressed for recovery to be considered complete.

Using this broad definition, treatment resistance affects a large minority of patients with FEP. A number of treatment-, patient-, and illness-related factors are known to be associated with treatment resistance. The key is to identify patients at increased risk as early as possible and tailor treatments accordingly. The remainder of Ch. 20 provides recommended guidelines with regards to pharmacological and non-pharmacological approaches to treatment resistance.

Finally, the last section of the book concludes with Ch. 21, which is authored by researchers from Australia (Meredith Harris), the UK (Tom Craig and Paddy Power), Canada (Donald Addington and Robert Zipursky) and Denmark (Merete Nordentoft). This chapter provides five international examples of the research and development of advanced early-psychosis service models. The services reviewed are the Early Psychosis Prevention and Intervention Centre (EPPIC) in Melbourne, Australia; the Lambeth Early Onset Service (LEO) in south London, UK; the First Episode Psychosis Program (FEPP) – Centre for Addiction and Mental Health (CAHM) in Toronto, Canada; the Calgary Early Psychosis Treatment Services (CEPTS) in Canada; and OPUS (intensive integrated treatment in the early phase of psychosis) in Copenhagen and Aarhus (and more recently, Odense), Denmark. These services have provided unequivocal evidence for the effectiveness of the early intervention model; however, one area that remains unresolved is the optimal duration of treatment, which does not extend beyond 18–24 months in most early-psychosis services owing to limited funding and high service demand. The optimal duration of specialized treatment requires further research in order to guide future service development.

The early psychosis mission

From the outset, what has attracted us, and indeed people all over the world, to clinical work with young people with early psychosis is the chance to develop and offer a preventive and personal focus aimed at maximizing recovery. This means timely intervention, a personal and family focus involving a formulation-based approach, and identifying and addressing factors that operate to maintain or even worsen the disorder and impede recovery. In essence, we have sought to develop and provide young people and their families with the best, most appropriate and most acceptable treatment with minimum stigma and adverse effects. We continue to be driven by the goals of maximizing positive outcomes for the individual and our goal is maximum recovery and social and economic participation, not merely symptom remission.

Our approach is entirely consistent with the International Clinical Practice Guidelines for Early Psychosis (International Early Psychosis Association Writing Group, 2005). These guidelines emphasize, amongst many other things, the need for early identification of people in the earliest stages of psychotic disorders, combined with phase-specific programmes of care. We need to provide our clients with the best evidence-based pharmacological and psychosocial treatments and, where there are gaps in our evidence base, use the best clinical and research expertise to provide our clients with the most appropriate treatments. We also need to encourage community-wide education about psychotic disorders and their treatment. This, in our view, is one way of tackling the vexed problem of stigma. Finally, it is imperative as clinicians that we work with consumers, families and other caregivers to provide them with information, support and assistance.

REFERENCES

International Early Psychosis Association Writing Group (2005). International clinical practice guidelines for early psychosis. *British Journal of Psychiatry*, **187**(Suppl 48), s120–4.

McGorry, P. D. & Jackson, H. J. (eds.) (1999). *The Recognition and Management of Early Psychosis: A Preventive Approach.* Cambridge, UK: Cambridge University Press.

Mrazek, P. J. & Haggerty, R. J. (eds.) (1994). *Reducing Risk for Mental Disorders: Frontiers for Preventive Intervention Research.* Washington, DC: National Academic Press.

Diagnosis and the staging model of psychosis

Patrick D. McGorry, Kelly Allott and Henry J. Jackson

Introduction

Just as with any medical or psychiatric condition, the primary aim of making a diagnosis of psychotic illness is to ensure that the person with the condition is treated with the most appropriate evidence-based intervention. Yet, researchers and clinicians within the psychosis field can claim to have advanced this aim further than in other psychiatric domains by implementing the early diagnosis strategy developed in the mainstream healthcare field for disorders such as cancer, stroke and diabetes. The intention here is to improve prognosis by reducing mortality and preventing progression or worsening of the disorder and to minimize the distress, morbidity, comorbidity, disability and costs associated with the diagnosis of psychosis. Since the first edition (McGorry & Jackson, 1999), we have observed a gradual lifting of the pessimism instilled by the conceptual framework of Kraepelin (1919) and a continued reform momentum in support of early intervention in psychosis. Evidence of this growing optimism is demonstrated by the emergence, worldwide, of more than 200 early psychosis services over the past 10–15 years (e.g. see Chs. 6, 7 and 21), with an increased recognition of the need for stage-of-illness approaches to psychosis. Clinical practice guidelines for the treatment of schizophrenia now typically have a section devoted to early psychosis (e.g. APA Steering Committee on Practice Guidelines, 2002; International Early Psychosis Writing Group, 2005; McGorry *et al.*, 2005). Also, as outlined in Ch. 1, there has been a dramatic increase in the literature on early psychosis. A further indication of the importance of early

intervention is the appearance in 2007 of a new international journal entitled *Early Intervention in Psychiatry*.

In the first edition of our book (McGorry & Jackson, 1999), we introduced the framework of preventive intervention put forward by Mrazek and Haggerty (1994) with its depiction of prevention lying on a spectrum or continuum of interventions ranging from *universal*, *selective* and *indicated* prevention through early case identification and ultimately treatment and rehabilitation. To briefly recap, at the *universal* level, we are applying interventions to whole populations (e.g. national anti-smoking public health campaigns, and immunization campaigns for influenza). At the *selective* level, intervention(s) are targeted at people who may have a higher than average risk for the emergence of disorder, but who at present are asymptomatic. One example would be females with a positive family history of breast cancer who are urged to undergo annual mammograms. The third concept – that of *indicated prevention* – focuses on people who are at high imminent risk for a disorder, for example with attenuated or subthreshold clinical symptoms plus a fall in daily functioning and a positive family history for the disorder of interest. More focused and intense interventions would be delivered to this group with the aim of preventing first onset of full-blown disorder. This would be analogous to intervening in people with transient ischaemic attacks in order to prevent a cerebrovascular accident or stroke. The aims of early detection and diagnosis of psychotic illness are outlined in Box 2.1.

In the first edition of the book (McGorry & Jackson, 1999), we commented that indicated prevention raised

The Recognition and Management of Early Psychosis: A Preventive Approach, ed. Henry J. Jackson and Patrick D. McGorry.
Published by Cambridge University Press. © Cambridge University Press 2009.

Box 2.1. The aims of early detection and diagnosis of psychotic illness

To reduce or prevent progression or worsening of symptoms/syndrome

To reduce or prevent progression or worsening of associated neurobiological changes and neuropathology

To reduce or prevent secondary psychiatric morbidity such as depression, anxiety, suicide and substance use

To reduce or prevent significant deterioration in, or failure to achieve, role functioning

To reduce or prevent the individual and/or family's experience of trauma and/or stress often associated with severe psychotic illness, involuntary hospital admissions, etc.

To reduce stigma and provide psychoeducation early

To reduce or minimize disruption to normal developmental processes

To reduce costs to the community and government

the genuine possibility of preventing the development of full-threshold psychotic disorder. Since then, considerable progress has been made. First, there has been an increased research focus on identifying early markers (e.g. biological markers, endophenotypes, clinical phenotypes) of psychotic illness and, importantly, better characterization of the early phases of psychotic disorder. Second, we have witnessed the emergence worldwide of a number of prodrome or 'ultra-high risk' (UHR) treatment clinics. Third, several randomized controlled trials have been conducted to ascertain the most effective pharmacological, psychological or combination treatments for this target population.

Further progress in research and clinical care may be catalysed by the development and elaboration of a heuristic concept, namely a *clinical staging model* – which builds upon and elaborates the preventive framework of Mrazek and Haggerty (1994). This staging model is underpinned by the premise that psychiatric (e.g. psychotic) disorder can be usefully divided into a series of stages similar to those described in cancer and other medical disorders. These stages require different treatment strategies, and treatment within each stage is intended not only to promote recovery but also to prevent progression to the next and more advanced

stage of disorder, from which recovery may be less likely. This is an ideal model for further research and treatment in relation to the detection and management of early psychosis. Before describing this model in detail, we will briefly discuss issues surrounding validity in the early diagnosis of psychotic 'disorder'.

Diagnosis of psychosis: issues of validity

The American Psychiatric Association (APA) *Diagnostic and Statistical Manual of Mental Disorders* (DSM-IV; APA, 1994) lists nine psychotic disorders: schizophrenia, schizophreniform disorder, schizoaffective disorder, delusional disorder, brief psychotic disorder, shared psychotic disorder, psychotic disorder due to a general medical condition, substance-induced psychotic disorder and psychotic disorder not otherwise specified (NOS). Additionally, congruent and incongruent psychotic or psychotic-like features may be present in other mental disorders, particularly mood and personality disorders.

Nosologies such as DSM (APA, 1994) or the World Health Organization (WHO) *International Statistical Classification of Diseases and Related Health Problems* (ICD; WHO, 1992) are based on crystallized forms of disorders with clear symptom pictures and with built-in duration criteria. They assume that a syndrome is 'concrete' and stable across all phases of a disorder, and this is not necessarily the case. Such 'classic' prototypes may not be accurate depictions or representations of disorders at the earliest stages, where symptoms may be undifferentiated and non-specific. If one follows patients forward in time then the symptoms may or may not coalesce, consolidate and differentiate from non-specific symptom mixtures. But even with the emergence of a florid psychotic episode (i.e. where the person meets 'caseness' for a given disorder for the first time), this does not necessarily guarantee that the symptomatology will remain stable over time. If relapse occurs, the patient may not necessarily present with the same phenotype and may attract another diagnostic label. It is only with repeated episodes, persistent symptoms and/or accumulating disability and time (i.e. chronicity) that the features may become more or less crystallized and stable. The problem, however, is that such chronic 'cases' represent end-stage disorder and are not typical of the complete sample or universe of psychotic disorder. Nevertheless, this view has been entrenched since Kraepelin's conceptualization of schizophrenia as an illness of chronic course and poor outcome (Kraepelin, 1919). Many of our psychiatric diagnoses beyond the schizophrenia spectrum are based on chronic patient populations, and this is an example of the clinician's illusion. Here, prognosis and diagnosis have become confused, leading to unfounded pessimism and an undermining of the confidence to intervene and change the pattern, course and outcomes of a disorder.

To further complicate matters, individuals at UHR and individuals with first-episode psychosis (FEP) present with a range of non-specific symptoms (e.g. anxiety, suicidal ideation, sleep disturbance) that do not come under the diagnostic criteria of psychosis but may represent a prodrome, psychiatric comorbidity or secondary morbidity. These individuals are characteristically diagnostically confusing. The presence of 'additional' symptoms may be sufficient in number and coherence to be considered a 'syndrome'. However, such symptoms are discounted by the application of current diagnostic systems, as they are not seen to be part and parcel of the focal syndrome, but clearly require treatment. It seems the case that DSM has reified 'syndromes' that naturally may be poorly defined at the boundaries and early in the course of the disorder where they can merge or overlap with other syndromes. It appears that we have shored up reliability without impacting on validity (Andreasen, 2007; McGorry, Copolov & Singh, 1989).

Earlier detection of psychotic disorders and the presence of less-stable psychotic syndromes with prominent comorbidity, including axis II traits and disorders, ensures that the clinical phenotype looks less typical and 'textbook-like'. Even though some patients may still technically meet criteria for DSM-IV (APA, 1994) categories such as schizophreniform disorder, clinicians may be reluctant to apply such terms or labels to patients who look 'atypical'. They suspect such patients may not be truly 'psychotic' or 'schizophrenic'. Others fall genuinely short of the threshold for schizophrenia or schizophreniform disorder and yet are psychotic, perhaps in a more focal way. This is a good thing and a success story for early intervention. However, the evidence base for treating them is not yet clear-cut. Many of these patients end up in the wastebasket diagnostic category of 'Psychotic Disorder NOS' (APA, 1994). We have tried to avoid the problems with this category by using a more generic term of 'early psychosis' with subtypes, including severe psychotic mood disorder. In general, however, we must remember that these diagnostic terms are all descriptive, syndromal and rather arbitrary.

These issues are further highlighted when we consider the role of clinical judgement in deciding whether the phenomena the patient experiences are abnormal or not (McGorry, Yung & Phillips, 2001; van Os et al., 2000). The problem is further amplified when one moves from a single phenomenon to multiple phenomena, as is the case in deciding whether or not one is confronted by a syndrome, that is a group of say five or more phenomena, each of which needs to be judged as being abnormal or not in its own right (Eaton, 2001).

Although there has been an explosion of research into identifying potential biological markers of psychotic illness, and aberrant neural mechanisms are accepted as underlying mental disorder, to date scientists have been unable to identify a specific gene, gene combination or specific brain pathology that is a unique marker of illness (Andreasen, 1997; Patel et al., 2007). At present, the underlying biological substrates and causal risk factors for psychotic disorder remain unknown. Nevertheless, there have been many breakthroughs in terms of neurological/biological risk factors and abnormalities associated with psychotic disorder (Chs. 3 to 5 discuss genetic and neurobiological factors). Yet, frequently, the same biological or neurocognitive deficits are found across a range of disorders (e.g. hypothalamus–pituitary–adrenal axis dysfunction, working memory deficits, reduced hippocampal volume; Jackson & McGorry, 2008).

We would argue that clinicians need to tolerate ambiguity in their practice. This ambiguity and uncertainty increases the further one goes back in terms of phase of illness, so at the earliest phases clinical symptoms may be less pronounced and less crystallized.

Similarly, biological changes may be subtle at the earliest stages, and in some cases they may precede the emergence of clinical symptoms, while in others they may emerge approximately contemporaneously with clinical symptoms, and in still others they may follow symptom emergence. We argue that a diagnostic approach should combine both 'clinical descriptions' and 'biological' variables, be phase-of-disorder focused, and treatment oriented (Jackson & McGorry, 2008). In the following section, we discuss the staging model as a useful heuristic for this approach to diagnosis, intervention and research in psychosis, with a particular focus on early psychosis.

The staging model and its application to early psychosis

Clinical staging is a refined diagnostic system that defines the extent of progression of illness in an individual at a particular point in time (i.e. stage). It emphasizes the description of where a person lies along the continuum of the course of illness. Milder initial clinical phenomena are differentiated from more severe and chronic phenomena, and subcategories are imposed on dimensional phenomena. Clinical staging guides the clinician in selecting treatments that are most appropriate to the specific stage of illness. Treatment based on clinical staging assumes that the appropriateness and effectiveness of treatment will be maximized and the harmfulness of the treatment will be minimized. Like diagnosis in general, while staging links treatment selection and prediction, its role in treatment selection is more crucial than its role in prediction, because early successful treatment may improve prognosis and even prevent progression to more severe stages of the disorder. Hence, the key driver behind the staging approach is to prevent progression of an 'illness' to a subsequent more severe stage, thus providing a preventively oriented framework of intervention. The two main assumptions of the staging model are first that patients in the early stages of an illness have a better response to treatment and prognosis than those in later stages and second that treatments offered/delivered in the early stages should be more benign and more effective than those offered in the later stages.

Clinical staging has traditionally been applied and proven within medical settings, most commonly in the treatment of malignancies (e.g. Jones, 1984; Kasimir-Bauer et al., 2003; Legorreta et al., 2004). However, it has recently been proposed that clinical staging can potentially be useful for any psychiatric disorder that tends to, or might, progress (Fava & Kellner, 1993; McGorry et al., 2006). In this regard, psychotic disorder, in particular, appears to be a prime candidate for the clinical staging model. Outcomes for psychosis are extremely heterogeneous but may be moderated by how early intervention strategies are applied (Harrison et al., 2001). The stages of psychosis can be defined by dimensions of severity, the impact of symptoms on the person's developing personal world and social environment (i.e. functioning and quality of life), and by the degree of persistence and recurrence of the disorder and related comorbidity (Table 2.1).

The clinical staging approach to diagnosis and intervention in early psychosis recognizes the need to conceptualize psychopathology within the context of a neurodevelopmental framework. The putative prodrome and first onset of disorder generally occur during adolescence or early adulthood, a critical period of development normally characterized by significant neurodevelopment and emotional and cognitive maturation, which is paralleled by social and educational/vocational achievements and increasing independence (Rice & Barone, 2000; Steinberg, 2005). This implies that approaches to diagnosis and intervention need to be specifically tailored to the individual's age and developmental stage. Given these neurodevelopmental considerations, psychological problems during adolescence and young adulthood can be diagnostically confusing and, therefore, require specialized therapeutic input (e.g. Berk et al., 2007; McCutcheon et al., 2007; McGorry, 2007a; McGorry, Killackey & Yung, 2007). Furthermore, the culture of care must be qualitatively different if young people are going to engage and persist with treatment. The whole treatment approach is radically different to treating an adult with later phases of illness, such as established schizophrenia (Edwards

Table 2.1. Clinical staging model[a] framework for psychotic disorders

Clinical stage	Definition	Target populations for recruitment	Potential interventions	Indicative biological and endophenotypic markers
0	Increased risk of psychotic disorder; no symptoms currently	First-degree teenage relatives of probands	Improved mental health literacy, family education, drug education, brief cognitive skills training	Trait marker candidates and endophenotypes, e.g. smooth pursuit eye movements, P50, niacin sensitivity, binocular rivalry, prepulse inhibition, mismatch negativity, olfactory deficits
1a	Mild or non-specific symptoms, including neurocognitive deficits, of psychotic disorder; mild functional change or decline	Screening of teenage populations Referral by primary care physicians or school counsellors	Formal mental health literacy, family psychoeducation, formal CBT, active substance-abuse reduction	Trait and state candidates where feasible according to sample size
1b	Ultra high risk: moderate but subthreshold symptoms, with moderate neurocognitive changes and functional decline to 'caseness' (GAF < 70)	Referral by educational agencies, primary care physicians, emergency departments, welfare agencies	Family psychoeducation, formal CBT, active substance-abuse reduction, low-dose atypical antipsychotic agents for episode, antidepressant agents or mood stabilizers for comorbid mood conditions	Niacin sensitivity, folate status, brain changes (magnetic resonance imaging and spectroscopy), hypothalamus–pituitary–adrenal axis dysregulation
2	First episode of psychotic disorder: full threshold disorder with moderate–severe symptoms, neurocognitive deficits and functional decline (GAF 30–50)	Referral by primary care physicians, emergency departments, welfare agencies, specialist care agencies, drug and alcohol services	Family psychoeducation, formal CBT, active substance-abuse reduction, atypical antipsychotic agents for episode, antidepressant agents or mood stabilizers, vocational rehabilitation	Continue with markers of illness state, trait and progression
3a	Incomplete remission from first episode of care (could be linked or fast-tracked to stage 4)	Primary and specialist care services	As for '2' with additional emphasis on medical and psychosocial strategies to achieve full remission	Continue with markers of illness state, trait and progression
3b	Recurrence or relapse of psychotic disorder, which stabilizes with treatment at a level of GAF, residual symptoms, or neurocognition below the best level achieved following remission from first episode	Primary and specialist care services	As for '3a' with additional emphasis on relapse-prevention and 'early warning signs' strategies	Continue with markers of illness state, trait and progression

Table 2.1. (cont.)

Clinical stage	Definition	Target populations for recruitment	Potential interventions	Indicative biological and endophenotypic markers
3c	Multiple relapses, provided worsening in clinical extent and impact of illness is objectively present	Specialist care services	As for '3b' with emphasis on long-term stabilization	Continue with markers of illness state, trait and progression
4[b]	Severe, persistent OR unremitting illness as judged on symptoms, neurocognition and disability criteria	Specialised care services	As for '3c' but with emphasis on clozapine, other tertiary treatments, social participation despite ongoing disability	Continue with markers of illness state, trait and progression

CBT, cognitive–behavioural therapy; GAF, Global Assessment of Functioning scale.

[a] The clinical staging model provides greater utility for testing efficacy, cost-effectiveness, risk–benefit ratios and feasibility of available interventions; clinicopathological correlates and predictors of illness stages can also be introduced within a neurodevelopmental framework.

[b] Could fast track to this stage at first presentation through specific clinical and functional criteria (from stage 2) or alternatively by failure to respond to treatment (from stage 3a)

Adapted with permission from McGorry *et al.* (2006).

et al., 1996; McGorry *et al.*, 1996, 2007). Recent trials and wider youth mental health reform strategies support the wisdom and effectiveness of this approach (Craig *et al.*, 2004; McGorry *et al.*, 2007; Petersen *et al.*, 2005a). The developmental and staging paradigms mesh quite well for epidemiological reasons – youth is the peak period for onset of the major disorders of adult life (Insel & Fenton, 2005).

Traditional diagnostic approaches (i.e. DSM) would argue that a 'real' diagnosis can only be made after development of eventual outcome. For example, a diagnosis of schizophreniform disorder requires the presence of continuous signs of the disorder for at least 1 month, or 6 months for a diagnosis of schizophrenia. This clearly confuses diagnosis with prognosis and may be harmful. By comparison, a clinical staging diagnostic approach recognizes that persistent subthreshold psychotic phenomena, depression or other clinical features, and/or early psychosocial decline, may represent an individual who is at UHR for, or in the prodrome of, a frank psychotic disorder (i.e. FEP).

Likewise, a patient with FEP is at risk for persistence and chronicity. Provision of appropriate intervention at this putative early or prodromal stage of illness may prevent progression to the stage of illness where criteria for schizophreniform disorder or schizophrenia are met.

Table 2.1 outlines the four-stage model and shows a worked-through example with regard to psychosis. In addition to the utility of the clinical staging model for applying treatment strategies, we may be able to move over time from a simple clinical staging model to a 'clinicopathological' staging model, as in other disorders. Staging may, therefore, provide a heuristic model for organizing and understanding the myriad biological research findings. A clinicopathological diagnostic approach, which takes into account symptom severity, intensity, coherence, persistence and duration (i.e. clinical phenomena), functioning and cognitive and biological variables, is central to the staging model (McGorry *et al.*, 2006). For example, intensity, persistence and frequency of psychotic symptoms form one element of the approach. The quality of the symptoms may also be informative, for example, bizarre or Schneiderian first-rank symptoms may reflect more serious illness progression. Neurocognitive impairment, neurological soft signs and other motor signs may also be incorporated. Non-invasive biological markers, such as changes in regional brain volume changes, olfactory deficits, genetic variation such as affecting catechol-*O*-methyltransferase and other potential phenotypic markers could also be incorporated to reflect stage of illness and may guide treatment selection and likely prognosis. Furthermore, indicators of psychosocial functioning, including degree of social isolation, educational/vocational failure or decline, could also indicate severity and degree of illness progression (McGorry *et al.*, 2006). In sum, the clinical staging model provides a useful heuristic from which to (1) assess the likely stage of psychosis that any one individual belongs to (i.e. ranging from no psychotic disorder present to chronic schizophrenia with significant disability); (2) guide the appropriate type(s) and intensity of intervention required for that specific stage (i.e. ranging from benign mental health literacy to clozapine medication and intensive psychosocial intervention); and (3) inform likely prognosis (i.e. ranging from a transient 'blip' or 'dip' in functioning to chronicity; see Table 2.1).

The four-stage model assumes that the phenotype is not necessarily stable or even coherent at a very early stage (stage 1a) and leaves open the notion that the phenotype, or a portion thereof, may be altered by treatment. Progression of the person from say stage 1 to stage 2 could, therefore, be prevented. From stage 0 to stage 1b we would see the emergence of non-differentiated symptoms, the intensification of existing features, the accretion of somewhat-more-specific features and a decrease in functioning (representing a smaller number of people at stage 1b than at stages 1a and 0). By stage 1b there would be evidence of a subthreshold syndrome with reduction in functioning. Stage 2 would represent the onset of a coherent or crystallized florid phenotype (i.e. FEP), while stages 3a to 3c would be characterized by incomplete remission, single and multiple relapses, and stage 4 would represent severe, persistent or unrelenting illness (i.e. chronic schizophrenia). The implications for treatment are different according to the specific stage. With relation to

psychosis, this book specifically focuses on stages 0 through 3a, which are explored in more detail below.

Stages 0–1a: increased risk for psychosis, mild non-specific symptoms, mild drop in functioning

Stages 0–1a represents the earliest stages when non-specific symptoms are manifested, the level of risk is low and the percentage of natural remission is large and widespread. At this early stage, it is not known whether these symptoms will resolve or crystallize, or even transmute into more serious subthreshold phenotypic forms. So, interventions at this earliest stage need to be easily delivered and benign (i.e. minimal side effects) because of the potentially large numbers of false positives. This could take the form of public health information messages and mental health literacy, for example leaflets, television advertisements and billboard messages for people to exercise, observe sleep hygiene and engage in positive activities involving mastery and pleasure (Jorm, 2000; see also Ch. 9). Such treatments are benign since they do not involve the ingestion of medications, and they are relatively cost-effective because they do not involve intensive one-to-one intervention requiring high levels of clinical expertise or equipment. They are also non-stigmatizing. Here, vulnerable people who are asymptomatic, such as relatives of people with mental illness, are likely to benefit from greater knowledge. In addition to generic mental health literacy programmes, specific educational programmes seeking to improve recognition and help-seeking have also been successfully implemented (e.g. Johannessen *et al.*, 2001; Kitchener & Jorm, 2002; Melle *et al.*, 2004; Wright *et al.*, 2005).

Stages 1a–1b: ultra-high risk or prodromal phase

Stages 1a–1b would include those individuals who are distressed, have manifested a drop in functioning and are seeking treatment (i.e. those we might identify as UHR). They may not meet 'caseness' for psychotic disorder, but they are at increased risk for the same owing to the presence of risk markers. For example, they may have attenuated paranoid ideation, perceptual changes, and/ or report a family history of schizophrenia. Stages 1a to 1b may represent a prolonged period requiring clinical care and monitoring, despite there being no diagnosis of a clear-cut psychotic disorder. These individuals require interventions that specifically target the presenting symptoms and dysfunction, with the aim of trying to reduce the risk that psychosis will worsen or fully emerge (Addington *et al.*, 2005). Treatment might include targeted cognitive-behaviour therapy (CBT) and perhaps low-dose antipsychotic medication. Moreover, functioning is equally worthy of intervention, for example skills training, structured activities and CBT aimed at return to school or vocational placement. At this stage, one has to weigh up the costs and benefits in terms of side effects. Some of these people will not go on to develop a full diagnostic psychotic disorder (i.e. 'false positives'). One argument has been that there is unnecessary exposure of some people to potentially serious side effects of treatment (Warner, 2005). This means that the benefits to the group as a whole must be significant and the risks to the entire group comparatively low (McGorry *et al.*, 2002). There are now a number of clinics worldwide that treat patients in the putative 'prodromal' phase of illness (Chs. 6 and 7). Service delivery includes informing patients of the risks and benefits of the range of available treatments, careful monitoring of mental states and functioning and a collaborative approach to treatment (McGlashan *et al.*, 2007). A small number of studies have found that transition to psychosis can be reduced by treating individuals who are identified as being at UHR for psychosis (McGlashan *et al.*, 2006; McGorry *et al.*, 2002; Morrison *et al.*, 2004; Nordentoft *et al.*, 2006).

Stage 2: first-episode psychosis

Stage 2 represents the stage at which full threshold psychotic disorder is reached; that is, when moderate to severe psychotic symptoms, neurocognitive deficits and functional decline are evident. The goal of detection and intervention at this stage is to minimize the duration of untreated psychosis (DUP) by delivering intensive biopsychosocial interventions that are aimed at maximizing symptom and functional recovery. The first 2–5 years after the onset of frank psychosis have been identified as a 'critical period' for intervention and the prevention of decline and 'collateral' damage (Birchwood & Fiorillo, 2000; Birchwood, Todd & Jackson, 1998). In support of this notion, two recent meta-analyses have reported a small to medium effect of DUP on a range of symptomatic and functional outcomes (Marshall *et al.*, 2005; Perkins *et al.*, 2005; see also Ch. 8). An intensive multidisciplinary approach to intervention is imperative and includes active engagement and assessment, individual and family psychoeducation, atypical antipsychotic medication, formal CBT, active substance-abuse reduction, group-based social interventions and vocational rehabilitation. Recent large-scale randomized controlled trials have demonstrated the effectiveness of specialized intensive treatment during the first episode (e.g. Garety *et al.*, 2006; Petersen *et al.*, 2005b). Chapters 8 and 10 focus on improving pathways to care and reducing DUP, while Chs. 11 and 13 are devoted to the assessment and intervention of the first psychotic and manic episode.

Stage 3a: incomplete recovery or treatment resistance

An individual enters Stage 3a when they have not experienced complete symptom remission and/or functional recovery from their first episode (say following the first 3 months of treatment) and where there may be a continued worsening or 'plateau' of illness impairment and disability. This may be a result of poor engagement, treatment reluctance (e.g. medication non-compliance), poor treatment efficacy, inadequate treatment delivery and/or treatment resistance. The timing of clozapine use and intensive psychosocial (e.g. CBT) and relapse-prevention strategies are key issues here. Chapters 12, 19 and 20 address in detail the approaches to relapse prevention, identification and management of individuals who have experienced incomplete recovery or treatment resistance from early psychosis.

Research implications

Clinical staging 'creates a prevention-oriented framework for understanding pathogenesis and evaluation of interventions' (McGorry, 2007b, p. 859). To emphasize, clinical staging is a framework for research, not just treatment. For example, the staging approach can help to distinguish vulnerability markers from sequelae of disease and it can aid us in attempting to increase the specificity of biological and environmental risk factors that indicate progression from one stage to the next. For example, what are state versus trait markers of illness, and which markers are stage specific? We can also investigate the relative potency of markers and the degree to which they are malleable by interventions.

The staging model also provides a framework for researching which factors are protective against stage progression (e.g. personality, coping style, shorter DUP, low expressed emotion, cognitive flexibility, medication adherence, etc.). It may be that particular combinations of factors provide better predictive validity than factors studied in isolation (e.g. gene–environment interactions; see Ch. 4).

The staging model supports the obvious tenet that a proportion of those with psychosis (many, but by no means all) will progress without timely and stage-linked treatment – but this needs to be empirically tested. Large, collaborative, longitudinal studies that span pre-onset to established phases of illness are needed, with sequential and nested treatment trials to build the evidence base at each stage for the same cohort.

Conclusions

Diagnosis should be treatment and outcome focused. Making a diagnosis of psychotic disorder based on current categorical diagnostic systems (e.g. DSM-IV) implies that an individual either has a psychotic disorder or does not. Traditionally, meeting full criteria for psychotic disorder has been conceptualized as representing a threshold for treatment (e.g. introduction of antipsychotic medication). This may, in fact, place too much faith in the current diagnostic system, which has been poor at defining thresholds for disorder and for treatment. In this chapter, we have highlighted the reasons for reduced validity and diffusion in the (categorical) diagnosis of psychotic disorders. We would argue that psychological phenomena, including psychotic-like phenomena, occur on a continuum ranging from not present to most severe. What is clinically important is whether an individual is help-seeking; how certain symptoms are experienced by the individual (e.g. level of distress); and what effect such symptoms are having on the individual's sense of well-being and day-to-day functioning, as well as the experience and functioning of those close to them. Based upon the tenet of the staging model, we would argue that early diagnostic markers or risk factors for psychotic illness, or isolated distressing and debilitating symptoms (which are not of sufficient range or number to meet full diagnosis), can and should be treated, and that such treatment may prevent the transition to full expression and/or subsequent stages of psychotic disorder. Studies like the UHR or prodromal trials and the greater effectiveness and acceptability of streamed FEP programmes provide real support for the staging model. However, the value of the model for the treatment and understanding of psychosis and, more broadly, psychiatry in general needs wider exploration. The early intervention strategy and a more flexible approach to diagnosis in psychiatry are key priorities for the future.

REFERENCES

Andreasen, N. C. (1997). Linking mind and brain in the study of mental illnesses: a project for a scientific psychopathology. *Science*, **275**, 1586–93.

Andreasen, N. C. (2007). DSM and the death of phenomenology in America: an example of unintended consequences. *Schizophrenia Bulletin*, **33**, 108–12.

APA (1994). *Diagnostic and Statistical Manual of Mental Disorders*, 4th edn. Washington, DC: American Psychiatric Press.

APA Steering Committee on Practice Guidelines (eds.) (2002). *American Psychiatric Association Practice Guidelines for the Treatment of Psychiatric Disorders Compendium 2002*. Washington, D.C: American Psychiatric Press.

Berk, M., Hallam, K., Lucas, N. *et al.* (2007). Early intervention in bipolar disorders: opportunities and pitfalls. *Medical Journal of Australia*, **187**(Suppl), S11–14.

Birchwood, M. & Fiorillo, A. (2000). The critical period for early intervention. *Psychiatric Rehabilitation Skills*, **4**, 182–98.

Birchwood, M., Todd, P. & Jackson, C. (1998). Early intervention in psychosis: the critical period hypothesis. *British Journal of Psychiatry*, **33**(Suppl), s53–9.

Craig, T., Garety, P., Power, P. *et al.* (2004). Lambeth Early Onset Service: a randomised controlled trial. *Schizophrenia Research*, **70**(Suppl), 145–6.

Eaton, W. W. (2001). *The Sociology of Mental Disorders*, 3rd edn. Westport, CT: Praeger.

Edwards, J., Francey, S. M., McGorry, P. D. & Jackson, H. J. (1996). Early psychosis prevention and intervention: evolution of a comprehensive community-based specialized service. *Behavior Change*, **11**, 223–33.

Fava, G. A. & Kellner, R. (1993). Staging: a neglected dimension in psychiatric classification. *Acta Psychiatrica Scandinavica*, **87**, 225–30.

Garety, P. A., Craig, T. K., Dunn, G. *et al.* (2006). Specialised care for early psychosis: symptoms, social functioning and patient satisfaction: randomised controlled trial. *British Journal of Psychiatry*, **188**, 37–45.

Harrison, G., Hopper, K., Craig, T., *et al.* (2001). Recovery from psychotic illness: a 15-and 25-year international follow-up study. *British Journal of Psychiatry*, **178**, 506–17.

Insel, T. R. & Fenton, W. S. (2005). Psychiatric epidemiology: it's not just about counting anymore. *Archives of General Psychiatry*, **62**, 590–2.

International Early Psychosis Writing Group (2005). International clinical practice guidelines for early psychosis. *British Journal of Psychiatry*, **187**(Suppl 48), s120–4.

Jackson, H. J. & McGorry, P. D. (2008). Psychiatric diagnoses: purposes, limitations and an alternative approach. In S. Wood, N. Allen & C. Pantelis (eds.), *Handbook of Neuropsychology in Mental Illness*. Cambridge, UK: Cambridge University Press, in press.

Johannessen, J. O., McGlashan, T. H., Larsen, T. K. *et al.* (2001). Early detection strategies for untreated first-episode psychosis. *Schizophrenia Research*, **51**, 39–46.

Jones, S. E. (1984). The staging of Hodgkin's disease revisited. *Medical Oncology and Tumor Pharmacotherapy*, **1**, 15–17.

Jorm, A. F. (2000). Mental health literacy: public knowledge and beliefs about mental disorders. *British Journal of Psychiatry*, **177**, 396–401.

Kasimir-Bauer, S., Schleucher, N., Weber, R., Neumann, R. & Seeber, S. (2003). Evaluation of different markers in non-small cell lung cancer: prognostic value of clinical staging, tumour cell detection and tumour marker analysis for tumour progression and overall survival. *Oncology Reports*, **10**, 475–82.

Kitchener, B. A. & Jorm, A. F. (2002). Mental health first aid training for the public: evaluation of effects on knowledge, attitudes and helping behaviour. *BMC Psychiatry*, **2**, 10. http://www.biomedcentral.com/1471-244X/2/10.

Kraepelin, E. (1919). *Dementia Praecox*. New York: Churchill Livingstone.

Legorreta, A. P., Chernicoff, H. O., Trinh, J. B. & Parker, R. G. (2004). Diagnosis, clinical staging, and treatment of breast cancer: a retrospective multiyear study of a large controlled population. *American Journal of Clinical Oncology*, **27**, 185–90.

Marshall, M., Lewis, S., Lockwood, A. *et al.* (2005). Association between duration of untreated psychosis and outcome in cohorts of first-episode patients: a systematic review. *Archives of General Psychiatry*, **62**, 975–93.

McCutcheon, L. K., Chanen, A. M., Fraser, R. J., Drew, L. & Brewer, W. (2007). Tips and techniques for engaging and managing the reluctant, resistant or hostile young person. *Medical Journal of Australia*, **187**(Suppl), S64–7.

McGlashan, T. H., Zipursky, R. B., Perkins, D. *et al.* (2006). Randomized, double-blind trial of olanzapine versus placebo in patients prodromally symptomatic for psychosis. *American Journal of Psychiatry*, **163**, 790–9.

McGlashan, T. H., Addington, J., Cannon, T. *et al.* (2007). Recruitment and treatment practices for help-seeking 'prodromal' patients. *Schizophrenia Bulletin*, **33**, 715–26.

McGorry, P. D. (2007a). The specialist youth mental health model: strengthening the weakest link in the public mental health system. *Medical Journal of Australia*, **187**(Suppl), S53–6.

McGorry, P. D. (2007b). Issues for DSM-V: clinical staging: a heuristic pathway to valid nosology and safer, more effective treatment in psychiatry. *American Journal of Psychiatry*, **164**, 859–60.

McGorry, P. D. & Jackson, H. J. (eds.) (1999). *The Recognition and Management of Early Psychosis: A Preventive Approach*. Cambridge, UK: Cambridge University Press.

McGorry, P. D., Copolov, D. L. & Singh, B. S. (1989). The validity of the assessment of psychopathology in the psychoses. *Australian and New Zealand Journal of Psychiatry*, **23**, 469–82.

McGorry, P. D., Edwards, J., Mihalopoulos, C., Harrigan, S. M. & Jackson, H. J. (1996). EPPIC: an evolving system of early detection and optimal management. *Schizophrenia Bulletin*, **22**, 305–26.

McGorry, P. D., Yung, A. & Phillips, L. (2001). Ethics and early intervention in psychosis: keeping up the pace and staying in step. *Schizophrenia Research*, **51**, 17–29.

McGorry, P. D., Yung, A. R., Phillips, L. J. *et al.* (2002). Randomized controlled trial of interventions designed to reduce the risk of progression to first-episode psychosis in a clinical sample with subthreshold symptoms. *Archives of General Psychiatry*, **59**, 921–8.

McGorry, P., Killackey, E., Lambert, T. & Lambert, M. (2005). Royal Australian and New Zealand College of Psychiatrists clinical practice guidelines for the treatment of schizophrenia and related disorders. *Australian and New Zealand Journal of Psychiatry*, **39**, 1–30.

McGorry, P. D., Hickie, I. B., Yung, A. R., Pantelis, C. & Jackson, H. J. (2006). Clinical staging of psychiatric disorders: a heuristic framework for choosing earlier, safer and more effective interventions. *Australian and New Zealand Journal of Psychiatry*, **40**, 616–22.

McGorry, P., Killackey, E. & Yung, A. (2007). Early intervention in psychotic disorders: detection and treatment of the first episode and the critical early stages. *Medical Journal of Australia*, **187**(Suppl), S8–10.

Melle, I., Larsen, T. K., Haahr, U. *et al.* (2004). Reducing the duration of untreated first-episode psychosis: effects on clinical presentation. *Archives of General Psychiatry*, **61**, 143–50.

Morrison, A. P., French, P., Walford, L. *et al.* (2004). Cognitive therapy for the prevention of psychosis in people at ultra-high risk: randomised controlled trial. *British Journal of Psychiatry*, **185**, 291–7.

Mrazek, P. J. & Haggerty, R. J. (eds.) (1994). *Reducing Risk for Mental Disorders: Frontiers for Preventive Intervention Research*. Washington, DC: National Academic Press.

Nordentoft, M., Thorup, A., Petersen, L. *et al.* (2006). Transition rates from schizotypal disorder to psychotic disorder for first-contact patients included in the OPUS trial. A randomized clinical trial of integrated treatment and standard treatment. *Schizophrenia Research*, **83**, 29–40.

Patel, V., Flisher, A. J., Hetrick, S. & McGorry, P. (2007). Mental health of young people: a global public-health challenge. *Lancet*, **369**, 1302–13.

Perkins, D. O., Gu, H., Boteva, K. & Lieberman, J. A. (2005). Relationship between duration of untreated psychosis and outcome in first-episode schizophrenia: a critical review and meta-analysis. *American Journal of Psychiatry*, **162**, 1785–804.

Petersen, L., Jeppesen, P., Thorup, A. *et al.* (2005a). A randomised multicentre trial of integrated versus standard treatment for patients with a first episode of psychotic illness. *British Medical Journal*, **331**, 602–5.

Petersen, L., Nordentoft, M., Jeppesen, P. *et al.* (2005b). Improving 1-year outcome in first-episode psychosis: OPUS trial. *British Journal of Psychiatry*, **187**(Suppl), s98–103.

Rice, D. & Barone, S. J. (2000). Critical periods of vulnerability for the developing nervous system: evidence from humans and animal models. *Environmental Health Perspectives*, **108** (Suppl 3), S511–33.

Steinberg, L. (2005). Cognitive and affective development in adolescence. *Trends in Cognitive Sciences*, **9**, 69–74.

van Os, J., Hanssen, M., Bijl, R. V. & Ravelli, A. (2000). Strauss (1969) revisited: a psychosis continuum in the general population? *Schizophrenia Research*, **45**, 11–20.

Warner, R. (2005). Problems with early and very early intervention in psychosis. *British Journal of Psychiatry*, **187** (Suppl), s104–7.

WHO (1992). *International Statistical Classification of Diseases and Related Health Problems*, Vol. 10 revision. Geneva: World Health Organization.

Wright, A., Harris, M. G., Wiggers, J. H. *et al.* (2005). Recognition of depression and psychosis by young Australians and their beliefs about treatment. *Medical Journal of Australia*, **183**, 18–23.

SECTION 2

Risk and vulnerability

Genetic vulnerability

Daniel Weinberger and Gregor Berger

Introduction

The current state of schizophrenia genetics might seem at first glance to be at odds with family, twin and adoption studies pointing towards a high genetic liability, with a point estimate of 81% (Sullivan, Kendler & Neale, 2003), because no single gene appears to carry by itself a major risk effect (Harrison & Weinberger, 2005). The molecular aetiology of schizophrenia remains enigmatic, pointing towards the involvement of multiple genes with small effects across diverse populations (acting like quantitative trait genes), aetiopathological heterogeneity, or the combination of both. Complex inheritance patterns are suggested where detrimental and protective gene effects interact and may define a threshold determining if the phenotype schizophrenia is expressed under certain environmental influences, and during critical developmental periods. Genes are turned on and off during critical developmental periods and may interact with particular environmental influences. We can think of those genes as the basic instruction blocks of human development and maintenance that encode protein products at the molecular level that will finally direct an organism's phenotypic characteristics (Prathikanti & Weinberger, 2005). In contrast to Mendelian disorders (e.g. cystic fibrosis), major psychosis does not behave in such a way, where one mutated gene and its product impacts on a range of developmental processes and finally translates into abnormal phenotypic characteristics that are defined as one particular 'disease'.

In the case of relatively common disorders such as schizophrenia or bipolar disorder, inheritance is more complex, and it is likely that single genetic variations do not substantially alter the protein structure. Susceptibility genes appear to increase the probability of illness, and they do so by acting in conjunction with other gene variations and environmental factors, until they finally manifest on a functional (clinical) level. The currently known candidate gene variations for schizophrenia identified through linkage and association studies (Table 3.1) are likely to behave in such a manner and pose one of the biggest challenges for applied psychiatric genetic research, as we have to deal with multiple small effects that interact in a very complex manner. A good example is the interaction between early heavy cannabis abuse, a functional polymorphism in the gene for catechol-O-methyltransferase (COMT) and the increased risk to develop schizophrenia (Caspi *et al.*, 2005). These complex interactions may increase the potential to find benign, preventive interventions that can modulate exactly these processes (e.g. targeted preventive cannabis abstinence programmes for young individuals at high risk to develop a psychotic disorder who are COMT Val158Met carriers).

In the previous chapter, the authors tried to map the onset of psychosis, highlighting the importance of the dimensional nature of its emergence and course. They introduced a staging model for psychotic disorders similar to models well known for cancer. Such staging models may have clinical implications and inform clinicians about treatment choices. For example, a stage 1 carcinoma in situ may need a minor procedure or even only monitoring compared with later stages, which may need more invasive procedures such as surgery or chemotherapy. Translated into psychiatry, a stage 1

The Recognition and Management of Early Psychosis: A Preventive Approach, ed. Henry J. Jackson and Patrick D. McGorry.
Published by Cambridge University Press. © Cambridge University Press 2009.

Table 3.1. Schizophrenia susceptibility genes and the strength of evidence in four domains: Strength of evidence (0 to 5+)

Candidate gene[a]	Location	Association with schizophrenia	Linkage to gene locus	Biological plausibility	Altered expression in schizophrenia
COMT	22q11	++++	++++	++++	Yes, +
DTNBP1	6p22	+++++	++++	++	Yes, ++
NRG1	8p12-21	+++++	++++	+++	Yes, +
RGS4	1q21-22	+++	+++	+++	Yes, ++
GRM3	7q21-22	+++	+	++++	No, ++
DISC1	1q42	+++	++	++	Not known
DAOA (G72/G30)	13q32-34	+++	++	++	Not known
DAAO	12q24	++	+	++++	Not known
PPP3CC	8p21	+	++++	++++	Yes, +
CHRNA7	15q13-14	+	++	+++	Yes, +++
PRODH2	22q11	+	++++	++	No, +
AKT1	14q22-32	+	+	++	Yes, ++
GAD1	2q31.1	++		++	Yes, +++
ERBB4	2q34	++			Yes, ++
FEZ1	11q24.2	++		+++	Yes, ++
MUTED	6p24.3	++++	++++	+++	Yes
MRDS1 (OFCC1)	6p24.3	++	++++	+	Not known

[a] See the text for discussion of the role of the gene products.
Revised from Harrison and Weinberger (2005), with permission.

psychotic disorder (prodrome) that has no or minimal genetic 'loading' may only need psychoeducation and a lifestyle change, whereas a stage 3 psychotic disorder may need lifelong antipsychotic treatment in conjunction with supportive therapy. The clinical implications of such potential staging models need to be rigorously tested in future research, but their promise is that they may inform clinicians about diagnostic specificity, prognosis and treatment choices. The great hope of molecular genetics in conjunction with other (intermediate) phenotypic information is that such models may finally support clinicians to make informed choices about what type of intervention will be necessary at what stage, what type of (side) effects we can expect and for how long the intervention will be necessary.

As schizophrenia is an end-stage-based concept, we do not know how the identified candidate gene variants map on to the onset of disorder and on the modification of its dimensional course. There is a great need for better understanding of the functional implications of those gene variations for the different stages of major psychosis, as well as to what extent they interact with environmental factors such as birth complications, high expressed emotion in the family environment, illicit substance abuse, or other factors not yet known.

This chapter tries to evaluate critically the extent to which molecular genetics may be informative in the understanding of vulnerability for psychotic disorders. In addition, the implications of gene–environment interactions for the emergence of psychosis will be discussed.

The phenotype called schizophrenia

Despite the continuous lack of specific neurobiological substrates for the phenotype schizophrenia, the commonly used classification systems (DSM-IV: APA, 1994; ICD 10: WHO, 1992) result in high diagnostic reliability (First *et al.*, 2002; van Os *et al.*, 2000) and result in similar incidence rates across different cultures, socioeconomic classes and races (Jablensky, 1999). The current state of research is suggestive that the prefrontal cortex, hippocampus, superior temporal cortex and thalamus are affected in schizophrenia, as demonstrated using neuroimaging techniques such as positron emission tomography and functional magnetic resonance imaging (fMRI), and neuropsychological testing. Furthermore, histological findings in postmortem tissue point towards subtle changes in the synaptic microcircuitry of these regions, ranging from alterations in the morphology of the dendritic tree to molecular changes at interneuronal synapses and including associated glial elements (Harrison & Weinberger, 2005). However, the results are not conclusive and they are likely to be confounded by clinical heterogeneity, effects of chronic illness and medication. Nevertheless, genome-wide linkage studies identifying loci in extended family pedigrees have resulted in the discovery of candidate genes with modest effects, such as those for dysbindin, neuregulin or a D-amino acid oxidase activator (*DAOA*; formerly G72). The identification of new genes using such approaches may finally help to dissect the illness not by phenomenology but by using genetic information, and this may help to reduce some of the uncertainties that have plagued the phenomenological study of these disorders.

Linkage studies

Traditional methods in family studies focus on large multiply affected pedigrees, under the assumption that affected families are segregating genes of major effect. Linkage studies rest on the principle that large blocks of DNA are inherited unchanged from each parent, and polymorphic DNA markers can trace the inheritance of these blocks to individual offspring. Linkage studies, therefore, can use a few hundred DNA markers to trace transmission of these blocks from parents to offspring, and to scan the entire genome to test if specific parental blocks are inherited

within a family by ill offspring. If such a block co-segregates with illness within the family, one can assume that a disease-causing gene is located in such a block. Linkage studies are usually conducted using the DNA from extended families and measures allele sharing within families. Such strategies have been successfully applied in a range of disorders and resulted in the successful identification of candidate genes such as that for presenilin 1, which explains a rare form of early-onset Alzheimer's disease (less than 5% of all those with Alzheimer's disease; Rocchi *et al.*, 2003). However, such single major effect genes have not yet been detected in schizophrenia and related disorders. The evidence from family segregation studies of the phenotype schizophrenia has suggested the presence of a limited number of genes with moderate effect size (1.5–3; Risch & Merikangas, 1996). Nevertheless, findings from early linkage studies provided important clues for the majority of the candidate genes now considered for schizophrenia (Table 3.1), and have shed some new light on the neurobiology of these conditions.

The low effect size of individual marker loci and the heterogeneity of the phenotype schizophrenia may be the core reasons why genome-wide linkage studies are difficult to replicate (Owen, Williams & O'Donovan, 2004). Meta-analyses of aggregated uncorrected data have been applied to deal with these problems, and three regions have reached genome-wide significance: 8p21-22, 13q32-34 and 22q11-12 (Badner & Gershon, 2002; Lewis *et al.*, 2003). Other promising regions include 1q21-22, 5q21-q33, 6q24-25, 6p24-22, 10p15-p11, and 1q42. Similar attempts have been made for bipolar disorder, where some new regions were identified (4p16, 4q32, 12q23-24, 15q14, 4q35, 9p22-21, 10q21-22, 14q24-32, 13q32-34), with some regions overlapping with those known for schizophrenia (6q22, 22q11-22). A more recent linkage meta-analysis produced a different set of loci linked to schizophrenia; in decreasing order, suggestive significance was reported on 5p, 3p, 11q, 2q, 1q, 22q, 8p, 6p, 20p and 14q. Interestingly, 8p and 22q were regions that were identified in both meta-analyses (Badner & Gershon, 2002; Lewis *et al.*, 2003) and they may, therefore, harbour a range of candidate genes for psychotic disorders in general.

Allelic association studies

Population-based association studies compare the frequency of allelic variations between (unrelated) patients and controls. Unfortunately, they are prone to statistical errors, largely as a result of population stratification and multiple testing (Owen, Holmans & McGuffin, 1997). Larger sample sizes, conservative significance levels, ethnic matching and family-based association methods (transmission disequilibrium test or haplotype relative risk; Slager & Schaid, 2001) are increasingly being used to avoid such errors. Allelic association studies consider specific genes believed to be involved in the pathogenesis of a disorder. In contrast to linkage studies, where the relationship between genetic loci and a phenotype is tested, association studies test the relationship of a specific allele, mostly a single nucleotide polymorphism (SNP) within a specific gene with a particular phenotype. Association studies are based on the assumption that an ancestral mutation in the DNA introduced the disease, or an increased risk for a particular disease, to that population. This DNA mutation would then be passed down across generations. These SNPs can be causal (functional SNPs) or can serve as potential markers for a nearby aetiological disease SNP. When a marker SNP serves as a proxy for a nearby aetiological SNP, the two SNPs are said to be in linkage disequilibrium, because they are inherited together on the same stretch of chromosome. Allelic association studies measure whether a hypothesized disease allele is more frequent in ill individuals relative to the control population. The big advantage of association studies is that they can detect weak gene effects, which are not easily detected with linkage. Association studies are also a strategy to test directly if mutations in a gene have any relationship with the investigated illness. Such genes are often selected for theoretical reasons, such as the pharmacological efficacy of antipsychotic drugs (e.g. dopamine receptor system), models of schizophrenia (e.g. such as the neurodevelopmental hypothesis of schizophrenia that pointed towards the potential importance of brain-derived neurotrophic factor (BDNF)), genes of conditions known to be associated with a high prevalence of psychosis (e.g. velo-cardio-facial syndrome) or, more recently, increasing accuracy of positional linkage studies and fine mapping of candidate loci (with dysbindin being a good example). The currently known candidate genes (Table 3.1) are likely to be part of a polygenic chorus rather than principal oligogenic markers, though work remains to be done before we understand precisely how genetic variations of these genes confer susceptibility for the onset of psychotic disorders (Owen *et al.*, 2004).

Dysbindin

The gene for dysbindin-1 (*DTNBP1*) was identified as a schizophrenia susceptibility gene based on a positional genetics approach and is located in the chromosome 6p22-24 region (Straub *et al.*, 2002). Of association studies reported to date, 12 of 15 have claimed association of SNPs in *DTNBP1* with schizophrenia (see Holliday *et al.*, 2006; Kendler, 2004; Tochigi *et al.*, 2006); this degree of positive results far exceeds what could be attributed simply to chance. The association remained true, even under very conservative family-based association methods for three-marker haplotypes ($p = 0.008$–0.0001; Straub *et al.*, 2002). However, it has not yet been possible to identify consistent individual SNPs or haplotypes across the different cohorts, suggesting allelic heterogeneity (Schwab *et al.*, 2003). Two other studies (Kohn *et al.*, 2004; Raybould *et al.*, 2005) also found associations with bipolar disorder with psychotic features. Interestingly, dysbindin-1 is part of the dystrophin-associated protein complex, located in both pre- and postsynaptic glutamatergic neurons (Talbot *et al.*, 2004); this neurotransmitter system has increasingly been linked with schizophrenia. However, it is not clear whether the relationship of dystrophin-1 to schizophrenia is based on its interaction with other dystrophin-related proteins or on its critical role in another protein system, the BLOC-1 system, which is involved in lysosomal trafficking (Harrison & Weinberger, 2005). Interestingly, two studies have found that dysbindin production in the schizophrenic brain is reduced (Talbot *et al.*, 2004; Weickert *et al.*, 2004), suggesting that its role in the pathophysiology of schizophrenia may extend beyond just genetic association.

Neuregulin

A number of genome-wide linkage studies have indicated that 8p22-p12 is a likely positive locus (Stefansson *et al.*, 2002, 2003; Tang *et al.*, 2004; Williams *et al.*, 2003; Yang *et al.*, 2003). Several genes that have been reported to be associated with schizophrenia map to this broad linkage region, but the most consistently confirmed and extensively studied is the gene for neuregulin (*NRG1*). A complex pattern of associations has been reported for this gene (Harrison & Law, 2006; Li, Collier & He, 2006; Norton, Williams & Owen, 2006); somewhat similar to dysbindin, the pattern of SNPs and haplotypes has differed across world populations, suggesting allelic heterogeneity within the gene. Two studies (Cassidy *et al.*, 2006; Green *et al.*, 2005) also found a similar association in bipolar disorder, with the greatest effect size in those patients showing mood-incongruent psychotic features, suggesting *NRG1* variants may, therefore, modulate mood-incongruent psychotic features, perhaps again similar to findings with dysbindin. The neuregulins are cell–cell signalling proteins acting as ligands for receptor tyrosine kinases of the ErbB family and are important for normal brain development and synaptic plasticity (Falls, 2003). Furthermore, neuregulins modulate the *N*-methyl-D-aspartate (NMDA) receptor systems, glial functioning (Hakak *et al.*, 2001) and myelination (Canoll *et al.*, 1999), which are also implicated in schizophrenia (Berger, Wood & McGorry, 2003; Davis *et al.*, 2003; Falls, 2003). Increased gene expression and the pattern of specific NRG1 isoforms in the dorsolateral prefrontal cortex and in the hippocampus of postmortem brain tissue of patients with schizophrenia (Hashimoto *et al.*, 2004; Law *et al.*, 2004) have been associated with variants in the original risk haplotype identified in Iceland (Law *et al.*, 2006). These findings at the level of brain expression further support the potential importance of *NRG1* as a susceptibility gene for schizophrenia and related disorders.

D-Amino acid oxidase activator

The gene *DAOA*, located on chromosome 13q22-34, is another candidate gene identified from genome-wide linkage studies (Owen *et al.*, 2004). Indeed, it is the only putative schizophrenia susceptibility gene identified entirely via positional cloning, in that no prior information about this gene was known prior to its identification from genome linkage scanning. Chumakov *et al.* (2002) investigated eight SNPs across DAOA and demonstrated that four intronic SNPs were associated with schizophrenia in French-Canadians, and one of these SNPs was positive in a Russian case–control sample. Several subsequent studies confirmed positive association with *DAOA* in other samples, though negative reports have also appeared. A recent meta-analysis has reported significant evidence for associations between several markers near *DAOA* with both schizophrenia and bipolar disorder (Detera-Wadleigh & McMahon, 2006), supporting the notion that both disorders share some common susceptibility genes. However, again, the associated alleles and haplotypes are not identical across studies. The protein product of *DAOA* (also known as PLG72) interacts with D-amino acid oxidase which is encoded by a gene located on chromosome 12q. Both gene products play a role in D-serine metabolism, which itself acts on the NMDA receptor known to be involved in memory and learning and implicated in psychosis. It has been proposed that DAAO may act as a detoxifying enzyme against exogenous D-amino acids. It also appears to modulate the levels of D-serine in the brain, which, in turn, is an endogenous modulator of NMDA receptors. These association findings are among the most compelling supporting genome-wide linkage analysis as a tool to identify completely unknown genes and their associated pathways, which is important for the understanding of disorders such as schizophrenia and bipolar disorder that are not fully understood yet and potentially could open up new treatment approaches to both disorders.

Regulator of G-protein signalling-4

The gene for regulator of G-protein signalling-4 (*RGS4*), a protein that negatively modulates signal transduction at G-protein-coupled receptors, has been proposed as a further candidate schizophrenia susceptibility gene based on a study of differential gene expression in the human brain (Mirnics *et al.*, 2001). This gene maps to a region showing strong prior linkage in several (Owen *et al.*, 2004), though not all (Levinson *et al.*, 2002), studies. A recent meta-analysis of genotype data (Talkowski *et al.*, 2006) on 2160 families did not confirm any significant associations with specific individual SNPs/haplotypes, but it did confirm weak association to genetic variation within the gene overall. This finding was unexpected given earlier positive findings from adequately powered studies (Chowdari *et al.*, 2002; Williams *et al.*, 2004). One possible explanation may be allele heterogeneity between the studies, with differing patterns of individual SNPs and haplotypes. Postmortem studies also found differential expression patterns of *RGS4* (Abi-Dargham *et al.*, 2000; Mirnics *et al.*, 2001). Interestingly, a recent study suggests that the COMT Val158Met form is associated with prefrontal and hippocampal *RGS4* mRNA expression in an allele dose-dependent manner, with carriers of the allele for COMT Val-158 showing significantly lower expression than in heterozygous individuals or in subjects homozygous for the Met-producing allele (Lipska *et al.*, 2006a).

Catechol-*O*-methyltransferase

The gene *COMT* (chromosome 22q11) encodes a key protein important for dopaminergic neurotransmission. A common coding SNP, causing a valine-to-methionine (Val158Met) substitution, alters the activity of this key enzyme. The gene *COMT* is a candidate gene not only because it encodes a key dopamine catabolic enzyme but also because velo-cardio-facial syndrome, which is associated with psychosis in up to 25% of patients (Egan *et al.*, 2001a), is caused by a 3 MB deletion affecting the *COMT* region. However, the positional support for 22q11 as a schizophrenia locus is conflicting (Glatt, Faraone & Tsuang, 2003; Kremer *et al.*, 2003; Lewis *et al.*, 2003). Meta-analyses (Munafo et al, 2005) only provide modest effect size estimates (~1.1) of the Val158Met allele substitution (Craddock, O'Donovan & Owen, 2006). Haplotype data (Shifman *et al.*, 2002) seem to be more promising (Chen *et al.*, 2004; Handoko *et al.*, 2005; Sanders *et al.*, 2005), with one negative report (Williams *et al.*, 2005). A recent imaging study suggested that multiple functional variants in COMT may combine to impact on the

likelihood of risk being increased in any given sample based on Val/Met carriage alone (Meyer-Lindenberg *et al.*, 2006a). This proposal has been partially confirmed in a case-control study that was negative for Val/Met (Nicodemus *et al.*, 2007). A large body of literature has associated *COMT* variations with cognitive impairment (Bilder *et al.*, 2002; Egan *et al.*, 2001a; Goldberg *et al.*, 2003; Meyer-Lindenberg *et al.*, 2006a; Tsai *et al.*, 2003); prefrontal P300 amplitude (Gallinat *et al.*, 2003) and signal-to-noise ratio (Winterer *et al.*, 2006); smooth eye pursuit disturbances (Rybakowski *et al.*, 2002); specific behavioural characteristics, such as aggressive or homicidal behaviour (Jones *et al.*, 2001; Strous *et al.*, 2003); and prognosis (Herken & Erdal, 2001), including response to antipsychotic drugs (Bertolino *et al.*, 2004). Interestingly, the Val158Met variation was also associated with higher scores for schizotypy and aggression in healthy volunteers (Avramopoulos *et al.*, 2002), opening up new genetically driven avenues for indicated prevention (Tsuang *et al.*, 2002). Furthermore, two studies also suggested that *COMT* may be important for manic–depressive illness (Funke *et al.*, 2005; Shifman *et al.*, 2004), in particular in bipolar patients with psychotic symptoms (Craddock *et al.*, 2006) and schizophrenia patients with manic symptoms (Funke *et al.*, 2005). Finally, in a dramatic study of potential interactions of COMT with environmental risk factors, Caspi *et al.* (2005), in a New Zealand South Island public health longitudinal cohort study, reported that early adolescent marijuana users who were Val/Val carriers had a 10-fold increase in risk for adult schizophrenia compared with the general population. The Met/Met type appeared to protect against the effect of early cannabis use. These results have potential public health implications. The gene *COMT* is a very good example of the complexity of gene–gene (Lipska *et al.*, 2006a) and gene–environment (Caspi *et al.*, 2005) interactions and in how understanding such molecular genetics may help us to dissect psychotic disorders further.

The 'disrupted in schizophrenia' genes

Another chromosomal abnormality of interest is the balanced chromosomal translocation (1;11)(q42.1:q14.3) that co-segregates with schizophrenia and other psychiatric disorders (Hennah *et al.*, 2003). This rare chromosomal defect was identified in a Scottish kindred that had a high prevalence of mental illness. A linkage analysis of the relationship of the translocation with psychiatric illness within the family generated a LOD (logarithm of the odds) score of 3.6 when the disease phenotype was restricted to schizophrenia, of 4.5 when the disease phenotype was restricted to affective disorders and of 7.1 when relatives with recurrent major depression, manic–depressive disorder or schizophrenia were included (Blackwood *et al.*, 2001), providing further support that some of the candidate genes may be shared across a range of diagnostic entities. The translocation directly disrupts two genes on chromosome 1 that have been coined as 'disrupted in schizophrenia' genes (*DISC1* and *DISC2*) (Millar *et al.*, 2000); however, only *DISC1* has been found to encode a protein. This protein appears to be important for cytoskeleton function, implying that variations of these genes may result in dysfunctional neuronal migration, pruning, neuronal architecture and intracellular transport mechanisms, all aspects proposed to be altered in psychotic disorders (Ozeki *et al.*, 2003). Evidence that *DISC1* is associated with psychosis has emerged from studies in several other samples. The gene is close to chromosome 1 markers that showed linkage in two Finnish studies (Ekelund *et al.*, 2001; Hennah *et al.*, 2003; Hovatta *et al.*, 1998). The same have reported two-point and haplotype associations to several SNPs and haplotypes in the gene (Hennah *et al.*, 2003). Several studies in American populations have reported associations with *DISC1*, but again the SNPs and haplotypes are not consistent across samples (Callicott *et al.*, 2005; Hodgkinson *et al.*, 2004). Callicott *et al.* (2005) also found that a coding SNP in *DISC1*, which showed associations in a family sample, was predictive of measures of hippocampal structure and function, assayed with MRI and with cognitive measures. So far, DISC1 has not been found to be abnormally produced in schizophrenic brain tissue, but there is evidence that some of its molecular partners may be downregulated in schizophrenia and related to risk-associated SNPs in *DISC1* (Lipska *et al.*, 2006b).

Brain-derived neurotrophic factor

A growing body of evidence suggests the importance of growth factors (neurotrophin-3, BDNF) and their receptors (e.g. TrkB) in both antipsychotic drug action and schizophrenia pathogenesis (Hong *et al.*, 2003). The development, regeneration, survival and maintenance of neurons and glial cells as well as their progenitor cells are promoted by BDNF (Seroogy *et al.*, 1994) and BDNF is critically involved in synaptic plasticity, and learning and memory (Iritani *et al.*, 2003). Studies in postmortem human brain have consistently found reductions in BDNF in schizophrenia, as well as reductions in its tyrosine kinase receptor, TrkB (Lewis, Hashimoto & Volk, 2005; Lewis *et al.*, 2006; Takahashi *et al.*, 2000; Weickert *et al.*, 2005). Recent genetic association studies investigating *BDNF* gene variations between patients with schizophrenia and normal controls found a polymorphism (C270T) in the 5′-noncoding region that was more prevalent in the patient groups (Nanko *et al.*, 2003; Szekeres *et al.*, 2003). Another common BDNF gene polymorphism (G196A), which results in an amino acid change (Val66Met), was also more frequent in schizophrenia and was associated with treatment response to clozapine in a Chinese patient cohort with schizophrenia (Hong *et al.*, 2003). However, at least as many studies have been negative for these SNPs and schizophrenia. Studies investigating the $(GT)_n$ dinucleotide repeat in *BDNF* (located 1.04 kb upstream from the transcription site) were less conclusive, with more studies finding no association between this polymorphism and schizophrenia (Hawi *et al.*, 1998; Sasaki *et al.*, 1997; Virgos *et al.*, 2001; Wassink *et al.*, 1999), compared with one family study demonstrating a moderate association (Muglia *et al.*, 2003) and another study finding an association with later onset of illness and treatment response (Krebs *et al.*, 2000). The Val66Met variant (G196A) in *BDNF* has also been shown to be more prevalent in sporadic Alzheimer's disease (Ventriglia *et al.*, 2002), bipolar disorder (Neves-Pereira *et al.*, 2002), restricted anorexia nervosa (Ribases *et al.*, 2003), obsessive-compulsive disorder (Hall *et al.*, 2003) and memory impairment in normal subjects (Egan *et al.*, 2003). This suggests that BDNF may be protective in subjects prone to mental disorders in general, and if it is dysfunctional this would be important for outcome in general, rather than for diagnostic entities per se.

Other candidate genes

A number of other candidate genes have been reported, including *PRODH2* (for proline dehydrogenase), *5HT2a* (for 5-hydroxytryptamine-2a), *PPP3CC* (for protein phosphatase 3 catalytic subunit), *CHRNA7* (for the nicotinic receptor) and *DRD3* (for dopamine receptor 3) (Table 3.1). Attempts at replications of these are continuing in a number of laboratories, and future research will show to what extent they will be relevant for psychosis (Harrison & Weinberger, 2005).

Intermediate phenotypes (endophenotypes)

The lack of consistency across genetic studies, especially in the early phase of linkage, was often interpreted as reflecting that the phenotype schizophrenia may be too complex or inadequate for traditional genetic approaches. Irving Gottesman suggested in the late 1960s that schizophrenia is a polygenic disorder and that we need to identify endophenotypes that might provide a stronger signal of gene action than the phenotype schizophrenia (Gottesman & Shields, 1967). The great hope has been that traits that are 'intermediate' between the biological substrate at the level of the cell and the phenomenological phenotype potentially could help to dissect complex disorders such as bipolar disorder or schizophrenia into biological meaningful subgroups (Gottesman & Gould, 2003). Such intermediate phenotypes should be measurable traits that are presumably causally closer to the pathogenic genotype than the clinical phenotype itself. Gottesman proposed criteria of such intermediate phenotypes (Box 3.1). The putative marker must be stable over time (trait-like) and should be found in (some) non-affected or mildly affected relatives, and be milder or less common in other disorders or in the relatives of individuals with other disorders.

Box 3.1. Definition of intermediate phenotype (endophenotype) according to Gottesman and Gould (2003) and Meyer-Lindenberg and Weinberger (2006)

1. The intermediate phenotype is associated with illness in the population
2. The intermediate phenotype is heritable
3. The intermediate phenotype is primarily state independent (manifests in an individual whether or not illness is active)
4. Within families, intermediate phenotypes and illness co-segregate
5. The intermediate phenotype found in affected family members is found in non-affected family members at a higher rate than in the general population

Alternatively, since genes do not encode for psychopathology, it would be expected that the penetrance (i.e. effect size) of a gene effect at the level of an intermediate biological trait related to the biology of the gene would be greater than at the level of the clinical diagnosis. It has been argued that intermediate phenotype is a better term for this association than is endophenotype, because the biological trait phenotype (e.g. cognition, electroencephalograph, imaging data) is not hidden and it may be a more direct reflection of the effect of the gene than is diagnosis (Meyer-Lindenberg, Mervis & Berman, 2006b). The identification of such traits may help to dissect neuropsychiatric disorders based on neurobiological deficits that may be more relevant for preventive and treatment choices than our phenomenological-based categorical concepts.

A good example of a potentially clinically useful intermediate phenotype is neuropsychological test performance. Beginning with several discordant monozygotic twin studies (Cannon *et al.*, 2000; Goldberg *et al.*, 1995) and then in family studies (Egan *et al.*, 2001b), cognitive deficits qualitatively similar to those associated with schizophrenia were found with increased prevalence in unaffected siblings of patients with schizophrenia. Egan *et al.* (2001a) reported that abnormal prefrontal brain function was impaired in those individuals who were carriers of the allele at codon 108 of

COMT that expressed valine in patients, their healthy siblings as well as in controls, an allele that is only weakly and inconsistently associated with schizophrenia. This was one of the first validated experiments using intermediate phenotypes and ascertaining genetic correlation in psychiatry to clarify how a particular gene variation may be related to the complex clinical diagnosis. Using a similar approach, Egan *et al.* (2004) demonstrated that *GRM3* gene variations (encoding metabotropic glutamate receptor 3) that were part of an over-transmitted haplotype had a weak effect on cognitive functioning. Focusing on their most positively associated SNP, they found significant effects of genotypes on verbal list learning in episodic memory and verbal fluency for letters in patients and siblings, and, to some extent, even normal subjects showed an association with the risk allele. In a follow-up study, the finding that prefrontal cortex function was associated with *GRM3* variants (SNP rs6465084) could be substantiated in healthy comparison subjects using magnetic resonance spectroscopic imaging at 3 T. The A/A genotype group exhibited a significant reduction of *N*-acetylaspartate/creatine levels in the right dorsolateral prefrontal cortex compared with the G carriers. A tendency in the same direction was seen in the left dorsolateral prefrontal cortex and in the white matter adjacent to the prefrontal cortex. These findings provide another example of how genotype information may be used as future markers to improve characterization of risk groups (e.g. A/A carriers of *GRM3* gene variant rs6465084 in ultra-high-risk cohorts).

Epigenetics

The term epigenetics generally refers to heritable changes in gene function unrelated to changes in DNA sequence. It encompasses a broad definition ranging from mechanisms that lead to the phenotypic expression of genetic information in an individual to a narrower definition concerned with the mechanisms through which cells become committed to a particular form or function and through which that functional or structural state is then transmitted in cell lineages

(Jablonka & Lamb, 2002). There are several proposed mechanisms involved in this process, such as the methylation of a cytosine (or guanine) nucleotide molecule in a DNA sequence as well as acetylation of histone and chromatin rearrangements (Fraga *et al.*, 2005). Methylation of DNA and histonal acetylation are dynamic processes that facilitate the turning on and off of gene transcription. Changes in chromatin configuration based on histones and DNA methylation can be passed on as stable heritable molecular traits. This may be an important mechanism to explain why identical twins can be discordant for schizophrenia (or other traits) despite the extremely high genetic liability associated with schizophrenia (Petronis *et al.*, 2003). Of particular interest is a study that found different methylation status at two CpG sites in the promoter region of *COMT*, another potential reason for the inconclusive results of *COMT* association studies (Mill *et al.*, 2006).

Discussion

One of the key difficulties in defining and categorizing mental illnesses is that we still do not have specific biological substrates as found in other areas of medicine, where we can directly study the abnormality associated with the disease. The phenotype 'schizophrenia' has been characterized by the presence of behavioural abnormalities, the related outcome and its longitudinal course, but not its fundamental biological substrate. The absence of a neuropathological basis for schizophrenia (e.g. in contrast to Alzheimer's dementia) was one reason that some researchers believed that the actual illness process has to occur in the prenatal developmental period where the brain does not respond with a major inflammatory reaction that would result in permanent gliotic changes. This suggestion has been the foundation of the neurodevelopmental hypothesis of schizophrenia put forward by Weinberger (1987). Evidence of obstetrical complications being associated with risk of schizophrenia (Murray & Lewis, 1987) and with early childhood developmental delay (Murray, Jones & O'Callaghan, 1991) added to the belief that developmental abnormalities were involved. If true, the postulated abnormal biological processes would happen during critical periods of brain development that finally manifest when particular brain regions are activated or under increased demand, as in adolescence. However, the premorbid risk factors associated with schizophrenia (e.g. motor and cognitive delay, obstetrical complications) are non-specific, their prevalence in the non-affected population is substantial and their positive predictive value for the development of schizophrenia is limited. When neuroimaging anomalies were found in samples of patients with first-episode psychosis (regarded, often erroneously, as close to 'onset'), this was interpreted as supportive of a static structural abnormality associated with schizophrenia that had originated early in neurodevelopment (Weinberger & McClure, 2002). One of the key questions is to clarify the timing and specificity of these changes. Progressive MRI changes in longitudinal studies in childhood-onset schizophrenia (Jacobsen *et al.*, 1998; Rapoport *et al.*, 1997), and differences in MRI measures before and after transition to psychosis (Pantelis *et al.*, 2003), in the course of early psychosis (DeLisi, 1999a,b,c; Gur *et al.*, 1998, Lieberman *et al.*, 2001), as well as in subgroups of patients with chronic schizophrenia (Davis *et al.*, 1998; Gur *et al.*, 1998; Mathalon *et al.*, 2001; Velakoulis *et al.*, 2001, 2000) indicate the need for revised explanatory models, integrating the presence of early neurodevelopmental abnormalities with more dynamic changes around the onset phase of psychosis (Weinberger & McClure, 2002). Unifying models have been formulated including two-hit (Bayer, Falkai & Maier, 1999) and three-hit (Keshavan, 1999, Velakoulis *et al.*, 2000) models of schizophrenia, suggesting illicit drug use and environmental stress as potential secondary triggers accompanying the onset and course of schizophrenia (Allin & Murray, 2002). The precise nature of the underlying biology of these MRI-based changes is unknown, and the lack of degenerative changes seen in postmortem examination argues against those being irreversible. Indeed, there is evidence that the MRI changes can reverse in some patients, raising the possibility that they reflect plasticity phenomena that may prove somewhat peripheral to understanding the disorder.

Recently, the association of molecular genetics with intermediate phenotypes such as cognitive impairment or abnormal brain functioning, as measured with functional neuroimaging, has generated a much more diverse understanding of major psychosis, and the combination of these fields of study have resulted in some provocative models. Research in Alzheimer's disease has demonstrated how powerful the integration of multiple levels of research can be in understanding complex disorders. Bookheimer *et al.* (2000) investigated *APOE4* alleles (encoding apolipoprotein E), and evaluated the effects of *APOE* genotypes on the fMRI response in the hippocampus during memory processing, and found that the risk allele affected memory processing even in healthy subjects. Similar findings were obtained for functional polymorphism in the gene for BDNF, which impacts on hippocampal learning and memory in animals, and in normal humans (Egan *et al.*, 2003). These publications illustrate the convergent use of different methodologies to improve the characterization of genetic mechanisms in the living human brain and, indeed, point out an important direction for future research. The combination of different levels may be of particular importance for longitudinal 'at-risk' studies. These studies address the important issue of whether we can identify individuals who are at true risk of developing major psychosis prior to its full clinical expression (Yung *et al.*, 2002), enabling us to treat 'at-risk' individuals prior to full manifestation of psychosis and prevent its appearance during critical developmental periods such as late adolescence.

Gene–environment interactions are likely to be at the heart of moving from vulnerability states to expression of the clinical phenotype (Chapter 4). The measurement of genetic profiles using groups of candidate genes in combination with psychosocial risk factors such as stress and illicit drug use in samples of patients with clinically significant but subthreshold features of psychosis and mood disorder is a key research strategy which is now feasible. Such a strategy may be useful in enhancing predictive power for transition to more established and severe psychotic disorders. It may also help in treatment selection and longer-term prognostic forecasting. In the research clinic, it may also be possible to investigate genetic variables with endophenotypic markers, such as imaging, neurocognition and psychophysiological indicators, in such crucial early psychosis samples.

Conclusions

In conclusion, linkage studies followed by confirmatory association studies paved the way for the discovery of an array of important candidate genes with modest effect size. Growing evidence suggests that diagnostic boundaries may be modified based on genetic information, and some genes such as *NRG1*, *DTNBP1*, *DISC1* and *BDNF* may relate to risk for both schizophrenia and mood disorders (Prathikanti & Weinberger, 2005). This should not be surprising because clearly genes do not encode for psychopathology per se, and the human genome did not evolve with the intention of reifying the DSM-IV criteria (APA, 1994). The list of susceptibility genes related to major psychosis is growing. The synergistic use of genotyping, with intermediate phenotypes characterizing brain functioning, will contribute to a better understanding of the mechanisms by which genes interact with other genes and/or environmental risk factors. Ultimately, this may help to determine if an individual carries a vulnerability for a major psychotic illness. The translation of the recent provocative findings of candidate genes for major psychosis into the clinic is still to come, but the progress in the last decade can provide us with optimism that the next decade will open up new ways to understand major psychosis and to translate the findings into daily clinical practice.

REFERENCES

Abi-Dargham, A., Rodenhiser, R. J., Printz, D. *et al.* (2000). Increased baseline occupancy of D$_2$ receptors by dopamine in schizophrenia. *Proceedings of the National Academy of Sciences USA*, **97**, 8104–9.

Allin, M. & Murray, R. M. (2002). Schizophrenia: a neurodevelopmental or neurodegenerative disorder? *Current Opinion in Psychiatry*, **15**, 9–15.

APA (1994). *Diagnostic and Statistical Manual of Mental Disorders*, 4th edn. Washington, DC: American Psychiatric Press.

Avramopoulos, D., Stefanis, N. C., Hantoumi, I. *et al.* (2002). Higher scores of self reported schizotypy in healthy young males carrying the COMT high activity allele. *Molecular Psychiatry*, **7**, 706–11.

Badner, J. A. & Gershon, E. S. (2002). Meta-analysis of whole-genome linkage scans of bipolar disorder and schizophrenia. *Molecular Psychiatry*, **7**, 405–11.

Bayer, T. A., Falkai, P. & Maier, W. (1999). Genetic and nongenetic vulnerability factors in schizophrenia: the basis of the 'two hit hypothesis'. *Journal of Psychiatric Research*, **33**, 543–8.

Berger, G., Wood, S. & McGorry, P. (2003). Incipient neurovulnerability and neuroprotection in early psychosis. *Psychopharmacology Bulletin*, **37**, 79–101.

Bertolino, A., Caforio, G., Blasi, G. *et al.* (2004). Interaction of COMT (Val(108/158)Met) genotype and olanzapine treatment on prefrontal cortical function in patients with schizophrenia. *American Journal of Psychiatry*, **161**, 1798–805.

Bilder, R. M., Volavka, J., Czobor, P. *et al.* (2002). Neurocognitive correlates of the COMT Val(158)Met polymorphism in chronic schizophrenia. *Biological Psychiatry*, **52**, 701–7.

Blackwood, D. H., Fordyce, A., Walker, M. T. *et al.* (2001). Schizophrenia and affective disorders: cosegregation with a translocation at chromosome 1q42 that directly disrupts brain-expressed genes: clinical and P300 findings in a family. *American Journal of Human Genetics*, **69**, 428–33.

Bookheimer, S. Y., Strojwas, M. H., Cohen, M. S. *et al.* (2000). Patterns of brain activation in people at risk for Alzheimer's disease. *New England Journal of Medicine*, **343**, 450–6.

Callicott, J. H., Straub, R. E., Pezawas, L. *et al.* (2005). Variation in DISC1 affects hippocampal structure and function and increases risk for schizophrenia. *Proceedings of the National Academy of Sciences USA*, **102**, 8627–32.

Cannon, T., Huttunen, M., Lonnqvist, J. *et al.* (2000). The inheritance of neuropsychological dysfunction in twins discordant for schizophrenia. *American Journal of Human Genetics*, **67**, 369–82.

Canoll, P. D., Kraemer, R., Teng, K. K., Marchionni, M. A. & Salzer, J. L. (1999). GGF/neuregulin induces a phenotypic reversion of oligodendrocytes. *Molecular and Cellular Neuroscience*, **13**, 79–94.

Caspi, A., Moffitt, T. E., Cannon, M. *et al.* (2005). Moderation of the effect of adolescent-onset cannabis use on adult psychosis by a functional polymorphism in the catechol-O-methyltransferase gene: longitudinal evidence of a gene X environment interaction. *Biological Psychiatry*, **57**, 1117–27.

Cassidy, F., Roche, S., Claffey, E. & McKeon, P. (2006). First family-based test for association of neuregulin with bipolar affective disorder. *Molecular Psychiatry*, **11**, 706–7.

Chen, X., Wang, X., O'Neill, A. F., Walsh, D. & Kendler, K. S. (2004). Variants in the catechol-*O*-methyltransferase (COMT) gene are associated with schizophrenia in Irish high-density families. *Molecular Psychiatry*, **9**, 962–7.

Chowdari, K. V., Mirnics, K., Semwal, P. *et al.* (2002). Association and linkage analyses of RGS4 polymorphisms in schizophrenia. *Human Molecular Genetics*, **11**, 1373–80.

Chumakov, I., Blumenfeld, M., Guerassimenko, O. *et al.* (2002). Genetic and physiological data implicating the new human gene *G72* and the gene for D-amino acid oxidase in schizophrenia. *Proceedings of the National Academy of Sciences USA*, **99**, 13675–80.

Craddock, N., O'Donovan, M. C. & Owen, M. J. (2006). Genes for schizophrenia and bipolar disorder? Implications for psychiatric nosology. *Schizophrenia Bulletin*, **32**, 9–16.

Davis, K. L., Buchsbaum, M. S., Shihabuddin, L. *et al.* (1998). Ventricular enlargement in poor-outcome schizophrenia. *Biological Psychiatry*, **43**, 783–93.

Davis, K. L., Stewart, D. G., Friedman, J. I. *et al.* (2003). White matter changes in schizophrenia: evidence for myelin-related dysfunction. *Archives of General Psychiatry*, **60**, 443–56.

Delisi, L. E. (1999a). Defining the course of brain structural change and plasticity in schizophrenia. *Psychiatry Research*, **92**, 1–9.

Delisi, L. E. (1999b). Regional brain volume change over the lifetime course of schizophrenia. *Journal of Psychiatric Research*, **33**, 535–41.

Delisi, L. E. (1999c). Structural brain changes in schizophrenia. *Archives of General Psychiatry*, **56**, 195–6.

Detera-Wadleigh, S. D. & McMahon, F. J. (2006). G72/G30 in schizophrenia and bipolar disorder: review and meta-analysis. *Biological Psychiatry*, **60**, 106–14.

Egan, M. F., Goldberg, T. E., Kolachana, B. S. *et al.* (2001a). Effect of COMT Val108/158 Met genotype on frontal lobe function and risk for schizophrenia. *Proceedings of the National Academy of Sciences USA*, **98**, 6917–22.

Egan, M. F., Goldberg, T. E., Gscheidle, T. *et al.* (2001b). Relative risk for cognitive impairments in siblings of patients with schizophrenia. *Biological Psychiatry*, **50**, 98–107.

Egan, M. F., Kojima, M., Callicott, J. H. *et al.* (2003). The BDNF val66met polymorphism affects activity-dependent secretion of BDNF and human memory and hippocampal function. *Cell*, **112**, 257–69.

Egan, M. F., Straub, R. E., Goldberg, T. E. *et al.* (2004). Variation in GRM3 affects cognition, prefrontal glutamate, and risk for schizophrenia. *Proceedings of the National Academy of Sciences USA*, **101**, 12604–9.

Ekelund, J., Hovatta, I., Parker, A. *et al.* (2001). Chromosome 1 loci in Finnish schizophrenia families. *Human Molecular Genetics*, **10**, 1611–17.

Falls, D. L. (2003). Neuregulins: functions, forms, and signaling strategies. *Experimental Cell Research*, **284**, 14–30.

First, M. B., Spitzer, R. L., Gibbon, M. & Williams, J. B. W. (2002). *Structured Clinical Interview for DSM-IV-TR Axis I Disorders*, research version, patient edn (SCID-I/P). New York: Biometrics Research, New York State Psychiatric Institute.

Fraga, M. F., Ballestar, E., Paz, M. F. *et al.* (2005). Epigenetic differences arise during the lifetime of monozygotic twins. *Proceedings of the National Academy of Sciences USA*, **102**, 10604–9.

Funke, B., Malhotra, A. K., Finn, C. T. *et al.* (2005). COMT genetic variation confers risk for psychotic and affective disorders: a case control study. *Behavioral and Brain Functions*, **1**, 19–27.

Gallinat, J., Bajbouj, M., Sander, T. *et al.* (2003). Association of the G1947A COMT (Val(108/158)Met) gene polymorphism with prefrontal P300 during information processing. *Biological Psychiatry*, **54**, 40–8.

Glatt, S. J., Faraone, S. V. & Tsuang, M. T. (2003). Association between a functional catechol *O*-methyltransferase gene polymorphism and schizophrenia: meta-analysis of case-control and family-based studies. *American Journal of Psychiatry*, **160**, 469–76.

Goldberg, T. E., Torrey, E. F., Gold, J. M. *et al.* (1995). Genetic risk of neuropsychological impairment in schizophrenia: a study of monozygotic twins discordant and concordant for the disorder. *Schizophrenia Research*, **17**, 77–84.

Goldberg, T. E., Egan, M. F., Gscheidle, T. *et al.* (2003). Executive subprocesses in working memory: relationship to catechol-*O*-methyltransferase Val158Met genotype and schizophrenia. *Archives of General Psychiatry*, **60**, 889–96.

Gottesman, I. I. & Gould, T. D. (2003). The endophenotype concept in psychiatry: etymology and strategic intentions. *American Journal of Psychiatry*, **160**, 1–10.

Gottesman, I. I. & Shields, J. (1967). A polygenic theory of schizophrenia. *Proceedings of the National Academy of Sciences USA*, **58**, 199–205.

Green, E. K., Raybould, R., MacGregor, S. *et al.* (2005). Operation of the schizophrenia susceptibility gene, neuregulin 1, across traditional diagnostic boundaries to increase risk for bipolar disorder. *Archives of General Psychiatry*, **62**, 642–8.

Gur, R. E., Cowell, P., Turetsky, B. I. *et al.* (1998). A follow-up magnetic resonance imaging study of schizophrenia. Relationship of neuroanatomical changes to clinical and neurobehavioral measures. *Archives of General Psychiatry*, **55**, 145–52.

Hakak, Y., Walker, J. R., Li, C. *et al.* (2001). Genome-wide expression analysis reveals dysregulation of myelination-related genes in chronic schizophrenia. *Proceedings of the National Academy of Sciences USA*, **98**, 4746–51.

Hall, D., Dhilla, A., Charalambous, A., Gogos, J. A. & Karayiorgou, M. (2003). Sequence variants of the brain-derived neurotrophic factor (BDNF) gene are strongly associated with obsessive-compulsive disorder. *American Journal of Human Genetics*, **73**, 370–6.

Handoko, H. Y., Nyholt, D. R., Hayward, N. K. *et al.* (2005). Separate and interacting effects within the catechol-*O*-methyltransferase (COMT) are associated with schizophrenia. *Molecular Psychiatry*, **10**, 589–97.

Harrison, P. J. & Law, A. J. (2006). Neuregulin 1 and schizophrenia: genetics, gene expression, and neurobiology. *Biological Psychiatry*, **60**, 132–40.

Harrison, P. J. & Weinberger, D. R. (2005). Schizophrenia genes, gene expression, and neuropathology: on the matter of their convergence. *Molecular Psychiatry*, **10**, 40–68.

Hashimoto, R., Straub, R. E., Weickert, C. S. *et al.* (2004). Expression analysis of neuregulin-1 in the dorsolateral prefrontal cortex in schizophrenia. *Molecular Psychiatry*, **9**, 299–307.

Hawi, Z., Straub, R. E., O'Neill, A. *et al.* (1998). No linkage or linkage disequilibrium between brain-derived neurotrophic factor (BDNF) dinucleotide repeat polymorphism and schizophrenia in Irish families. *Psychiatry Research*, **81**, 111–16.

Hennah, W., Varilo, T., Kestila, M. *et al.* (2003). Haplotype transmission analysis provides evidence of association for DISC1 to schizophrenia and suggests sex-dependent effects. *Human Molecular Genetics*, **12**, 3151–9.

Herken, H. & Erdal, M. E. (2001). Catechol-*O*-methyltransferase gene polymorphism in schizophrenia: evidence for association between symptomatology and prognosis. *Psychiatric Genetics*, **11**, 105–9.

Hodgkinson, C. A., Goldman, D., Jaeger, J. *et al.* (2004). Disrupted in schizophrenia 1 (DISC1): association with schizophrenia, schizoaffective disorder, and bipolar disorder. *American Journal of Human Genetics*, **75**, 862–72.

Holliday, E. G., Handoko, H. Y., James, M. R. *et al.* (2006). Association study of the dystrobrevin-binding gene with schizophrenia in Australian and Indian samples. *Twin Research and Human Genetics*, **9**, 531–9.

Hong, C. J., Yu, Y. W., Lin, C. H. & Tsai, S. J. (2003). An association study of a brain-derived neurotrophic factor Val66Met polymorphism and clozapine response of schizophrenic patients. *Neuroscience Letters*, **349**, 206–8.

Hovatta, I., Lichtermann, D., Juvonen, H. *et al.* (1998). Linkage analysis of putative schizophrenia gene candidate regions on chromosomes 3p, 5q, 6p, 8p, 20p and 22q in a population-based sampled Finnish family set. *Molecular Psychiatry*, **3**, 452–7.

Iritani, S., Niizato, K., Nawa, H., Ikeda, K. & Emson, P. C. (2003). Immunohistochemical study of brain-derived neurotrophic factor and its receptor, TrkB, in the hippocampal formation of schizophrenic brains. *Progress in Neuropsychopharmacology and Biological Psychiatry*, **27**, 801–7.

Jablensky, A. (1999). The concept of schizophrenia: pro et contra. *Epidemiologia e Psichiatria Sociale*, **8**, 242–7.

Jablonka, E. & Lamb, M. J. (2002). The changing concept of epigenetics. *Annals of the New York Academy of Sciences*, **981**, 82–96.

Jacobsen, L. K., Giedd, J. N., Castellanos, F. X. *et al.* (1998). Progressive reduction of temporal lobe structures in childhood-onset schizophrenia. *American Journal of Psychiatry*, **155**, 678–85.

Jones, G., Zammit, S., Norton, N. *et al.* (2001). Aggressive behaviour in patients with schizophrenia is associated with catechol-*O*-methyltransferase genotype. *British Journal of Psychiatry*, **179**, 351–5.

Kendler, K. S. (2004). Schizophrenia genetics and dysbindin: a corner turned? *American Journal of Psychiatry*, **161**, 1533–6.

Keshavan, M. S. (1999). Development, disease and degeneration in schizophrenia: a unitary pathophysiological model. *Journal of Psychiatric Research*, **33**, 513–21.

Kohn, Y., Danilovich, E., Filon, D. *et al.* (2004). Linkage disequilibrium in the DTNBP1 (dysbindin) gene region and on chromosome 1p36 among psychotic patients from a genetic isolate in Israel: findings from identity by descent haplotype sharing analysis. *American Journal of Medical Genetics Part B: Neuropsychiatric Genetics*, **128**, 65–70.

Krebs, M. O., Guillin, O., Bourdell, M. C. *et al.* (2000). Brain derived neurotrophic factor (BDNF) gene variants association with age at onset and therapeutic response in schizophrenia. *Molecular Psychiatry*, **5**, 558–62.

Kremer, I., Pinto, M., Murad, I. *et al.* (2003). Family-based and case-control study of catechol-*O*-methyltransferase in schizophrenia among Palestinian Arabs. *American Journal of Medical Genetics*, **119B**, 35–9.

Law, A. J., Shannon Weickert, C., Hyde, T. M., Kleinman, J. E. & Harrison, P. J. (2004). Neuregulin-1 (NRG-1) mRNA and protein in the adult human brain. *Neuroscience*, **127**, 125–36.

Law, A. J., Lipska, B. K., Weickert, C. S. *et al.* (2006). Neuregulin 1 transcripts are differentially expressed in schizophrenia and regulated by 5′ SNPs associated with the disease.

Proceedings of the National Academy of Sciences USA, **103**, 6747–52.

Levinson, D. F., Holmans, P. A., Laurent, C. *et al.* (2002). No major schizophrenia locus detected on chromosome 1q in a large multicenter sample. *Science*, **296**, 739–41.

Lewis, C. M., Levinson, D. F., Wise, L. H. *et al.* (2003). Genome scan meta-analysis of schizophrenia and bipolar disorder, part II: schizophrenia. *American Journal of Human Genetics*, **73**, 34–48.

Lewis, D. A., Hashimoto, T. & Volk, D. W. (2005). Cortical inhibitory neurons and schizophrenia. *Nature Reviews Neuroscience*, **6**, 312–24.

Lewis, M. A., Hunihan, L., Franco, D. *et al.* (2006). Identification and characterization of compounds that potentiate NT-3-mediated Trk receptor activity. *Molecular Pharmacology*, **69**, 1396–404.

Li, D., Collier, D. A. & He, L. (2006). Meta-analysis shows strong positive association of the neuregulin 1 (NRG1) gene with schizophrenia. *Human Molecular Genetics*, **15**, 1995–2002.

Lieberman, J., Chakos, M., Wu, H. *et al.* (2001). Longitudinal study of brain morphology in first episode schizophrenia. *Biological Psychiatry*, **49**, 487–99.

Lipska, B. K., Mitkus, S., Caruso, M. *et al.* (2006a). RGS4 mRNA expression in postmortem human cortex is associated with COMT Val158Met genotype and COMT enzyme activity. *Human Molecular Genetics*, **15**, 2804–12.

Lipska, B. K., Peters, T., Hyde, T. M. *et al.* (2006b). Expression of DISC1 binding partners is reduced in schizophrenia and associated with DISC1 SNPs. *Human Molecular Genetics*, **15**, 1245–58.

Mathalon, D. H., Sullivan, E. V., Lim, K. O. & Pfefferbaum, A. (2001). Progressive brain volume changes and the clinical course of schizophrenia in men: a longitudinal magnetic resonance imaging study. *Archives of General Psychiatry*, **58**, 148–57.

Meyer-Lindenberg, A. & Weinberger, D. R. (2006). Intermediate phenotypes and genetic mechanisms of psychiatric disorders. *Nature Reviews Neuroscience*, **7**, 818–27.

Meyer-Lindenberg, A., Nichols, T., Callicott, J. H. *et al.* (2006a). Impact of complex genetic variation in COMT on human brain function. *Molecular Psychiatry*, **11**, 867–77.

Meyer-Lindenberg, A., Mervis, C. B. & Berman, K. F. (2006b). Neural mechanisms in Williams' syndrome: a unique window to genetic influences on cognition and behaviour. *Nature Reviews Neuroscience*, **7**, 380–93.

Mill, J., Dempster, E., Caspi, A. *et al.* (2006). Evidence for monozygotic twin (MZ) discordance in methylation level at two CpG sites in the promoter region of the catechol-*O*-methyltransferase (COMT) gene. *American Journal of Medical Genetics Part B: Neuropsychiatric Genetics*, **141**, 421–5.

Millar, J. K., Wilson-Annan, J. C., Anderson, S. *et al.* (2000). Disruption of two novel genes by a translocation co-segregating with schizophrenia. *Human Molecular Genetics*, **9**, 1415–23.

Mirnics, K., Middleton, F. A., Stanwood, G. D., Lewis, D. A. & Levitt, P. (2001). Disease-specific changes in regulator of G-protein signaling 4 (RGS4) expression in schizophrenia. *Molecular Psychiatry*, **6**, 293–301.

Muglia, P., Vicente, A. M., Verga, M. *et al.* (2003). Association between the *BDNF* gene and schizophrenia. *Molecular Psychiatry*, **8**, 146–7.

Munafo, M. R, Bowes, L., Clark, T. G. & Flint, J. (2005). Lack of association of the COMT (Val(158/108) Met) gene and schizophrenia: a meta-analysis of case-control studies. *Molecular Psychiatry*, **10**, 765–70.

Murray, R. M. & Lewis, S. W. (1987). Is schizophrenia a neurodevelopmental disorder? *British Medical Journal (Clinical Research Edition)*, **295**, 681–2.

Murray, R. M., Jones, P. & O'Callaghan, E. (1991). Fetal brain development and later schizophrenia. *Ciba Foundation Symposium*, **156**, 155–70.

Nanko, S., Kunugi, H., Hirasawa, H. *et al.* (2003). Brain-derived neurotrophic factor gene and schizophrenia: polymorphism screening and association analysis. *Schizophrenia Research*, **62**, 281–3.

Neves-Pereira, M., Mundo, E., Muglia, P. *et al.* (2002). The brain-derived neurotrophic factor gene confers susceptibility to bipolar disorder: evidence from a family-based association study. *American Journal of Human Genetics*, **71**, 651–5.

Nicodemus, K. K., Kolachana, B. S., Vakkalanka, R. *et al.* (2007). Evidence for statistical epistasis between catechol-*O*-methyltransferase (COMT) and polymorphisms in RGS4, G72 (DAOA), GRM3, and DISC1: influence on risk of schizophrenia. *Human Genetics*, **120**, 889–906.

Norton, N., Williams, H. J. & Owen, M. J. (2006). An update on the genetics of schizophrenia. *Current Opinion in Psychiatry*, **19**, 158–64.

Owen, M. J., Holmans, P. & McGuffin, P. (1997). Association studies in psychiatric genetics. *Molecular Psychiatry*, **2**, 270–3.

Owen, M. J., Williams, N. M. & O'Donovan, M. C. (2004). The molecular genetics of schizophrenia: new findings promise new insights. *Molecular Psychiatry*, **9**, 14–27.

Ozeki, Y., Tomoda, T., Kleiderlein, J. *et al.* (2003). Disrupted-in-schizophrenia-1 (DISC-1): mutant truncation prevents binding to NudE-like (NUDEL) and inhibits neurite outgrowth. *Proceedings of the National Academy of Sciences USA*, **100**, 289–94.

Pantelis, C., Velakoulis, D., McGorry, P. D. *et al.* (2003). Neuroanatomical abnormalities before and after onset of psychosis: a cross-sectional and longitudinal MRI comparison. *Lancet*, **361**, 281–8.

Petronis, A., Gottesman, I. I., Kan, P. *et al.* (2003). Monozygotic twins exhibit numerous epigenetic differences: clues to twin discordance? *Schizophrenia Bulletin*, **29**, 169–78.

Prathikanti, S. & Weinberger, D. R. (2005). Psychiatric genetics – the new era: genetic research and some clinical implications. *British Medical Bulletin*, **73–74**, 107–22.

Rapoport, J. L., Giedd, J., Kumra, S. *et al.* (1997). Childhood-onset schizophrenia. Progressive ventricular change during adolescence. *Archives of General Psychiatry*, **54**, 897–903.

Raybould, R., Green, E. K., MacGregor, S. *et al.* (2005). Bipolar disorder and polymorphisms in the dysbindin gene (DTNBP1). *Biological Psychiatry*, **57**, 696–701.

Ribases, M., Gratacos, M., Armengol, L. *et al.* (2003). Met66 in the brain-derived neurotrophic factor (BDNF) precursor is associated with anorexia nervosa restrictive type. *Molecular Psychiatry*, **8**, 745–51.

Risch, N. & Merikangas, K. (1996). The future of genetic studies of complex human diseases. *Science*, **273**, 1516–17.

Rocchi, A., Pellegrini, S., Siciliano, G. & Murri, L. (2003). Causative and susceptibility genes for Alzheimer's disease: a review. *Brain Research Bulletin*, **61**, 1–24.

Rybakowski, J. K., Borkowska, A., Czerski, P. M. & Hauser, J. (2002). Eye movement disturbances in schizophrenia and a polymorphism of catechol-*O*-methyltransferase gene. *Psychiatry Research*, **113**, 49–57.

Sanders, A. R., Rusu, I., Duan, J. *et al.* (2005). Haplotypic association spanning the 22q11.21 genes *COMT* and *ARVCF* with schizophrenia. *Molecular Psychiatry*, **10**, 353–65.

Sasaki, T., Dai, X. Y., Kuwata, S. *et al.* (1997). Brain-derived neurotrophic factor gene and schizophrenia in Japanese subjects. *American Journal of Medical Genetics*, **74**, 443–4.

Schwab, S. G., Knapp, M., Mondabon, S. *et al.* (2003). Support for association of schizophrenia with genetic variation in the 6p22.3 gene, dysbindin, in sib-pair families with linkage and in an additional sample of triad families. *American Journal of Human Genetics*, **72**, 185–90.

Seroogy, K. B., Lundgren, K. H., Tran, T. M. *et al.* (1994). Dopaminergic neurons in rat ventral midbrain express brain-derived neurotrophic factor and neurotrophin-3 mRNAs. *Journal of Comprehensive Neurology*, **342**, 321–34.

Shifman, S., Bronstein, M., Sternfeld, M. *et al.* (2002). A highly significant association between a COMT haplotype and schizophrenia. *American Journal of Human Genetics*, **71**, 1296–302.

Shifman, S., Bronstein, M., Sternfeld, M. *et al.* (2004). COMT: a common susceptibility gene in bipolar disorder and schizophrenia. *American Journal of Medical Genetics Part B: Neuropsychiatric Genetics*, **128**, 61–4.

Slager, S. L. & Schaid, D. J. (2001). Evaluation of candidate genes in case–control studies: a statistical method to account for related subjects. *American Journal of Human Genetics*, **68**, 1457–62.

Stefansson, H., Sigurdsson, E., Steinthorsdottir, V. *et al.* (2002). Neuregulin 1 and susceptibility to schizophrenia. *American Journal of Human Genetics*, **71**, 877–92.

Stefansson, H., Sarginson, J., Kong, A. *et al.* (2003). Association of neuregulin 1 with schizophrenia confirmed in a Scottish population. *American Journal of Human Genetics*, **72**, 83–7.

Straub, R. E., Jiang, Y., MacLean, C. J. *et al.* (2002). Genetic variation in the 6p22.3 gene *DTNBP1*, the human ortholog of the mouse dysbindin gene, is associated with schizophrenia. *American Journal of Human Genetics*, **71**, 337–48.

Strous, R. D., Nolan, K. A., Lapidus, R. *et al.* (2003). Aggressive behaviour in schizophrenia is associated with the low enzyme activity COMT polymorphism: a replication study. *American Journal of Medical Genetics*, **120B**, 29–34.

Sullivan, P. F., Kendler, K. S. & Neale, M. C. (2003). Schizophrenia as a complex trait: evidence from a meta-analysis of twin studies. *Archives of General Psychiatry*, **60**, 1187–92.

Szekeres, G., Juhasz, A., Rimanoczy, A., Keri, S. & Janka, Z. (2003). The C270T polymorphism of the brain-derived neurotrophic factor gene is associated with schizophrenia. *Schizophrenia Research*, **65**, 15–18.

Takahashi, M., Shirakawa, O., Toyooka, K. *et al.* (2000). Abnormal expression of brain-derived neurotrophic factor and its receptor in the corticolimbic system of schizophrenic patients. *Molecular Psychiatry*, **5**, 293–300.

Talbot, K., Eidem, W. L., Tinsley, C. L. *et al.* (2004). Dysbindin-1 is reduced in intrinsic, glutamatergic terminals of the hippocampal formation in schizophrenia. *Journal of Clinical Investigation*, **113**, 1353–63.

Talkowski, M. E., Seltman, H., Bassett, A. S. *et al.* (2006). Evaluation of a susceptibility gene for schizophrenia: genotype based meta-analysis of RGS4 polymorphisms from thirteen independent samples. *Biological Psychiatry*, **60**, 152–62.

Tang, J. X., Chen, W. Y., He, G. *et al.* (2004). Polymorphisms within 5′ end of the *neuregulin 1* gene are genetically associated with schizophrenia in the Chinese population. *Molecular Psychiatry*, **9**, 11–12.

Tochigi, M., Zhang, X., Ohashi, J. *et al.* (2006). Association study of the dysbindin (*DTNBP1*) gene in schizophrenia from the Japanese population. *Neuroscience Research*, **56**, 45–7.

Tsai, S. J., Yu, Y. W., Chen, T. J. *et al.* (2003). Association study of a functional catechol-*O*-methyltransferase gene polymorphism and cognitive function in healthy females. *Neuroscience Letters*, **338**, 123–6.

Tsuang, M. T., Stone, W. S., Tarbox, S. I. & Faraone, S. V. (2002). An integration of schizophrenia with schizotypy: identification of schizotaxia and implications for research on treatment and prevention. *Schizophrenia Research*, **54**, 169–75.

van Os, J., Gilvarry, C., Bale, R. *et al.* (2000). Diagnostic value of the DSM and ICD categories of psychosis: an evidence-based approach. UK700 Group. *Social Psychiatry and Psychiatric Epidemiology*, **35**, 305–11.

Velakoulis, D., Wood, S. J., McGorry, P. D. & Pantelis, C. (2000). Evidence for progression of brain structural abnormalities in schizophrenia: beyond the neurodevelopmental model. *Australian and New Zealand Journal of Psychiatry*, **34**, 113–26.

Velakoulis, D., Stuart, G. W., Wood, S. J. *et al.* (2001). Selective bilateral hippocampal volume loss in chronic schizophrenia. *Biological Psychiatry*, **50**, 531–9.

Ventriglia, M., Bocchio Chiavetto, L., Benussi, L. *et al.* (2002). Association between the BDNF 196 A/G polymorphism and sporadic Alzheimer's disease. *Molecular Psychiatry*, **7**, 136–7.

Virgos, C., Martorell, L., Valero, J. *et al.* (2001). Association study of schizophrenia with polymorphisms at six candidate genes. *Schizophrenia Research*, **49**, 65–71.

Wassink, T. H., Nelson, J. J., Crowe, R. R. & Andreasen, N. C. (1999). Heritability of *BDNF* alleles and their effect on brain morphology in schizophrenia. *American Journal of Medical Genetics*, **88**, 724–8.

Weickert, C. S., Straub, R. E., McClintock, B. W. *et al.* (2004). Human dysbindin (*DTNBP1*) gene expression in normal brain and in schizophrenic prefrontal cortex and midbrain. *Archives of General Psychiatry*, **61**, 544–55.

Weickert, C. S., Ligons, D. L., Romanczyk, T. *et al.* (2005). Reductions in neurotrophin receptor mRNAs in the prefrontal cortex of patients with schizophrenia. *Molecular Psychiatry*, **10**, 637–50.

Weinberger, D. R. (1987). Implications of normal brain development for the pathogenesis of schizophrenia. *Archives of General Psychiatry*, **44**, 660–9.

Weinberger, D. R. & McClure, R. K. (2002). Neurotoxicity, neuroplasticity, and magnetic resonance imaging morphometry: what is happening in the schizophrenic brain? *Archives of General Psychiatry*, **59**, 553–8.

Williams, H. J., Glaser, B., Williams, N. M. *et al.* (2005). No association between schizophrenia and polymorphisms in COMT in two large samples. *American Journal of Psychiatry*, **162**, 1736–8.

Williams, N. M., Preece, A., Spurlock, G. *et al.* (2003). Support for genetic variation in neuregulin 1 and susceptibility to schizophrenia. *Molecular Psychiatry*, **8**, 485–7.

Williams, N. M., Preece, A., Spurlock, G. *et al.* (2004). Support for RGS4 as a susceptibility gene for schizophrenia. *Biological Psychiatry*, **55**, 192–5.

Winterer, G., Egan, M. F., Kolachana, B. S. *et al.* (2006). Prefrontal electrophysiologic 'noise' and catechol-*O*-methyltransferase genotype in schizophrenia. *Biological Psychiatry*, **60**, 578–84.

WHO (1992). *The ICD-10 Classification of Mental and Behavioural Disorders: Clinical Descriptions and Diagnostic Categories*. Geneva: World Health Organization.

Yang, J. Z., Si, T. M., Ruan, Y. *et al.* (2003). Association study of neuregulin 1 gene with schizophrenia. *Molecular Psychiatry*, **8**, 706–9.

Yung, A. R., Yuen, H. P., Berger, G. *et al.* (2002). Declining transition rate in ultra high risk (prodromal) services: dilution or reduction of risk? *Schizophrenia Bulletin*, **33**, 673–81.

4

Environmental vulnerability and genetic–environmental interactions

Jim van Os and Richie Poulton

Introduction

Attempts to discover genes that relate directly to psychotic disorder (i.e. the simple 'main effects' approach) have been frustrating and often disappointing, resulting in methodological concerns (Harrison & Weinberger, 2005; Norton, Williams & Owen, 2006; Straub & Weinberger, 2006). Exciting findings in other areas of psychiatry have motivated researchers to turn their attention to improving their understanding of the complex ways in which nature interacts with nurture to produce psychosis. This genotype – environmental interaction ($G \times E$) approach differs from the linear gene–phenotype approach by positing *a causal role for the environmental risk factor and a moderating role for genes*. This seems a particularly suitable approach for understanding the development of psychosis because it is known to be associated with environmentally mediated risks (Cannon & Clarke, 2005; van Os *et al.*, 2005), yet people display considerable heterogeneity in their response to those environmental risks (i.e. not all people exposed succumb; Fig. 4.1). The issue of heterogeneity is particularly relevant for the topic of first-episode psychosis, as the greatest challenge is to identify as early as possible those at risk of making the transition from early, non-specific psychotic experiences to full-blown psychotic disorder, and current approaches towards reducing this heterogeneity with an aim to enhance predictive power are clearly limited (van Os & Delespaul, 2005). Therefore, combining genetic risks, either measured directly as genetic polymorphisms or indirectly as genetically mediated traits (endophenotypes), with environmental

exposures in order to create more robust predictions of transition is arguably the best hope for improving strategies of early identification and treatment in psychosis.

Gene–environment relationships

If genetic and environmental factors work together to determine outcomes, (i.e. $G \times E$), differences in genetic endowment explain why people respond differently to the same environment. Most evidence for $G \times E$ in psychosis has come indirectly from twin and adoption studies, and a variety of naturalistic designs in which non-specific genetic contributions have been assessed. More recently, researchers have obtained information about how variation in specific measured genes interacts with specific measured environments (Moffitt, Caspi & Rutter, 2005). Both sets of findings are reviewed below.

In contrast to $G \times E$, gene–environment correlation (hereafter *rGE*) refers to how differences in an individual's genotype can 'drive' differential environmental exposure (Fig. 4.2). Exposure to environmental events is not a random phenomenon; rather it stems (at least partly) from differences in genetic make-up (Plomin, De Fries & Loehlin, 1977). There are three main types of *rGE*. *Passive rGE* refers to environmental influences linked to genetic effects external to the person. For example, parents create the early child rearing environment, as well as providing genetic material to their offspring. In contrast *active rGE* (e.g. selection of specific environments or 'niche picking') and *evocative rGE* arise largely as a result of genetic factors nested within the individual (Rutter, Moffitt & Caspi, 2006). Examples

The Recognition and Management of Early Psychosis: A Preventive Approach, ed. Henry J. Jackson and Patrick D. McGorry. Published by Cambridge University Press. © Cambridge University Press 2009.

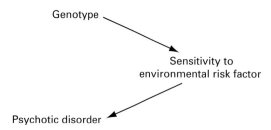

Fig. 4.1. Gene–environment interaction: genes controlling environmental sensitivity. In the figure, genes impact on psychotic disorder indirectly by making an individual more sensitive to the psychotogenic effect of an environmental pathogen.

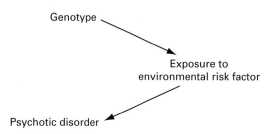

Fig. 4.2. Gene–environment correlation: genes controlling environmental exposure. In the figure, genes impact on psychotic disorder indirectly by influencing the probability that an individual becomes exposed to an environmental pathogen.

of active *rGE* can be seen in one person's preference for sporting activities over another person's penchant for artistic endeavours, thus selecting themselves into different environments. The different responses elicited from the social environment by gregarious versus shy individuals provide an example of evocative *rGE*. Combining the two, *rGE* might manifest as arguments and disagreements preceding marital dissolution, yet $G \times E$ will determine who becomes depressed as a result of that relationship breakdown.

First-generation gene–environment interaction studies in psychosis

Until recently, the conventional wisdom within psychiatry and behavioural genetics was that $G \times E$ occurrences

were exceedingly rare and difficult to demonstrate. The revival of interest in $G \times E$ derives largely from (1) failures of direct gene–phenotype association studies to uncover genes related to susceptibility for psychiatric disorders and the realization that their multifactorial aetiology likely includes many complicated interactive effects requiring more advanced approaches (Hamer, 2002; Rutter, 2006); (2) work demonstrating the operation of $G \times E$ in many other branches of medicine; and (3) recent evidence of $G \times E$ within psychiatry (see review by Moffitt *et al.*, 2005).

The recent $G \times E$ findings in psychiatry suggest that genes are likely to influence disorder only indirectly, via their impact upon physiological pathways, and work to increase (or decrease) the likelihood of developing a psychiatric disorder rather than as direct *causes* of disorder per se. Thus, the notion of 'a gene for . . .' is misleading and diverts attention from more important issues (Kendler, 2005, 2006). Further, some theorists now suggest that (1) additive, non-interactive genetic effects may be less common than previously assumed (cf. Colhoun, McKeigue & Davey-Smith, 2003); (2) studying genes in isolation from known environmental risks may fail to detect important genetic influences; and (3) traditional notions of multiplicative interaction are probably not appropriate for 'real-world' interactions (Darroch, 1997), particularly given the ubiquity of some environmental exposures (Moffitt *et al.*, 2005; Rutter *et al.*, 2006). Thus, biological synergism (co-participation of causes to some outcome) between environmental exposure and background genetic vulnerability is thought to be common in multifactorial disorders such as psychosis. The classic problem, however, is how co-participation between causes in nature (biological synergism) can be inferred from statistical manipulations with research data (statistical interaction), in particular with regard to the choice of additive (change in risk occurs by adding a quantity) or multiplicative (change in risk occurs by multiplying by a quantity) models. It has been shown that the true degree of biological synergism can be better estimated from – but is not the same as – the additive statistical interaction rather than the much more often used multiplicative interaction (Darroch, 1997).

Epidemiological findings

Two related epidemiological 'facts' suggest that 'genes' and 'environments' operate interactively to produce schizophrenia. First, there is widespread geographic, temporal, ethnic and other demographic variation in the incidence of schizophrenia (Kirkbride *et al.*, 2006; McGrath *et al.*, 2004), reinforcing the aetiological role played by environmental factors. Second, there is marked variability in people's responses to these environmental risk factors, ranging from obvious vulnerability to extreme resilience. This well-recognized heterogeneity in response points to the operation of $G \times E$.

Findings from twin, adoption and family studies

Twin and adoption studies provide strong but non-specific evidence for the involvement of both genes and environmental factors in the aetiology of schizophrenia (Gottesman & Shields, 1976). Both have shown moderate to high heritability for schizophrenia, but even monozygotic twins show only 50% concordance, thereby underscoring the importance of environmental influences. Therefore, it is most likely that genetic endowment and environmental factors work synergistically to produce psychotic symptoms and disorder (van Os & Sham, 2003). Findings from several adoption studies are consistent with $G \times E$ in the development of psychotic disorders. For example, Carter *et al.* (2002), in a 25-year longitudinal study, compared 212 children of schizophrenic mothers with 99 children of normal parents in terms of exposure to environmental risk (i.e. institutional care and family instability). Very few cases of psychosis were identified in those families without a history of schizophrenia, but strong environmental effects were observed among those with a family history. Tienari *et al.* (2004) compared adopted-away offspring ($n = 145$) of mothers with a history of psychotic illness with those without illness ($n = 158$). Measures of the rearing environment in the adoptive home were obtained (measures on scales of 'critical/conflictual', 'constricted' and 'boundary problems') and revealed strong effects for those with a biological predisposition (odds ratio approximately 10) that were absent in those with low genetic risk (odds ratio approximately 1).

Findings in support of $G \times E$ also come from migration designs, which, for example, have demonstrated a higher risk of psychosis among Caribbean immigrants to the UK compared with the majority population in the UK (e.g. Harrison *et al.*, 1997). Further, family studies of UK-born Afro-Caribbeans have demonstrated a particularly high risk of schizophrenia among the siblings of young Afro-Caribbean patients (15.9% compared with 1.8% in siblings of white patients), whereas the rates of schizophrenia among the white and Afro-Caribbean parents were similar (8.4% and 8.9%, respectively; Sugarman & Craufurd, 1994).

Further indirect evidence for $G \times E$ comes from studies by van Os and colleagues (e.g. van Os *et al.*, 2003; van Os, Pedersen & Mortensen, 2004). For example, in a follow-up of a cohort of 1 020 063 Danish individuals, yielding 3364 patients with schizophrenia, they demonstrated a significant interaction between living in an urban environment and a history of schizophrenia in a first-degree relative. Thus, the increase in risk for schizophrenia associated with one unit change in urbanicity, measured on a five-point scale, was 0.054%, for those without a family history of schizophrenia and 0.22% for individuals with a positive family history (van Os *et al.*, 2004). The findings are consistent with the operation of $G \times E$, especially as they were unlikely to be confounded by rGE (the phenomenon that some genes make exposure to an environmental risk factor more likely) owing to selective drift to urban areas by those most vulnerable to psychosis (van Os *et al.*, 2004).

Studies using psychometric psychosis liability approach

Operationalizing G and E in a different way, Henquet *et al.* (2005) showed that a psychometric measure of psychosis proneness interacted with cannabis use to predict the likelihood of developing psychotic symptoms. In this study, rGE via self-medication with cannabis was unlikely to have been a confounder since no association between baseline psychosis proneness and subsequent use of cannabis was observed. Nonetheless, confounding cannot be ruled out entirely because the proxy genetic measure (a psychometric scale of psychosis proneness) may itself be a combination of both genetic and environmental factors. As a nice complement to the observational designs described above, Verdoux *et al.* (2003) used a quasi-experimental 'experience sampling' method and obtained similar findings, showing that psychosis liability moderated the effect of cannabis in terms of 'switching on' psychotic symptoms in the flow of daily life. The measure of psychometric psychosis liability is interesting in terms of first-episode psychosis, as it has been shown that this measure predicts future psychotic disorder, albeit with widely different magnitude of effect across different studies (van Os & Delespaul, 2005). Reducing the heterogeneity in predictive power by studying environmental moderators may contribute to the science of early prediction and treatment. For example, other studies using psychometric psychosis liability as a proxy measure for genetic risk were able to demonstrate $G \times E$ with childhood urbanicity (Spauwen *et al.*, 2006a) and childhood trauma (Spauwen *et al.*, 2006b).

Studies of environmental impact on DNA sequence and methylation

Apart from genes impacting on sensitivity for environmental risk factors, $G \times E$ in psychotic disorder may also take the form of environmental factors impacting on either the DNA sequence (causing de novo mutations) or DNA methylation (causing altered gene expression). The best evidence for such mechanisms comes from studies linking advanced paternal age to the risk of schizophrenia in the offspring (Byrne *et al.*, 2003; Malaspina *et al.*, 2001; Sipos *et al.*, 2004; Zammit *et al.*, 2003). Paternal age varies as a function of the sociocultural environment. The observed paternal age effect on schizophrenia may arise from mutagenesis, causing de novo spontaneous mutations, which would then propagate and accumulate in successive generations of sperm-producing cells. Alternatively, the mechanism underlying the paternal age effect may be imprinting (Flint, 1992). Genomic imprinting is the phenomenon whereby a small subset of all the genes

in the genome are expressed according to their parent of origin. Some imprinted genes are expressed from a maternally inherited chromosome and silenced on the paternal chromosome, while other imprinted genes show the opposite expression pattern. One of the mechanisms for gene silencing is DNA methylation. The inherited methylation pattern is maintained in somatic cells but is erased and reestablished late in spermatogenesis for paternally imprinted genes, a process that could become impaired as age advances. Although it is early days, DNA methylation as a mechanism underlying $G \times E$ in psychiatry appears a promising field. For example, early maternal behaviour in animals can affect offspring stress sensitivity through DNA methylation of key neuronal receptor systems involved in the stress response (Meaney & Szyf, 2005; Weaver *et al.*, 2004).

The main environmental factors that investigators have focused on are summarized in Table 4.1. Table 4.2 summarizes the different first-generation $G \times E$ studies. For each study, the proxy genetic factor, the proxy environmental factor and the main findings as well as main limitations are given.

Table 4.1. Environmental exposures investigated in studies of gene–environment interactions

Likely period of impact	Environmental variable
Fetal life	Maternal pregnancy complications, in particular, fetal hypoxia
Early life	Quality of early rearing environment (institutional care, school, parents) Childhood trauma (abuse or neglect)
Late childhood/ adolescence	Urban environment during development: a variable indicating the level of population density, or size of a city within a country, of the place where the individual was growing up (between the ages of 5 and 15 years) Cannabis use Traumatic head injury Ethnic minority group membership status Stressful life events

Table 4.2. First-generation studies of proxy gene–environment interaction in psychotic disorder

Proxy genetic variable	Proxy environmental variable	Findings	Remarks
Positive family history	Ethnic group	Familial morbid risk for psychotic disorder higher in siblings of Afro-Caribbean probands than in siblings of white probands (Hutchinson *et al.*, 1996; Sugarman & Craufurd, 1994).	May be informative; however, preferably environmental exposure status and clinical status is measured in both cases *and* all first-degree relatives and analyses are adjusted for age, sex and number of relatives
	Urban birth	No association between urban birth and a positive family history for psychotic disorder (Mortensen *et al.*, 1999); however, interaction was tested on multiplicative rather than additive scale (see below)	Level of misclassification may be high because many unaffected relatives may carry the high-risk genotype
	Obstetric complications	Mostly inconclusive findings with regard to family history (Kunugi *et al.*, 1996; Nimgaonkar, Wessely & Murray, 1988; O'Callaghan *et al.*, 1992)	*Absence* of an association between positive family history and environmental exposure does *not* rule out $G \times E$ and *presence* of an association does not rule out *lack* of $G \times E$ (Marcelis *et al.*, 1998)
	Birth in winter/spring	Positive, negative and inconclusive associations with family history (Baron & Gruen, 1988; Dassa *et al.*, 1996; Pulver *et al.*, 1992; Shur, 1982)	Evidence can be considered stronger if replicated (e.g. urbanicity findings)
	Stressful life events	Positive association with family history (van Os *et al.*, 1994)	Testing for interaction on an additive scale is likely to be more informative (Darroch, 1997)
	Urbanicity	Evidence for synergism between urban environment (proxy environmental risk) and family history (proxy genetic risk) when tested on additive scale (van Os *et al.* 2003)	
Having an identical twin with psychotic disorder	Being discordant for psychotic disorder	Children of both affected and non-affected twin in discordant pair have higher rate of psychotic disorder (Fischer, 1971; Gottesman & Bertelsen, 1989; Kringlen & Cramer, 1989)	Suggests environmental factor is necessary for expression of high-risk genotype in affected twin or inhibition of protective genotype in unaffected twin

Table 4.2. (cont.)

Proxy genetic variable	Proxy environmental variable	Findings	Remarks
Biological parent with psychotic disorder	Growing up in dysfunctional adoptive family environment	Risk of psychotic disorder spectrum disorder or psychotic disorder-associated thought disorder higher in high-risk adoptees who had been brought up in dysfunctional adoptive family environment (Tienari et al., 1994, 2004; Wahlberg et al., 1997, 2004)	Risk of psychotic disorder spectrum disorder 3% in absence of environmental risk, and 62% in presence of environmental risk; this difference seems extremely high Children destined to develop psychotic disorder may have contributed to dysfunctional family environment rather than the other way round
	Institutional care, family instability	Very few cases of psychosis were identified in those families without a history of psychotic disorder, but among those with a family history, strong environmental effects were observed (Carter et al., 2002)	Case-control comparison difficult as many other factors may be involved
	Having positive relationships with father and mother	High-risk children with positive parental relationships had lower risk for developing psychotic disorder (Carter et al., 1999)	May suggest negative $G \times E$
Having neither, one or two parents with psychotic disorder	Obstetric complications	The greater the proxy genetic risk, the greater the effect of obstetric complications, in particular fetal hypoxia, on ventricular enlargement (the psychotic disorder endophenotype) (Cannon et al., 1993, 2002)	Genetic risk may increase risk of obstetric complication (rGE) Genetic risk may increase risk of heavy alcohol consumption or head injury resulting in greater obstetric complications effect sizes
Having a parent with psychotic disorder and additionally having an electrodermal abnormality as a child	Paternal absence	Higher rate of paternal absence in children who subsequently developed psychotic disorder (Walker, 1981)	Status of electrodermal abnormality as a marker of genetic risk for psychotic disorder unclear
Having a monozygotic twin with psychotic disorder	Sharing the same chorion with the co-twin	Concordance rate was higher for monozygotic twins whose marker suggested they were monochorionic than those whose marker indicated they were dichorionic (Davis & Phelps, 1995)	These results are compatible with an environmental factor in the prenatal environment facilitating expression of genetic risk for psychotic disorder

Genotype	Environment	Evidence	Comments
Having expression of genetically influenced psychometric psychosis liability (Hanssen et al. 2006; Linney et al., 2003)	Early trauma	Evidence that trauma and psychometric psychosis liability synergistically increase the risk for psychosis persistence over time (Spauwen et al., 2006b)	Difficult to disentangle rGE from G × E Psychometric psychosis liability very indirect measure of genetic risk
	Cannabis use	Evidence that cannabis and psychometric psychosis liability synergistically increase the risk for psychosis persistence over time (Henquet et al., 2005; see also Verdoux et al., 2003)	
	Growing up in urban environment	Evidence that urbanicity and psychometric psychosis liability synergistically increase the risk for psychosis persistence over time (Spauwen et al., 2006a)	
Being a member of a schizophrenia pedigree	Traumatic head injury	Within the schizophrenia pedigrees but not bipolar pedigrees, traumatic brain injury was associated with a greater risk of schizophrenia, consistent with synergistic effects between genetic vulnerability for schizophrenia and traumatic brain injury	Similar comments as for positive family history
None	Having an older father	Having an older father is associated with an increased risk of schizophrenia in the offspring (Byrne et al., 2003; Malaspina et al., 2001; Sipos et al., 2004; Zammit et al., 2003)	The underlying mechanism of this association may represent a special case of G × E whereby the environment impacts on DNA sequence (de novo mutation) or DNA methylation (affecting gene expression); thus, age of the father is a variable that is partly under control from the sociocultural environment, and older age may have an effect on DNA methylation in the sex cells (the inherited methylation pattern in humans is maintained in somatic cells but is erased and reestablished late in spermatogenesis for paternally imprinted genes, a process that could become impaired as age advances). Alternatively, advanced paternal age may lead to an increased rate of de novo mutations in gametes

$G \times E$, gene–environment interaction; rGE, gene–environment correlation.

Second-generation gene–environment interaction studies in psychosis

To date, most evidence in support of $G \times E$ in psychotic disorders comes from first-generation studies using either non-specific or indirect (proxy) measures of genes and environments. However, more recent second-generation epidemiological and human experimental studies have directly tested for interactions between specific measured genes and environments, in particular the interaction between the gene for catechol-O-methyltransferase (COMT) and cannabis (Fig. 4.3). In perhaps the first successful attempt to move beyond indirect measures of $G \times E$, Caspi *et al.* (2005) investigated whether the relationship between adolescent cannabis use and the development of psychosis in adulthood was moderated by genotype, in this case the *COMT* gene. The gene *COMT* was chosen because of its putative links to both schizophrenia and cognitive symptoms associated with cannabis use, and its importance in the prefrontal cortex (Craddock, Owen & O'Donovan, 2006; Fergusson *et al.*, 2006;

Tunbridge, Harrison & Weinberger, 2006). Evidence about the influence of COMT on prefrontal cortex function suggested that the *COMT* allele that expresses valine in the protein at locations 108 and 158 should interact with cannabis use to predict psychosis. Findings showed a significant main effect for cannabis use, no main effect for genotype by itself, and a significant interaction between adolescent cannabis use and *COMT*. The robustness of this $G \times E$ was confirmed by several 'internal' replications using alternative measures of the phenotype, including self-reported psychotic symptoms, diagnosis of schizophreniform disorder, evidence of hallucinatory experiences and informant reports of psychotic symptoms. Further, these $G \times Es$ survived adjustment for (1) adult cannabis use; (2) adolescent use of drugs other than cannabis; (3) adult use of amphetamines and hallucinogens; (4) childhood intelligence quotient (IQ); and (5) adolescent conduct disorder. Gene–environment correlation was ruled out because cannabis use during adolescence did not differ by genotype. Furthermore, the $G \times E$ survived adjustment of prodromal psychotic symptoms measured at age 11 years, before cannabis

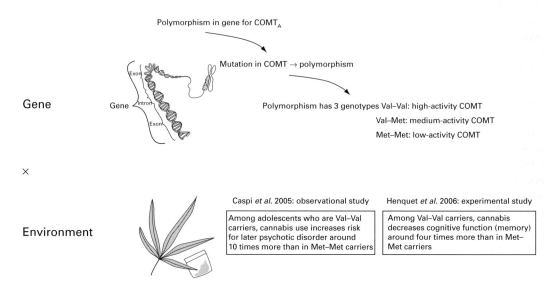

Fig. 4.3. Second-generation studies of the gene–environment interaction in psychosis. The gene encodes catechol-O-methyltransferase (COMT), which catabolizes monoamines in the brain. The environmental factor is tetrahydrocannabinol (THC), the main psychotropic component of cannabis. The high-activity Val–Val form of COMT is associated with greater breakdown of dopamine.

use began. Interestingly, the cannabis–COMT interaction only applied to cannabis use during adolescence. That is, when cannabis use beginning in adulthood was examined, the $G \times E$ was no longer apparent, implying that adolescence is a particularly vulnerable period for brain development and risk associated with cannabis use.

This study also sought to establish the specificity of the relationship between the exposure (adolescent cannabis use), COMT genotype and the psychosis outcome. Analyses showed that the interaction applied to cannabis use but not to substances other than cannabis (e.g. opiates, psychedelics) or other environmental risks (e.g. childhood maltreatment), nor did other genes interact with cannabis use to predict psychosis, e.g. genes for monoamine oxidase A (Caspi et al., 2002) or that for the serotonin transporter, 5-HTTLPR (Caspi et al., 2003). Finding the relationship was specific to cannabis as opposed to 'harder' drugs points toward a biochemical basis for the association rather than psychosocial explanations emphasizing high levels of stress and social isolation/rejection that often accompany 'hard' drug use. Interestingly, the COMT – cannabis interaction predicted psychosis and depression (but not anxiety, alcohol dependence or cannabis dependence), implying that the mechanisms underlying this interaction might involve neurobiological processes that are shared to some degree by affective and psychotic disorders.

In what appears to be the first replication of the COMT – cannabis finding, Henquet et al. (2006) used a double-blind, placebo crossover design, enrolling patients with a psychotic disorder ($n = 30$), relatives of patients with a psychotic disorder ($n = 12$) and healthy controls ($n = 32$). Subjects were exposed to delta-9-tetrahydrocannabinol (THC; the main psychoactive compound in cannabis) or placebo, followed by a cognitive assessment and assessment of current psychotic experiences; previous psychosis was also assessed (Henquet et al., 2006). Consistent with Caspi et al. (2005), they found that the allele encoding Val carriage moderated sensitivity to the effects of THC on psychotic symptoms as well as for several cognitive measures including verbal and recognition memory, and reaction time. This significant $G \times E$ survived adjustment for age, sex, age of onset of cannabis use, frequency of cannabis use, use of stimulants or cocaine, and psychosis proneness. The study went further by showing that, in

addition to COMT genotype, sensitivity to THC was also partly conditional upon additional evidence of psychosis liability (i.e. other 'unmeasured' genes). Valine carriers with psychosis liability experienced more THC-induced transient psychotic symptoms than Val carriers without additional liability, although the authors rightly urged caution when interpreting these findings owing to limited power for tests of three-way interactions. There was little evidence that rGE affected the moderating role of COMT val158Met polymorphism because COMT genotype was unrelated to psychosis liability, cognitive functioning or cannabis use.

It is unlikely that the moderating effect of psychometrically assessed psychosis liability and COMT on the association between cannabis and psychosis are the result of the same underlying process, because psychometric psychosis liability is strongly associated with psychotic disorder whereas COMT is not. Therefore, although psychometric psychosis liability and COMT genotype may confer different vulnerabilities, both impact upon the final common pathway of developing psychosis following cannabis use. It is attractive to hypothesize that these separate moderating mechanisms show synergistic effects to the extent that psychometric psychosis liability represents a genetic influence (Hanssen et al., 2006; Jacobs et al., 2005; Linney, Peters & Ayton, 1998). Synergism between COMT genotype and psychometric psychosis liability supports the hypothesis of underlying gene–gene interaction rather than additive gene involvement.

More recently, Stefanis and colleagues (2007) investigated whether the COMT Val158Met polymorphism also moderates the psychosis-inducing effects of 'stress' using a quasi-experimental design. They found that stress exposure at army induction (306 men aged 19–24 years) was associated with an increased level of psychotic symptoms. Critically, carriers of the COMT allele encoding valine were more susceptible to stress in terms of psychotic symptoms than inductees with the Met/Met genotype (test for direction $\chi^2 = 4.85$, degrees of freedom, 1; $p = 0.028$).

The combined results of Caspi et al. (2005), Henquet et al. (2006) and Stefanis et al. (2007) suggest that $G \times E$ interactions, in which the dopamine system plays an important role, partly underlie the complex aetiology of psychotic symptoms.

Discussion

To date, the study of $G \times E$ has largely been epidemiological, where genotype, risk exposure and disorder are studied as they occur in the population (Khoury *et al.*, 2004). A key contribution of a robust $G \times E$ comes from knowing that three apparently unconnected factors (gene, environmental risk factor and disorder) are, in fact, causally linked (Moffitt *et al.*, 2005). However, there are a number of methodological concerns that continue to challenge genetic–epidemiological research, mainly because the observational method struggles to achieve the degree of control that is possible using experimental designs (reviewed by Caspi & Moffitt, 2006). The following are some concerns.

1. *The ideal sample size for genetics research.* Clearly the optimal sample size required to detect $G \times E$ will vary according to the design used. For example, case–control studies will generally require very large sample sizes simply because the genetic effects are expected to be small. However, even with prospective cohort studies, large sample sizes may be required when the environmental risk factor(s) and/or disorder of interest occur at low frequencies. However, large sample sizes are not always necessary, or desirable given the costs of amassing large samples. Indeed, sample size requirements can be substantially reduced with high-quality measurement of environmental risk factors, especially when measures are repeated over time (Wong *et al.*, 2003).

2. *Which endophenotypes to study?* Within psychiatry, there are a plethora of endophenotypes (i.e. intermediate phenotypes) from which to choose. These include neuropsychological, neurophysiological, neurohormonal, neuroanatomical and biochemical correlates of a disorder. The appeal of studying endophenotypes is obvious: with compared clinical diagnoses, which are often characterized by substantial heterogeneity, endophenotypes appear to be cleaner, simpler constituents of psychopathology and promise (maybe falsely) improved odds of detecting true gene effects. Nonetheless, questions remain about which endophenotypes, for which disorder, are most worthy of study in a $G \times E$ framework.

3. *Confounding by gene–environment correlation.* Such correlation describes how genes can increase or decrease environmental risk exposure. As stated earlier, *rGE* can operate in three ways (Plomin *et al.*, 1977). Passive *rGE* occurs when parental behaviour, which is partly under genetic control, influences the nature of the early child-rearing environment. Thus, parental genes can exert an influence upon the child via the child's environment, but the effects are independent of the child. Active and evocative *rGE* differ because they are a result of the child's behaviour. Specifically, active *rGE* occurs when children, by virtue of their temperament or behaviour, select and/or shape their environment. Evocative *rGE* refers to the impact of the child's behaviour on their social environment, in particular the responses they elicit from people around them. In studies aimed at detecting $G \times E$, *rGE* is noise and must be ruled out. In other words, the *E* in $G \times E$ must be shown to be a true environmentally mediated effect. Experimental paradigms effectively deal with this problem by randomly assigning participants to the exposed and unexposed conditions.

4. *How to measure the environment well?* There are legitimate concerns about how to capture faithfully the environmental risk exposure history of participants. This task is particularly challenging when measuring psychosocial risk factors, where the negative effects may act cumulatively across long periods of the life course. Equally challenging are the inherent difficulties in precisely measuring 'unit exposure' for illicit substances such as cannabis, which can be ingested in different forms, with different THC levels, using different methods. Measuring tobacco intake is comparatively straightforward, but even this presents problems with accuracy of recall over long periods. Experimental paradigms, like those of van Os and colleagues described above, have obvious advantages: (1) randomization precludes confounding by not only known but, critically, also unknown confounders; (2) *rGE*, which may plague observational studies, is not an issue if *G* is randomly allocated to *E* and (3) it is relatively easy to make the sample size match the required power.

5. *Multiple tests.* There are legitimate concerns about low prior probability testing for associations between a large number of polymorphisms (e.g. via single nucleotide polymorphism chips) and specific disorders in the absence of some guiding theory that will allow researchers to sort true- from false-positive associations. Guarding against 'fishing-trips' is important if we are to advance in our understanding of how $G \times E$ operates in the development of schizophrenia.

Future research needs to improve the integration of epidemiological and experimental paradigms (Caspi & Moffitt, 2006). This is desirable because traditional genetic epidemiology cannot tell us much about the biological mechanisms involved in an interaction. These approaches are complementary, with each informing the other, and ideally should be used in unison for best effect. Many (but by no means all) of the challenges confronting genetic epidemiology listed above can be addressed using experimental designs, with their advantages of greater control and precision. However, these benefits have to be balanced against the loss of ecological validity that can sometimes result. Epidemiologists should be encouraged to incorporate more physiological (i.e. mechanistic) measures in their studies and to move beyond two-way interactions to models involving multiple genes and environments as well as gene–gene and environment–environment interactions. The work by Henquet *et al.* (2006) is a good step in this direction. Embracing a $G \times E$ approach, which assumes a 'causal' role for environment factors but where the likelihood of disorder ultimately depends upon genotype, has implications for gene discovery. That is, selecting and/or stratifying samples based on documented environmental risk exposure may not only help in the quest to identify new susceptibility genes for psychotic disorders but also help in unravelling the pathway to the onset of first-episode psychosis.

REFERENCES

Baron, M. & Gruen, R. (1988). Risk factors in schizophrenia. Season of birth and family history. [See comments.] *British Journal of Psychiatry*, **152**, 460–5.

Byrne, M., Agerbo, E., Ewald, H., Eaton, W. W. & Mortensen, P. B. (2003). Parental age and risk of schizophrenia: a case–control study. *Archives of General Psychiatry*, **60**, 673–8.

Cannon, M. & Clarke, M. C. (2005). Risk for schizophrenia: broadening the concepts, pushing back the boundaries. *Schizophrenia Research*, **79**, 5–13.

Cannon, T. D., Mednick, S. A., Parnas, J. *et al.* (1993). Developmental brain abnormalities in the offspring of schizophrenic mothers. I. Contributions of genetic and perinatal factors [see comments]. *Archives of General Psychiatry*, **50**, 551–64.

Cannon, T. D., van Erp, T. G., Rosso, I. M. *et al.* (2002). Fetal hypoxia and structural brain abnormalities in schizophrenic patients, their siblings, and controls. *Archives of General Psychiatry*, **59**, 35–41.

Carter, J. W., Parnas, J., Cannon, T. D., Schulsinger, F. & Mednick, S. A. (1999). MMPI variables predictive of schizophrenia in the Copenhagen High-Risk Project: a 25-year follow-up. *Acta Psychiatrica Scandinavica*, **99**, 432–40.

Carter, J. W., Schulsinger, F., Parnas, J., Cannon, T. & Mednick, S. A. (2002). A multivariate prediction model of schizophrenia. *Schizophrenia Bulletin*, **28**, 649–82.

Caspi, A. & Moffitt, T. E. (2006). Gene–environment interactions in psychiatry: joining forces with neuroscience. *Nature Review Neuroscience*, **7**, 583–90.

Caspi, A., McClay, J., Moffitt, T. E. *et al.* (2002). Role of genotype in the cycle of violence in maltreated children. *Science*, **297**, 851–4.

Caspi, A., Sugden, K., Moffitt, T. E. *et al.* (2003). Influence of life stress on depression: moderation by a polymorphism in the $5\text{-}HT_T$ gene. *Science*, **301**, 386–9.

Caspi, A., Moffitt, T. E., Cannon, M. *et al.* (2005). Moderation of the effect of adolescent-onset cannabis use on adult psychosis by a functional polymorphism in the *COMT* gene: longitudinal evidence of a gene × environment interaction. *Biological Psychiatry*, **57**, 1117–27.

Colhoun, H. M., McKeigue, P. M. & Davey-Smith, G. (2003). Problems of reporting genetic associations with complex outcomes. *Lancet*, **361**, 865–72.

Craddock, N., Owen, M. J. & O'Donovan, M. C. (2006). The catechol-*O*-methyltransferase (*COMT*) gene as a candidate for psychiatric phenotypes: evidence and lessons. *Molecular Psychiatry*, **11**, 446–58.

Darroch, J. (1997). Biologic synergism and parallelism. [See comments.] *American Journal of Epidemiology*, **145**, 661–8.

Dassa, D., Sham, P. C., van Os, J. *et al.* (1996). Relationship of birth season to clinical features, family history, and obstetric complication in schizophrenia. *Psychiatry Research*, **64**, 11–17.

Davis, J. O. & Phelps, J. A. (1995). Twins with schizophrenia: genes or germs? *Schizophrenia Bulletin*, **21**, 13–18.

Fergusson, D. M., Poulton, R., Smith, P. F. & Boden, J. M. (2006). Cannabis and psychosis. *British Medical Journal*, **332**, 172–5.

Fischer, M. (1971). Psychoses in the offspring of schizophrenic monozygotic twins and their normal co-twins. *British Journal of Psychiatry*, **118**, 43–52.

Flint, J. (1992). Implications of genomic imprinting for psychiatric genetics. *Psychological Medicine*, **22**, 5–10.

Gottesman, I. I. & Bertelsen, A. (1989). Confirming unexpressed genotypes for schizophrenia. Risks in the offspring of Fischer's Danish identical and fraternal discordant twins. [See comments.] *Archives of General Psychiatry*, **46**, 867–72.

Gottesman, I. I. &, Shields, J. (1976). A critical review of recent adoption, twin, and family studies of schizophrenia: behavioral genetics perspectives. *Schizophrenia Bulletin*, **2**, 360–401.

Hamer, D. (2002). Genetics. Rethinking behavior genetics. *Science*, **298**, 71–2.

Hanssen, M., Krabbendam, L., Vollema, M., Delespaul, P. & van Os, J. (2006). Evidence for instrument and family-specific variation of subclinical psychosis dimensions in the general population. *Journal of Abnormal Psychology*, **115**, 5–14.

Harrison, G., Glazebrook, C., Brewin, J. *et al.* (1997). Increased incidence of psychotic disorders in migrants from the Caribbean to the United Kingdom. *Psychological Medicine*, **27**, 799–806.

Harrison, P. J. & Weinberger, D. R. (2005). Schizophrenia genes, gene expression, and neuropathology: on the matter of their convergence. *Molecular Psychiatry*, **10**, 40–68.

Henquet, C., Krabbendam, L., Spauwen, J. *et al.* (2005). Prospective cohort study of cannabis use, predisposition for psychosis, and psychotic symptoms in young people. *British Medical Journal*, **330**, 11–14.

Henquet, C., Rosa, A., Krabbendam, L. *et al.* (2006). An experimental study of catechol-*O*-methyltransferase Val158Met moderation of delta-9-tetrahydrocannabinol-induced effects on psychosis and cognition. *Neuropsychopharmacology*, **31**, 2748–57.

Hutchinson, G., Takei, N., Fahy, T. A. *et al.* (1996). Morbid risk of schizophrenia in first-degree relatives of white and African-Caribbean patients with psychosis. *British Journal of Psychiatry*, **169**, 776–80.

Jacobs, N., Myin-Germeys, I., Derom, C., Vlietinck, R & van Os, J. (2005). Deconstructing the familiality of the emotive component of psychotic experiences in the general population. *Acta Psychiatrica Scandinavica*, **112**, 394–401.

Kendler, K. S. (2005). 'A gene for . . .': the nature of gene action in psychiatric disorders. *American Journal of Psychiatry*, **162**, 1243–52.

Kendler, K. S. (2006). Reflections on the relationship between psychiatric genetics and psychiatric nosology. *American Journal of Psychiatry*, **163**, 1138–46.

Khoury, M. J., Millikan, R., Little, J. & Gwinn, M. (2004). The emergence of epidemiology in the genomics age. *International Journal of Epidemiology*, **33**, 936–44.

Kirkbride, J. B., Fearon, P., Morgan, C. *et al.* (2006). Heterogeneity in incidence rates of schizophrenia and other psychotic syndromes: findings from the 3-center AeSOP study. *Archives of General Psychiatry*, **63**, 250–8.

Kringlen, E. & Cramer, G. (1989). Offspring of monozygotic twins discordant for schizophrenia. *Archives of General Psychiatry*, **46**, 873–7.

Kunugi, H., Nanko, S., Takei, N. *et al.* (1996). Perinatal complications and schizophrenia. Data from the Maternal and Child Health Handbook in Japan. *Journal of Nervous and Mental Disease*, **184**, 542–6.

Linney, Y. M., Peters, E. R. & Ayton, P. (1998). Reasoning biases in delusion-prone individuals. *British Journal of Clinical Psychology*, **37**(Pt 3), 285–302.

Linney, Y. M., Murray, R. M., Peters, E. R. *et al.* (2003). A quantitative genetic analysis of schizotypal personality traits. *Psychological Medicine*, **33**, 803–16.

Malaspina, D., Harlap, S., Fennig, S. *et al.* (2001). Advancing paternal age and the risk of schizophrenia. *Archives of General Psychiatry*, **58**, 361–7.

Marcelis, M., van Os, J., Sham, P. *et al.* (1998). Obstetric complications and familial morbid risk of psychiatric disorders. *American Journal of Medical Genetics*, **81**, 29–36.

McGrath, J., Saha, S., Welham, J. *et al.* (2004). A systematic review of the incidence of schizophrenia: the distribution of rates and the influence of sex, urbanicity, migrant status and methodology. *BMC Medicine*, **2**, 13.

Meaney, M. J. & Szyf, M. (2005). Environmental programming of stress responses through DNA methylation: life at the interface between a dynamic environment and a fixed genome. *Dialogues in Clinical Neuroscience*, **7**, 103–23.

Moffitt, T. E., Caspi, A. & Rutter, M. (2005). Strategy for investigating interactions between measured genes and measured environments. *Archives of General Psychiatry*, **62**, 473–81.

Mortensen, P. B., Pedersen, C. B., Westergaard, T. *et al.* (1999). Effects of family history and place and season of birth on the risk of schizophrenia. [See comments.] *New England Journal of Medicine*, **340**, 603–8.

Nimgaonkar, V. L., Wessely, S. & Murray, R. M. (1988). Prevalence of familiality, obstetric complications, and structural brain damage in schizophrenic patients. *British Journal of Psychiatry*, **153**, 191–7.

Norton, N., Williams, H. J. & Owen, M. J. (2006). An update on the genetics of schizophrenia. *Current Opinion in Psychiatry*, **19**, 158–64.

O'Callaghan, E., Gibson, T., Colohan, H. A. *et al.* (1992). Risk of schizophrenia in adults born after obstetric complications and their association with early onset of illness: a controlled study. [See comments.] *British Medical Journal*, **305**, 1256–9.

Plomin, R., DeFries, J. C. & Loehlin, J. C. (1977). Genotype-environment interaction and correlation in the analysis of human behavior. *Psychological Bulletin*, **84**, 309–22.

Pulver, A. E., Liang, K. Y., Brown, C. H. *et al.* (1992). Risk factors in schizophrenia. Season of birth, gender, and familial risk [see comments]. *British Journal of Psychiatry*, **160**, 65–71.

Rutter, M. (2006). *Genes and Behavior: Nature–Nurture Interplay Explained*. Malden, MA: Blackwell.

Rutter, M., Moffitt, T. E. & Caspi, A. (2006). Gene-environment interplay and psychopathology: multiple varieties but real effects. *Journal of Child Psychology and Psychiatry*, **47**, 226–61.

Shur, E. (1982). Season of birth in high and low genetic risk schizophrenics. *British Journal of Psychiatry*, **140**, 410–15.

Sipos, A., Rasmussen, F., Harrison, G. *et al.* (2004). Paternal age and schizophrenia: a population based cohort study. *British Medical Journal*, **329**, 1070–3.

Spauwen, J., Krabbendam, L., Lieb, R., Wittchen, H. U. & van Os, J. (2006a). Evidence that the outcome of developmental expression of psychosis is worse for adolescents growing up in an urban environment. *Psychological Medicine*, **36**, 407–15.

Spauwen, J., Krabbendam, L., Lieb, R., Wittchen, H. U. & van Os, J. (2006b). Impact of psychological trauma on the development of psychotic symptoms: relationship with psychosis proneness. *British Journal of Psychiatry*, **188**, 527–33.

Stefanis, N. C., Henquet, C., Avramopoulos, D. *et al.* (2007). COMT Val158Met moderation of stress-induced psychosis. *Psychological Medicine*, **37**, 1–6.

Straub, R. E. & Weinberger, D. R. (2006). Schizophrenia genes; famine to feast. *Biological Psychiatry*, **60**, 81–3.

Sugarman, P. A. & Craufurd, D. (1994). Schizophrenia in the Afro-Caribbean community. *British Journal of Psychiatry*, **164**, 474–80.

Tienari, P., Wynne, L. C., Moring, J. *et al.* (1994). The Finnish adoptive family study of schizophrenia. Implications for family research [see comments]. *British Journal of Psychiatry*, **164** (Suppl), s20–6.

Tienari, P., Wynne, L. C., Sorri, A. *et al.* (2004). Genotype-environment interaction in schizophrenia-spectrum disorder. Long-term follow-up study of Finnish adoptees. *British Journal of Psychiatry*, **184**, 216–22.

Tunbridge, E. M., Harrison, P. J. & Weinberger, D. R. (2006). Catechol-*O*-methyltransferase, cognition, and psychosis: val (158)met and beyond. *Biological Psychiatry*, **60**, 141–51.

van Os, J. & Delespaul, P. (2005). Toward a world consensus on prevention of schizophrenia. *Dialogues in Clinical Neuroscience*, **7**, 53–67.

van Os, J. & Sham, P. (2003). Gene-environment correlation and interaction in schizophrenia. In R. M.. Murray, P. B. Jones, E. Susser, J. van Os & M. Cannon (eds.), *The Epidemiology of Schizophrenia*. Cambridge, UK: Cambridge University Press, pp. 235–53.

van Os, J., Hanssen, M., Bak, M., Bijl, R. V. & Vollebergh, W. (2003). Do urbanicity and familial liability coparticipate in causing psychosis? *American Journal of Psychiatry*, **160**, 477–82.

van Os, J., Pedersen, C. B. & Mortensen, P. B. (2004). Confirmation of synergy between urbanicity and familial liability in the causation of psychosis. *American Journal of Psychiatry*, **161**, 2312–14.

van Os, J., Krabbendam, L., Myin-Germeys, I. & Delespaul, P. (2005). The schizophrenia environment and its genomic impact. *Current Opinion in Psychiatry*, **18**, 141–5.

Verdoux, H., Gindre, C., Sorbara, F., Tournier, M. & Swendsen, J. D. (2003). Effects of cannabis and psychosis vulnerability in daily life: an experience sampling test study. *Psychological Medicine*, **33**, 23–32.

Wahlberg, K. E., Wynne, L. C., Oja, H. *et al.* (1997). Gene-environment interaction in vulnerability to schizophrenia: findings from the Finnish Adoptive Family Study of Schizophrenia. *American Journal of Psychiatry*, **154**, 355–62.

Wahlberg, K. E., Wynne, L. C., Hakko, H. *et al.* (2004). Interaction of genetic risk and adoptive parent communication deviance: longitudinal prediction of adoptee psychiatric disorders. *Psychological Medicine*, **34**, 1531–41.

Walker, E. (1981). Attentional and neuromotor functions of schizophrenics, schizoaffectives, and patients with other affective disorders. *Archives of General Psychiatry*, **38**, 1355–8.

Weaver, I. C., Cervoni, N., Champagne, F. A. *et al.* (2004). Epigenetic programming by maternal behavior. *Nature Neuroscience*, **7**, 847–54.

Wong, M. Y., Day, N. E., Luan, J. A., Chan, K. P. & Wareham, N. J. (2003). The detection of gene-environment interaction for continuous traits: should we deal with measurement error by bigger studies or better measurement? *International Journal of Epidemiology*, **32**, 51–7.

Zammit, S., Allebeck, P., Dalman, C. *et al.* (2003). Paternal age and risk for schizophrenia. *British Journal of Psychiatry*, **183**, 405–8.

5

Neurobiological endophenotypes of psychosis and schizophrenia: are there biological markers of illness onset?

Christos Pantelis, Murat Yücel, Stephen J. Wood, Warrick J. Brewer, Alex Fornito, Gregor Berger, Tyrone Cannon and Dennis Velakoulis

Introduction

In this chapter, we describe neuropsychological, psychophysiological and brain imaging findings in the early stages of psychosis and schizophrenia, with a particular focus on the recent high-risk studies, and consider whether the evidence supports these as potential endophenotypic markers of illness. We argue that few potential markers meet criteria to be considered true endophenotypes of schizophrenia. Rather, the evidence supports the notion that there are a number of processes relevant to the onset of psychosis, which influence the phenotypic expression of the disorder at its different illness stages. Further, potential markers are non-specific and actively changing as the psychosis evolves and the illness progresses. Concurrently, these same potential indices are also dynamically changing as part of normal maturation during the adolescent and early adult period. Consequently, we suggest that these potential markers are not stable attributes of schizophrenia, nor psychosis more generally. A more parsimonious model needs to take account of the dynamic changes occurring in the brain (especially in frontal and temporal cortices) during adolescence – the period of life during which the illness typically manifests itself. Studies have not taken account of such changes, particularly in assessing the stability of proposed endophenotypes. We suggest that there is an interaction of genetic and environmental aetiological factors with stage of brain maturation at illness onset, leading to the phenotypic characteristics of the illness. Accordingly, we assert that the current conceptualizations of 'endophenotypes' for schizophrenia may need to be reconsidered in the context of 'early' versus 'late' brain maturational processes.

Background

For a neurobiological marker to be considered an endophenotype for psychosis, it needs to (1) differentiate people with and without psychosis; (2) be seen at all stages of the disorder (i.e. independent of state), including premorbidly; and (3) be heritable and, therefore, present in first-degree relatives at higher rates than the general population (Braff *et al.*, 2007; Gottesman & Gould, 2003). These include neuropsychological, neurophysiological, neuroimaging and neuropathological markers (Benes, 2007; Glahn, Thompson & Blangero, 2007; Gur, Keshavan & Lawrie, 2007a; Snitz, MacDonald & Carter, 2006).

Most studies looking for such markers have focused on patients with established schizophrenia, often restricted to patients with a chronic unremitting course and poor response to medication. While these investigations have been informative in identifying potential endophenotypes (Braff *et al.*, 2007; Glahn *et al.*, 2007; Gottesman & Gould, 2003; Weinberger, 2002), it remains unclear if these markers are apparent early in the course of the illness.

The most consistent neuroanatomical findings, which may represent potential endophenotypes, are enlarged ventricles and reduced medial temporal and prefrontal cortical (PFC) volume (Lawrie & Abukmeil,

The Recognition and Management of Early Psychosis: A Preventive Approach, ed. Henry J. Jackson and Patrick D. McGorry.
Published by Cambridge University Press. © Cambridge University Press 2009.

1998; Liddle & Pantelis, 2003; Van Horn & McManus, 1992). However, these structural abnormalities are usually subtle – the psychophysiological and functional deficits are often more profound. Psychophysiological measures, such as event-related potentials (ERPs) can track changes in brain function over short epochs, thereby providing dynamic information about the progression of brain activity (Keshavan *et al.*, 2005; Turetsky *et al.*, 2007), while neuropsychological deficits provide information about higher cognitive functions. Deficits in psychomotor speed, attention, memory and executive function are consistently identified in schizophrenia (Dickinson, Ramsey & Gold, 2007; Heinrichs, 2005; Keefe *et al.*, 2006) and have been considered as central to its neurobiology (Pantelis & Maruff, 2002). Such deficits are often present at the first onset (Bilder *et al.*, 2000), are related more to negative rather than positive symptomatology (Pantelis *et al.*, 2001; Rhinewine *et al.*, 2005), have been considered stable and persistent (Hoff *et al.*, 2005) and are proposed as endophenotypic markers (Gur *et al.*, 2007b; Snitz *et al.*, 2006), though the evidence is limited.

Overall, the findings in patients with established forms of schizophrenia and related disorders are complicated by the effects of chronic illness, such as a history of acute relapses and hospitalizations, the impact of multiple biological treatments, as well as substance abuse and an abnormal psychosocial trajectory, which make it nearly impossible to distinguish if these markers are truly related to the underlying disease process or its impact (Keshavan *et al.*, 2005). Further, these patients are usually not representative of all patients developing a schizophreniform illness, being biased to those with the poorest outcome, usually with the prominent negative symptoms that are associated with more severe neuropsychological impairments. For these reasons, abnormalities present in those with established illness may not reflect neurobiological processes at earlier illness or pre-illness stages, and provide limited information about how the illness progresses over time. Consequently, while it has been suggested that these structural and functional abnormalities have their basis in early brain development (Murray & Lewis, 1987; Weinberger, 1987), elucidating the nature, timing and course of the underlying neurobiological changes has proved difficult (Harrison & Lewis, 2003).

To truly understand the neurobiological processes underlying the emergence of psychotic disorders, and the nature of progressive changes over time, as well as determine which indices represent illness endophenotypes versus predictive markers of the illness or its course, longitudinal studies from before illness onset and over the initial stages of psychosis are required.

Biological markers at psychosis onset

While most neurobiological studies examine patients with established illness or during the first-episode of illness, as well as family members, the recent 'high risk for psychosis' strategies examining the prodrome provide the means to validate the sensitivity and specificity of potential endophenotypes.

High-risk strategies

The traditional approach to investigating individuals considered at high risk for psychotic illness has been to follow children and adolescents with a positive family history (usually of schizophrenia; for discussion about high-risk strategies see Cannon (2005a)). There have been a number of such 'genetic' high-risk studies that have identified early predictors of later schizophrenia (e.g. Cannon & Mednick, 1993; Erlenmeyer-Kimling *et al.*, 2000; Ingraham *et al.*, 1995), such as deficits in attention, working memory and executive function, particularly in the verbal domain (Cornblatt & Keilp, 1994; Stone *et al.*, 2005; Wolf & Cornblatt, 1996). However, in these studies, the number of individuals who make the transition to psychosis and schizophrenia has been small and the studies have required a lengthy follow-up period of at least 20–30 years. In that time, there has been considerable development in our understanding of schizophrenia and psychosis, and technological advances in imaging, cognitive neuroscience and genetics, that could not be incorporated into the investigations.

More recently, two alternative 'high-risk' strategies have been helpful in assessing brain structural and functional changes surrounding the onset of psychosis and schizophrenia. Akin to the earlier genetic high-risk studies that follow individuals with at least one family member having schizophrenia, Johnstone and colleagues in Edinburgh have established a cohort of adolescents with at least two affected first-degree family members (the Edinburgh High Risk Study (EHRS); Johnstone *et al.*, 2005). This has the advantage of giving a putative transition rate of about 10% over a 10-year period. However, the focus on a sample with a high genetic loading may not be representative of schizophrenia, and the low transition rate still requires large cohorts and long follow-up intervals.

A novel strategy has been the Australian (Melbourne-based) approach of identifying those at 'ultra-high risk' (UHR) for psychosis using a 'close-in' strategy (Chapter 6) that maximizes the number of participants who make the transition to psychosis (30 to 40%) over a 12-month period (Yung & McGorry, 1996). This strategy does not imply that a full-threshold psychotic illness such as schizophrenia is inevitable, but it suggests that an individual is displaying a 'need-for-care' and is at increased risk of developing a psychotic disorder by virtue of his or her mental state. A related approach has been applied by a German group in Cologne that has used the historic concept of 'basic symptoms' (Klosterkötter *et al.*, 2001; see Chapter 6). Because of the high rate of transition to illness over a relatively short follow-up interval, these strategies provide a unique opportunity to examine potential endophenotypes of psychosis and schizophrenia. Below we examine the evidence supporting potential illness markers in the context of these and related high-risk studies.

Evidence for neurobiological markers from the recent 'high-risk' studies

Neuropsychological studies

The early 'genetic' high-risk studies have provided some information about potential endophenotypic markers that are apparent premorbidly (discussed in special issues of *Schizophrenia Bulletin*: volume 11, issue 1 (1985) and volume 13, issue 3 (1987)). In neuropsychology, these earlier studies focused on motor function, behaviour and attention, with more limited information available with respect to other cognitive domains, such as working memory (Mirsky, 1995; Weintraub, 1987; Wolf *et al.*, 2002). The New York High-Risk Study has been most informative in this respect, showing that childhood deficits in attention, motor skills and short-term memory at 7 to 12 years of age predicted a high proportion of those who later developed a schizophrenia-related psychosis (Erlenmeyer-Kimling *et al.*, 2000). Further, Wolf *et al.* (2002) demonstrated that subjects at genetic high-risk for schizophrenia, but not affective psychoses, had impaired performance on the Wisconsin Card Sorting Test (a set-shifting task probing prefrontal functioning) although performance did not discriminate those at risk for schizophrenia who converted versus those who did not.

Another approach has been to identify cases from long-term population-based follow-up studies, such as in the Dunedin Multidisciplinary Health and Development Study (Poulton *et al.*, 2000), the Finnish birth cohort study (Murray *et al.*, 2006; Taanila *et al.*, 2005), the Israeli draft registry study (Reichenberg *et al.*, 2005) and the British birth cohort study (Jones *et al.*, 1994; Murray *et al.*, 2007). Though difficult to set up and undertake, and while the number of individuals developing schizophrenia is small, such population-based approaches are particularly informative as they do not focus only on the offspring of patients with schizophrenia.

The findings from these birth cohort studies suggest that general cognitive domains, including non-verbal and verbal educational achievement, and organizational and reading ability, are impaired early in development of individuals who later acquire schizophrenia (Cannon *et al.*, 1997, 2000; David *et al.*, 1997; Davidson *et al.*, 1999; Kremen *et al.*, 1998). These domains include relatively more specific problems in mathematical and vocabulary skills, mechanical knowledge and lower intelligence (IQ) (David *et al.*, 1997; Davidson *et al.*, 1999; Jones *et al.*, 1994). However, there is also evidence that developmental delay is associated with poorer development of intellectual abilities in a normal healthy population and vice versa (Murray *et al.*, 2007; Taanila *et al.*, 2005), suggesting that such risk factors may not be specific and represent poor predictors of schizophrenia. Few studies have examined the developmental trajectory of these abilities from childhood through adolescence, which would assist in determining if such deficits represent static (developmental arrest) or progressive (neurodegenerative) processes, or a combination of both (for discussion see Testa & Pantelis (2007)).

The more recent high-risk studies have comprehensively assessed neuropsychological function, though not all data have been published as yet. In initial reports from the EHRS, slightly lower levels of global cognitive function were identified in a high-risk cohort than in a matched control group (Byrne *et al.*, 1999). When this difference was controlled for, the high-risk group was significantly impaired only on a global memory test and on a sentence completion test that implicates executive functions. However, none of the subjects in that study had become acutely psychotic at the time of publication. In subsequent reports from the EHRS, investigators assessed the relationship to symptom severity in the high-risk cohort as few had converted to psychosis. Cosway *et al.* (2000, 2002) found that IQ, verbal memory and executive function did distinguish between young relatives with subthreshold psychotic symptoms and those without such symptoms during follow-up, while attentional measures did not differ between high-risk subjects and controls. A small number of individuals have now developed schizophrenia in the EHRS, allowing comparison of converters and non-converters. Initial neuropsychological findings (Whyte *et al.*, 2006) were consistent with the earlier studies in identifying memory impairments in their high-risk cohort, with deficits in immediate and delayed story recall in the high-risk group as a whole, while there was a suggestion that those converting to illness showed poorer baseline verbal learning performance. There were no significant group-by-time interactions observed, suggesting that the deficits were stable. While the deficits in memory in the high-risk group are consistent with other studies discussed below, the numbers of individuals converting to psychosis (13 out of 118) are too small to draw any firm conclusions.

The literature investigating neuropsychological and brain activity using the UHR strategy has gained momentum, with several groups adopting the approach (reviewed by Brewer *et al.* (2006a); Wood *et al.* (2008)). However, apart from the Melbourne studies, many of these investigations remain preliminary, with few UHR subjects having converted to psychosis.

The most consistent cognitive findings from studies in which adequate numbers of UHR individuals have converted to psychosis are impairments on executive tasks tapping PFC function, such as on a self-ordered spatial working memory task (Wood *et al.*, 2003a) or antisaccade eye movements (Nieman *et al.*, 2007); olfactory identification (Brewer *et al.*, 2003); and tasks requiring rapid processing and organization of information such as story recall (Brewer *et al.*, 2005; Lencz *et al.*, 2006). Individuals who were UHR and who later developed psychosis showed specific deficits on these tasks when compared with those who did not become ill. To date, only premorbid olfactory identification deficits have been specifically associated with the later onset of schizophrenia (Brewer *et al.*, 2003).

More recently, the Cologne group have reported on prodromal subjects converting to psychosis (Pukrop *et al.*, 2007). Those developing psychosis were impaired across a number of domains of neuropsychological function compared with controls, while in comparison with non-converters, they were more impaired on a working memory task (the Subject Ordered Pointing Task (SOPT), a non-spatial *self-ordered* task) (Petrides, 1995), verbal IQ and processing speed. These tests were predictive of illness onset in this clinically prodromal group, with a positive predictive value of 0.80 and negative predictive value of 0.74. Interestingly, while the delayed response task of spatial working memory did not discriminate the groups, the findings of the SOPT are consistent with the results described above from the Melbourne group on the self-ordered spatial working memory task from the CANTAB (Wood *et al.*, 2003a). Together, these findings suggest that pre-onset working memory impairments may not be related to stimulus modality but rather reflect a difficulty conducting a self-ordered search through the contents of working memory.

The two largest UHR studies (Brewer *et al.*, 2005; Lencz *et al.*, 2006) both found that UHR subjects had significantly lower performance IQ than the comparison subjects, regardless of outcome, along with lower pre-morbid functioning. However, whereas Brewer *et al.* (2005) found impairments specific to the UHR patients who developed psychosis, using visual reproduction and story recall tasks, Lencz *et al.* (2006) found that only a composite verbal memory measure predicted psychosis outcome. No other memory, attentional or executive tasks discriminated between any of the groups in either study.

While these studies, together with similar findings from the EHRS described above (Whyte *et al.*, 2006), suggest that verbal memory deficits might be an impor-tant risk factor for the development of schizophrenia-spectrum psychotic disorders, the fact that they were assessed using fairly complex tasks requiring organiza-tional and strategic ability as well as memory implic-ates a prefrontal–hippocampal system abnormality. Therefore, these deficits may be more akin to the self-ordered working memory deficits cited above (Pukrop *et al.*, 2007; Wood *et al.*, 2003a); however, further examination of the subprocesses involved in performance of these tasks is required.

Interestingly, the one predictive cognitive marker identified in previous genetic high-risk studies (atten-tional deficits assessed with the identical pairs version of the continuous performance task (Cornblatt & Keilp, 1994; Erlenmeyer-Kimling *et al.*, 2000; Rutschmann, Cornblatt & Erlenmeyer-Kimling, 1977)) has not pro-ven predictive in more recent studies. Both Francey *et al.* (2005) and Lencz *et al.* (2004) found non-specific deficits in separate UHR cohorts. Similarly, Cosway *et al.* (2002) found no association between attentional deficits on the task and genetic vulnerability to schizo-phrenia. These findings suggest that such attentional tasks are not useful endophenotypes of schizophrenia or psychosis.

Potential neuropsychological trait markers should be stable over time. There have been few longitudinal studies in high-risk groups to inform this issue. Wood and colleagues recently examined progressive changes in cognitive function over the transition to psychosis as part of the Melbourne UHR studies (Wood *et al.*, 2007). Neuropsychological functioning of 16 UHR patients (seven of whom developed psychosis) was assessed at baseline and after transition to psychosis (or after 12

months). While performance on most tests was stable or improved, visuospatial memory, verbal fluency and attentional switching showed significant decline over the transition to psychosis. These progressive impair-ments were not seen in the non-psychotic UHR group. These data would seem consistent with progressive brain structural changes over transition to psychosis (Pantelis *et al.*, 2005, 2007; Wood *et al.*, 2008) and suggest that some biological markers proposed to be endophenotypes may not be stable over the transition to illness (and, therefore, not meet the criteria for true endophenotypes).

The notion that deficits may be progressive is also supported by the large cross-sectional study from the Cologne group. Pukrop and colleagues (2006) found deficits in verbal executive functions and verbal mem-ory in the prodromal group. In particular, those who were 'late' prodromal showed additional attentional deficits, while comparison with the other patient groups suggested that neurocognitive deficits may be progressive.

Taken together, the findings of research conducted prior to psychosis onset contradict work in chronically ill samples in failing to identify pervasive cognitive deficits. Rather the data are consistent with relatively subtle impairments in specific cognitive domains, which may show a progression during the transition to a first psychotic episode. The domains that appear to be affected most in the prodromal period are self-ordered working memory tasks (perhaps reflecting increased demand on the executive system), certain types of memory requiring rapid and complex organ-ization of material, and olfactory identification ability. However, as we discuss below, the status of such defi-cits as endophenotypes may need revision in the con-text of the maturational trajectory of these cognitive abilities, and in light of the longitudinal changes in brain structure and function known to occur during the period of highest risk for psychosis onset.

Psychophysiological studies: event-related potentials

Few studies have examined ERPs in individuals at high-risk for psychosis, though ERPs have been proposed to be potential endophenotypes. Mismatch negativity (MMN) is a negative auditory ERP, occurring 150–250 milliseconds (ms) after presentation of 'deviant' stimuli, which are elicited by interspersing infrequent sounds (differing in pitch, duration, intensity or spatial location) in a sequence of repetitive sounds. The MMN is evoked automatically, is preconscious and is thought to have generators in auditory cortices, but it may also have a prefrontal generator (Salisbury, Krljes & McCarley, 2003). It is reduced in patients with established schizophrenia (Javitt, Shelley & Ritter, 2000), with some degree of specificity (Catts *et al.*, 1995). In contrast, patients with first-episode schizophrenia early in their course of illness are unimpaired (Salisbury *et al.*, 2002), while those within the first 3 years of illness show a mild deficit (Javitt *et al.*, 2000). Further, longitudinal findings provide evidence of progressive changes associated with reductions in the volume of the left hemisphere Heschl gyrus grey matter (Salisbury *et al.*, 2007). The limited available data from pre-psychotic subjects support the notion of progressive changes in this measure with increasing chronicity (Brockhaus-Dumke *et al.*, 2005). These findings suggest that MMN may be a marker of progression rather than an endophenotype in the traditional sense.

In contrast to MMN, which is pre-attentive, the P300 ERP is elicited when subjects actively attend to a rare occurrence of an infrequent target, using the 'oddball' paradigm (Salisbury *et al.*, 2003). Typically, patients with chronic schizophrenia show reduced P300 amplitude and these deficits are considered to reflect impairments in sustained attention and higher-level cognitive abilities, including working memory (Jeon & Polich, 2001; Kimble *et al.*, 2000). The evidence suggests that the P300 is reduced over the midline and left temporal regions, is associated with reduced volume of the left posterior superior temporal gyrus, tracks symptom changes (Ford *et al.*, 1994; Mathalon, Ford & Pfefferbaum, 2000) and shows specificity for schizophrenia rather than affective psychosis (McCarley *et al.*, 2002; McCarley *et al.*, 1993). Moreover, P300 abnormality has been associated with longer duration of untreated psychosis (Wang *et al.*, 2005) and is found in neuroleptic-naive (Hirayasu *et al.*, 1998) and unmedicated patients (Faux *et al.*, 1993). Recent findings in patients with

first-episode psychosis did not identify an abnormality, although there was an association with positive symptoms (Renoult *et al.*, 2007). Therefore, while suggestive, it is not entirely clear that P300 is a stable trait marker of illness. However, there is no clear evidence of progressive abnormality as with MMN, which may suggest that the P300 may index poorer prognosis.

The early studies of P300 abnormalities in individuals at genetic high risk for developing schizophrenia (review by Friedman & Squires-Wheeler (1994)) found prolonged P300 latencies in these individuals (Blackwood *et al.*, 1991; Frangou *et al.*, 1997), with evidence to suggest this particularly involves frontal P300 (Turetsky *et al.*, 2000) or fronto-parietal networks (Sponheim, McGuire & Stanwyck, 2006). A very recent study of 35 UHR individuals (of whom seven later developed psychosis) found significantly lower P300 amplitudes, but no difference in latency (Bramon *et al.*, 2008). The notion of P300 measures as an endophenotype were not supported by the finding of no differences between the group who developed psychosis and those who did not; however, further longitudinal research from prodromal to late stages is needed.

Other potential ERP markers of interest include auditory P50 inhibition deficits, which are consistently reported in schizophrenia and considered to reflect a sensory gating deficit (Freedman *et al.*, 2000; Jin *et al.*, 1998). This marker is also reported in individuals with schizotypal personality disorder, especially in those with a family history of schizophrenia (Cadenhead *et al.*, 2000), and has been linked to a candidate gene (Freedman *et al.*, 2000). As such, it may represent a more promising endophenotype for further investigation. This notion is supported by a recent study of individuals at clinical high risk for schizophrenia using inclusion criteria similar to those of the Melbourne group (Cadenhead *et al.*, 2005), as well as in a group of genetically defined high-risk adolescents (Myles-Worsley *et al.*, 2004). These data suggest that P50 may be a more stable ERP marker, although a recent study failed to identify such deficits in early schizophrenia or their unaffected relatives (de Wilde *et al.*, 2007). The authors of this study propose that such deficits may be developmentally dependent, a notion we consider further below.

Functional neuroimaging studies

Functional imaging studies have consistently identified abnormalities in the PFC in patients with established schizophrenia (Carter *et al.*, 1998; Davidson & Heinrichs, 2003; Fusar-Poli *et al.*, 2007a; Velakoulis & Pantelis, 1996), as well as in those with first-episode psychosis, including unmedicated patients (Harrison *et al.*, 2006; MacDonald *et al.*, 2005), which may be specific to schizophrenic psychosis (MacDonald *et al.*, 2005; Molina *et al.*, 2005). While both hypo- and hyper-frontality have been found during cognitive activation tasks, leading to concerns surrounding the reproducibility of the findings, such inconsistencies can be explained in terms of methodological factors that, once controlled for, may still be construed as reflecting an abnormally functioning PFC (Manoach *et al.*, 2000; Manoach *et al.*, 1999). While some have argued that these abnormalities are robust to treatment status (Snitz *et al.*, 2005), other studies (Brewer *et al.*, 2007; Fusar-Poli *et al.*, 2007b; Jones *et al.*, 2004) demonstrate that prefrontal metabolism may be modified by neuroleptic treatment. This suggests that examination of the value of neural circuitry integrity as an endophenotype of schizophrenia should be conducted in neuroleptic-naive subjects.

These findings are of interest given that abnormalities such as working memory deficits, which rely on the integrity of PFC, have shown promise as markers of schizophrenia in neuropsychological studies. It has been suggested that identifying the genes coding for working memory ability and functional integrity of prefrontal systems, such as that for catechol-*O*-methyltransferase (COMT), may be relevant to the genetics of schizophrenia (Harrison & Weinberger, 2005; Rapoport *et al.*, 2005). While early findings related to *COMT* looked promising (Egan *et al.*, 2001) the evidence linking such genes to the disorder remains unconvincing (Testa & Pantelis, 2007). As discussed below, a link to brain maturation, including synaptic plasticity and cortical development (Harrison & Weinberger, 2005; Rapoport *et al.*, 2005; Walker & Bollini, 2002), may be more consistent with the available evidence relevant to late neurodevelopment and psychosis onset (Cannon *et al.*, 2003; Pantelis *et al.*, 2005). Consequently, genes coding for brain maturation may prove to be more useful, including candidates such as the genes for dysbindin (Gornick *et al.*, 2005), glutamic acid decarboxylase 1 (Addington *et al.*, 2005; Straub *et al.*, 2007), neuregulin/erbB4 (Law *et al.*, 2007; Silberberg *et al.*, 2006; Stefansson *et al.*, 2002) and the disrupted in schizophrenia 1 gene (*DISC1*) (Callicott *et al.*, 2005; Camargo *et al.*, 2007; Cannon *et al.*, 2005). Therefore, assessing the evidence for functional imaging abnormalities in high-risk individuals is of particular importance.

In their recent review of functional imaging studies in genetic high-risk subjects, Whalley, Harris & Lawrie (2007) concluded that the relatively small number of studies, combined with methodological differences, do not allow firm conclusions. However, some of the evidence points to dorsolateral hyperfrontality, particularly on the right and especially for tasks requiring working memory, as well as increased activity in parietal regions (Whalley *et al.*, 2007). Whether these are state- or trait-related is not entirely clear. For example, Marjoram *et al.* (2006), using theory of mind tasks, found a complex pattern of differences of prefrontal function when comparing symptomatic with non-symptomatic relatives of patients, depending on whether current versus lifetime history of symptoms was examined. Interestingly, the parietal response premorbidly has been shown to distinguish individuals at genetic risk who converted to psychosis from non-converters (Whalley *et al.*, 2006). However, only four subjects converted to psychosis in this study. Involvement of the neural circuitry relevant to working memory ability is interesting given the findings from the neuropsychological studies described above, as well as the structural evidence described below. In a further investigation linking genes to brain function from the EHRS, Hall and colleagues (2006) showed that a variant of the gene *NRG1* (coding neuregulin 1) was associated with decreased premorbid IQ, psychotic symptoms and hypo-activity of frontal and temporal regions. The dynamic interaction of genes and brain function during adolescent brain development remains to be assessed.

Only one study to date has used functional imaging to assess a UHR group experiencing prodromal symptoms (Morey *et al.*, 2005). In this cross-sectional functional magnetic resonance imaging (fMRI) study, fronto-striatal function was assessed using an attentional task (visual oddball paradigm) in 10 UHR individuals, 15 patients early in the course of schizophrenia, 11 patients with chronic schizophrenia and 16 control subjects. Both patient groups manifested abnormal function, while the UHR group did not differ significantly from controls, though they did manifest behavioural deficits. A linear trend analysis of the fMRI findings indicated that there was a progressive decline in frontal and striatal activation, from pre-psychosis to chronic illness. While a longitudinal study is needed, these data are consistent with the structural imaging results outlined below and with the notion of progressive changes across illness stages. Such findings indicate that potential functional imaging markers of illness may not be static but, rather, may need to be viewed dynamically over time, and ideally within a brain maturational context.

Structural neuroimaging studies

The most consistent structural neuroimaging findings in schizophrenia appear to be ventricular enlargement; smaller brain volume; smaller volumes of frontal lobes, temporal lobes and hippocampi; and reduced asymmetry (Boos *et al.*, 2007; Liddle & Pantelis, 2003; Wright *et al.*, 2000). Further, there is evidence for specificity as differences are reported between schizophrenia and bipolar affective disorder, at least for some structures, including hippocampi, amygdala (Hirayasu *et al.*, 2001; Kuroki *et al.*, 2006; McDonald *et al.*, 2004a; Velakoulis *et al.*, 2006) and corpus callosum (Walterfang *et al.*, 2008). Currently, it is not clear that all of these volumetric abnormalities are apparent from illness onset (e.g. temporal lobe reduction not confirmed) (Vita *et al.*, 2006) and the resolution of the techniques may be at the limits for identifying subtle volume differences (Steen *et al.*, 2006). However, other abnormalities may be more readily detected, such as anomalies in cortical folding patterns, observed in the anterior cingulate (Fornito *et al.*, 2006; Yücel *et al.*, 2002), PFC (Bonnici *et al.*, 2007; Harris *et al.*, 2007; Narr *et al.*, 2004; Stanfield *et al.*, 2007; Wiegand *et al.*, 2005), temporal lobe (Cachia *et al.*, 2008; Harris *et al.*, 2004) and

speech-related brain areas (Wisco *et al.*, 2007). These last anomalies are consistent with an early neurodevelopmental anomaly, given that cortical folding patterns are primarily determined pre- and perinatally (Armstrong *et al.*, 1995; Chi, Dooling & Gilles, 1977).

Cortical folding patterns like these were recently examined in the EHRS. Specifically, the gyrification of the PFC was compared between those high-risk subjects who subsequently developed schizophrenia and those who did not. As has previously been found for a sample with chronic schizophrenia (Vogeley *et al.*, 2000) as well as unaffected family members (Vogeley *et al.*, 2001), the group who went on to develop the illness had *hyper*gyrification of the PFC specific to the right hemisphere (Harris *et al.*, 2007). Although the precise mechanisms by which this confers risk are unclear, one possibility is that this pattern of gyrification is a result of altered cortical connectivity.

The findings from twin studies have been informative in discriminating genetic from non-genetic influences (Cannon, 2005b). Twin studies assessing regions of interest have reported decreases in intracranial, whole-brain and hippocampal volume to be associated with genetic vulnerability to schizophrenia, with additional effects of illness and/or environmental factors on certain structures, including hippocampus (Baaré *et al.*, 2001; van Erp *et al.*, 2004; van Haren *et al.*, 2004). In a voxel-wise structural study of the lateral cortical surface in twins with schizophrenia, Cannon *et al.* (2002) found illness-related reductions in grey matter density in the dorsolateral PFC, superior temporal gyrus and superior parietal lobule. Neuroanatomical changes associated with genetic liability to schizophrenia were restricted to a frontal lobe region encompassing the dorsolateral PFC and the frontal poles. Medial wall and subcortical structures were not investigated in this study, limiting any conclusions regarding the diagnostic or predictive relevance of changes in these regions. Hulshoff Pol *et al.* (2006) assessed all brain regions using a voxel-based morphometry approach, and identified left-sided anterior hemisphere changes, including decreased grey matter and increased white matter in the region of the left medial orbito-frontal region, which they suggest may be useful as endophenotypes in genetic studies. However, such a conclusion does not adequately account for the existing evidence for progressive changes in this region during psychosis onset (Pantelis *et al.*, 2003), as discussed below.

Attempts to demonstrate that these abnormalities are apparent prior to illness onset in high-risk populations are still nascent (Lawrie, 2004; Pantelis *et al.*, 2005, 2007; Whalley *et al.*, 2007). In a recent review of imaging studies in schizophrenia, Keshavan, Prasad & Pearlson (2007) concluded that brain structural measures were stable trait characteristics that were heritable and associated with cognitive and behavioural phenotypes and thereby met criteria as endophenotypes in major psychoses; however, the issue of specificity was less clear. McDonald and colleagues (2004b) assessed the question of specificity by examining bipolar disorder and schizophrenia and found some specificity but also areas of overlap between the disorders. The situation is further complicated by the heterogeneity of the findings, their relationship to non-genetic aetiological factors and evidence for progressive structural changes, especially in the earliest illness stages (Pantelis *et al.*, 2005, 2007; Woods *et al.*, 2005).

Initial studies from the Melbourne group focused on medial temporal structures, particularly the hippocampus, as smaller hippocampi have been found consistently in schizophrenia (Lawrie & Abukmeil, 1998; Nelson *et al.*, 1998; Steen *et al.*, 2006; Wright *et al.*, 2000), making them potential candidate endophenotypes.

In the largest published study of hippocampal and amygdala volumes (examined separately) in psychosis, involving 473 individuals with first-episode psychosis, chronic schizophrenia and UHR, Velakoulis and colleagues (2006) confirmed that those UHR subjects who converted to psychosis had normal hippocampal volumes, and also had normal size of amygdala. In contrast, patients with first-episode schizophrenia had smaller left hippocampal volumes, while patients with chronic schizophrenia had bilaterally smaller hippocampi. Further, patients with schizophrenia-spectrum disorders had normal amygdala size, while those with affective psychoses or psychosis not otherwise specified exhibited larger amygdalae but normal hippocampal size – suggesting diagnostic differences in these brain structures. Magnetic resonance spectroscopy (MRS) studies in these patients supported these findings, in

that levels of *N*-acetylaspartate (NAA; a marker of neuronal integrity) in the hippocampus were normal at the earliest stages of psychosis and schizophrenia (Wood *et al.*, 2003b), which contrasts with the findings of lower NAA levels in established schizophrenia (Bertolino *et al.*, 1998; Heckers, 2001). Therefore, while smaller hippocampal volumes may show some degree of specificity to schizophrenic psychoses, they are not premorbid illness markers; rather, they may be related to illness progression.

The few available longitudinal structural MRI studies of individuals at high risk for schizophrenia and psychosis have provided insights into brain changes during the period of transition from the at-risk state to the illness/psychosis state. Studies from our group as well as those from the EHRS have been the first to follow subjects through the period of transition to illness (Job *et al.*, 2005; Pantelis *et al.*, 2003) (reviewed by Cannon *et al.*, 2003; Lawrie, 2004; Pantelis *et al.*, 2005, 2007; Seidman *et al.*, 2003). In their voxel-based morphometric study, Pantelis *et al.* (2003) found that UHR individuals who developed a psychotic disorder showed left-sided grey matter loss in left inferior frontal, medial temporal and inferior temporal regions, and the mid-cingulate bilaterally. In a subsequent longitudinal voxel-based morphometric study from the EHRS, Job and colleagues (2005) also found reductions in the left inferior temporal lobe, left uncus and right cerebellum, as well as hippocampal changes. Importantly, their subjects were all naive for neuroleptic drugs, indicating that medication did not explain these findings. These longitudinal results provide further evidence that changes in temporal (as well as frontal) structures are progressive and may not necessarily represent premorbid markers of psychosis.

Following on from work demonstrating progressive changes in medial temporal structures, studies have examined pituitary size as a proxy measure of hypothalamic–pituitary–adrenal axis dysregulation, which may be associated with stress-related damage to structures like the hippocampus (Phillips *et al.*, 2006). Studies from the Melbourne group demonstrated that pituitary size was larger in those with first-episode schizophrenia compared with those with chronic schizophrenia (Pariante *et al.*, 2004). Pariante *et al.* (2005) confirmed that these changes in those with first-episode psychosis were not explained by neuroleptic medication. Using the same methodology to study 94 previously never-medicated UHR individuals, Garner and colleagues (2005) found that 31 converters to psychosis had significantly larger (+12%) baseline pituitary volumes compared with subjects who did not develop a psychotic disorder. Further, the risk of developing psychosis during the follow-up period was significantly increased (20% for every 10% increase in baseline pituitary volume), and increased size of pituitary was significantly associated with shorter time to psychosis onset. This work indicates that abnormal function of the hypothalamic–pituitary–adrenal axis around the time of transition to psychosis is highly predictive of psychosis onset, but this is temporally dependent on proximity to illness onset; therefore, pituitary size likely represents a state rather than a trait marker.

In a cross-sectional study examining the surface morphology of the anterior cingulate cortex, Yücel *et al.* (2003) compared 63 males at UHR for the development of psychosis (21 subsequently developed psychosis) and 75 healthy male subjects. Compared with healthy controls, the UHR group had more interruptions in the course of the cingulate sulcus and were less likely to have a well-developed paracingulate sulcus in the left hemisphere, with a loss of the normal leftward asymmetry of the sulcus (see Yücel *et al.*, 2001, 2002). However, these surface morphological measures did not discriminate those who progressed to psychosis from those who did not. While these findings suggest that UHR individuals show abnormalities in anterior cingulate morphology, the presence of such abnormalities may not be specific to schizophrenia or psychosis but rather reflect a more general vulnerability to psychopathology or other aetiological factors.

More recently, Fornito *et al.* (2008) assessed thickness, surface area and depth of the anterior cingulate in first-episode and UHR subjects. In first-episode patients, they found evidence for a bilateral reduction in cortical thickness extending across the paralimbic region of the anterior cingulate cortex. In UHR individuals who went on to develop psychosis, these reductions were restricted to a rostral subdivision of the paralimbic

anterior cingulate cortex. Together, these data suggest that thickness reductions begin focally in the rostral paralimbic anterior cingulate cortex prior to psychosis onset and extend across to include the dorsal and subcallosal portions of the paralimbic area during the first episode. This suggestion is supported by longitudinal work, which shows that the earliest grey matter reductions are apparent in paralimbic areas, and then spread to engulf limbic areas with ongoing illness (Vidal *et al.*, 2006). Pantelis *et al.* (2003) also demonstrated progressive bilateral cingulate grey matter loss in UHR subjects subsequently developing psychosis. Further evidence for a premorbid cingulate abnormality comes from a small MRS study of 19 UHR patients, which found a significant reduction in NAA in the cingulate region bilaterally (Jessen *et al.*, 2006). While NAA reductions did not predict transition to psychosis, trimethylamines were higher in the later-psychotic group, indicative of higher rates of cell membrane turnover (Miller *et al.*, 1996). Taken together, these data point to the anterior cingulate as a key region relevant to the onset of psychosis, with possible progressive changes following transition. Additional studies with other modalities, such as phosphorus MRS, are required to elucidate the nature of these findings.

In a study investigating genetic influences on brain structure in schizophrenia and bipolar disorders, genetic risk for schizophrenia was not associated with anterior cingulate volume or with hippocampal volume (McDonald *et al.*, 2004b). These findings received support in a further elaboration of our UHR studies in which we examined hippocampal volume and anterior cingulate surface morphology in the UHR individuals according to familial risk of schizophrenia (Wood *et al.*, 2005). Compared with those UHR individuals having a positive family history of schizophrenia, those without such a family history had significantly smaller left hippocampal volume and a trend towards anomalous left cingulate surface morphology, with reduced paracingulate sulcus folding and a greater incidence of cingulate sulcus interruptions. These findings are consistent with the notion of an early insult of non-genetic origin, which may render these regions susceptible to later progressive changes. The findings also suggest that such abnormalities are poor candidates as illness-related markers.

We have also recently examined changes at the neo-cortical surface in UHR individuals as well as in patients with first-episode schizophrenia (Sun *et al.*, 2008). In these studies, we have used an approach that assesses expansion or retraction at every point on the cerebral hemisphere and combined this with the cortical pattern-matching techniques developed by Toga and Thompson (Thompson *et al.*, 2000). Preliminary find-ings from these studies have identified changes in PFC regions, indicative of an accelerated rate of grey matter retraction at the earliest stages of psychosis, including in pre-psychotic UHR individuals during the transition to psychosis. The changes appear consistent with accel-eration of the normal maturational processes occurring in schizophrenia from its earliest stages. Further, the rate of grey matter retraction was significantly associ-ated with proximity to the transition point to psychosis. Such work awaits replication with larger cohorts.

Similar to the findings from neuropsychology, psy-chophysiology and functional imaging, while there have been a number of brain structural abnormalities identified that were potential endophenotypes of schiz-ophrenia and psychosis, a review of the studies in pre-psychotic individuals at high risk for transition to illness has not provided compelling evidence to sup-port these abnormalities as illness-related markers (although some, such as gyrification indices, may prove promising). Rather, it would seem that many of the findings represent state-related abnormalities or changes that occur dynamically over the course of the illness. In this respect, identifying stable trait markers may need to be reconsidered in the context of a dynam-ically changing system. In this context, the dynamic brain changes occurring in adolescence and early adulthood may provide a context for interpreting some of the findings reviewed above.

Conclusions

The neurobiology of schizophrenia and related psy-chotic disorders has challenged us to develop novel approaches and methodologies to elucidating the causes of this illness. The endophenotype approach is potentially useful as it provides a way forward in linking features of the disorder to underlying brain mecha-nisms, as well as to potential illness-related genes. While a number of potential endophenotypic markers seem promising, it is clear that few have met all the criteria to be considered true endophenotypes of the illness. In particular, we have reviewed the available studies at the earliest stages of the disorder and many of the potential markers are either less apparent or nor-mal in individuals at high risk for developing psychosis and schizophrenia. Further, a number of these markers either lack specificity or may be changing over the initial stages of the illness, indicating that they do not represent stable or even enduring trait markers. The most promising markers, such as certain executive functions (e.g. measured with self-ordered working memory tasks) and more direct measures of frontal lobe integrity (derived from psychophysiology as well as functional and structural imaging), relate to frontal and perhaps temporal cortices, which are the brain regions that are changing dynamically during adoles-cence and early adulthood (Giedd, 2004; Paus, 2005). Cannon (2005a) observed that the behavioural expres-sion of schizophrenia-related neural disturbances becomes apparent with maturation, especially in ado-lescence. These changes may represent an accelerated process of late brain maturation, involving ongoing myelination and synaptic pruning (Feinberg, 1982; Huttenlocher, 1984). Therefore, one possibility is that potential endophenotypes represent abnormalities in the normal maturational process.

In this context, the disparate findings from the vari-ous studies discussed above may be understood by considering how these various measures change during normal or anomalous brain maturation, especially dur-ing adolescence and early adulthood when psychotic disorders develop (Brewer *et al.*, 2006b; Wood *et al.*, 2004). Few investigations have taken account of normal changes in these measures during adolescent brain development (i.e. 'late' neurodevelopment), though maturational changes in certain aspects of neuropsy-chological function and in inhibitory control have been examined. For example, as well as P50 mentioned above, other markers of inhibitory control have been associated with risk of schizophrenia, including pre-pulse inhibition and antisaccade eye movements

(Ettinger *et al.*, 2006; Smyrnis *et al.*, 2003; Swerdlow *et al.*, 2006; Turetsky *et al.*, 2007). While each of these have been identified as potential endophenotypes it is likely that adolescent brain maturation influences these functions, as demonstrated in developmental studies (Asato, Sweeney & Luna, 2006; Luna & Sweeney, 2001, 2004). Working memory has also been examined in this regard and shown to be developing well into the mid-twenties (De Luca *et al.*, 2003), while evidence for progressive brain structural changes involving PFC (Nakamura *et al.*, 2007; Sun *et al.*, 2008) has been shown to represent an acceleration of the normal pattern across the brain (D.-Q. Sun, P. D. McGorry, G. W. Stuart *et al.*, unpublished data).

The relevant approach may be to view these potential markers as part of a dynamically changing system and to consider how the onset of an illness like schizophrenia interacts with this process. Therefore, studies of proposed endophenotypes should be examined in the context of brain maturation during the period of heightened risk for psychosis and schizophrenia, including longitudinal studies. This will assist in ascertaining what these potential markers are indexing in the context of psychosis and schizophrenia: that is, illness-related markers, indices of transition to illness or prognosis, or markers of anomalous maturation. The genes relevant to prefrontal systems and brain maturation of these systems are likely to be particularly interesting in this regard.

Cannon (2005a) summarized the evidence for potential genes that would be consistent with the findings above. For example, *DISC1* has been associated with schizophrenia (Harrison & Weinberger, 2005) and is relevant to neurodevelopment, including neuritic outgrowth, neuronal migration, synaptogenesis and glutamatergic transmission (Camargo *et al.*, 2007). Further, *DISC1* and the adjacent *TRAX* genes have been associated with altered PFC function and altered working memory performance in patients with schizophrenia and their relatives, including impaired working memory and reduced grey matter volume (Cannon *et al.*, 2005; Hennah *et al.*, 2005), and decreased P300 (Blackwood *et al.*, 2001). Therefore, dynamic understanding and approaches are needed in future studies to elucidate the nature and progression of the disease from before onset, and prediction may need a longitudinal perspective.

ACKNOWLEDGEMENTS

This work was supported by project grants from the National Health and Medical Research Council (NHMRC; grant IDs: 145627, 145737, 970598, 981112, 970391), NHMRC Program Grant (ID: 350241). Drs Yücel, Wood, Brewer and Fornito are supported by fellowships from NHMRC. Dr Fornito was supported by a J. N. Peters Fellowship from the University of Melbourne and Dr Wood is also supported by a NARSAD Young Investigator Award. Dr Cannon is supported by NIH grant MH65078.

REFERENCES

Addington, A. M., Gornick, M., Duckworth, J. *et al.* (2005). GAD1 (2q31.1), which encodes glutamic acid decarboxylase (GAD(67)), is associated with childhood-onset schizophrenia and cortical gray matter volume loss. *Molecular Psychiatry*, **10**, 581–8.

Armstrong, E., Schleicher, A., Omran, H., Curtis, M. & Zilles, K. (1995). The ontogeny of human gyrification. *Cerebral Cortex*, **5**, 56–63.

Asato, M. R., Sweeney, J. A. & Luna, B. (2006). Cognitive processes in the development of TOL performance. *Neuropsychologia*, **44**, 2259–69.

Baaré, W. F., van Oel, C. J., Hulshoff Pol, H. E. *et al.* (2001). Volumes of brain structures in twins discordant for schizophrenia. *Archives of General Psychiatry*, **58**, 33–40.

Benes, F. M. (2007). Searching for unique endophenotypes for schizophrenia and bipolar disorder within neural circuits and their molecular regulatory mechanisms. *Schizophrenia Bulletin*, **33**, 932–6.

Bertolino, A., Callicott, J. H., Elman, I. *et al.* (1998). Regionally specific neuronal pathology in untreated patients with schizophrenia: a proton magnetic resonance spectroscopic imaging study. *Biological Psychiatry*, **43**, 641–8.

Bilder, R. M., Goldman, R. S., Robinson, D. *et al.* (2000). Neuropsychology of first-episode schizophrenia: initial characterization and clinical correlates. *American Journal of Psychiatry*, **157**, 549–59.

Blackwood, D. H., St Clair, D. M., Muir, W. J. & Duffy, J. C. (1991). Auditory P300 and eye tracking dysfunction in schizophrenic pedigrees. *Archives of General Psychiatry*, **48**, 899–909.

Blackwood, D. H., Fordyce, A., Walker, M. T. *et al.* (2001). Schizophrenia and affective disorders – cosegregation with a translocation at chromosome 1q42 that directly disrupts brain-expressed genes: clinical and P300 findings in a family. *American Journal of Human Genetics*, **69**, 428–33.

Bonnici, H. M., William, T., Moorhead, J. *et al.* (2007). Prefrontal lobe gyrification index in schizophrenia, mental retardation and comorbid groups: an automated study. *Neuroimage*, **53**, 648–54.

Boos, H. B., Aleman, A., Cahn, W., Pol, H. H. & Kahn, R. S. (2007). Brain volumes in relatives of patients with schizophrenia: a meta-analysis. *Archives of General Psychiatry*, **64**, 297–304.

Braff, D. L., Freedman, R., Schork, N. J. & Gottesman, II. (2007). Deconstructing schizophrenia: an overview of the use of endophenotypes in order to understand a complex disorder. *Schizophrenia Bulletin*, **33**, 21–32.

Bramon, E., Shaikh, M., Broome, M. *et al.* (2008). Abnormal P300 in people with high risk of developing psychosis. *Neuroimage*, **41**, 553–60.

Brewer, W. J., Wood, S. J., McGorry, P. D. *et al.* (2003). Impairment of olfactory identification ability in individuals at ultra-high risk for psychosis who later develop schizophrenia. *American Journal of Psychiatry*, **160**, 1790–4.

Brewer, W. J., Francey, S. M., Wood, S. J. *et al.* (2005). Memory impairments identified in people at ultra-high risk for psychosis who later develop first-episode psychosis. *American Journal of Psychiatry*, **162**, 71–8.

Brewer, W. J., Wood, S. J., Phillips, L. J. *et al.* (2006a). Generalized and specific cognitive performance in clinical high-risk cohorts: a review highlighting potential vulnerability markers for psychosis. *Schizophrenia Bulletin*, **32**, 538–55.

Brewer, W. J., Pantelis, C., De Luca, C. R. & Wood, S. J. (2006b). Olfactory processing and brain maturation. In W. J. Brewer, D. J. Castle & C. Pantelis (eds.), *Olfaction and the Brain*. Cambridge, UK: Cambridge University Press, pp. 103–18.

Brewer, W. J., Yucel, M., Harrison, B. J. *et al.* (2007). Increased prefrontal cerebral blood flow in first-episode schizophrenia following treatment: longitudinal positron emission tomography study. *Australian and New Zealand Journal of Psychiatry*, **41**, 129–35.

Brockhaus-Dumke, A., Tendolkar, I., Pukrop, R. *et al.* (2005). Impaired mismatch negativity generation in prodromal subjects and patients with schizophrenia. *Schizophrenia Research*, **73**, 297–310.

Byrne, M., Hodges, A., Grant, E., Owens, D. G. & Johnstone, E. C. (1999). Neuropsychological assessment of young people at high genetic risk for developing schizophrenia compared with controls: preliminary findings of the Edinburgh High Risk Study (EHRS). *Psychological Medicine*, **29**, 1161–73.

Cachia, A., Paillere-Martinot, M. L., Galinowski, A. *et al.* (2008). Cortical folding abnormalities in schizophrenia patients with resistant auditory hallucinations. *Neuroimage*, **39**, 927–35.

Cadenhead, K. S., Light, G. A., Geyer, M. A. & Braff, D. L. (2000). Sensory gating deficits assessed by the P50 event-related potential in subjects with schizotypal personality disorder. *American Journal of Psychiatry*, **157**, 55–9.

Cadenhead, K. S., Light, G. A., Shafer, K. M. & Braff, D. L. (2005). P50 suppression in individuals at risk for schizophrenia: the convergence of clinical, familial, and vulnerability marker risk assessment. *Biological Psychiatry*, **57**, 1504–9.

Callicott, J. H., Straub, R. E., Pezawas, L. *et al.* (2005). Variation in DISC1 affects hippocampal structure and function and increases risk for schizophrenia. *Proceedings of the National Academy of Sciences USA*, **102**, 8627–32.

Camargo, L. M., Collura, V., Rain, J. C. *et al.* (2007). Disrupted in schizophrenia 1 interactome: evidence for the close connectivity of risk genes and a potential synaptic basis for schizophrenia. *Molecular Psychiatry*, **12**, 74–86.

Cannon, M., Jones, P., Gilvarry, C. *et al.* (1997). Premorbid social functioning in schizophrenia and bipolar disorder: similarities and differences. *American Journal of Psychiatry*, **154**, 1544–50.

Cannon, T. D. (2005a). Clinical and genetic high-risk strategies in understanding vulnerability to psychosis. *Schizophrenia Research*, **79**, 35–44.

Cannon, T. D. (2005b). The inheritance of intermediate phenotypes for schizophrenia. *Current Opinion in Psychiatry*, **18**, 135–40.

Cannon, T. D. & Mednick, S. A. (1993). The schizophrenia high-risk project in Copenhagen: three decades of progress. *Acta Psychiatrica Scandinavica*, **370**(Suppl), 33–47.

Cannon, T. D., Bearden, C. E., Hollister, J. M. *et al.* (2000). Childhood cognitive functioning in schizophrenia patients and their unaffected siblings: a prospective cohort study. *Schizophrenia Bulletin*, **26**, 379–93.

Cannon, T. D., Thompson, P. M., van Erp, T. G. *et al.* (2002). Cortex mapping reveals regionally specific patterns of genetic and disease-specific gray-matter deficits in twins discordant for schizophrenia. *Proceedings of the National Academy of Sciences, USA*, **99**, 3228–33.

Cannon, T. D., van Erp, T. G., Bearden, C. E. *et al.* (2003). Early and late neurodevelopmental influences in the prodrome to schizophrenia: contributions of genes, environment, and their interactions. *Schizophrenia Bulletin*, **29**, 653–69.

Cannon, T. D., Hennah, W., van Erp, T. G. *et al.* (2005). Association of DISC1/TRAX haplotypes with schizophrenia, reduced prefrontal gray matter, and impaired short- and long-term memory. *Archives of General Psychiatry*, **62**, 1205–13.

Carter, C. S., Perlstein, W., Ganguli, R. *et al.* (1998). Functional hypofrontality and working memory dysfunction in schizophrenia. *American Journal of Psychiatry*, **155**, 1285–7.

Catts, S. V., Shelley, A. M., Ward, P. B. *et al.* (1995). Brain potential evidence for an auditory sensory memory deficit in schizophrenia. *American Journal of Psychiatry*, **152**, 213–19.

Chi, J., Dooling, E. & Gilles, F. (1977). Gyral development of the human brain. *Annals of Neurology*, **1**, 86–93.

Cornblatt, B. A. & Keilp, J. G. (1994). Impaired attention, genetics, and the pathophysiology of schizophrenia. *Schizophrenia Bulletin*, **20**, 31–46.

Cosway, R., Byrne, M., Clafferty, R. *et al.* (2000). Neuropsychological change in young people at high risk for schizophrenia: results from the first two neuropsychological assessments of the Edinburgh High Risk Study. *Psychological Medicine*, **30**, 1111–21.

Cosway, R., Byrne, M., Clafferty, R. *et al.* (2002). Sustained attention in young people at high risk for schizophrenia. *Psychological Medicine*, **32**, 277–86.

David, A. S., Malmberg, A., Brandt, L., Allebeck, P. & Lewis, G. (1997). IQ and risk for schizophrenia: a population-based cohort study. *Psychological Medicine*, **27**, 1311–23.

Davidson, L. L. & Heinrichs, R. W. (2003). Quantification of frontal and temporal lobe brain-imaging findings in schizophrenia: a meta-analysis. *Psychiatry Research*, **122**, 69–87.

Davidson, M., Reichenberg, A., Rabinowitz, J. *et al.* (1999). Behavioral and intellectual markers for schizophrenia in apparently healthy male adolescents. *American Journal of Psychiatry*, **156**, 1328–35.

De Luca, C. R., Wood, S. J., Anderson, V. *et al.* (2003). Normative data from the CANTAB. I: development of executive function over the lifespan. *Journal of Clinical and Experimental Neuropsychology*, **25**, 242–54.

de Wilde, O. M., Bour, L. J., Dingemans, P. M., Koelman, J. H. & Linszen, D. H. (2007). Failure to find p50 suppression deficits in young first-episode patients with schizophrenia and clinically unaffected siblings. *Schizophrenia Bulletin*, **33**, 1319–23.

Dickinson, D., Ramsey, M. E. & Gold, J. M. (2007). Overlooking the obvious: a meta-analytic comparison of digit symbol coding tasks and other cognitive measures in schizophrenia. *Archives of General Psychiatry*, **64**, 532–42.

Egan, M. F., Goldberg, T. E., Kolachana, B. S. *et al.* (2001). Effect of COMT Val108/158 Met genotype on frontal lobe function and risk for schizophrenia. *Proceedings of the National Academy of Sciences, USA*, **98**, 6917–22.

Erlenmeyer-Kimling, L., Rock, D., Roberts, S. A. *et al.* (2000). Attention, memory, and motor skills as childhood predictors of schizophrenia-related psychoses: the New York High-risk Project. *American Journal of Psychiatry*, **157**, 1416–22.

Ettinger, U., Picchioni, M., Hall, M. H. *et al.* (2006). Antisaccade performance in monozygotic twins discordant for schizophrenia: the Maudsley twin study. *American Journal of Psychiatry*, **163**, 543–5.

Faux, S. F., McCarley, R. W., Nestor, P. G. *et al.* (1993). P300 topographic asymmetries are present in unmedicated schizophrenics. *Electroencephalography and Clinical Neurophysiology*, **88**, 32–41.

Feinberg, I. (1982). Schizophrenia: caused by a fault in programmed synaptic elimination during adolescence? *Journal of Psychiatric Research*, **17**, 319–34.

Ford, J. M., White, P. M., Csernansky, J. G. *et al.* (1994). ERPs in schizophrenia: effects of antipsychotic medication. *Biological Psychiatry*, **36**, 153–70.

Fornito, A., Yücel, M., Wood, S. J. *et al.* (2006). Morphology of the paracingulate sulcus and executive cognition in schizophrenia. *Schizophrenia Research*, **88**, 192–7.

Fornito, A., Yücel, M., Wood, S. J. *et al.* (2008). Surface-based morphometry of the anterior cingulate cortex in first episode schizophrenia. *Human Brain Mapping*, **29**, 478–89.

Francey, S. M., Jackson, H. J., Phillips, L. J. *et al.* (2005). Sustained attention in young people at high risk of psychosis does not predict transition to psychosis. *Schizophrenia Research*, **79**, 127–36.

Frangou, S., Sharma, T., Alarcon, G. *et al.* (1997). The Maudsley Family Study, II: Endogenous event-related potentials in familial schizophrenia. *Schizophrenia Research*, **23**, 45–53.

Freedman, R., Adams, C. E., Adler, L. E. *et al.* (2000). Inhibitory neurophysiological deficit as a phenotype for genetic investigation of schizophrenia. *American Journal of Medical Genetics*, **97**, 58–64.

Friedman, D. & Squires-Wheeler, E. (1994). Event-related potentials (ERPs) as indicators of risk for schizophrenia. *Schizophrenia Bulletin*, **20**, 63–74.

Fusar-Poli, P., Perez, J., Broome, M. *et al.* (2007a). Neurofunctional correlates of vulnerability to psychosis: a systematic review and meta-analysis. *Neurosciences and Biobehavioral Reviews*, **31**, 465–84.

Fusar-Poli, P., Broome, M. R., Matthiasson, P. *et al.* (2007b). Effects of acute antipsychotic treatment on brain activation in first episode psychosis: an fMRI study. *European Neuropsychopharmacology*, **17**, 492–500.

Garner, B., Pariante, C. M., Wood, S. J. *et al.* (2005). Pituitary volume predicts future transition to psychosis in individuals at ultra-high risk of developing psychosis. *Biological Psychiatry*, **58**, 417–23.

Giedd, J. N. (2004). Structural magnetic resonance imaging of the adolescent brain. *Annals of the New York Academy of Science*, **1021**, 77–85.

Glahn, D. C., Thompson, P. M. & Blangero, J. (2007). Neuroimaging endophenotypes: strategies for finding genes influencing brain structure and function. *Human Brain Mapping*, **28**, 488–501.

Gornick, M. C., Addington, A. M., Sporn, A. *et al.* (2005). Dysbindin (DTNBP1, 6p22.3) is associated with childhood-onset psychosis and endophenotypes measured by the Premorbid Adjustment Scale (PAS). *Journal of Autism and Developmental Disorders*, **35**, 831–8.

Gottesman, I. I. & Gould, T. D. (2003). The endophenotype concept in psychiatry: etymology and strategic intentions. *American Journal of Psychiatry*, **160**, 636–45.

Gur, R. E., Keshavan, M. S. & Lawrie, S. M. (2007a). Deconstructing psychosis with human brain imaging. *Schizophrenia Bulletin*, **33**, 921–31.

Gur, R. E., Calkins, M. E., Gur, R. C. *et al.* (2007b). The consortium on the genetics of schizophrenia: neurocognitive endophenotypes. *Schizophrenia Bulletin*, **33**, 49–68.

Hall, J., Whalley, H. C., Job, D. E. *et al.* (2006). A neuregulin 1 variant associated with abnormal cortical function and psychotic symptoms. *Nature Neurosciences*, **9**, 1477–8.

Harris, J. M., Yates, S., Miller, P. *et al.* (2004). Gyrification in first-episode schizophrenia: a morphometric study. *Biological Psychiatry*, **55**, 141–7.

Harris, J. M., Moorhead, T. W., Miller, P. *et al.* (2007). Increased prefrontal gyrification in a large high-risk cohort characterizes those who develop schizophrenia and reflects abnormal prefrontal development. *Biological Psychiatry*, **62**, 722–9.

Harrison, B. J., Yücel, M., Shaw, M. *et al.* (2006). Dysfunction of dorsolateral prefrontal cortex in antipsychotic-naive schizophreniform psychosis. *Psychiatry Research*, **148**, 23–31.

Harrison, P. J. & Lewis, D. A. (2003). Neuropathology of schizophrenia. In S. R. Hirsch & D. R. Weinberger (eds.), *Schizophrenia*. Oxford: Blackwell Science, pp. 310–25.

Harrison, P. J. & Weinberger, D. R. (2005). Schizophrenia genes, gene expression, and neuropathology: on the matter of their convergence. *Molecular Psychiatry*, **10**, 40–68; image 5.

Heckers, S. (2001). Neuroimaging studies of the hippocampus in schizophrenia. *Hippocampus*, **11**, 520–8.

Heinrichs, R. W. (2005). The primacy of cognition in schizophrenia. *American Psychologist*, **60**, 229–42.

Hennah, W., Tuulio-Henriksson, A., Paunio, T. *et al.* (2005). A haplotype within the *DISC1* gene is associated with visual memory functions in families with a high density of schizophrenia. *Molecular Psychiatry*, **10**, 1097–103.

Hirayasu, Y., Asato, N., Ohta, H. *et al.* (1998). Abnormalities of auditory event-related potentials in schizophrenia prior to treatment. *Biological Psychiatry*, **43**, 244–53.

Hirayasu, Y., Tanaka, S., Shenton, M. E. *et al.* (2001). Prefrontal gray matter volume reduction in first episode schizophrenia. *Cerebral Cortex*, **11**, 374–81.

Hoff, A. L., Svetina, C., Shields, G., Stewart, J. & DeLisi, L. E. (2005). Ten year longitudinal study of neuropsychological functioning subsequent to a first episode of schizophrenia. *Schizophrenia Research*, **78**, 27–34.

Hulshoff Pol, H. E., Schnack, H. G., Mandl, R. C. *et al.* (2006). Gray and white matter density changes in monozygotic and same-sex dizygotic twins discordant for schizophrenia using voxel-based morphometry. *Neuroimage*, **31**, 482–8.

Huttenlocher, P. (1984). Synapse elimination and plasticity in developing human cerebral cortex. *American Journal of Mental Deficiency*, **88**, 488–96.

Ingraham, L. J., Kugelmass, S., Frenkel, E., Nathan, M. & Mirsky, A. F. (1995). Twenty-five-year followup of the Israeli High-Risk Study: current and lifetime psychopathology. *Schizophrenia Bulletin*, **21**, 183–92.

Javitt, D. C., Shelley, A. & Ritter, W. (2000). Associated deficits in mismatch negativity generation and tone matching in schizophrenia. *Clinical Neurophysiology*, **111**, 1733–7.

Jeon, Y. W. & Polich, J. (2001). P300 asymmetry in schizophrenia: a meta-analysis. *Psychiatry Research*, **104**, 61–74.

Jessen, F., Scherk, H., Träber, F. *et al.* (2006). Proton magnetic resonance spectroscopy in subjects at risk for schizophrenia. *Schizophrenia Research*, **87**, 81–8.

Jin, Y., Bunney, W. E., Jr, Sandman, C. A. *et al.* (1998). Is p50 suppression a measure of sensory gating in schizophrenia? *Biological Psychiatry*, **43**, 873–8.

Job, D. E., Whalley, H. C., Johnstone, E. C. & Lawrie, S. M. (2005). Grey matter changes over time in high risk subjects developing schizophrenia. *Neuroimage*, **25**, 1023–30.

Johnstone, E. C., Ebmeier, K. P., Miller, P., Owens, D. G. & Lawrie, S. M. (2005). Predicting schizophrenia: findings from the Edinburgh High-Risk Study. *British Journal of Psychiatry*, **186**, 18–25.

Jones, H. M., Brammer, M. J., O'Toole, M. *et al.* (2004). Cortical effects of quetiapine in first-episode schizophrenia: a preliminary functional magnetic resonance imaging study. *Biological Psychiatry*, **56**, 938–42.

Jones, P., Rodgers, B., Murray, R. & Marmot, M. (1994). Child development risk factors for adult schizophrenia in the British 1946 birth cohort. *Lancet*, **344**, 1398–402.

Keefe, R. S., Bilder, R. M., Harvey, P. D. *et al.* (2006). Baseline neurocognitive deficits in the CATIE schizophrenia trial. *Neuropsychopharmacology*, **31**, 2033–46.

Keshavan, M. S., Berger, G., Zipursky, R. B., Wood, S. J. & Pantelis, C. (2005). Neurobiology of early psychosis. *British Journal of Psychiatry Supplement*, **48**, s8–18.

Keshavan, M. S., Prasad, K. M. & Pearlson, G. (2007). Are brain structural abnormalities useful as endophenotypes in schizophrenia? *International Review of Psychiatry*, **19**, 397–406.

Kimble, M., Lyons, M., O'Donnell, B. *et al.* (2000). The effect of family status and schizotypy on electrophysiologic measures of attention and semantic processing. *Biological Psychiatry*, **47**, 402–12.

Klosterkötter, J., Hellmich, M., Steinmeyer, E. M. & Schultze-Lutter, F. (2001). Diagnosing schizophrenia in the initial prodromal phase. *Archives of General Psychiatry*, **58**, 158–64.

Kremen, W. S., Buka, S. L., Seidman, L. J. *et al.* (1998). IQ decline during childhood and adult psychotic symptoms in a community sample: a 19-year longitudinal study. *American Journal of Psychiatry*, **155**, 672–7.

Kuroki, N., Shenton, M. E., Salisbury, D. F. *et al.* (2006). Middle and inferior temporal gyrus gray matter volume abnormalities in first-episode schizophrenia: an MRI study. *American Journal of Psychiatry*, **163**, 2103–10.

Law, A. J., Kleinman, J. E., Weinberger, D. R. & Weickert, C. S. (2007). Disease-associated intronic variants in the *ErbB4* gene are related to altered *ErbB4* splice-variant expression in the brain in schizophrenia. *Human Molecular Genetics*, **16**, 129–41.

Lawrie, S. M. (2004). Premorbid structutral abnormalities in schizophrenia. In M. S. Keshavan, J. L. Kennedy & R. M. Murray (eds.), *Neurodevelopment and Schizophrenia*. Cambridge, UK: Cambridge University Press, pp. 347–72.

Lawrie, S. M. & Abukmeil, S. S. (1998). Brain abnormality in schizophrenia: a systematic and quantitative review of volumetric magnetic resonance imaging studies. *British Journal of Psychiatry*, **172**, 110–20.

Lencz, T., Smith, C. W., Auther, A., Correll, C. U. & Cornblatt, B. (2004). Nonspecific and attenuated negative symptoms in patients at clinical high-risk for schizophrenia. *Schizophrenia Research*, **68**, 37–48.

Lencz, T., Smith, C. W., McLaughlin, D. *et al.* (2006). Generalized and specific neurocognitive deficits in prodromal schizophrenia. *Biological Psychiatry*, **59**, 863–71.

Liddle, P. F. & Pantelis, C. (2003). Brain imaging in schizophrenia. In S. R. Hirsch & D. R. Weinberger (eds.), *Schizophrenia*. Oxford, UK: Blackwell Science, pp. 403–17.

Luna, B. & Sweeney, J. A. (2001). Studies of brain and cognitive maturation through childhood and adolescence: a strategy for testing neurodevelopmental hypotheses. *Schizophrenia Bulletin*, **27**, 443–55.

Luna, B. & Sweeney, J. A. (2004). The emergence of collaborative brain function: fMRI studies of the development of response inhibition. *Annals of the New York Academy of Science*, **1021**, 296–309.

MacDonald, A. W., III, Carter, C. S., Kerns, J. G. *et al.* (2005). Specificity of prefrontal dysfunction and context processing deficits to schizophrenia in never-medicated patients with first-episode psychosis. *American Journal of Psychiatry*, **162**, 475–84.

Manoach, D. S., Press, D. Z., Thangaraj, V. *et al.* (1999). Schizophrenic subjects activate dorsolateral prefrontal cortex during a working memory task, as measured by fMRI. *Biological Psychiatry*, **45**, 1128–37.

Manoach, D. S., Gollub, R. L., Benson, E. S. *et al.* (2000). Schizophrenic subjects show aberrant fMRI activation of dorsolateral prefrontal cortex and basal ganglia during working memory performance. *Biological Psychiatry*, **48**, 99–109.

Marjoram, D., Job, D. E., Whalley, H. C. *et al.* (2006). A visual joke fMRI investigation into theory of mind and enhanced risk of schizophrenia. *Neuroimage*, **31**, 1850–8.

Mathalon, D. H., Ford, J. M. & Pfefferbaum, A. (2000). Trait and state aspects of P300 amplitude reduction in schizophrenia: a retrospective longitudinal study. *Biological Psychiatry*, **47**, 434–49.

McCarley, R. W., Shenton, M. E., O'Donnell, B. F. *et al.* (1993). Auditory P300 abnormalities and left posterior superior temporal gyrus volume reduction in schizophrenia. *Archives of General Psychiatry*, **50**, 190–7.

McCarley, R. W., Salisbury, D. F., Hirayasu, Y. *et al.* (2002). Association between smaller left posterior superior temporal gyrus volume on magnetic resonance imaging and smaller left temporal P300 amplitude in first-episode schizophrenia. *Archives of General Psychiatry*, **59**, 321–31.

McDonald, C., Zanelli, J., Rabe-Hesketh, S. *et al.* (2004a). Meta-analysis of magnetic resonance imaging brain morphometry studies in bipolar disorder. *Biological Psychiatry*, **56**, 411–17.

McDonald, C., Bullmore, E. T., Sham, P. C. *et al.* (2004b). Association of genetic risks for schizophrenia and bipolar disorder with specific and generic brain structural endophenotypes. *Archives of General Psychiatry*, **61**, 974–84.

Miller, B. L., Chang, L., Booth, R. *et al.* (1996). In vivo ^{1}H MRS choline: correlation with *in vitro* chemistry/histology. *Life Sciences*, **58**, 1929–35.

Mirsky, A. F. (1995). Israeli High Risk Study: editor's introduction. *Schizophrenia Bulletin*, **21**, 179–82.

Molina, V., Sanz, J., Reig, S. *et al.* (2005). Hypofrontality in men with first-episode psychosis. *British Journal of Psychiatry*, **186**, 203–8.

Morey, R. A., Inan, S., Mitchell, T. V. *et al.* (2005). Imaging frontostriatal function in ultra-high-risk, early, and chronic schizophrenia during executive processing. *Archives of General Psychiatry*, **62**, 254–62.

Murray, G. K., Jones, P. B., Moilanen, K. *et al.* (2006). Infant motor development and adult cognitive functions in schizophrenia. *Schizophrenia Research*, **81**, 65–74.

Murray, G. K., Jones, P. B., Kuh, D. & Richards, M. (2007). Infant developmental milestones and subsequent cognitive function. *Annals of Neurology*, **62**, 128–36.

Murray, R. M. & Lewis, S. W. (1987). Is schizophrenia a neuro-developmental disorder? *British Medical Journal* (*Clinical Research Edition*), **295**, 681–2.

Myles-Worsley, M., Ord, L., Blailes, F., Ngiralmau, H. & Freedman, R. (2004). P50 sensory gating in adolescents from a Pacific island isolate with elevated risk for schizophrenia. *Biological Psychiatry*, **55**, 663–7.

Nakamura, M., Salisbury, D. F., Hirayasu, Y. *et al.* (2007). Neocortical gray matter volume in first-episode schizophrenia and first-episode affective psychosis: a cross-sectional and longitudinal MRI study. *Biological Psychiatry*, **62**, 773–83.

Narr, K. L., Bilder, R. M., Kim, S. *et al.* (2004). Abnormal gyral complexity in first-episode schizophrenia. *Biological Psychiatry*, **55**, 859–67.

Nelson, M. D., Saykin, A. J., Flashman, L. A. & Riordan, H. J. (1998). Hippocampal volume reduction in schizophrenia as assessed by magnetic resonance imaging: a meta-analytic study. *Archives of General Psychiatry*, **55**, 433–40.

Nieman, D., Becker, H., van de Fliert, R. *et al.* (2007). Antisaccade task performance in patients at ultra high risk for developing psychosis. *Schizophrenia Research*, **95**, 54–60.

Pantelis, C. & Maruff, P. (2002). The cognitive neuropsychiatric approach to investigating the neurobiology of schizophrenia and other disorders. *Journal of Psychosomatic Research*, **53**, 655–64.

Pantelis, C., Stuart, G. W., Nelson, H. E., Robbins, T. W. & Barnes, T. R. E. (2001). Spatial working memory deficits in schizophrenia: relationship with tardive dyskinesia and negative symptoms. *American Journal of Psychiatry*, **158**, 1276–85.

Pantelis, C., Velakoulis, D., McGorry, P. D. *et al.* (2003). Neuroanatomical abnormalities before and after onset of psychosis: a cross-sectional and longitudinal MRI comparison. *Lancet*, **361**, 281–8.

Pantelis, C., Yücel, M., Wood, S. J. *et al.* (2005). Structural brain imaging evidence for multiple pathological processes at different stages of brain development in schizophrenia. *Schizophrenia Bulletin*, **31**, 672–96.

Pantelis, C., Velakoulis, D., Wood, S. J. *et al.* (2007). Neuroimaging and emerging psychotic disorders: the Melbourne Ultra-High Risk Studies. *International Review of Psychiatry*, **19**, 371–9.

Pariante, C. M., Vassilopoulou, K., Velakoulis, D. *et al.* (2004). Pituitary volume in psychosis. *British Journal of Psychiatry*, **185**, 5–10.

Pariante, C. M., Dazzan, P., Danese, A. *et al.* (2005). Increased pituitary volume in antipsychotic-free and antipsychotic-treated patients of the AEsop first-onset psychosis study. *Neuropsychopharmacology*, **30**, 1923–31.

Paus, T. (2005). Mapping brain maturation and cognitive development during adolescence. *Trends in Cognitive Science*, **9**, 60–8.

Petrides, M. (1995). Impairments on nonspatial self-ordered and externally ordered working memory tasks after lesions of the mid-dorsal part of the lateral frontal cortex in the monkey. *Journal of Neuroscience*, **15**(Pt 1), 359–75.

Phillips, L. J., McGorry, P. D., Garner, B. *et al.* (2006). Stress, the hippocampus and the hypothalamic–pituitary–adrenal axis: implications for the development of psychotic disorders. *Australian and New Zealand Journal of Psychiatry*, **40**, 725–41.

Poulton, R., Caspi, A., Moffitt, T. E. *et al.* (2000). Children's self-reported psychotic symptoms and adult schizophreniform disorder: a 15-year longitudinal study. *Archives of General Psychiatry*, **57**, 1053–8.

Pukrop, R., Schultze-Lutter, F., Ruhrmann, S. *et al.* (2006). Neurocognitive functioning in subjects at risk for a first episode of psychosis compared with first- and multiple-episode schizophrenia. *Journal of Clinical and Experimental Neuropsychology*, **28**, 1388–407.

Pukrop, R., Ruhrmann, S., Schultze-Lutter, F. *et al.* (2007). Neurocognitive indicators for a conversion to psychosis: comparison of patients in a potentially initial prodromal state who did or did not convert to a psychosis. *Schizophrenia Research*, **92**, 116–25.

Rapoport, J. L., Addington, A. M., Frangou, S. & Psych, M. R. (2005). The neurodevelopmental model of schizophrenia: update 2005. *Molecular Psychiatry*, **10**, 434–49.

Reichenberg, A., Weiser, M., Rapp, M. A. *et al.* (2005). Elaboration on premorbid intellectual performance in schizophrenia: premorbid intellectual decline and risk for schizophrenia. *Archives of General Psychiatry*, **62**, 1297–304.

Renoult, L., Prevost, M., Brodeur, M. *et al.* (2007). P300 asymmetry and positive symptom severity: a study in the early stage of a first episode of psychosis. *Schizophrenia Research*, **93**, 366–73.

Rhinewine, J. P., Lencz, T., Thaden, E. P. *et al.* (2005). Neurocognitive profile in adolescents with early-onset schizophrenia: clinical correlates. *Biological Psychiatry*, **58**, 705–12.

Rutschmann, J., Cornblatt, B. & Erlenmeyer-Kimling, L. (1977). Sustained attention in children at risk for schizophrenia. Report on a continuous performance test. *Archives of General Psychiatry*, **34**, 571–5.

Salisbury, D. F., Shenton, M. E., Griggs, C. B., Bonner-Jackson, A. & McCarley, R. W. (2002). Mismatch negativity in chronic schizophrenia and first-episode schizophrenia. *Archives of General Psychiatry*, **59**, 686–94.

Salisbury, D. F., Krljes, S. & McCarley, R. W. (2003). Electrophysiology of schizophrenia. In S. R. Hirsch & D. R. Weinberger (eds.), *Schizophrenia*. Oxford: Blackwell Science, pp. 298–309.

Salisbury, D. F., Kuroki, N., Kasai, K., Shenton, M. E. & McCarley, R. W. (2007). Progressive and interrelated functional and structural evidence of post-onset brain reduction in schizophrenia. *Archives of General Psychiatry*, **64**, 521–9.

Seidman, L. J., Pantelis, C., Keshavan, M. S. *et al.* (2003). A review and new report of medial temporal lobe dysfunction as a vulnerability indicator for schizophrenia: a magnetic resonance imaging morphometric family study of the parahippocampal gyrus. *Schizophrenia Bulletin*, **29**, 803–30.

Silberberg, G., Darvasi, A., Pinkas-Kramarski, R. & Navon, R. (2006). The involvement of ErbB4 with schizophrenia: association and expression studies. *American Journal of Medical Genetics Part B: Neuropsychiatry Genetics*, **141**, 142–8.

Smyrnis, N., Evdokimidis, I., Stefanis, N. C. *et al.* (2003). Antisaccade performance of 1273 men: effects of schizotypy, anxiety, and depression. *Journal of Abnormal Psychology*, **112**, 403–14.

Snitz, B. E., MacDonald, A., III, Cohen, J. D. *et al.* (2005). Lateral and medial hypofrontality in first-episode schizophrenia: functional activity in a medication-naive state and effects of short-term atypical antipsychotic treatment. *American Journal of Psychiatry*, **162**, 2322–9.

Snitz, B. E., Macdonald, A. W., III, & Carter, C. S. (2006). Cognitive deficits in unaffected first-degree relatives of schizophrenia patients: a meta-analytic review of putative endophenotypes. *Schizophrenia Bulletin*, **32**, 179–94.

Sponheim, S. R., McGuire, K. A. & Stanwyck, J. J. (2006). Neural anomalies during sustained attention in first-degree biological relatives of schizophrenia patients. *Biological Psychiatry*, **60**, 242–52.

Stanfield, A. C., Moorhead, T. W., Harris, J. M. *et al.* (2007). Increased right prefrontal cortical folding in adolescents at risk of schizophrenia for cognitive reasons. *Biological Psychiatry*, **63**, 80–5.

Steen, R. G., Mull, C., McClure, R., Hamer, R. M. & Lieberman, J. A. (2006). Brain volume in first-episode schizophrenia: systematic review and meta-analysis of magnetic resonance imaging studies. *British Journal of Psychiatry*, **188**, 510–18.

Stefansson, H., Sigurdsson, E., Steinthorsdottir, V. *et al.* (2002). Neuregulin 1 and susceptibility to schizophrenia. *American Journal of Human Genetics*, **71**, 877–92.

Stone, W. S., Faraone, S. V., Seidman, L. J., Olson, E. A. & Tsuang, M. T. (2005). Searching for the liability to schizophrenia: concepts and methods underlying genetic high-risk studies of adolescents. *Journal of Child and Adolescent Psychopharmacology*, **15**, 403–17.

Straub, R. E., Lipska, B. K., Egan, M. F. *et al.* (2007). Allelic variation in GAD1 (GAD(67)) is associated with schizophrenia and influences cortical function and gene expression. *Molecular Psychiatry*, **12**, 854–69.

Sun, D.-Q., Phillips, L. J., Velakoulis, D. *et al.* (2008). Progressive brain structural changes mapped as psychosis develops in 'at risk' individuals. *Schizophrenia Research*, epub PMID 18262769.

Swerdlow, N. R., Light, G. A., Cadenhead, K. S. *et al.* (2006). Startle gating deficits in a large cohort of patients with schizophrenia: relationship to medications, symptoms, neurocognition, and level of function. *Archives of General Psychiatry*, **63**, 1325–35.

Taanila, A., Murray, G. K., Jokelainen, J., Isohanni, M. & Rantakallio, P. (2005). Infant developmental milestones: a 31-year follow-up. *Developmental Medicine and Child Neurology*, **47**, 581–6.

Testa, R. & Pantelis, C. (2007). The role of executive functions in psychiatric disorders. In S. J. Wood, N. Allen & C. Pantelis, (eds.), *Neuropsychology of Mental Disorders*. Cambridge, UK: Cambridge University Press,

Thompson, P. M., Woods, R. P., Mega, M. S. & Toga, A. W. (2000). Mathematical/computational challenges in creating deformable and probabilistic atlases of the human brain. *Human Brain Mapping*, **9**, 81–92.

Turetsky, B. I., Cannon, T. D. & Gur, R. E. (2000). P300 subcomponent abnormalities in schizophrenia: III. Deficits in unaffected siblings of schizophrenic probands. *Biological Psychiatry*, **47**, 380–90.

Turetsky, B. I., Calkins, M. E., Light, G. A. *et al.* (2007). Neurophysiological endophenotypes of schizophrenia: the viability of selected candidate measures. *Schizophrenia Bulletin*, **33**, 69–94.

van Erp, T. G., Saleh, P. A., Huttunen, M. *et al.* (2004). Hippocampal volumes in schizophrenic twins. *Archives of General Psychiatry*, **61**, 346–53.

van Haren, N. E., Picchioni, M. M., McDonald, C. *et al.* (2004). A controlled study of brain structure in monozygotic twins concordant and discordant for schizophrenia. *Biological Psychiatry*, **56**, 454–61.

Van Horn, J. D. & McManus, I. C. (1992). Ventricular enlargement in schizophrenia. A meta-analysis of studies of the ventricle:brain ratio (VBR). *British Journal of Psychiatry*, **160**, 687–97.

Velakoulis, D. & Pantelis, C. (1996). What have we learned from functional imaging studies in schizophrenia? The role of frontal, striatal and temporal areas. *Australian and New Zealand Journal of Psychiatry*, **30**, 195–209.

Velakoulis, D., Wood, S. J., Wong, M. T. *et al.* (2006). Hippocampal and amygdala volumes according to psychosis stage and diagnosis: a magnetic resonance imaging study of chronic schizophrenia, first-episode psychosis, and ultra-high-risk individuals. *Archives of General Psychiatry*, **63**, 139–49.

Vidal, C. N., Rapoport, J. L., Hayashi, K. M. *et al.* (2006). Dynamically spreading frontal and cingulate deficits mapped in adolescents with schizophrenia. *Archives of General Psychiatry*, **63**, 25–34.

Vita, A., de Peri, L., Silenzi, C. & Dieci, M. (2006). Brain morphology in first-episode schizophrenia: a meta-analysis of quantitative magnetic resonance imaging studies. *Schizophrenia Research*, **82**, 75–88.

Vogeley, K., Schneider-Axmann, T., Pfeiffer, U. *et al.* (2000). Disturbed gyrification of the prefrontal region in male schizophrenic patients: a morphometric postmortem study. *American Journal of Psychiatry*, **157**, 34–9.

Vogeley, K., Tepest, R., Pfeiffer, U. *et al.* (2001). Right frontal hypergyria differentiation in affected and unaffected siblings from families multiply affected with schizophrenia: a morphometric MRI study. *American Journal of Psychiatry*, **158**, 494–6.

Walker, E. & Bollini, A. M. (2002). Pubertal neurodevelopment and the emergence of psychotic symptoms. *Schizophrenia Research*, **54**, 17–23.

Walterfang, M., Wood, A., Reutens, D. C. *et al.* (2008). Morphology of the corpus callosum at different stages of schizophrenia: a cross-sectional study in first-episode and chronic illness. *British Journal of Psychiatry*, **192**, 429–34.

Wang, J., Hirayasu, Y., Hokama, H. *et al.* (2005). Influence of duration of untreated psychosis on auditory P300 in drug-naive and first-episode schizophrenia. *Psychiatry and Clinical Neuroscience*, **59**, 209–14.

Weinberger, D. R. (1987). Implications of normal brain development for the pathogenesis of schizophrenia. *Archives of General Psychiatry*, **44**, 660–9.

Weinberger, D. R. (2002). Biological phenotypes and genetic research on schizophrenia. *World Psychiatry*, **1**, 2–6.

Weintraub, S. (1987). Risk factors in schizophrenia: the Stony Brook High-Risk Project. *Schizophrenia Bulletin*, **13**, 439–50.

Whalley, H. C., Simonotto, E., Moorhead, W. *et al.* (2006). Functional imaging as a predictor of schizophrenia. *Biological Psychiatry*, **60**, 454–62.

Whalley, H. C., Harris, J. C. & Lawrie, S. M. (2007). The neurobiological underpinnings of risk and conversion in relatives of patients with schizophrenia. *International Review of Psychiatry*, **19**, 383–97.

Whyte, M. C., Brett, C., Harrison, L. K. *et al.* (2006). Neuropsychological performance over time in people at high risk of developing schizophrenia and controls. *Biological Psychiatry*, **59**, 730–9.

Wiegand, L. C., Warfield, S. K., Levitt, J. J. *et al.* (2005). An in vivo MRI study of prefrontal cortical complexity in first-episode psychosis. *American Journal of Psychiatry*, **162**, 65–70.

Wisco, J. J., Kuperberg, G., Manoach, D. *et al.* (2007). Abnormal cortical folding patterns within Broca's area in schizophrenia: evidence from structural MRI. *Schizophrenia Research*, **94**, 317–27.

Wolf, L. E. & Cornblatt, B. A. (1996). Neuropsychological functioning in children at risk for schizophrenia. In C. Pantelis, H. E. Nelson & T. R. E. Barnes (eds.), *Schizophrenia: A Neuropsychological Perspective*. London: John Wiley, pp. 161–179.

Wolf, L. E., Cornblatt, B. A., Roberts, S. A., Shapiro, B. M. & Erlenmeyer-Kimling, L. (2002). Wisconsin card sorting deficits in the offspring of schizophrenics in the New York High-Risk Project. *Schizophrenia Research*, **57**, 173–82.

Wood, S. J., Pantelis, C., Proffitt, T. *et al.* (2003a). Spatial working memory ability is a marker of risk-for-psychosis. *Psychological Medicine*, **33**, 1239–47.

Wood, S. J., Berger, G., Velakoulis, D. *et al.* (2003b). Proton magnetic resonance spectroscopy in first episode psychosis and ultra high-risk individuals. *Schizophrenia Bulletin*, **29**, 831–43.

Wood, S. J., De Luca, C. R., Anderson, V. & Pantelis, C. (2004). Cognitive development in adolescence: cerebral underpinnings, neural trajectories and the impact of aberrations. In M. S. Keshavan, J. L. Kennedy & R. M. Murray, (eds.), *Neurodevelopment and Schizophrenia*. Cambridge, UK: Cambridge University Press, pp. 69–88.

Wood, S. J., Yücel, M., Velakoulis, D. *et al.* (2005). Hippocampal and anterior cingulate morphology in subjects at ultra-high-risk for psychosis: the role of family history of psychotic illness. *Schizophrenia Research*, **75**, 295–301.

Wood, S. J., Brewer, W. J., Koutsouradis, P. *et al.* (2007). Cognitive decline following psychosis onset: Data from the PACE clinic. *British Journal of Psychiatry*, **191**(Suppl 51), s52–7.

Wood, S. J., Pantelis, C., Velakoulis, D. *et al.* (2008). Progressive changes in the development towards schizophrenia: studies in subjects at increased symptomatic risk. *Schizophrenia Bulletin*, **34**, 322–9.

Woods, B. T., Ward, K. E. & Johnson, E. H. (2005). Meta-analysis of the time-course of brain volume reduction in schizophrenia: implications for pathogenesis and early treatment. *Schizophrenia Research*, **73**, 221–8.

Wright, I. C., Rabe-Hesketh, S., Woodruff, P. W. *et al.* (2000). Meta-analysis of regional brain volumes in schizophrenia. *American Journal of Psychiatry*, **157**, 16–25.

Yücel, M., Stuart, G. W., Maruff, P. *et al.* (2001). Hemispheric and gender-related differences in the gross morphology of the anterior cingulate/paracingulate cortex in normal volunteers: an MRI morphometric study. *Cerebral Cortex*, **11**, 17–25.

Yücel, M., Stuart, G. W., Maruff, P. *et al.* (2002). Paracingulate morphological differences in males with established schizophrenia: a magnetic resonance imaging morphometric study. *Biological Psychiatry*, **52**, 15–23.

Yücel, M., Wood, S. J., Phillips, L. J. *et al.* (2003). Morphology of the anterior cingulate cortex in young men at ultra-high risk of developing a psychotic illness. *British Journal of Psychiatry*, **182**, 518–24.

Yung, A. R. & McGorry, P. D. (1996). The prodromal phase of first-episode psychosis: past and current conceptualizations. *Schizophrenia Bulletin*, **22**, 353–70.

At-risk mental state

6

At-risk mental state and prediction

Alison R. Yung, Joachim Klosterkötter, Barbara Cornblatt
and Frauke Schultze-Lutter

Introduction

Recently, the area of 'prodromal' research in schizophrenia and related disorders has grown considerably. From initial retrospective studies of this phase, dating back to the early twentieth century, the last decade of the century has seen the beginning and expansion of prospective studies aiming to identify the earliest manifestations of psychotic illnesses. From identification of these prodromal or 'ultra-high-risk' (UHR) individuals, the area has also developed to include intervention studies aiming to prevent, delay or ameliorate the onset of a full-blown psychotic disorder and to investigate underlying processes that cause or contribute to the onset. This chapter discusses the rationale behind this field of research, reviews the literature on the detection of prodromal or UHR individuals, summarizes the findings on the prediction of psychosis in these people and provides an up-to-date overview of progress and future directions in the field. We start by briefly reviewing the background.

Background: the prodrome of psychotic disorders

The fact that psychotic disorders, such as schizophrenia, begin with a prodromal phase prior to the onset of frank psychotic symptoms has been known since the first descriptions of the illness were documented (Conrad, 1958; Kraepelin, 1919). Although there is great variability between patients in how their prodromes manifest, certain symptoms and signs have

been frequently described. These include depressed mood, anxiety, irritability and aggressive behaviour, suicidal ideation and attempts, and substance use. The most commonly occurring prodromal symptoms, according to retrospective studies of patients with schizophrenia and schizophreniform disorder, are shown in Box 6.1. Two things emerge from studying this list of prodromal symptoms. First, many of them are non-specific. That is, they occur frequently in the prodromes and threshold syndromes of non-psychotic disorders (Häfner et al., 2005). Second, a considerable amount of psychiatric symptoms, disability, self-harming and other health-damaging behaviours occur during this prodromal phase, even in the earliest stages (Häfner et al., 1999; Yung et al., 2003, 2004a).

Subtle self-experienced deficits, including cognitive, affective and social disturbances are also commonly described in the early prodromal phase. These are known as 'basic symptoms' (Gross, 1989; see the Appendix). The term 'basic symptoms' was originally chosen to express two assumptions: first, that these symptoms form the psychopathological base from which Schneiderian first-rank symptoms develop, and second, that they were more closely related to the underlying schizophrenic-disease process than positive psychotic symptoms. This concept of basic symptoms, developed in the 1960s, has significantly influenced thinking about schizophrenia in German-speaking countries for decades. More recently, it is influencing the newer area of prodromal research (Klosterkötter et al., 1997a; 2001; Schultze-Lutter, 2004).

Closer to the onset of frank psychotic symptoms, people often experience attenuated or subthreshold

The Recognition and Management of Early Psychosis: A Preventive Approach, ed. Henry J. Jackson and Patrick D. McGorry.
Published by Cambridge University Press. © Cambridge University Press 2009.

Box 6.1. Common prodromal symptoms.

Reduced concentration and attention

Reduced drive and motivation

Depression

Sleep disturbance

Anxiety

Social withdrawal

Suspiciousness

Deterioration in role functioning

Irritability

forms of psychotic symptoms, which can also have deleterious effects (Docherty *et al.*, 1978; Donlon & Blacker, 1973; Yung & McGorry, 1996). For example, the belief that others may be thinking badly about, or laughing at, a person may result in social withdrawal; non-attendance at school, work or university; and suspiciousness and altered behaviour towards family and friends.

Neurocognitive abnormalities are also evident in the prodromal phase. Individuals diagnosed as 'prodromal' (or UHR) display a range of neurocognitive deficits similar to those found in first-degree relatives of patients with schizophrenia (Seidman *et al.*, 2006; Snitz, Macdonald & Carter, 2006). These deficits are consistent with those displayed by fully affected patients, but at a lower degree of severity (Heinrichs & Zakzanis, 1998). In particular, impaired attention, spatial and verbal memory, and speeded information processing have been consistently reported in UHR individuals compared with various control groups (Cornblatt *et al.*, 2003; Francey *et al.*, 2005; Hawkins *et al.*, 2004; Lencz *et al.*, 2006; Niendam *et al.*, 2006; Wood *et al.*, 2003). In addition to lowered specific impairments, there is some (although less consistent) indication that cognitive dysfunctions may be less widespread in UHR individuals than in patients with fully expressed illness. Brewer *et al.* (2006) reported little evidence for global pre-psychosis cognitive deficits and suggested that measuring overall cognition may result in missing true vulnerability markers. In contrast, support for a generalized or global deficit has been reported by both Hawkins *et al.* (2004) and

Lencz *et al.* (2006). Both theories may be correct. A global cognitive impairment may be present that represents a necessary, but not sufficient, biological core of illness, one which is not related directly to conversion from UHR state to psychosis but, rather, to overall functional impairment (Cornblatt *et al.*, 2003). Specific deficits, by comparison, may be related more directly to affected brain structures and candidate genes, and thus may be more directly predictive of psychosis.

Neurobiological changes may also be occurring during the prodromal and onset phase of psychotic disorders. Magnetic resonance imaging (MRI) brain scans were obtained on some UHR patients (that is, prior to onset of frank psychosis). Some were re-scanned after the onset of psychotic disorder. There was evidence of significant bilateral reduction in grey matter volume in the cingulate region as well as in the left para-hippocampal gyrus, left fusiform gyrus, left orbito-frontal cortex and one region of the left cerebellar cortex (Pantelis *et al.*, 2003). These brain changes were not present in the UHR group who did not go on to develop psychosis. This finding suggests that neurobiological changes can occur during the process of transition to psychosis.

Rationale: why focus on the prodrome?

Our knowledge that many symptoms and a great deal of disability develop during the prodrome, coupled with the finding of possible neurobiological and neurocognitive damage during this period, has added impetus for renewed efforts at attempting to intervene at this early stage. If the prodrome can be recognized prospectively and treatment provided at this stage, then disability could be minimized, some recovery may be possible before symptoms and poor functioning become entrenched, and the possibility of preventing, delaying or ameliorating the onset of diagnosable psychotic disorder arises.

The findings of both global and specific neurocognitive changes in those at high risk of psychosis support the need for early intervention to slow or possibly stop further deterioration associated with impaired cognition. In the first case, intervention is essential to reduce the poor functional outcome characterizing many vulnerable individuals, whether or not psychosis actually develops. In the second, intervention targeting specific deficits may slow or even stop further progression to psychosis. This idea of intervening during the prodrome is not new. The following quotation (in Sullivan 1994, p. 135) comes from 1927: 'I feel certain that many incipient cases might be arrested before the efficient contact with reality is completely suspended, and a long stay in institutions made necessary.'

However, early attempts at prodromal intervention were hampered, mainly by the problem of 'false positives' and their implication for preventive intervention. 'False positives' refers to those who are identified as being prodromal, that is, at risk of developing a psychotic disorder in the near future, but who do not do so. Some of these people were in fact never 'destined' to develop a psychotic disorder (the 'true false positives'). These individuals may be harmed by being labelled as 'prodromal' or 'high risk of psychosis' and may receive treatment unnecessarily (Corcoran, Malaspina & Hercher, 2005; Heinssen *et al.*, 2001; Yung, 2003). In contrast are those individuals who would have developed a psychotic disorder were it not for some alteration in their circumstances, such as a treatment intervention, stress reduction or cessation of illicit drug use, that prevented this from occurring. This latter group has been termed 'false false positive' (Yung *et al.*, 2003). Clearly, it is impossible to distinguish between these two groups phenotypically at both baseline and follow-up.

The non-specific nature of the most common prodromal features (Box 6.1) adds to the likelihood of detecting false positives. This had seemed like an insurmountable burden for progressing the idea of pre-psychotic intervention. However, two factors have added optimism to this idea of prodromal or very early intervention. First, the development of different methods of identifying people likely to be experiencing a prodrome. In other words, an improvement in our ability to detect those truly at high risk of a psychotic disorder and a concomitant reduction in false positives. Second, the growth of optimism that the course of schizophrenia and other psychotic disorders is not inevitably deteriorating, and that early intervention may improve outcome.

The idea of prodromal or very early intervention was originally formulated and trialled in a population-based manner by Falloon (1992), with a project that encouraged primary care physicians in the English county of Buckinghamshire to refer patients suspected of having a 'schizophrenic prodrome' to a mental health service for treatment. A reduction in the incidence of first-episode schizophrenia compared with historical figures was found and cited as possible evidence for the effectiveness of such targeted preventive intervention. Falloon acknowledged methodological difficulties with this approach and the fact that some people not actually at risk of schizophrenia would have been unnecessarily labelled and treated. However, this study opened the way for early intervention strategies in psychosis to consider the prodromal phase as a potential focus for treatment.

Identification of the population

Prodromal research: early intervention and basic symptom research meet genetic high-risk studies

Three strands of research were pivotal for forming the basis of prodromal research: the field of early intervention in psychotic disorders, schizophrenic basic symptoms research and the genetic high-risk studies investigating causes of schizophrenia. All three approaches are now used in attempting to identify individuals at imminent risk of psychosis onset. This is reflected in the criteria that many studies around the world use for defining the 'prodromal' population. In the following section, we expand on the different approaches to defining and codifying UHR or prodromal criteria.

Ultra-high-risk criteria: the Melbourne PACE approach

Owing to their non-specific nature, there are problems with using prodromal symptoms and signs alone to identify people thought to be at incipient risk of onset of psychotic disorder. Even psychotic-like experiences (attenuated or subthreshold psychotic symptoms) have been found to occur commonly in the general population, especially amongst adolescents and young adults (Johns *et al.*, 2004; Tien, 1991; van Os *et al.*, 2001). Using symptoms alone would result in a high false-positive rate. Consequently, some added criteria were needed to focus on those most likely to be in the prodromal phase of a psychotic disorder. In order to address this issue, we proposed a sequential screening approach or 'close-in strategy' (Bell, 1992), which require multiple risk factors to be combined. This had the effect of concentrating the level of risk in the selected sample to create an enriched cohort. Using this approach, however, meant that some people who were genuinely at risk may not meet the criteria, that is, specificity was given priority over sensitivity. Despite this issue, we considered it a legitimate strategy, given that we needed to establish that it was possible to identify individuals who would develop psychosis within a brief time period, such as 12 months.

The close-in strategy that we applied required that symptoms and signs be combined with other risk factors. One risk factor was age. It is known that the age of highest incidence of psychotic disorder is adolescence and young adulthood (Häfner *et al.*, 1993; Verdoux *et al.*, 1998). Another important factor is that of clinical need for care. In order to test our model, we established a specialized service for the UHR group in 1994, the Personal Assessment and Crisis Evaluation (PACE) Clinic (Yung *et al.*, 1995, 1996).

The PACE Clinic recruits those with a perceived need for psychiatric help. A two-stage screening procedure is applied: recognition of need for care, then recognition of UHR criteria within the help-seeker. This method reduces the chance that a well person who happens to have psychotic-like experiences, but who is otherwise functioning adequately, will be identified as UHR.

The PACE UHR criteria require that a young person aged between 14 and 30 is referred for healthcare to the service and meets criteria for one or more of the following groups.

1. *Attenuated psychotic symptoms group (APS)*: have experienced subthreshold, attenuated positive psychotic symptoms during the past year.
2. *Brief limited intermittent psychotic symptoms group (BLIPS)*: have experienced episodes of frank psychotic symptoms that have not lasted longer than a week and have spontaneously abated.
3. *Trait and state risk factor group*: have a first-degree relative with a psychotic disorder or the identified client has a schizotypal personality disorder and they have experienced a significant decrease in functioning during the previous year (Yung *et al.*, 2003, 2004a).

The basis for the primarily symptom-based criteria is the assumption that psychotic symptoms are dimensional (Strauss, 1969) and that they lie on three continua: intensity, frequency and duration. Obviously any cutoff points are arbitrary, imposing categorical distinctions on dimensional phenomena. As well as meeting the criteria for at least one of these groups, subjects must not have experienced a previous psychotic episode. Thus, the UHR criteria identify young people who are in the age range of peak incidence of onset of a psychotic disorder (late adolescence/early adulthood) who additionally describe mental state changes that are suggestive of an emerging psychotic process, or who may have a strong family history of psychosis accompanied by evidence of mental ill health. They must be help-seeking or have been identified by someone else as being in need of a clinical service.

Necessarily, criteria have also been developed to define the onset of frank psychotic disorder. These are not identical to DSM-IV criteria (APA, 1994) but are designed to define the minimal point at which antipsychotic treatment is indicated. This definition is arbitrary, but it does at least have clear treatment implications and applies equally well to substance-related symptoms, symptoms that have a mood component – either depression or mania – and schizophrenia-spectrum disorders. The predictive target is first-episode psychosis that is judged to require antipsychotic medication, arbitrarily defined by the persistence of frank psychotic symptoms for over 1 week (Yung *et al.*, 2003).

The criteria for each of the UHR groups were originally operationalized using the Brief Psychiatric Rating Scale (BPRS: Overall & Gorham, 1962) and the Comprehensive Assessment of Symptoms and History interview (CASH: Andreasen, 1987), which could be used to specify the intensity of a psychotic symptom. Additionally, criteria specifying the frequency and duration of the experiences were needed, as this degree of fine detail in relation to subthreshold symptoms is missing from the BPRS and CASH. Prospectively, the recency of these symptoms also needed to be assessed as degree of risk may fluctuate depending on current or recent symptomatology. Subsequently, a new instrument, the Comprehensive Assessment of At Risk Mental States (CAARMS) was designed so that all relevant domains (intensity, frequency, duration and recency) could be assessed with the one tool (Yung et al., 2005).

Using these UHR criteria, we found that it was possible to detect and engage a subset of young people who were subthreshold for fully fledged psychotic disorder yet who had demonstrable clinical needs and other syndromal diagnoses, and who appeared to be at incipient risk of frank psychosis (Yung et al., 1996, 1998, 2003, 2004a). The rate of transition to psychosis within 12 months in this cohort was about 35% (Yung et al., 2003, 2004a), a rate several thousand-fold over the expected incidence rate for first-episode psychosis in the general population. This occurred despite the provision of minimal supportive counselling, case management and antidepressant medication if required. The primary diagnostic outcome of the group who developed psychosis was schizophrenia (65%; Yung et al., 2003). These results cannot be easily generalized to the wider population as a whole, or even to individuals with a family history of psychosis but who are asymptomatic. Participants recruited to research at the PACE Clinic are a selected sample, characterized by high help-seeking characteristics or other non-specific factors. It undoubtedly includes only a minority of those who proceed to a first episode of psychosis, and an unstable proportion of false positives, depending on sampling and detection factors. These factors can affect the base rate of true positives in the sample (McGorry, Yung & Phillips, 2003).

The PACE UHR criteria have been adopted and adapted in a number of other settings around the world (Haroun et al., 2006; Olsen & Rosenbaum, 2006). For example, the Prevention through Risk Identification, Management and Education (PRIME) Clinic at Yale University, USA, developed their own instrument, the Structured Interview for Prodromal Symptoms (SIPS: Miller et al., 2003a) based on the PACE UHR criteria.

They reported a 54% transition rate (7 of 13 subjects) within 12 months (Miller et al., 2002). The PRIME Clinic has now expanded to include other North American sites (Miller et al., 2003b; Woods et al., 2003). The Psychological Assistance Service (PAS) in Newcastle, Australia, using criteria similar to that of PACE, described a 50% transition rate over 12 months (Mason et al., 2004), the TOPP Clinic in Norway reported a 12-month transition rate of 43% (Larsen, 2002), the Early Identification and Intervention Evaluation (EDIE) Clinic in Manchester, UK, described a 22% transition rate (Morrison et al., 2002) and the Cognitive Assessment and Risk Evaluation (CARE) Clinic in San Diego, USA, reported a 15% transition rate at 12 months (Haroun et al., 2006). Combining these and other studies, an average annual transition rate of 36.7% in subjects not receiving special antipsychotic treatment has been found (Ruhrmann, Schultze-Lutter & Klosterkötter, 2003).

To explore the effect of sampling on transition rate further, we applied the UHR criteria to a sample of young people seeking help for non-psychotic disorders who were referred to a youth mental health service (Yung et al., 2006a). We aimed to apply the UHR criteria to all young people referred and to determine psychosis status at follow-up 6 months later for those meeting and those not meeting the criteria. Because many in the group were not specifically identified as being 'prodromal' or at high risk of psychosis, we expected the transition rate to be lower than that of the original PACE cohort. However, we hypothesized that those meeting UHR criteria would have a higher risk of transition to psychosis over the 6-month follow-up period than those not meeting UHR criteria. Consecutive referrals to ORYGEN Youth Health (OYH) over the period from April to October 2003 were recruited into the study. This is a public mental health programme for young people aged between 15 and 24 years living in metropolitan Melbourne, Australia. The clinical service has three components: EPPIC (the Early Psychosis Prevention and Intervention Centre, a service for people with first-episode psychotic disorder), PACE (described above) and Youthscope (a service for non-psychotic individuals). Referrals to OYH are taken from a range of sources including primary care physicians and other primary care services, school and university counselling services, drug and alcohol services, as well as from families/carers and young people themselves. A central triage service takes referrals for all three service components and refers to a specific component based on clinical judgement. At the time that this study took place, the triage system did not routinely enquire about attenuated psychotic symptoms or brief self-limiting psychotic symptoms if these were not the focus of the young person's presenting complaint. Therefore, it was possible that someone could meet UHR criteria but not be referred to PACE if he or she did not volunteer that they were having psychotic-like experiences and these were not enquired about by the clinician. Determination of UHR status for this study was done by researchers independent of clinical decision making. Hence, a proportion of young people meeting UHR criteria were not referred to the PACE clinic.

There were 292 participants in the sample, 119 of whom (40.7%) met the UHR criteria at baseline. Of these, 12 (10.1%) became psychotic within 6 months and 107 did not. Of the 173 individuals who did not meet UHR criteria at baseline, only one developed psychosis in the follow-up period. These findings indicate that although the young people who met UHR criteria were at significantly increased risk of psychosis compared with those who did not meet criteria (odds ratio, 19.3; 95% confidence interval, 2.5–150.5), the transition rate was much lower than in the previous PACE sample (Yung *et al.*, 2006a).

There are likely to be several reasons for this apparent reduction in transition rate. First, the members of this study group were not necessarily identified as possibly 'prodromal' or at high risk of psychosis by triage clinicians. Therefore, they differed in some way from previous PACE cohorts, who were thought by clinicians to be at high risk. However, the transition rate was similar in those who were not thought to be prodromal (those referred to Youthscope; 11.6%) and those thought to be prodromal (those referred to PACE; 9.2%). One possible relevant factor is that some members of the PACE subsample (25 out of 76 (33%)) received an intervention targeting their psychotic-like experience through a separate study conducted at PACE. This could have

included an antipsychotic medication, cognitive therapy or general case management.

Another possible contributing factor is referral source. In the original cohort, many participants were referred to PACE by mental health facilities. Young people were referred to these services as possibly psychotic. When they were assessed and found to be below the psychosis threshold, they were referred on to PACE. A change has occurred in referral pattern, however, since the mid 1990s. As the work of the PACE Clinic has become more well known around its geographical area, the formal and informal use of the UHR criteria has spread to other mental health teams, private psychiatrists, primary care physicians and even schools. Thus, consequently, psychotic-like experiences are being detected when previously they may not have been. It is also likely that they are being detected earlier (Yung *et al.*, 2007). This could result in referrals to OYH of individuals who may previously not have been referred and possibly in earlier referrals. For those referred earlier, this means that onset of psychosis would be expected to occur later than 6 or even 12 months, or possibly prevented altogether. However, more false positives could also be referred: that is, those who would previously not have been detected and referred and who may never be at risk of psychosis.

In other words, sampling from different populations may be contributing to the drop in transition rate. Hence, although the PACE UHR criteria have been used and adapted in a number of other settings around the world (Haroun *et al.*, 2006; Olsen & Rosenbaum, 2006), they need ongoing evaluation in these different settings.

Basic symptoms criteria

In line with the German tradition of the basic symptoms concept, the Cologne Early Recognition (CER) study (Klosterkötter *et al.*, 2001; Schultze-Lutter, Ruhrmann & Klosterkötter, 2006) sought to investigate the validity of these basic symptoms for the prediction of schizophrenia. In this study, 385 patients who were thought to be in the prodromal phase of schizophrenia were prospectively followed up after an average of 9.6 (±7.6) years. Nearly half (49.4%) of the sample of 160 who were contacted at follow-up had developed schizophrenia. Only two patients who subsequently developed schizophrenia had not reported any basic symptom at baseline. Therefore, the presence/absence of any basic symptom correctly predicted later presence/absence of conversion to schizophrenia in 78.1% of participants.

Analysis of the most predictive clusters of basic symptoms was undertaken. From these results, 10 cognitive-perceptive basic symptoms of 'information processing disturbances' were found (1) to have been reported at baseline by at least a quarter of later schizophrenia patients and (2) to show a good positive predictive value of at least 0.70. These symptoms included thought interferences, perseveration, pressure or blockages; disturbances of receptive language; decreased ability to discriminate between ideas and perception or fantasy and true memories; unstable ideas of reference; derealization; and visual or auditory perceptual disturbances.

It was concluded that it should be possible to identify subjects at risk of developing schizophrenia using this subgroup of basic symptoms and, therefore, to base an early intervention on these symptoms. Because basic symptoms were frequently found before any subthreshold or attenuated psychotic symptoms, these criteria were thought to be detecting the very beginning of the initial prodromal phase (Häfner et al., 1995).

Based on these findings, the first European centre for the early detection and treatment of psychoses was established in 1997, at the psychiatric department of the University of Cologne, Germany: the Früh-Erkennungs und Therapie-Zentrum für Psychische Krisen (FETZ). Subsequently, three other early detection and intervention centres were established in Germany based on the FETZ model, at Bonn, Düsseldorf and Munich. Additional early detection services are being established elsewhere in Germany and the German-speaking part of Switzerland.

The FETZ services use a close-in strategy to define criteria for 'at risk' or prodromal individuals. However, unlike the PACE clinic, they distinguish between the 'early initial prodromal state' (EIPS) and the 'late initial prodromal state' (LIPS). The EIPS criteria attempt to define a group at incipient but not imminent or immediate risk of psychosis. The criteria consist of the 10 predictive basic symptoms, of which one or more is required, plus the PACE' trait and state risk UHR criterion (see above). The LIPS criterion attempts to identify those at more immediate risk and is based on the PACE APS and BLIPS criteria (Ruhrmann et al., 2003). The EIPS and LIPS criteria are summarized in Table 6.1. This two-stage definition of the prodromal state guides the treatment approach, that is, psychological or pharmacological therapy (Bechdolf et al., 2005a; Ruhrmann et al., 2003, 2005).

In addition to clinical service delivery, FETZ is also involved in a public relations and awareness campaign targeting the local general population as well as potential referral sources who might be contacted by at-risk persons. This campaign includes audience-oriented informative events, regular newsletters with information about recent developments in the field and press coverage in local and national papers, radio and television. As a result, FETZ has established a broad network of cooperation with primary care physicians, psychiatrists, psychologists and psychotherapists, as well as with counselling services, self-help groups, schools and draft boards.

Following the introduction of basic symptoms into the definition of the prodrome, a phase-specific intervention strategy was developed and assessed in Cologne, Bonn, Düsseldorf and Munich as part of the German Research Network on Schizophrenia (GRNS; Häfner et al., 2004; Wölwer et al., 2003). The process of recruitment into the trials involved the initial use of a brief checklist that had a low threshold for identifying those in need of further assessment. Individuals who underwent this first step but who did not report any of the inclusion criteria were then given a tentative diagnosis and referred to appropriate services. Those who reported relevant prodromal symptoms or risk factors without fulfilling EIPS or LIPS criteria were offered further supportive and observational contacts with the FETZ. Individuals fulfilling EIPS criteria were offered participation in the GRNS early intervention trial comparing a specially designed cognitive–behavioural programme with a control condition of supportive counselling (Bechdolf et al., 2005b, c). Those fulfilling LIPS criteria were asked to participate in the GRNS pharmacological early intervention trial comparing

Table 6.1. Inclusion criteria for an early and late initial prodromal state

Initial prodromal state	Criteria
Early (EIPS)	One or more of the following basic symptoms that have occurred at least a year ago and appeared several times a week within the last 3 months: thought interferences; thought perseveration; thought pressure; thought blockages; disturbances of receptive language, either heard or read; decreased ability to discriminate between ideas and perception, fantasy and true memories; unstable ideas of reference; derealization; visual perception disturbances; auditory perceptual disturbances *and/or* Reduction in the Global Assessment of Functioning Score (DSM-IV) of at least 30 points (within the past year) and at least one of the following risk factors: first-degree relative with a lifetime diagnosis of schizophrenia or a schizophrenia-spectrum disorder and/or pre- or perinatal complications *and* absence of attenuated or transient psychotic symptoms
Late (LIPS)	Presence of at least one of the following attenuated positive symptoms (APS) present within the last 3 months, appearing several times per week for a period of at least 1 week, but no longer in the same severity than 1 year: ideas of reference; odd beliefs or magical thinking; unusual perceptual experiences; odd thinking and speech; suspiciousness or paranoid ideation *and/or* Brief limited intermittent psychotic symptoms (BLIPS), defined as appearance of one of the following frank psychotic symptoms for less than 1 week (interval between episodes at least 1 week) and resolving spontaneously: hallucinations; delusions; formal thought disorder; gross disorganized or catatonic behaviour

the combination of clinical management and low-dose atypical neuroleptic drugs with clinical management alone (Ruhrmann *et al.*, 2005). Both intervention studies were carried out as multicentre randomized controlled trials. The rationale for this design was that the psychotic-like LIPS criteria denote an imminent risk of transition to psychotic disorder within the next 12 months. Therefore, an antipsychotic medication appeared justified. Membership of the EIPS group implies that there is more time to intervene and a less imminent risk of transition.

During the 5-year term of the GRNS projects, 1348 individuals were screened for the EIPS and 1599 persons for LIPS criteria. Of these, 232 (17.2%) fulfilled EIPS and 382 (23.9%) LIPS criteria. Those who met any one criterion and agreed to participate in an intervention study were further assessed with the Early Recognition Inventory (ERI) based on the Instrument for the Retrospective Assessment of the Onset of Schizophrenia (IRAOS, Häfner *et al.*, 1992, 2004). This instrument consists of 110 items, including non-specific

symptoms such as anxiety or sleep disturbance as well as basic and negative symptoms and attenuated and frank psychotic symptoms. In addition, other psychopathological data (e.g. of comorbidity or personality) and neurobiological parameters were collected.

Of the patients meeting EIPS criteria, mainly the basic symptom one, 128 (55%) agreed to participate in the psychological intervention trial and were randomized to either the cognitive–behavioural therapy or the supportive control condition (Bechdolf *et al.*, 2006). Follow-up assessments occurred at the end of the 12-month treatment phase and again at 24 and 36 months. Outcomes included transition to frank psychotic symptoms for more than 1 week (i.e. the transition to a psychotic disorder) as well as – following the two-stage model – the occurrence of APS and BLIPS (i.e. the transition to a LIPS state from EIPS). At 12 months, only 3 (4.8%) of the 63 patients in the intervention group, but 11 (16.9 %) of the 65 patients in the control condition, made a transition; only one of the intervention group developing a psychotic disorder compared with eight in the control group (Bechdolf *et al.*, 2006). Therefore, the intervention appeared successful in preventing further progression of the illness. Its long-term effects will be assessed after analyses of the follow-up data at 24 and 36 months.

Of the persons meeting LIPS criteria, 124 (32.5%) participated in the pharmacological open-label study and were randomized to two treatment conditions. One condition featured a needs-focused intervention comprising crisis intervention ($n=59$), including psycho-education, family counselling and assistance with education or work-related difficulties. The other condition ($n=65$) combined this intervention with the second-generation neuroleptic amisulpride. An initial analysis of acute symptomatic treatment results during the first 12 weeks of intervention revealed superior treatment effects of the combination regarding basic symptoms, attenuated and full-blown psychotic symptoms, negative and affective symptoms, and global functioning (Ruhrmann *et al.*, 2007).

Another research approach that resulted from earlier studies, especially the CER study (Klosterkötter *et al.*, 2001), has aimed at the validation and, if possible, improvement of the prediction of psychosis by basic symptoms. A new instrument, the Schizophrenia Proneness Instrument, adult version (SPI-A; Schultze-Lutter *et al.*, 2004, 2007a), has been developed based on the Bonn Scale for the Assessment of Basic Symptoms (BSABS; Klosterkötter *et al.*, 1997b). Rather than assessing only the presence or absence of basic symptoms, the SPI-A includes assessment of the severity, frequency and recency of basic symptoms. It has reduced the original 98 items of the BSABS to 34. The SPI-A comprises six subscales containing five to six items each:

- 'affective–dynamic disturbances', including an impaired tolerance to certain stressors, a change in general mood and a decrease in emotional responsiveness in general, as well as towards significant others or special events
- 'cognitive–attentional impediments', for example an inability to divide attention between tasks relying on different senses (such as between talking and preparing a sandwich), feeling overly distracted by all kinds of stimuli, difficulties with short-term

memory and concentration as well as slowed-down thinking and lack of purposive thoughts
- 'cognitive disturbances', for example an increased indecisiveness with regard to making minor decisions, disturbances of immediate recall, thought blockages and disturbances of receptive and expressive speech
- 'disturbances in experiencing the self and surroundings', including unstable ideas of reference, decreased capacity to distinguish between different kinds of emotion and an increased emotional reactivity in response to routine social interactions
- 'body perception disturbances' involving various coenaesthetic phenomena such as skin numbness, muscle stiffness, peculiar isolated pains, feelings of being electrified, feelings of the body shrinking or enlarging
- 'perception disturbances', including hypersensitivity to light/optic stimuli and/or to sounds, changes in the perception of the intensity or quality of acoustic stimuli.

In a prospective evaluation of the SPI-A, a transition to psychosis rate of 24.6% within the first year following baseline assessment was found in a group who met EIPS criteria (however, 80% had also APS; Schultze-Lutter *et al.*, 2007b). Furthermore, in a cross-sectional evaluation of the SPI-A (Schultze-Lutter *et al.*, 2007c), comparable expressions of basic symptoms in first-episode schizophrenia and potentially prodromal subjects were found for all subscales of the SPI-A, and these were more severe than in non-psychotic depressive subjects. This was true even for the more depressive-like complaints described in the affective–dynamic disturbances section. This supports the notion that basic symptoms are specific to the schizophrenia spectrum.

Additionally, slightly altered basic symptom criteria (two of nine basic symptoms required; Schultze-Lutter *et al.*, 2006) were employed alongside the UHR criteria in the multisite European Prediction of Psychosis Study (EPOS: Klosterkötter *et al.*, 2005). This multi-centre, international prospective follow-up study involved 246 putatively prodromal subjects in six regions in four countries (Germany (Cologne and Berlin), Finland (Turku), the Netherlands (Amsterdam), UK

(Birmingham and Manchester)). Subjects have been followed for 18 months so far and assessed for psycho-pathological, psychosocial and neurobiological variables at baseline, 9 and 18 months. A preliminary analysis of the distribution of the four inclusion criteria across the first 153 subjects showed that APS (75.2%) and cognitive basic symptoms (72.6%) were the most frequently met criteria, with a significant overlap of between 19% and 50% depending on the region (Graf von Reventlow *et al.*, 2004). Final analyses will show the predictive value of each as well as for possible combinations of the four criteria, and the impact of potentially influential other variables on transition or non-transition to psychosis within the follow-up period.

Clinical high-risk criteria: the New York RAP programme

A different approach to identifying UHR individuals has been undertaken at the Hillside Recognition and Prevention (Hillside-RAP) programme in New York (Cornblatt, 2002). Investigators at this site, who bring their expertise from genetic high-risk studies to the area of pre-psychotic research, have schizophrenia as their target syndrome, rather than just psychosis. Accordingly, some of their intake and outcome criteria have been modified from the PACE and PRIME criteria. The RAP Clinic has two categories of what are dubbed 'clinical high-risk' (CHR) patients. This terminology is used to contrast these putatively prodromal individuals from subjects recruited through the traditional high-risk projects that use family history as the sole intake criterion (such as the Copenhagen High-risk Project: Mednick *et al.*, 1987). The three intake groups in the RAP Clinic are (1) the CHR-negative group, which includes young people displaying attenuated negative symptoms such as social isolation, avolition, and deterioration of role or academic functioning; (2) the CHR-positive group, which consists of adolescents with attenuated positive psychotic symptoms (according to SIPS scores); and (3) the 'schizophrenia-like psychosis' group (those with psychotic symptoms but not meeting criteria for schizophrenia). The CHR-negative group is thought to be at heightened risk of developing schizophrenia because of cognitive impairments, which are

hypothesized to precede the onset of schizophrenia. All three groups had high levels of non-specific and negative symptoms at baseline: cognitive deficits, affective complaints, social isolation and school failure. The RAP investigators theorize that the developmental course of schizophrenia follows a progression from CHR-negative to CHR-positive to schizophrenia-like psychosis to schizophrenia. The transition rate from CHR-positive status to psychotic disorder was 26.5% (9 of 34 patients) within 6 months (Lencz *et al.*, 2003). The transition rate to schizophrenia in the schizophrenia-like psychosis group was 33% (Cornblatt *et al.*, 2002).

Disadvantages of 'prodromal' identification

The methods developed to identify people at risk of psychosis have improved identification from the general population rate of 1% to a rate of approximately 30%, which represents an encouraging development towards more accurate identification. However, these developments have not been without criticism. One is that the screening process would not be effective in the general population because of the lower base rate of psychotic illness in that population (Warner, 2005). While this is true, pre-onset identification is predicated on indicated, high-risk samples rather than general population samples. Indeed, screening for UHR criteria at a population level would not be supported at this stage (Yung, 2003). The second criticism is that there is a high false-positive rate in all of these studies, with the majority of participants not developing psychotic disorder within a brief time frame (although some may be false false positives as discussed above). Consequently, some individuals will be 'diagnosed', followed up and treated as if they were at high risk of developing a psychotic disorder, when this may not be true. These falsely identified individuals may be harmed by being labelled, and/or receiving treatment at this stage. For example, they may become anxious or depressed about the possibility of developing schizophrenia, stigmatized by others or themselves or both (Yung, Philips & McGorry, 2004b), and they may avoid developmentally appropriate challenges (Heinssen *et al.*, 2001) for fear of increasing their 'stress' level and risking precipitation of psychosis. Similarly, these falsely identified individuals may be exposed to drug or other therapies, with potential adverse reactions without gaining any benefit. These issues have been reviewed in detail previously (Cornblatt, Lencz & Kane, 2001; McGlashan, 2001; McGorry, Yung & Phillips, 2001; Yung & McGorry, 1997; Yung *et al.*, 2004b) and are discussed in Ch. 7. Concerns about the risk benefit balance of early intervention strategies lie at the heart of this controversy and need to be addressed by an evidence-based approach (Bentall & Morrison, 2002; Yung & McGorry, 2003).

Predictors of psychotic disorder in high-risk groups

The predictive validity of the different *criteria* from different research groups has briefly been described. In this section we summarize the findings from various different services and research projects with respect to prediction of psychotic disorder, including variables that are not directly related to the inclusion criteria.

Psychopathological and clinical variables

Clinical variables that predict onset of psychosis have now been identified and will be discussed in turn.

Schizotypal personality features

Schizotypal personality disorder, if accompanied by recent and marked impairment in functioning, forms part of the PACE 'trait and state' UHR criteria (Yung *et al.*, 2003; see above). In the PAS UHR group, having schizotypal personality characteristics at baseline, as measured by the International Personality Disorder Examination (Loranger *et al.*, 1994), predicted onset of psychosis after follow-up of 1 to 2 years (Mason *et al.*, 2004). In particular, odd beliefs and magical thinking at baseline were significant predictors of psychosis at follow-up.

It is not clear, of course, whether schizotypal personality in this study truly preceded the onset of the psychotic disorder or if, in retrospect, the schizotypal features were prodromal manifestations of the illness. Another factor to consider is that these measures of

schizotypy and schizotypal personality consist of a mixture of items assessing positive psychotic-like experiences, magical thinking ('schizotypal cognition', e.g. belief in lucky charms) and negative symptoms. Where possible, we attempt to tease out the individual items of significance and include them in the relevant section.

Positive psychotic phenomena

Attenuated or subthreshold psychotic symptoms form the basis of most of the UHR and prodromal intake criteria in centres throughout the world. 'Odd beliefs' at baseline were predictive of psychosis in the PAS group (see above), as was level of auditory hallucinations (Mason *et al.*, 2004). The PACE UHR study (Yung *et al.*, 2003) also found that a high score on the BPRS psychotic subscale (comprising unusual thought content, suspiciousness, perceptual disturbance and conceptual disorganization) was a significant predictor of psychosis at 12-month follow-up. Similarly, in the CARE study (Haroun *et al.*, 2006), those who developed psychosis within 12 months had significantly higher scores of unusual thought content, suspiciousness and disorganized communication, as measured by the SIPS (Miller *et al.*, 2002), compared with those who remained non-psychotic. They also had a higher score on the Scale for Assessment of Positive Symptoms and higher levels of formal thought disorder as measured by both this and the BPRS.

Negative symptoms

High levels of negative symptoms have been found at baseline in several different UHR or prodromal samples, including the PACE group (Yung *et al.*, 2003, 2004a) and all RAP cohorts (Lencz *et al.*, 2004), despite not being part of the inclusion criteria. Negative symptoms have also been found to be predictive of psychosis in a number of studies. The negative subscales of the CAARMS were found to be significant predictors of onset of psychosis in the PACE UHR sample. These symptoms were impaired concentration and attention, subjectively abnormal emotional experiences, blunted affect, impaired energy and impaired tolerance to stress

(Yung *et al.*, 2005). Impaired attention, as assessed by the Scale for Assessment of Negative Symptoms (Andreasen, 1983) was also a significant predictor in this sample (Yung *et al.*, 2003). In the PAS UHR cohort, marked impairment in role functioning, flat or inappropriate affect, anhedonia and asociality were all found at significantly higher levels at baseline in those who went on to develop psychosis than in those who did not (Mason *et al.*, 2004). The CARE group also found that some negative symptoms were significant predictors of psychosis. In their sample, the total SIPS negative scale score, the SIPS individual items of decreased experience of the self and decreased ideational richness, and the BPRS item withdrawal/retardation were significantly higher in the group that made the transition compared with those who did not (Haroun *et al.*, 2006).

Basic symptoms

Two, partially overlapping basic symptom-based criteria for defining the initial prodrome of psychosis have been developed on the data from the CER study (Klosterkötter *et al.*, 2001). One is based on the findings regarding the predictive accuracy of individual basic symptoms and included in the EIPS criteria (Table 6.1). The second is based on a methodological study on the same data (Schultze-Lutter, 2001). This found that a cluster of nine cognitive basic symptoms was repeatedly selected as the most predictive of all seven examined clusters. This cluster was called 'cognitive disturbances'. The two criteria lists have five symptoms in common and, in fact, differ little in their general predictive accuracy. The most favourable cutoff was 1 out of the 10 symptom selections (COPER) and two of the 'cognitive disturbances' cluster (COGDIS). At these cut-offs, the two selection criteria showed satisfactory accuracy values, with the COGDIS selection tending to be more conservative than the COPER selection. The COGDIS criterion was more accurate at predicting subsequent schizophrenia than the COPER criterion (positive predictive values of 0.79 and 0.65, respectively). However, the COGDIS criterion performed less well at excluding subsequent schizophrenia (negative predictive values of 0.72 and 0.82, respectively). The COGDIS criterion also seemed to indicate a more imminent risk

of psychosis, with 23.9% of those meeting the COGDIS criterion converting to frank psychosis within the first year following baseline assessment, 22.4% within the second, 14.9% within the third and 17.9% within more than 3 years. In contrast, these figures were only 19.8%, 17.0%, 13.2%, and 15.1%, respectively, for the COPER criterion.

Within the PACE UHR group, the basic symptoms of reduced energy and impaired tolerance to normal stress, as measured by the CAARMS, significantly predicted onset of psychotic disorder within 12 months (Yung *et al.*, 2005).

Depression, anxiety and distress

Depression and anxiety are common prodromal symptoms (Yung & McGorry, 1996). Depression has been found to be a significant predictor of psychosis in the PACE UHR group (Yung *et al.*, 2003) and the Edinburgh High Risk Study (Johnstone *et al.*, 2005). Indeed, in community samples, individuals who experience distress or depression related to their psychotic-like experiences are more likely to seek help compared with those who do not have distress and depression associated with their symptoms (Bak *et al.*, 2003; Krabbendam *et al.*, 2005). Distress and depression in relation to psychotic experiences have also been found to be associated with poor psychosocial functioning (Yung *et al.*, 2006b). These findings have led several researchers to propose that distress, anxiety, depression and other forms of affective disturbance may play a major role in determining whether young people with psychotic symptoms progress to develop psychotic disorder (Broome *et al.*, 2005; Escher *et al.*, 2002; Freeman & Garety, 2003; Yung *et al.*, 2006b).

Poor functioning

Poor functioning at intake as assessed by the Global Assessment of Functioning significantly predicted onset of psychosis in the two separate PACE cohorts (Yung *et al.*, 2003, 2006a), and in a more general help-seeking sample of young people with non-psychotic disorders who met UHR criteria (Yung *et al.*, 2006a). Impairment in role functioning also significantly predicted development of psychosis in the PAS UHR group (Mason *et al.*, 2004).

Substance use

Longitudinal studies to date report contrasting findings related to the predictive ability of substance use in UHR groups. History of substance abuse was present in significantly more subjects who developed psychosis than in those who did not in the CARE study (Haroun *et al.*, 2006). In contrast, against expectations, in the PACE UHR cohort, neither cannabis use nor dependence in the year prior to contact with the service was associated with a higher risk of developing psychosis over the following year (Phillips *et al.*, 2002a). This may be because the PACE sample included mainly help-seeking individuals, who may not be typical of the whole population of people at risk of psychosis. Individuals with high levels of cannabis use may well be less highly motivated to seek treatment than our subjects. Hence, the PACE research was biased against finding cannabis as a risk factor for psychosis. Additionally, this study was able to report analysis of cannabis use at intake only. Changes in cannabis use over the study period were, therefore, not identified, and these may have been important in influencing outcome more proximal to the timing of psychosis onset. While this study did not support a role for cannabis in the development of first-episode psychosis, it is too early to exclude it completely as a candidate risk factor for onset of psychosis. Indeed, these seemingly contrasting findings may indicate that cannabis is neither necessary nor sufficient to cause psychosis, but may be dependent on other risk factors to influence onset (Linszen & van Amelsvoort, 2007).

Stress

The finding that stressful life events may precede onset of psychotic illnesses (Bebbington *et al.*, 1993; Brown & Birley, 1968; Canton & Fraccon, 1985; Chung, Langeluddecke & Tennant, 1986; Day *et al.*, 1987; Malla & Norman, 1992) and psychotic relapses in established disorders (Hirsch *et al.*, 1996; Leff *et al.*, 1983; Malla *et al.*, 1990; Nuechterlein *et al.*, 1994;

Ventura *et al.*, 1989) has led to the hypothesis that adverse life experiences may actually precipitate onset of psychotic episodes in vulnerable individuals. Some researchers have suggested that 'minor' life events or day-to-day 'hassles' cause more stress than major, yet infrequent, events such as deaths or separations (Malla & Norman, 1992). This has led to the development of the Hassles Scale (Kanner *et al.*, 1981) and investigation into the role of frequent, but more minor, stressful situations on the development of psychosis.

It is also likely that the subjective experiences of stress, rather than stressful events per se, may be relevant to outcome. The role of the ability to tolerate stress was demonstrated in one study, which found that prodromal subjects reported a decreased stress tolerance in comparison with their premorbid phase. This intolerance of stress was more pronounced than in patients with depressive disorder (Schultze-Lutter *et al.*, 2007c), though not specific to psychosis (Klosterkötter *et al.*, 2001). Another longitudinal study related subjectively perceived stress to objective measures, including cortisol level, and is discussed in more detail below.

Neurocognitive variables

Cognitive deficits are recognized as one of the core features of schizophrenia (Pantelis, Wood & Maruff, 2002) and have been associated with functional outcome (Green, 1996). Recent research has attempted to detect the presence of such deficits prior to illness onset, as they may represent neurocognitive trait markers for schizophrenia. In particular, a promising marker is working memory, which is consistently impaired throughout the course of the illness (Goldman-Rakic, 1994; Pantelis *et al.*, 1997; Park *et al.*, 1999). It has been demonstrated that working memory is impaired prior to the onset of psychotic disorder in two separate UHR samples, and that deficits in working memory were predictive of subsequent transition to psychotic disorder (Brewer *et al.*, 2005). Immediate verbal recall deficits were also identified prior to illness onset. Rapid registration and efficient recall may be the cognitive processes that indicate compromised prefrontal functioning (Brewer *et al.*, 2005).

A further promising marker is olfactory identification where deficits have been found to occur prior to psychosis onset. They were also found to be worse in those who were later diagnosed with schizophrenia (Brewer *et al.*, 2001).

In another recent German study, abnormal sensory gating was compared in patients with UHR, first-episode schizophrenia and chronic schizophrenia as well as healthy controls (Brockhaus-Dumke *et al.*, 2008). The N100 suppression, but not P50 suppression, was significantly reduced in all three patient groups compared with controls and lowest in both psychotic groups. Furthermore, UHR patients with BLIPS or APS exhibited significantly more severe suppression deficits compared with those with basic symptoms only. The lack of significant differences between 'prodromal' patients and those with schizophrenia supported the hypothesis that suppression of mid-latency auditory event-related potentials reflects an endophenotype of schizophrenia that is already present in prodromal stages of the illness and, as such, might facilitate prediction of transition to psychosis in patients at risk.

Neurobiological variables

Another promising area of study is the hypothalamic–pituitary–adrenal (HPA) axis dysfunction which may play a role in the development of psychotic disorders. This theory is supported by the finding of higher cortisol levels (plasma, salivary or urinary) and abnormal circadian cortisol rhythms in patients with psychotic disorders compared with healthy control subjects (Altamura, Guercetti & Percudani, 1989; Kaneko *et al.*, 1992). Results of the dexamethasone suppression test (Carroll, 1985) in patients with schizophrenia are consistent with this. The test measures the response of the adrenal glands to adrenocorticotrophic hormone, produced by the pituitary. Those with schizophrenia show non-suppression compared with the normal suppression seen in healthy controls. The level of non-suppression is less than that seen in depressed patients (Asnis *et al.*, 1987; Hubain, Simonnet & Mendlewicz, 1986; Kaneko *et al.*, 1992).

In a recent study of 23 UHR subjects at the PACE Clinic, a strong association was found between the number of minor stressful events ('hassles') experienced and plasma cortisol level ($r = 0.53$; $p = 0.051$;

$n = 14$) and between the level of anxiety and depression and plasma cortisol level ($r = 0.87$; $p = 0.000$; $n = 23$). However, level of psychotic-like symptoms was not correlated with plasma cortisol level. Unexpectedly, UHR subjects who developed psychosis had significantly lower plasma cortisol levels at intake than the UHR cohort who did not develop psychosis (t (16) = 3.29; $p = 0.005$). This may have been because cortisol was measured at baseline, with the development of psychosis occurring a considerable time after this measurement (between 104 and 527 days; $n = 5$), or it may reflect the low number in the sample (L. J. Phillips, unpublished data).

Studies of brain structure may also be relevant to the HPA axis dysfunction model of psychotic disorders. The hippocampus and pituitary gland are two brain structures that are integral to the HPA axis. It is hypothesized that abnormal HPA axis responses to stress might result in hippocampal damage. This might then compromise attention, memory and other cognitive skills and ultimately influence the development of psychotic symptoms such as delusional thoughts, hallucinations and thought disorder. Reduced hippocampal volume (Bogerts *et al.*, 1990, 1993; Velakoulis *et al.*, 1999) and hippocampal glucocorticoid receptor numbers (Webster *et al.*, 2002) have been reported in association with psychotic illnesses. A longitudinal study of non-patient subjects at genetic high risk of schizophrenia found that those who developed psychotic symptoms had significantly smaller temporal lobe volumes than those who did not develop psychotic symptoms (Lawrie *et al.*, 2002).

In the light of these findings, it was hypothesized that UHR subjects would have reduced hippocampal volume. In an UHR study at PACE, hippocampal volumes of subjects at intake lay midway between those of normal controls and patients with chronic schizophrenia or first-episode psychosis (Phillips *et al.*, 2002b). However, in one study, reduced hippocampal volumes in the UHR cohort at baseline were not shown to be associated with a heightened risk of later development of psychosis. In fact, UHR subjects who developed psychosis had larger hippocampi at baseline than those who did not develop psychosis within a 12-month period. This was because the UHR subjects who did not develop psychosis (the false positives) had smaller than average hippocampal volumes. It must be remembered that these false positives are not normal healthy controls. They are help-seeking and symptomatic, with a range of symptoms and psychiatric syndromes. The reduced hippocampal volume in this subsample of patients may reflect this non-psychotic psychopathology.

The pituitary gland contains corticotrophs, the cells that produce and secrete adrenocorticotrophic hormone, which, in turn, activates the secretion of cortisol. A recent study found increased pituitary volumes in patients with first-episode psychosis while individuals with established schizophrenia of at least 5 years duration had smaller pituitary volumes than controls (Pariante *et al.*, 2004). In a longitudinal investigation of UHR subjects at the PACE Clinic, subjects who developed psychosis had larger pituitary volumes compared with UHR individuals who did not develop psychosis (Garner *et al.*, 2005). This increased volume is thought to reflect an increase in the size and number of corticotrophs.

Reduced grey matter volume in frontal regions may also be a risk factor for psychotic disorder. In the PACE UHR group, individuals who subsequently developed psychotic disorder had less grey matter in the inferior frontal cortex on baseline MRI scans compared with UHR individuals who did not develop psychosis (Pantelis *et al.*, 2003). In a subsample of UHR patients who developed psychosis, MRI brain scans were obtained at baseline (that is, prior to onset of frank psychotic disorder) and 1 year later (post-psychosis). Scans showed a significant bilateral reduction in grey matter volume in the cingulate region as well as in the left para-hippocampal gyrus, left fusiform gyrus, left orbito-frontal cortex and one region of the left cerebellar cortex (Pantelis *et al.*, 2003). These findings were not present in a group of UHR patients scanned at baseline and 1 year later who did not develop psychosis. This finding suggests that brain changes can occur during the transition to psychosis. While the basis of this remains uncertain, it opens up the possibility that, with sufficiently early treatment, such changes could be minimized or prevented.

Another potential neurobiological area to study is the gyrification index, which is defined as the ratio of the inner and outer surface contours of the brain (Kulynych *et al.*, 1997). One study found a reduced left cortical index in an adolescent high-risk group compared with controls (Jou, Hardan & Keshavan, 2005). However, a recent study found that potentially prodromal subjects fulfilling UHR or the basic symptoms 'cognitive disturbances' criteria showed higher frontal and parietal gyrification indices in both hemispheres when compared with healthy controls, but the indices did not differ from those for patients with first-episode psychosis (S. Ruhrmann *et al.*, unpublished data).

Intervention

Current studies suggest that intervention may be able to delay or even prevent onset of psychosis in the UHR or prodromal group. The first randomized controlled trial was conducted at the PACE Clinic from 1996 to 1999 (McGorry *et al.*, 2002). This study compared the effect of intensive cognitive-behaviourally oriented psychotherapy plus low-dose neuroleptic (risperidone) with supportive therapy alone on the development of psychotic disorder. There was a significantly higher rate of transition to psychosis in the control (supportive therapy) group ($n = 28$) than in the intervention group ($n = 31$) at the end of the 6-month treatment phase ($p = 0.026$). This difference was no longer significant at the 12-month follow-up point. This result is thought to indicate a delay in the onset of psychosis in the intervention group. Both groups experienced a reduction in global psychopathology and functioning over the treatment phase. Because psychological treatment and medication were combined in this trial, it was not possible to determine which was the active intervention, or whether they were synergistic.

A trial of cognitive therapy versus monitoring only conducted by the Early Detection and Intervention Evaluation group in Manchester, UK, showed a significant effect of this treatment (Morrison *et al.*, 2004). A multimodal cognitive–behavioural therapy was also effective at the end of the 12-month intervention period in EIPS subjects compared with the supportive control condition (Bechdolf *et al.*, 2005c; see above).

A double-blind randomized controlled trial of olanzapine versus supportive therapy and monitoring showed a non-significant trend for the intervention to be effective in preventing or delaying psychosis (McGlashan *et al.*, 2006). Additionally, the prodromal (UHR) patients who received olanzapine reported lower levels of 'prodromal' symptomatology (according to the SIPS: Miller *et al.*, 2002) compared with the UHR patients who received placebo medication. Similarly, a comparison was made of needs-focused intervention with ($n = 65$) or without ($n = 59$) amisulpride in individuals meeting the FETZ LIPS criteria. Those receiving the amisulpride showed a marked symptomatic benefit, with reductions in attenuated and full-blown psychotic symptoms, and basic, depressive and negative symptoms, and an improvement in global functioning (Ruhrmann *et al.*, 2007).

In all, results of these first treatment trials suggest that both antipsychotic medication and psychological interventions might have a role in treating the difficulties and problems that UHR young people experience, as well as delaying or preventing the onset of psychosis. There is scope for the investigation of a wide range of other approaches, including neuroprotective agents, in the treatment of the UHR population. Chapter 7 has a detailed account of the management of individuals with an 'at risk mental state'.

Conclusions and future directions

Since the establishment of the first pre-onset clinic in the mid 1990s, great advances have been made in devising criteria to identify those at risk of developing psychosis. Treatments for this identified group have been developed, which a majority of studies have shown can significantly reduce the rate of transition to psychosis and reduce symptomatology. Further research is required to determine which treatment strategies are most effective and for how long they should be continued. While work to date is promising, critics raise some valid concerns, such as the issue of false positives and the problems of mislabelling and stigma. In order to address these concerns, two key developments are required: first, the continued improvement of the accuracy of predictive tools, thereby reducing the false-positive rate as much as possible; second, developing a knowledge of which interventions are required at what stage, to reduce the exposure of individuals to unnecessary iatrogenic damage.

Another important consideration is that psychotic disorder per se may not be the only target of clinical relevance. Deterioration in psychosocial functioning and persistent disability are also outcomes of interest. Additionally, the development of non-psychotic disorders in those apparently at risk of a psychotic disorder is also worthy of attention. Recent research suggests that psychotic-like experiences may be risk factors for major depression (e.g. Verdoux *et al.*, 1999). Overall, this field of research and clinical care is still in its early years and needs ongoing development in an ethical and evidence-based manner.

Appendix: Short definition of basic symptoms included in the two basic symptom criteria of the initial prodrome, COPER and COGDIS

Basic symptom: general definition Subjective disturbance not known in current quantity/quality from what the patient considers the premorbid phase; not caused by substance use/intoxication or somatic causes/illness; mainly not observable; insight into pathological character of disturbance intact.

Thought interference Completely insignificant thoughts intrude on and disturb the person's thinking that are unrelated to the current thoughts. Such thoughts are *emotionally neutral* and have no special meaning for the individual and no association to the intended topic or affective state at that time

Thought perseveration Obsessive-like recapitulation of daily *unimportant, past events, conversations, etc. of no special affective meaning*; a mental fixation that occupies the patient's attention, is hard to terminate and hinders or inhibits work performance or sleep

Thought pressure A great number of random, different, completely unrelated thoughts or thought fragments – *not involving a common topic* – enter the mind and disappear again in quick succession without the patient being able to suppress or guide them

Thought blockages Subjective blocking of thought that can also be experienced as a sudden emptiness of thoughts, interruption of thoughts, fading (slipping) of thoughts or losing the thread/train of thoughts

Disturbance of receptive language Disturbance in immediately understanding everyday speech that is either read (visual) or heard (auditory); when reading or listening, the patient has difficulties or is unable to comprehend and recognize the meaning of words, word sequences or sentences

Disturbance of expressive speech Self-experienced difficulty with verbal expression, with a particular problem in producing adequate words, experienced as an impairment in verbal fluency; precision and availability of language with the correct words not recalled or only after a delay; sometimes words are recalled that are only slightly associated with the correct word and are, therefore, imprecise

Disturbance of abstract language Deficits in the comprehension of any kind of abstract or symbolic phrases or contents as well as self-reported phenomena of concretism including comprehension of visual signs; this is the only basic symptom that can be *tested* (e.g. by asking the patient to explain the meaning of idioms)

Inability to divide attention Difficulty in dealing with demands involving more than one sense; individuals have particular difficulties with integrating sensory input from more than one sense, such as visual and auditory stimuli, e.g. patient may not be able to listen and pay attention to an oral presentation and take down notes at the same time

Captivation of attention by details of the visual field A domination of the visual field by a random single aspect of it; a visual stimulus or a part of it stands out strikingly, seems almost isolated from the rest of the environment and is emphasized so that it catches and captures the whole attention; unintendedly, the patient has to look at this detail, is transfixed, spell-bound and has problems in turning away

Unstable ideas of reference Subjective dim feelings of self-reference that are almost immediately rectified by cognition; vague feeling that certain events, comments and actions by others were related to him/her but knows at the same time that this is impossible or at least highly improbable; other than in ideas or delusions of reference, no intellectual processes such as reasoning or searching for an explanation are involved, and reality testing is still completely intact

Derealization Change in affective bonding with the surrounding, either as (1) an estrangement and alienation so that the environment appears unreal, changed and strange, or, as (2) an increase in affective bonding, often coupled with positive or euphoric feelings

Decreased ability to discriminate between ideas and perception, fantasy and true memories Difficulties in distinguishing between internal–mental and external–perceived everyday events; no amnestic, dissociative memory gaps

Visual perception disturbances Disturbances related to his/her perception and not to real changes in his/her surroundings

- *partial seeing, including tubular vision*: only parts of a certain object are perceived
- *photopsia*: elementary, not concretized, optic 'pseudo-hallucinations' related to own seeing
- *near and tele-vision*: objects seem to be closer or farther away, but unchanged in size
- *micropsia, macropsia*: objects are perceived as smaller or bigger than they really are
- *metamorphopsia*: shape of objects is perceived as changed or distorted
- *changes in colour perception*: qualitative changes in colour vision, increase/decrease of colour intensity, perception of the whole visual field in one or more colours
- *changed perception of the face or body of others*
- *changed perception of the patient's own face*
- *pseudomovements of optic stimuli*: fixed objects seem to move; spontaneously often described as dizziness, vertigo or staggering
- *diplopia, oblique vision*: objects are perceived two- or three-fold, lopsided or crooked

- *disturbances of the estimation of distances or sizes*: distances or sizes of objects are misjudged but not perceived as different in size
- *disturbance of the perception of straight lines/contours*: only affecting the outer part of an object
- *maintenance of optic stimuli*: perception of images that had really been seen minutes up to hours before, 'visual echo'

Acoustic perception disturbances Disturbances related to his/her perception and not to real changes in his/her surrounding

- *acoasms*: simple non-verbal auditory 'pseudo-hallucinations', often referred to as tinnitus
- *changed intensity or quality of acoustic stimuli*
- *maintenance of acoustic stimuli*: 'acoustic echo', abnormally long-lasting remains of auditory stimuli or subsequent hearing of sounds that had really been heard minutes or even hours before

Source: Based on SPI-A; Schulze-Lutter *et al.* 2007a.

REFERENCES

Altamura, C., Guercetti, G. & Percudani, M. (1989). Dexamethasone suppression test in positive and negative schizophrenia. *Psychiatry Research*, **30**, 69–75.

APA (1994). *Diagnostic and Statistical Manual of Mental Disorders*, 4th edn. Washington, DC: American Psychiatric Press.

Andreasen, N. C. (1983). *The Scale for the Assessment of Negative Symptoms (SANS)*. Iowa City: University of Iowa.

Andreasen, N. C. (1987). *The Comprehensive Assessment of Symptoms and History (CASH) Interview*. Iowa City: University of Iowa.

Asnis, G. M., Halbreich, U., Ryan, N. D. *et al.* (1987). The relationship of the dexamethasone suppression test (1-mg and 2-mg) to basal plasma cortisol levels in endogenous depression. *Psychoneuroendocrinology*, **12**, 295–301.

Bak, M., Myin-Germeys, I., Hanssen, M. *et al.* (2003). When does experience of psychosis result in a need for care? A prospective general population study. *Schizophrenia Bulletin*, **29**, 349–58.

Bebbington, P., Wilkins, S., Jones, P. *et al.* (1993). Life events and psychosis: initial results from the Camberwell Collaborative Psychosis Study. *British Journal of Psychiatry*, **162**, 72–9.

Bechdolf, A., Ruhrmann, S., Wagner, M. *et al.* (2005a). Interventions in the initial prodromal states of psychosis in Germany: concept and recruitment. *British Journal of Psychiatry*, **187**, s45–8. [*Special Issue: Early Psychosis: A Bridge to the Future.*]

Bechdolf, A., Kohn, D., Knost, B., Pukrop, R. & Klosterkötter, J. (2005b). A randomized comparison of group cognitive-behavioural therapy and group psychoeducation in acute patients with schizophrenia: outcome at 24 months. *Acta Psychiatrica Scandinavica*, **112**, 173–9.

Bechdolf, A., Veith, V., Schwarzer, D. *et al.* (2005c). Cognitive-behavioral therapy in the pre-psychotic phase: an exploratory study. *Psychiatry Research*, **136**, 251–5.

Bechdolf, A., Phillips, L. J., Francey, S. M. *et al.* (2006). Recent approaches to psychological interventions for people at risk of psychosis. *European Archives of Psychiatry and Clinical Neuroscience*, **256**, 159–73.

Bell, R. Q. (1992). Multiple-risk cohorts and segmenting risk as solutions to the problem of false positives in risk for the major psychoses. *Psychiatry*, **55**, 370–81.

Bentall, R. P. & Morrison, A. P. (2002). More harm than good: the case against using antipsychotic drugs to prevent severe mental illness. *Journal of Mental Health*, **11**, 351–6.

Bogerts, B., Ashtari, M., Degreef, G. *et al.* (1990). Reduced temporal limbic structure volumes on magnetic resonance images in first episode schizophrenia. *Psychiatry Research*, **35**, 1–13.

Bogerts, B., Lieberman, J. A., Ashtari, M. *et al.* (1993). Hippocampus–amygdala volumes and psychopathology in chronic schizophrenia. *Biological Psychiatry*, **33**, 236–46.

Brewer, W. J., Pantelis, C., Anderson, V. *et al.* (2001). Stability of olfactory identification deficits in neuroleptic-naive patients with first-episode psychosis. *American Journal of Psychiatry*, **158**, 107–15.

Brewer, W. J., Francey, S. M., Wood, S. J. *et al.* (2005). Memory impairments identified in people at ultra-high risk for psychosis who later develop first-episode psychosis. *American Journal of Psychiatry*, **162**, 71–8.

Brewer, W. J., Wood, S. J., Phillips, L. J. *et al.* (2006). Generalised and specific cognitive performance in clinical high-risk cohorts: a review highlighting potential vulnerability markers for psychosis. *Schizophrenia Bulletin*, **32**, 538–55.

Brockhaus-Dumke, A., Schultze-Lutter, F., Müller, R. *et al.* (2008). Sensory gating in schizophrenia: P50 and N100 gating in antipsychotic-free subjects at risk, first-episode and chronic patients. *Biological Psychiatry*, Epub: 10.1016/j.biopsych.2008.02.006.

Broome, M. R., Woolley, J. B., Tabraham, P. *et al.* (2005). What causes the onset of psychosis? *Schizophrenia Research*, **79**, 23–34.

Brown, G. & Birley, J. (1968). Crises and life changes and the onset of schizophrenia. *Journal of Health and Social Behaviour*, **9**, 203–14.

Canton, G. & Fraccon, I. G. (1985). Life events and schizophrenia: a replication. *Acta Psychiatrica Scandanivica*, **71**, 211–16.

Carroll, B. J. (1985). Dexamethasone suppression test: a review of contemporary confusion. *Journal of Clinical Psychiatry*, **46**, 13–24.

Chung, R. K., Langeluddecke, P. & Tennant, C. (1986). Threatening life events in the onset of schizophrenia, schizophreniform psychosis and hypomania. *British Journal of Psychiatry*, **148**, 680–5.

Conrad, K. (1958). *Die Beginnende Schizophrenie*. Stuttgart: Georg Thieme.

Corcoran, C., Malaspina, D. & Hercher, L. (2005). Prodromal interventions for schizophrenia vulnerability: the risks of being 'at risk'. *Schizophrenia Research*, **73**, 173–84.

Cornblatt, B. A. (2002). The New York High Risk Project to the Hillside Recognition and Prevention (RAP) program. *American Journal of Medical Genetics*, **114**, 956–66.

Cornblatt, B. A., Lencz, T. & Kane, J. M. (2001). Treatment of the schizophrenia prodrome: it is presently ethical? *Schizophrenia Research*, **51**, 31–8.

Cornblatt, B. A., Lencz, T., Correll, C., Auther, A. & Smith, C. (2002). Treating the prodrome: naturalistic findings from the RAP program. *Acta Psychiatrica Scandinavica*, **106**, 44.

Cornblatt, B. A., Lencz, T., Smith, C. W. *et al.* (2003). The schizophrenia prodrome revisited: a neurodevelopmental perspective. *Schizophrenia Bulletin*, **29**, 633–51.

Day, R., Nielsen, J. A., Korten, A. *et al.* (1987). Stressful life events preceding the acute onset of schizophrenia: a cross-national study from the World Health Organization. *Culture, Medicine and Psychiatry*, **11**, 123–205.

Docherty, J. P., van Kammen, D. P., Siris, S. G. & Marder, S. R. (1978). Stages of onset of schizophrenic psychosis. *American Journal of Psychiatry*, **135**, 420–6.

Donlon, P. T. & Blacker, K. H. (1973). Stages of schizophrenic decompensation and reintegration. *Journal of Nervous and Mental Disease*, **157**, 200–9.

Escher, S., Romme, M., Buiks, A., Delespaul, P. & van Os, J. (2002). Formation of delusional ideation in adolescents hearing voices: a prospective study. *American Journal of Medical Genetics*, **114**, 913–20.

Falloon, I. R. H. (1992). Early intervention for first episodes of schizophrenia: a preliminary exploration. *Psychiatry*, **55**, 4–15.

Francey, S. M., Jackson, H. J., Phillips, L. J. *et al.* (2005). Sustained attention in young people at high risk of psychosis does not predict transition to psychosis. *Schizophrenia Research*, **79**, 127–36.

Freeman, D. & Garety, P. A. (2003). Connecting neurosis and psychosis: the direct influence of emotion on delusions and hallucinations. *Behaviour Research and Therapy*, **41**, 923–47.

Garner, B., Pariante, C. M., Wood, S. J. *et al.* (2005). Pituitary volume predicts future transition to psychosis in individuals at ultra-high risk of developing psychosis. *Biological Psychiatry*, **58**, 417–23.

Goldman-Rakic, P. S. (1994). Working memory in schizophrenia. *Journal of Neuropsychiatry and Clinical Neurosciences*, **6**, 348–57.

Graf von Reventlow, H., Ruhrmann, S., Klosterkötter, J. *et al.* (2004). Comparison of inclusion criteria for an early detection of psychosis study across different countries: first results from the European Prediction of Psychosis Study, EPOS. *Schizophrenia Research*, **67**(Suppl 1), 37.

Green, M. F. (1996). What are the functional consequences of neurocognitive deficits in schizophrenia? *American Journal of Psychiatry*, **153**, 321–30.

Gross, G. (1989). The 'basic' symptoms of schizophrenia. *British Journal of Psychiatry*, **155**(Suppl 7), s21–5.

Häfner, H., Riecher, R. A., Hambrecht, M. *et al.* (1992). IRAOS: an instrument for the assessment of onset and early course of schizophrenia. *Schizophrenia Research*, **6**, 209–23.

Häfner, H., Maurer, K., Loffler, W. & Riecher-Rossler, A. (1993). The influence of age and sex on the onset and early course of schizophrenia. *British Journal of Psychiatry*, **162**, 80–6.

Häfner, H., Maurer, W., Loffler, B. *et al.* (1995). Onset and early course of schizophrenia. In H. Häfner & W. F. Gattaz (eds.), *Search for the Causes of Schizophrenia*. New York: Springer, pp. 43–66.

Häfner, H., Loffler, W., Maurer, K., Hambrecht, M. & van der Heiden, W. (1999). Depression, negative symptoms, social stagnation and social decline in the early course of schizophrenia. *Acta Psychiatrica Scandinavica*, **100**, 105–18.

Häfner, H., Maurer, K., Ruhrmann, S. *et al.* (2004). Early detection and secondary prevention of psychosis: facts and visions. *European Archives of Psychiatry and Clinical Neuroscience*, **254**, 117–28.

Häfner, H., Maurer, K., Trendler, G., van der Heiden, W. & Schmidt, M. (2005). The early course of schizophrenia and depression. *European Archives of Psychiatry and Clinical Neuroscience*, **255**, 167–73.

Haroun, N., Dunn, L., Haroun, A. & Cadenhead, K. (2006). Risk and protection in prodromal schizophrenia: ethical implications for clinical practice and future research. *Schizophrenia Bulletin*, **32**, 166–78.

Hawkins, K. A., Addington, J., Keefe, R. S. E. *et al.* (2004). Neuropsychological status of subjects at high risk for a first episode of psychosis. *Schizophrenia Research*, **67**, 115–22.

Heinrichs, R. W. & Zakzanis, K. K. (1998). Neurocognitive deficit in schizophrenia: a quantitative review of the evidence. *Neuropsychology*, **12**, 426–45.

Heinssen, R. K., Perkins, D. O., Appelbaum, P. S. & Fenton, W. S. (2001). Informed consent in early psychosis research: National Institute of Mental Health Workshop, November 15, 2000. *Schizophrenia Bulletin*, **27**, 571–84.

Hirsch, S., Bowen, J., Emmani, J. *et al.* (1996). A one year prospective study of the effects of life events and medication in the aetiology of schizophrenic relapse. *British Journal of Psychiatry*, **168**, 49–56.

Hubain, P. P., Simonnet, M. P. & Mendlewicz, J. (1986). The dexamethasone suppression test in affective illnesses and schizophrenia: relationship with psychotic symptoms. *Neuropsychobiology*, **16**, 57–60.

Johns, L. C., Cannon, M., Singleton, N. *et al.* (2004). Prevalence and correlates of self-reported psychotic symptoms in the British population. *British Journal of Psychiatry*, **185**, 298–305.

Johnstone, E. C., Ebmeier, K. P., Miller, P., Owens, D. G. & Lawrie, S. M. (2005). Predicting schizophrenia: findings from the Edinburgh High-Risk Study. *British Journal of Psychiatry*, **186**, 18–25.

Jou, R. J., Hardan, A. Y. & Keshavan, M. S. (2005). Reduced cortical folding in individuals at high risk for schizophrenia: a pilot study. *Schizophrenia Research*, **75**, 309–13.

Kaneko, M., Yokoyama, F., Hoshino, Y. *et al.* (1992). Hypothalamic–pituitary–adrenal axis function in chronic schizophrenia: association with clinical features. *Neuropsychobiology*, **25**, 1–7.

Kanner, A. D., Coyne, J. C., Scharfer, C. & Lazarus, R. (1981). Comparison of two modes of stress measurement: daily hassles and uplifts vs major life events. *Journal of Behavioural Medicine*, **4**, 1–39.

Klosterkötter, J., Schultze-Lutter, F., Gross, G., Huber, G. & Steinmeyer, E. M. (1997a). Early self-experienced neuropsychological deficits and subsequent schizophrenic diseases: an 8-year average follow-up prospective study. *Acta Psychiatrica Scandinavica*, **95**, 396–404.

Klosterkötter, J., Gross, G., Huber, G. *et al.* (1997b). Evaluation of the 'Bonn Scale for the Assessment of Basic Symptoms – BSABS' as an instrument for the assessment of schizophrenia proneness: a review of recent findings. *Neurology, Psychiatry and Brain Research*, **5**, 137–50.

Klosterkötter, J., Hellmich, M., Steinmeyer, E. M. & Schultze-Lutter, F. (2001) Diagnosing schizophrenia in the initial prodromal phase. *Archives of General Psychiatry*, **58**, 158–64.

Klosterkötter, J., Birchwood, M., Linzen, D. *et al.* (2005). Overview on the recruitment, sample characteristics, and distribution of inclusion criteria of the European Prediction of Psychosis Study (EPOS). *European Psychiatry*, **20**(Suppl 1), s48.

Krabbendam, L., Myin-Germeys, I., Hanssen, M. *et al.* (2005). Development of depressed mood predicts onset of psychotic disorder in individuals who report hallucinatory experiences. *British Journal of Clinical Psychology*, **44**, 113–25.

Kraepelin, E. (1919). *Dementia Praecox*. New York: Churchill Livingstone.

Kulynych, J. J., Luevano, L. F., Jones, D. W. & Weinberger, D. R. (1997). Cortical abnormality in schizophrenia: an in vivo application of the gyrification index. *Biological Psychiatry*, **41**, 995–9.

Larsen, T. K. (2002). The transition from premorbid period to psychosis: how can it be described? *Acta Psychiatrica Scandinavica*, **106**(Suppl), S10–11.

Lawrie, S. M., Whalley, H., Abukmeil, S. S. *et al.* (2002). Temporal lobe volume changes in people at high risk of schizophrenia with psychotic symptoms. *British Journal of Psychiatry*, **181**, 138–43.

Leff, J., Kuipers, L., Berkowitz, R., Vaughn, L. & Sturgeon, D. (1983). Life events, relatives expressed emotion and maintenance neuroleptics in schizophrenic relapse. *Psychological Medicine*, **13**, 799–806.

Lencz, T., Smith, C. W., Auther, A. M., Correll, C. U. & Cornblatt, B. A. (2003). The assessment of 'prodromal schizophrenia': unresolved issues and future directions. *Schizophrenia Bulletin*, **29**, 717–28.

Lencz, T., Smith, C. W., Auther, A., Correll, C. U. & Cornblatt, B. (2004). Nonspecific and attenuated negative symptoms in patients at clinical high-risk for schizophrenia. *Schizophrenia Research*, **68**, 37–48.

Lencz, T., Smith, C. W., McLaughlin, D. *et al.* (2006). Generalized and specific neurocognitive deficits in prodromal schizophrenia. *Biological Psychiatry*, **59**, 863–71.

Linzen, D. & van Amelsvoort, T. (2007). Cannabis and psychosis: an update on course and biological plausible mechanisms. *Current Opinion in Psychiatry*, **20**, 116–20.

Loranger, A. W., Sartorius, N., Andreoli, A. *et al.* (1994). The International Personality Disorder Examination. The World Health Organization Alcohol, Drug Abuse and Mental Health Administration pilot study of personality disorders. *Archives of General Psychiatry*, **51**, 215–24.

Malla, A. K. & Norman, R. M. G. (1992). Relationship of life events and daily stressors to symptomatology in schizophrenia. *Journal of Nervous and Mental Disease*, **180**, 664–7.

Malla, A. K., Cortese, L., Shaw, T. S. & Ginsberg, B. (1990). Life events and relapse in schizophrenia: a one year prospective study. *Social Psychiatry and Psychiatric Epidemiology*, **25**, 221–4.

Mason, O., Startup, M., Halpin, S. *et al.* (2004). State and trait predictors of transition to first episode psychosis among individuals with at risk mental states. *Schizophrenia Research*, **71**, 227–37.

McGlashan, T. H. (2001). Psychosis treatment prior to psychosis onset: ethical issues. *Schizophrenia Research*, **51**, 47–54.

McGlashan, T. H., Zipursky, R. B., Perkins, D. *et al.* (2006). Randomized, double-blind trial of olanzapine versus placebo in patients prodromally symptomatic for psychosis. *American Journal of Psychiatry*, **163**, 790–9.

McGorry, P. D., Yung, A. & Phillips, L. (2001). Ethics and early intervention in psychosis: keeping up the pace and staying in step. *Schizophrenia Research*, **51**, 17–29.

McGorry, P. D., Yung, A. R., Phillips, L. J. *et al.* (2002). Randomized controlled trial of interventions designed to reduce the risk of progression to first episode psychosis in a clinical sample with subthreshold symptoms. *Archives of General Psychiatry*, **59**, 921–8.

McGorry, P. D., Yung, A. R. & Phillips, L. J. (2003). The 'close-in' or ultra high risk model: a safe and effective strategy for research and clinical intervention in prepsychotic mental disorder. *Schizophrenia Bulletin*, **29**, 771–90.

Mednick, S. A., Parnas, J., Schulsinger, F. & Mednick, B. (1987). The Copenhagen High-Risk Project, 1962–1986. *Schizophrenia Bulletin*, **13**, 485–96.

Miller, T. J., McGlashan, T. H., Rosen, J. L. *et al.* (2002). Prospective diagnosis of the initial prodrome for schizophrenia based on the Structured Interview for Prodromal Syndromes: preliminary evidence of interrater reliability and predictive validity. *American Journal of Psychiatry*, **159**, 863–5.

Miller, T. J., McGlashan, T. H., Rosen, J. L. *et al.* (2003a). Prodromal assessment with the structured interview for prodromal syndromes and the scale of prodromal symptoms: predictive validity, interrater reliability, and training to reliability. *Schizophrenia Bulletin*, **29**, 703–15.

Miller, T. J., Zipursky, R. B., Perkins, D. *et al.* (2003b). The PRIME North America randomized double-blind clinical trial of olanzapine versus placebo in patients at risk of being prodromally symptomatic for psychosis. II. Baseline characteristics of the 'prodromal' sample. *Schizophrenia Research*, **61**, 19–30.

Morrison, A. P., Bentall, R. P., French, P. *et al.* (2002). Randomised controlled trial of early detection and cognitive therapy for preventing transition to psychosis in high-risk individuals: study design and interim analysis of transition rate and psychological risk factors. *British Journal of Psychiatry*, **181**(Suppl), s78–84.

Morrison, A. P., French, P., Walford, L. *et al.* (2004). Cognitive therapy for the prevention of psychosis in people at ultra-high risk: randomised controlled trial. *British Journal of Psychiatry*, **185**, 291–7.

Niendam, T. A., Bearden, C. E., Johnson, J. K. *et al.* (2006). Neurocognitive performance and functional disability in the psychosis prodrome. *Schizophrenia Research*, **84**, 100–11.

Nuechterlein, K. H., Dawson, M. E., Ventura, J. *et al.* (1994). The vulnerability/stress model of schizophrenic relapse: a longitudinal study. *Acta Psychiatrica Scandanivica*, **89**, 58–64.

Olsen, K. A. & Rosenbaum, B. (2006). Prospective investigations of the prodromal state of schizophrenia: review of studies. *Acta Psychiatrica Scandinavica*, **113**, 247–72.

Overall, J. E. & Gorham, D. R. (1962). The Brief Psychiatric Rating Scale. *Psychological Reports*, **10**, 799–812.

Pantelis, C., Barnes, T. R., Nelson, H. E. *et al.* (1997). Frontal – striatal cognitive deficits in patients with chronic schizophrenia. *Brain*, **120**, 1823–43.

Pantelis, C., Wood, S. J. & Maruff, P. (2002). Schizophrenia. In A. M. Owen & J. Harrison (eds.), *Cognitive Deficits in Brain Disorders*. London: Martin Dunitz, pp. 217–48.

Pantelis, C., Velakoulis, D., McGorry, P. D. *et al.* (2003). Neuroanatomical abnormalities before and after onset of psychosis: a cross-sectional and longitudinal MRI comparison. *Lancet*, **361**, 281–8.

Pariante, C. M., Vassilopoulou, K., Velakoulis, D. *et al.* (2004). Abnormal pituitary volume in psychosis. *British Journal of Psychiatry*, **185**, 5–10.

Park, S., Püschel, J., Sauter, B. H., Rentsch, M. & Hell, D. (1999). Spatial working memory deficits and clinical symptoms in schizophrenia: a 4-month follow-up study. *Biological Psychiatry*, **46**, 392–400.

Phillips, L., Curry, C., Yung, A. *et al.* (2002a). Cannabis use is not associated with the development of psychosis in an 'ultra' high-risk group. *Australian and New Zealand Journal of Psychiatry*, **36**, 800–6.

Phillips, L. J., Velakoulis, D., Pantelis, C. *et al.* (2002b). Non-reduction in hippocampal volume is associated with risk for psychosis. *Schizophrenia Research*, **58**, 145–58.

Ruhrmann, S., Schultze-Lutter, F. & Klosterkötter, J. (2003). Early detection and intervention in the initial prodromal phase of schizophrenia. *Pharmacopsychiatry*, **36**(Suppl), s162–7.

Ruhrmann, S., Schultze-Lutter, F., Maier, W. & Klosterkötter, J. (2005). Pharmacological intervention in the initial prodromal phase of psychosis. *European Psychiatry*, **20**, 1–6.

Ruhrmann, S., Bechdolf, A., Kühn, K. *et al.* (2007). Acute effects of treatment for prodromal symptoms in persons putatively in a late initial prodromal state of psychosis. *British Journal of Psychiatry*, **191**(Suppl 51), s88–95.

Schultze-Lutter, F. (2001). Früherkennung der Schizophrenie anhand subjektiver Beschwerdeschilderungen: ein methodenkritischer Vergleich der Vorhersageleistung nonparametrischer statistischer und alternativer Verfahren zur Generierung von Vorhersagemodellen. Ph.D. thesis, University of Cologne (http://www.ub.uni-koeln.de/ediss/archiv/2001/11w1210.pdf).

Schultze-Lutter, F. (2004). Prediction of psychosis is necessary and possible. In C. McDonald, K. Schultz, R. Murray & P. Wright (eds.), *Schizophrenia: Challenging the Orthodox*. London: Taylor & Francis, pp. 81–90.

Schultze-Lutter, F., Wieneke, A., Picker, H. *et al.* (2004). The Schizophrenia Prediction Instrument, Adult Version (SPI-A). *Schizophrenia Research*, **70**(Suppl 1), s76–7.

Schultze-Lutter, F., Ruhrmann, S. & Klosterkötter, J. (2006). Can schizophrenia be predicted phenomenologically? In J. O. Johannessen, B. V. Martindale & J. Cullberg (eds.), *Evolving Psychosis*. New York: Routledge/Taylor & Francis, pp. 104–23.

Schultze-Lutter, F., Addington, J., Klosterkötter, J. & Ruhrmann, S. (2007a). *Schizophrenia Proneness Instrument, Adult version (SPI-A)*. Rome: Giovanni Fioriti Editore s.r.l.

Schultze-Lutter, F., Klosterkötter, J., Picker, H., Steinmeyer, E. M. & Ruhrmann, S. (2007b). Predicting first-episode psychosis by basic symptom criteria. *Clinical Neuropsychiatry*, **4**, 11–22.

Schultze-Lutter, F., Ruhrmann, S., Picker, H. *et al.* (2007c). Basic symptoms in early psychotic and depressive disorders. *British Journal of Psychiatry*, **191**(Suppl 51), s31–7.

Seidman, L. J., Giuliano, A. J., Smith, C. W. *et al.* (2006). Neuropsychological functioning in adolescents and young adults at genetic risk for schizophrenia and affective psychoses: results from the Harvard and Hillside Adolescent High Risk Studies. *Schizophrenia Bulletin*, **32**, 507–24.

Snitz, B. E., Macdonald, A. W. III, & Carter, C. S. (2006). Cognitive deficits in unaffected first-degree relatives of schizophrenia patients: a meta-analytic review of putative endophenotypes. *Schizophrenia Bulletin*, **32**, 179–94.

Strauss, J. S. (1969). Hallucinations and delusions as points on continua function. *Archives of General Psychiatry*, **21**, 581–6.

Sullivan, H. S. (1994). The onset of schizophrenia. *American Journal of Psychiatry*, **151**, 135–9.

Tien, A. Y. (1991). Distributions of hallucinations in the population. *Social Psychiatry and Psychiatric Epidemiology*, **26**, 287–92.

van Os, J., Hanssen, M., Bijl, R. V. & Vollebergh, W. (2001). Prevalence of psychotic disorder and community level of psychotic symptoms: an urban-rural comparison. *Archives of General Psychiatry*, **58**, 663–8.

Velakoulis, D., Pantelis, C., McGorry, P. D. *et al.* (1999). Hippocampal volume in first-episode psychoses and chronic schizophrenia: a high resolution magnetic resonance imaging study. *Archives of General Psychiatry*, **56**, 133–41.

Ventura, J., Nuechterlein, K. H., Lukoff, D. & Hardesty, J. P. (1989). A prospective study of stressful life events and schizophrenic relapse. *Journal of Abnormal Psychology*, **98**, 407–11.

Verdoux, H., van Os, J., Maurice-Tison, S. *et al.* (1998). Is early adulthood a critical developmental stage for psychosis proneness? A survey of delusional ideation in normal subjects. *Schizophrenia Research*, **29**, 24.

Verdoux, H., van Os, J., Maurice-Tison, S. *et al.* (1999). Increased occurrence of depression in psychosis-prone subjects: a follow-up study in primary care settings. *Comprehensive Psychiatry*, **40**, 462–8.

Warner, R. (2005). Problems with early and very early intervention in psychosis. *British Journal of Psychiatry*, **48** (Suppl), s104–7.

Webster, M. J., Knable, M. B., O'Grady, J., Orthmann, J. & Weickert, C. S. (2002). Regional specificity of brain glucocorticoid receptor mRNA alterations in subjects with schizophrenia and mood disorders. *Molecular Psychiatry*, **7**, 985–94.

Wölwer, W., Buchkremer, G., Häfner, H. *et al.* (2003). German research network on schizophrenia. Bridging the gap between research and care. *European Archives of Psychiatry and Clinical Neuroscience*, **253**, 321–9.

Wood, S. J., Pantelis, C., Proffitt, T. *et al.* (2003). Spatial working memory ability is a marker of risk-for-psychosis. *Psychological Medicine*, **33**, 1239–47.

Woods, S. W., Brier, A., Zipursky, R. B. *et al.* (2003). Randomized trial of olanzapine versus placebo in the symptomatic acute treatment of the schizophrenic prodrome. *Biological Psychiatry*, **54**, 453–64.

Yung, A. R. (2003). Commentary: the schizophrenia prodrome: a high-risk concept. *Schizophrenia Bulletin*, **29**, 859–65.

Yung, A. R. & McGorry, P. D. (1996). The prodromal phase of first-episode psychosis: past and current conceptualizations. *Schizophrenia Bulletin*, **22**, 353–70.

Yung, A. R. & McGorry, P. D. (1997). Is pre-psychotic intervention realistic in schizophrenia and related disorders? *Australian and New Zealand Journal of Psychiatry*, **31**, 799–805.

Yung, A. R. & McGorry, P. (2003). Keeping an open mind: investigating options for treatment of the pre-psychotic phase. *Journal of Mental Health*, **12**, 341–3.

Yung, A. R., McGorry, P. D., McFarlane, C. A. & Patton, G. (1995). The PACE Clinic: development of a clinical service for young people at high risk of psychosis. *Australasian Psychiatry*, **3**, 345–9.

Yung, A. R., McGorry, P. D., McFarlane, C. A. *et al.* (1996). Monitoring and care of young people at incipient risk of psychosis. *Schizophrenia Bulletin*, **22**, 283–303.

Yung, A. R., Phillips, L. J., McGorry, P. D. *et al.* (1998). The prediction of psychosis: a step towards indicated prevention of schizophrenia? *British Journal of Psychiatry*, **173**(Suppl 33), 14–20.

Yung, A. R., Phillips, L. J., Yuen, H. P. *et al.* (2003). Psychosis prediction: 12-month follow up of a high-risk ('prodromal') group. *Schizophrenia Research*, **60**, 21–32.

Yung, A. R., Phillips, L. J. & McGorry, P. D. (2004a). *Treating Schizophrenia in the Pre-Psychotic Phase*. London: Dunitz.

Yung, A. R., Phillips, L. J., Yuen, H. P. & McGorry, P. D. (2004b). Risk factors for psychosis in an ultra high-risk group: psychopathology and clinical features. *Schizophrenia Research*, **67**, 131–42.

Yung, A. R., Yuen, H. P., McGorry, P. D. *et al.* (2005). Mapping the onset of psychosis: the Comprehensive Assessment of At Risk Mental States (CAARMS). *Australian and New Zealand Journal of Psychiatry*, **39**, 964–71.

Yung, A. R., Stanford, C., Cosgrave, E. *et al.* (2006a). Testing the ultra high risk (prodromal) criteria for the prediction of psychosis in a clinical sample of young people. *Schizophrenia Research*, **84**, 57–66.

Yung, A. R., Buckby, J. A., Cotton, S. M. *et al.* (2006b). Psychotic-like experiences in non-psychotic help-seekers: associations with distress, depression and disability. *Schizophrenia Bulletin*, **32**, 352–9.

Yung, A. R., Yuen, H. P., Berger, G. *et al.* (2007). Declining transition rate in ultra high risk (prodromal) services: dilution or reduction of risk? *Schizophrenia Bulletin*, **33**, 673–81.

7

At-risk mental state: management

Lisa J. Phillips, Jean Addington and Anthony P. Morrison

Introduction

The potential benefits of providing effective treatment for young people at ultra-high risk (UHR) of developing a psychotic disorder have been recognized for some time. Early last century, Harry Stack Sullivan (1927) speculated that a full-blown psychotic illness might be preventable if it were possible to identify high-risk individuals during the early-onset phase of illness (known as the *prodrome*) and to provide them with appropriate and effective treatment. Even if it were not completely possible to prevent the development of a psychotic episode, it was thought that such early intervention might minimize the impact that the episode has on functioning, as the development of disability during the prodromal phase of illness creates a ceiling for eventual recovery (Häfner *et al.*, 1995a).

As outlined in Chapter 6, the at-risk mental state (ARMS) criteria were first developed at the Personal Assessment and Crisis Evaluation (PACE) Clinic in Melbourne, Australia, but they have subsequently been adopted at many other sites, such as Outreach and Support in South London (OASIS: Broome *et al.*, 2005); Early Detection and Intervention Evaluation, Manchester, UK (EDIE: Morrison *et al.*, 2004); Psychological Assistance Service in Newcastle, Australia (PAS: Mason *et al.*, 2004) and the North American Prevention through Risk Identification, Management and Education study (PRIME: McGlashan *et al.*, 2003). These criteria reliably identify young people who are at heightened risk or UHR for psychosis – or who are in the early stages of the onset of illness. The 12-month transition rate to full-blown psychosis of young people who meet these

criteria approaches 40% despite the provision of supportive psychotherapy and, where appropriate, antidepressant or anxiolytic medication (Cadenhead, 2002; Larsen, 2002; Mason *et al.*, 2004; Miller *et al.*, 2003a; Morrison *et al.*, 2004; Yung *et al.*, 2003). This rate of progression to illness is much higher than the incidence rate in the general population – between 0.2 and 0.5 new cases per 1000 population per year (Jablensky *et al.*, 1992) – and the 10–12% statistical risk a child of a parent with schizophrenia has of developing the illness later in life (Jablensky & Eaton, 1995).

Studies with UHR cohorts have shown that individuals who meet ARMS criteria experience an extremely diverse array of symptoms and behaviours. These experiences extend beyond the subthreshold psychotic symptoms that form the basis of the ARMS criteria, with depression, anxiety, substance-use problems and personality disorder traits commonly reported (Meyer *et al.*, 2005; Svirkis *et al.*, 2005). Although these symptoms do not always reach diagnostic thresholds, two studies have indicated that the American Psychiatric Association's DSM-IV non-psychotic diagnostic criteria (APA, 1994) are met by up to 50% of young people who meet ARMS criteria when they are first assessed (Meyer *et al.*, 2005; Yung, Phillips & McGorry, 2004).

Retrospective studies of patients with schizophrenia have reported that significant psychosocial decline occurs even before the onset of frank psychosis (Agerbo *et al.*, 2003; Häfner *et al.*, 1995b; Yung & McGorry, 1996). The vast majority of young people who meet ARMS criteria describe difficulty maintaining their usual activities and routines. They are also often highly distressed by their symptoms and compromised functioning.

The Recognition and Management of Early Psychosis: A Preventive Approach, ed. Henry J. Jackson and Patrick D. McGorry. Published by Cambridge University Press. © Cambridge University Press 2009.

In light of the above, treatment for young people who meet ARMS criteria should not only focus on the symptoms that constitute the ARMS criteria but also address the broader range of difficulties with which the young person might present. In this chapter, we aim to provide a critical overview of some of the approaches to treatment of ARMS that have been evaluated to date. Four clinical programmes for young people meeting ARMS criteria and a case study are described to illustrate current treatment approaches.

Ethics

Ethical considerations associated with treatment of young people who meet ARMS criteria have been widely debated (Corcoran, Malaspina & Hercher, 2005; Cornblatt, Lencz & Kane, 2001; Haroun *et al.*, 2006; Lencz *et al.*, 2003; McGlashan, 2001; McGorry, 2005; McGorry, Yung & Phillips, 2001; Post, 2001; Warner, 2005; Yung & McGorry, 2003). Contentious issues include concerns about the stigma associated with being identified as having a label of ARMS; concerns about the provision of treatment to individuals who meet ARMS criteria but are in fact 'false positives' (i.e. met ARMS criteria but in fact are never going to develop full-blown psychosis); what should be said to young people and their families regarding their 'at risk' status; and for how long should treatment be provided (in other words, how long is the period of risk). Many of these issues remain unresolved, even though clinical research into ARMS has now been conducted for over a decade, and further discussion is encouraged. Specific ethical issues related to the provision of medication and psychological treatments are outlined below.

Interventions

Antipsychotic medication

The case supporting antipsychotic medication

There are very few published studies to date that have studied the use of medications with an ARMS population. The first intervention trial at this early stage was

carried out by McGorry and colleagues in Melbourne, Australia. In this study, 59 individuals who met ARMS criteria were randomized to 6 months of active treatment (risperidone 1–2 mg/day plus a modified cognitive–behavioural therapy (CBT) or needs-based intervention alone (McGorry *et al.*, 2002). The mean daily dosage of risperidone for the active treatment group was 1.3 mg. The CBT followed a manual that incorporated a number of 'modules'. In reflection of the stress–vulnerability model of psychosis (Zubin & Spring, 1977), which influenced the CBT approach, all clients received treatment based on a 'stress management' module. The other treatment modules that were developed reflected the wide range of symptoms that can be experienced by individuals during the onset phase of a psychotic disorder (Yung & McGorry, 1996). Therefore, in response to the unique presentation of each client in the active treatment group, CBT-based treatment was provided that addressed positive psychotic symptoms, negative psychotic symptoms and depression or other symptoms (such as anxiety and substance use). The needs-based intervention was provided to all clients involved in the trial, regardless of the group to which they were randomized. Essentially, this treatment incorporated case management (addressing practical issues such as crisis management and difficulties with housing, education or employment), and symptom monitoring. There was a significant difference in the number of psychological sessions attended by clients in the two treatment groups: the active treatment groups attended an average of 11.3 sessions (standard deviation (SD) = 8.4) while the control group attended an average of 5.9 sessions (SD = 4.3). This difference reflects the more intensive nature of the CBT approach.

By the end of the treatment, significantly fewer individuals in the active treatment group had progressed to a first-episode of psychosis than in the needs-based group (9.7% versus 36%). Six months after treatment ended, the differences were no longer significant as more of the active treatment group converted to psychosis (19% versus 36%). Adherence to medication suggested a sustained effect as participants in the active treatment group who were compliant with antipsychotic medication were less likely to develop psychosis than those who were less compliant. Follow-up 3 to 4 years after intake to the study also showed no difference in transition rate to psychosis between the groups (Phillips *et al.*, 2007). These results suggest that a combination of antipsychotic medication and CBT may delay but not necessarily prevent the onset of psychosis in symptomatic high-risk subjects. Furthermore, McGorry *et al.* (2002) reported that high-risk individuals who did not progress to psychosis showed improvement in a range of symptoms and functioning when they received the combination of risperidone and CBT. This was a landmark study in considering the possibility of delaying or even preventing psychosis. However, as with many early studies, there were some methodological limitations that should be acknowledged. First, there was no blinding of subjects or raters to group assignment. Second, combining pharmacological and psychological treatments in the active treatment group does not allow the relative contribution of medication or CBT to be determined. Third, it was difficult to control for adherence to medication.

A second trial with a more rigorous design was initiated in 1999 by Thomas McGlashan at Yale University and included additional sites at the University of Calgary, the University of Toronto and the University of North Carolina (principal investigators J. Addington, R. Zipursky and D. Perkins, respectively). The PRIME study was a randomized double-blind parallel study of 60 prodromal subjects comparing the efficacy of a low-dose antipsychotic drug (5–15 mg/day olanzapine) with placebo in preventing or delaying the onset of psychosis (McGlashan *et al.*, 2003). These individuals were help-seeking and were between the ages of 12 and 45 years, with a mean age of 17 years. The Structured Interview for Prodromal Syndromes (Hawkins *et al.*, 2004; Miller *et al.*, 2002, 2003b) was used to determine if subjects met the criteria for prodromal symptoms (Miller *et al.*, 2002). These criteria operationally define the three prodromal syndromes (attenuated positive symptoms, genetic risk and deterioration and brief intermittent psychotic state) of Yung and McGorry (1996; see Ch. 6). Subjects were randomized to medication or placebo for 1 year and then in the second year did not receive any medications. Efficacy measures included the conversion-to-psychosis rate and the scores on the Scale of Prodromal Symptoms (SOPS).

A range of psychosocial interventions were available to all patients (drug and placebo). These included case management, supportive therapy, education regarding symptoms and medication and problem-solving strategies. The nature of the different interventions varied across sites, but all sites attempted to apply their particular treatments in a uniform fashion to all of their patients as needed.

At initial presentation, these subjects were help-seeking and symptomatic with a wide range of attenuated positive and negative symptoms. On average, they were rated at study entry as 'moderately ill' on the Clinical Global Impression scale. They demonstrated significant impairment in functioning having a mean rating of 42 on the Global Assessment of Functioning scale (Miller *et al.*, 2003a). Short-term analyses of this study at 8 weeks suggested that olanzapine was associated with significantly greater symptomatic improvement in prodromal symptoms than placebo (Woods *et al.*, 2002). At the 1-year follow-up, 16% of olanzapine-treated subjects converted to psychosis compared with 38% of placebo-treated subjects. Furthermore, the hazard of conversion to psychosis among placebo-treated patients was approximately 2.5 times that of the olanzapine-treated patients, a trend-level difference (McGlashan *et al.*, 2006). Interpretation of these findings may be limited by the small sample size. In year two, the conversion-to-psychosis rate did not differ significantly between the groups. Of the former olanzapine-treated subjects, three converted (33%) compared with two (25%) of the former placebo-treated subjects.

The groups did not differ significantly in mean changes from baseline to the 'last observation carried forward' endpoint with the exception of the positive symptom scores on the SOPS. There were significant baseline-to-endpoint improvement for the olanzapine-treated group in SOPS total ($p = 0.04$) and SOPS positive symptoms ($p < 0.002$) (McGlashan *et al.*, 2006). For example, changes on the positive symptoms items on the SOPS were on average 9.6 to 9.9 for the placebo group and 10.7 to 17.2 for the olanzapine-treated group. Although the primary objective in this study of demonstrating a significant treatment difference in the conversion-to-psychosis rate – was not met, the trend-level differences ($p = 0.08$; Fisher's exact test) between treatment groups in the conversion-to-psychosis rate point to the possibility that olanzapine might reduce the rate of conversion to psychosis and delay the onset of psychosis.

Overall, these medication trials suggest some benefits for those with early attenuated psychotic symptoms. Patients receiving medications showed significantly greater improvement in positive and total prodromal symptom severity over the first year in the PRIME study, a finding not seen in the placebo group (McGlashan *et al.*, 2006). In the PACE study, there was symptomatic and functional improvement in the treatment group as well as in the control group who received supportive, needs-based counselling (McGorry *et al.*, 2002). Medication seems to alleviate the early symptoms in those who may be prodromal for schizophrenic psychosis and to delay onset. These at-risk individuals entering medication trials (McGorry *et al.*, 2002; Miller *et al.*, 2003a) are usually in the late pre-onset period, reflected in their high rate of attenuated psychotic symptoms, poor level of functioning and high rates of conversion to psychosis.

Consequently, in support of medication trials, it should be noted that those being randomized for treatment are highly symptomatic and in these trials several individuals convert in the first few weeks, indicating that they were on the cusp of developing a full-blown psychotic illness. Furthermore, there seems to be some self-selection process occurring. In a recent publication of recruitment and decision data from the Calgary PRIME Clinic, it was reported that 95 individuals were identified as potentially eligible for the study during a 24-month recruitment period (Addington & Addington, 2005). After an assessment to determine if study criteria were met, it was found that 36 (38%) were definitely eligible for entry to the trial. However, 30 (83%) of these eligible persons refused to enter the trial, with 12 (39%) of these refusers stating that they were troubled by their symptoms, wanted active treatment as soon as possible and did not want to risk randomization to the placebo group. They were offered treatment in the Calgary Early Psychosis Program. Of the 36 eligible subjects 17 (47%) said they often felt debilitated by their symptoms but did not want to take medication. This group chose

either monitoring or education or both. The remaining five (14%) consented to enter the medication trial. An assessment of presenting symptoms with SOPS (Miller *et al.*, 2002, 2003b) demonstrated that those who wanted treatment and those who entered the trial had significantly higher scores on both the positive and negative symptom scales compared with those who did not want active treatment (Miller *et al.*, 2003a). This suggests that, in fact, patients themselves support a phased approach, where education and support or a psychological treatment may be preferred in the earlier phases of the high-risk period and medications seen as a preferred choice in the later phases when symptoms become more intense and have more impact. This supports suggestions that there is a role for medications at some point in the prepsychotic phase.

The case against antipsychotic medication

There are a number of reasons why providing antipsychotic medication to people at risk of developing psychosis may not be desirable (Bentall & Morrison, 2002). Probably most importantly, there are potentially serious side effects associated with all antipsychotic medications. These include extrapyramidal side effects such as tardive dyskinesia, which is often irreversible, although such problems are less common with the newer, atypical antipsychotics (Kane, 2004; Margolese *et al.*, 2005). However, even the most recent developments in antipsychotic medications are associated with distressing side effects; for example, olanzapine, the medication used in the PRIME study, is commonly associated with weight gain, diabetes and sexual dysfunction (none of which are likely to appeal to young people) (Eder-Ischia, Ebenbichler & Fleischhacker, 2005; Kinon *et al.*, 2005, Newcomer, 2005). Risperidone, used in the PACE study, has been associated with sexual dysfunction and insomnia (Jayaram, Hosalli & Stroup, 2006). There is also the remote risk of fatal adverse reactions, such as neuroleptic malignant syndrome (Caroff *et al.*, 2002; Sachdev, 2005). Emerging evidence also suggests that certain antipsychotics – particularly the older medications such as haloperidol – may actually damage the brain, with a recent study demonstrating that antipsychotic medication reduced grey matter volume in the brains of patients with a first episode of psychosis (Lieberman *et al.*, 2005). It is noted that the newer second-generation antipsychotic medications that have been used in trials with young people at risk of psychosis may, in fact, have neuro-protective qualities.

Another factor that may reduce the desirability of using antipsychotic medication with this population is that the vast majority of ARMS patients are concerned that they are going 'mad' (French & Morrison, 2004). If someone is concerned that they are losing mental control and have worries that perhaps they are going 'mad', or in fact are 'mad' (although, by definition, they are not), and this causes them distress, being prescribed medication designed for psychosis and schizophrenia may not disabuse them of this concern, especially if this occurs without the provision of information about the potential benefits of taking the medication. Other problems that people at risk of psychosis may have, also mean antipsychotic medication may be unsuitable. For example, 29% of the sample in the PACE intervention study received a diagnosis of a non-psychotic axis I disorder at completion (McGorry *et al.*, 2002), suggesting that treatments that target emotional disorders may be more useful in particular to the clients who are false positives. Many of the problems identified by people meeting ARMS criteria are to do with anxiety, depression and social relationships (French & Morrison, 2004), which are unlikely to respond to all antipsychotic drugs. Although there is some recent evidence supporting the use of atypical antipsychotic medication in the treatment of anxiety and depressive disorders (Nemeroff, 2005; Stathis, Martin & McKenna, 2005), there are many other treatment options for such difficulties – treatments that possess greater evidence bases and have less-severe side effects.

Psychosis is not always distressing, and there is evidence that psychotic experiences can be pleasurable or functional; for example, voice hearers often cite advantages such as the provision of companionship (Miller, O'Connor & DiPasquale, 1993), and paranoia may be viewed as a useful survival strategy (Morrison *et al.*, 2005). There are also demonstrable links between creativity and psychosis (Andreasen, 1987; O'Reilly, Dunbar & Bentall, 2001). Therefore, treatments that

seek to eradicate psychotic experiences may not be desirable for people whose psychotic experiences are not immediately associated with corresponding distress or disability.

Finally, it would appear that antipsychotic medications are less acceptable to service users themselves. For example, the dropout rates in studies using antipsychotic medications (McGorry *et al.*, 2002; Woods *et al.*, 2003) appear higher than in those using non-pharmacological intervention (Morrison *et al.*, 2004). For the PACE study, in addition to the 54% in the treatment group who were not at all or only partially compliant with risperidone, 23% of participants in the active treatment group dropped out and were not able to be followed up over the course of the study, while only 14% in the control group were lost to follow-up. In the PRIME trial (McGlashan *et al.*, 2006), of the 31 olanzapine-treated subjects, 17 dropped out with 5 converting, and of the 29 placebo-treated subjects, 10 dropped out with 11 converting. In the EDIE study, which involved psychological intervention alone, the consent to randomization rate was 95% and the dropout rate was only 14% (Morrison *et al.*, 2004).

Psychological interventions

The case supporting psychological interventions

There is one published trial of psychological intervention alone, which was completed in Manchester, UK. The EDIE study was a single-blind randomized controlled trial of cognitive therapy with individuals at high risk of psychosis (Morrison *et al.*, 2004). In this study, 58 individuals were randomized to either cognitive therapy or monitoring. The therapy was provided for the first 6 months and all patients were monitored on a monthly basis for 12 months. Cognitive therapy was shown to significantly reduce the likelihood of making progression to psychosis over 12 months, as defined on the Positive and Negative Syndrome Scale (Kay, Fiszbein & Opler, 1987) (6% versus 22%); being prescribed antipsychotic medication (6% versus 30%); and meeting criteria for a DSM-IV diagnosis of a psychotic disorder (APA, 1994) (6% versus 26%). Cognitive therapy also improved positive symptoms in the sample. It is of note that 95% of subjects consented to participate in this trial. Follow-up 3 years after entry to the trial indicated that cognitive therapy was associated with a significantly lower rate of transition to psychosis (when baseline cognitive factors were controlled for) and significantly reduced the likelihood of being prescribed antipsychotic medication (Morrison *et al.*, 2007).

The cognitive therapy utilized in this trial was based on an empirically validated cognitive model of psychosis (Morrison, 2001). The therapy adhered to the structure and principles of cognitive therapy (Beck, 1976), being time limited (up to a maximum of 26 sessions over 6 months; average number of sessions 12), problem orientated, collaborative and involving the use of homework tasks and guided discovery. Initial stages of therapy included a cognitive–behavioural assessment, the development of a shared list of problems and goals, and the generation of a case formulation based on the cognitive model. Common techniques, which were collaboratively selected on the basis of a shared case formulation, included the examination of advantages and disadvantages associated with particular ways of thinking and behaving, consideration of evidence, generations of alternative explanations and the use of behavioural experiments to evaluate beliefs. A comprehensive description of the therapy is provided in the treatment manual utilized in the trial (French & Morrison, 2004).

It may be that antipsychotic drugs are potentially useful in the later phases of the prodromal period when attenuated psychotic symptoms are clearly evident and the individual is potentially on the edge of a conversion to full threshold psychosis. Psychological interventions might be expected to be most promising at earlier and less-symptomatic stages of the prodrome. In fact, in the early stages of the putatively prodromal period, the presenting symptoms are not only less severe but also less specific. These individuals present with a wider range of concerns. They need and want to understand their perceptual difficulties; to manage the stress, depression, anxiety, sleep disturbance and decline in functioning; and to be supported through this difficult period of their lives (Yung *et al.*, 2003). These symptoms and concerns may actually be more modifiable with a psychological intervention than with

medication. French and Morrison (2004) presented several arguments to support why CBT may be a beneficial psychological intervention for this UHR group, including that it addresses the range of symptoms and concerns present in the UHR period and teaches potentially effective strategies to protect against the impact of environmental stressors that may contribute to the emergence of psychosis. For example, CBT was developed for mood disorders and has an extensive evidence base for treating anxiety disorders as well, and these problems are very common in the ARMS population (Yung & McGorry, 1996). Additionally, CBT is effective for the treatment of drug-resistant psychotic symptoms and relapse prevention (Valmaggia *et al.*, 2005; Zimmermann *et al.*, 2005), so it should be effective for the concerns of people with attenuated psychotic symptoms or with brief limited intermittent psychotic symptoms (Yung, Phillips & McGorry, 2004). It is also worth considering that the collaborative nature of CBT and the fact that it is problem orientated and involves working towards shared goals should ensure that it is useful and acceptable to clients who are 'false positives'. Finally, these young people themselves often express a preference for psychological interventions and will participate in trials of psychological interventions (Addington & Addington, 2005; Morrison *et al.*, 2004).

The case against psychological interventions

There are a number of factors that may question the desirability of utilizing psychological interventions to prevent psychosis (Warner, 2003). For example, fear and stigma may be associated with being labelled as at risk of developing psychosis, regardless of the type of intervention, although this hypothesis is not supported by any direct evidence to date. It may also be stigmatizing to receive psychological therapy; however, there is evidence that a psychological explanation of mental distress is less stigmatizing than a biological one (Read & Haslam, 2004). For example, a recent study found that young adults with biological causal beliefs, in comparison with those with psychosocial causal beliefs, view patients with mental health problems as more dangerous and unpredictable

(Read & Harre, 2001). It has also been suggested that people may impose restrictions upon themselves, avoiding stress because they identify themselves as being at risk of psychosis (Warner, 2003). However, if this belief was held by an individual, it could be challenged during the course of cognitive therapy. It is also possible that being treated for risk of developing psychosis may increase hopelessness about the future, which could lead to an increase in suicidal ideation. Again, if this is recognized then steps can be taken to prevent it, such as setting goals and providing normalizing information.

Other potential interventions

In addition to the specific treatment options for at-risk cohorts that are outlined above, there are other potential treatment options: social interventions, monitoring and no intervention at all.

Social interventions

Although there has been little research evaluating the effectiveness of social interventions for the prevention of psychosis, or the reduction of distress and improvement in quality of life for people who meet ARMS criteria, it would seem sensible to offer such approaches. For example, ensuring that people have adequate housing, meaningful social roles and satisfactory social networks is likely to contribute towards achieving these goals. There is certainly evidence that factors such as employment, vocational training and educational opportunities contribute to recovery from psychosis (Warner, 1985), as do social relationships and empowerment of an individual within society (Deegan, 1988). Therefore, it would seem relatively uncontroversial to provide such interventions to young people at risk of developing psychosis. Other than the arguments that can be levelled at all preventive approaches (such as the risk of self-imposed restrictions or unnecessary stigmatization), the only disadvantage of the social approaches is economic cost, since many of these components are expensive. However, if the personal, familial and societal costs (including inpatient hospital care, involvement with criminal justice systems

and loss of employment days) are included in calculations, it may be that the provision of such interventions may be cost-effective in the long term. It should be noted that such treatment has been incorporated within the PACE, EDIE and PRIME models but has not been tested on its own.

Monitoring

Regular monitoring at least ensures that appropriate treatment can be commenced reasonably rapidly if a full-blown psychotic episode develops. The contact and engagement the young person and their family have had with a clinical service during the phase of monitoring may also assist in the process of commencing treatment, as a therapeutic relationship has already been established. A clear rationale for the need for treatment can be given to the young person and their family, reflecting on the changes in symptomatology and functioning that have occurred and have been documented over the monitoring period.

No intervention

Currently, most young people who meet ARMS criteria receive no treatment or monitoring unless they are fortunate enough to reside within the catchment area for an 'at risk' clinic and actively seek treatment. Clearly, we do not think that this is the optimal situation – young people who meet ARMS criteria describe a range of psychological difficulties and problems (as reported above), are often distressed by their experiences and seek treatment and support – or at least an explanation for what is occurring. Their families are also often distressed and upset. The other risk of no intervention is that frank psychosis may develop and progress undetected and untreated for some time. As longer durations of untreated psychosis have been repeatedly associated with poorer outcomes (Carbone et al., 1999; Harrigan, McGorry & Krstev, 2003; Harris et al., 2005; Norman, Lewis & Marshall, 2005), this scenario is not ideal. However, providing no intervention at all avoids any possible stigmatizing effect that might result from even minimal involvement in a clinical service.

Table 7.1. Common problems experienced by young people with an at-risk mental state, and possible interventions

Problem	Possible interventions
Suspiciousness/paranoia	Antipsychotic medication
	Reality testing/behavioural experiments (Siddle & Haddock, 2004)
	Normalization techniques (Kingdon & Turkington, 1994)
Perceptual abnormalities	Antipsychotic medication
	Cognitive restructuring (Chadwick *et al.*, 1996; Fowler *et al.*, 1995)
	Coping enhancement (e.g. distraction; Tarrier *et al.*, 1990)
Delusional thinking	Cognitive therapy (Chadwick *et al.*, 1996; Fowler *et al.*, 1995)
Negative symptoms	Psychosocial approaches (Falzer, Stayner & Davidson, 2004)
Anxiety	Anxiolytic medication
	Relaxation training (Bernstein & Borkovec, 1973; Ost, 1987)
	Psychoeducation about stress and coping
	Cognitive restructuring
	Mindfulness techniques (Germer, 2005)
Anger, irritability	Problem solving
	Assertiveness training
	Cognitive restructuring (Deffenbacher & McKay, 2000)
Depression	Antidepressant medication
	Cognitive restructuring (Beck *et al.*, 1979; Meichenbaum, 1975)
	Behavioural activation
	Mindfulness techniques (Roemer & Orsillo, 2002; Ramel *et al.*, 2004)
Sleep disturbance	Anxiolytic medication
	Psychoeducation about sleep hygiene
Social withdrawal	Cognitive restructuring (Fowler *et al.*, 1995)
Reduced concentration and attention	Cognitive remediation therapy (Wykes & van der Gaaz, 2001)
Reduced motivation and interest	Activity scheduling and goal setting (Fowler *et al.*, 1995)
Interpersonal/family difficulties	Cognitive analytic therapy (Ryle & Kerr, 2002)
	Family support and counselling (Addington & Burnett, 2004)
	Family group treatment (McFarlane *et al.*, 2003)
Alcohol and substance use	Motivational interviewing (Miller & Rollnick, 1991)
	Psychoeducation and counselling re substance use (Barrowclough *et al.*, 2001, Elkins *et al.*, 2004)
	Detox (inpatient/outpatient)
Housing/occupation/education difficulties	Problem solving
	Case management

Summary

There are clearly valid arguments both for and against psychological treatment and medication trials with at-risk cohorts. Many of the problems described by young people who meet at-risk criteria and treatment techniques that can address them are shown in Table 7.1. However, it is imperative that clinicians and researchers alike realize that these interventions are still in the very early stages of testing with this specific population. More studies are required to assess the benefits and the risks of different treatments, particularly with respect to biological treatments. In terms of psychological treatments, they may be not only necessary but sufficient for some of these putatively prodromal patients. In a recently published text *Working with People at High Risk of Developing Psychosis* (Addington, Francey & Morrison, 2006), issues such as formulation development, engagement, managing stress, substance use, family work and group work with this population are addressed with the most up to date information. However, many of these innovative ideas require further testing and validation. From an ethical viewpoint, if there is a 'need for care' and treatment is sought by a young person who meets at-risk criteria, then some care should be provided. As further research is required regarding the efficacy and effectiveness of specific psychological and pharmacological treatments, a more conservative approach (such as regular monitoring or supportive psychotherapy) should be taken at the present time in clinical services that do not have a specific at-risk mental state focus.

Current treatment approaches

To illustrate the approaches that are described above, the current treatment approaches for young people meeting ARMS criteria at four sites are described below. A comprehensive case study is also provided.

The Toronto Prevention Risk Identification, Management and Education Clinic

The Toronto PRIME Clinic is dedicated to the early identification and treatment of young people aged 16–30 years who are at risk of developing psychosis. Through the research protocols, assessments, monitoring, psychiatric management as required, case management and psychological interventions are offered. On referral to the clinic, everyone receives a comprehensive assessment. If they meet ARMS criteria they are invited to participate in a longitudinal study that offers randomization to CBT or supportive therapy plus monitoring. All participants have access to a psychiatrist and case manager as needed. Supportive therapy is available to those who participated in the non-therapy study. For those who develop a psychotic illness, there is an easy transition to the First Episode of Psychosis Programme and the First Episode Bipolar Program. The model of CBT used is based on the work of French and Morrison (2004). It is through such clinics that one day evidence-based practices may be translated into routine practices.

The Australian Personal Assessment and Crisis Evaluation Clinic

The PACE Clinic has completed its second randomized controlled intervention trial with young people. The design of this trial has taken into consideration shortcomings associated with the previous trial (McGorry et al., 2002), which have been described above. First, participants have been randomized into three treatment groups. The first received antipsychotic medication (up to 2 mg risperidone) and CBT; the second received placebo medication plus CBT; and the third received placebo medication and supportive therapy. Thus, it will be possible to determine the relative contributions of medication, CBT and supportive therapy. Second, clinicians (with the obvious exception of psychologists), research interviewers and participants were blinded to the type of treatment provided. Finally, in this second trial, treatment has been provided for 12 months to determine if the longer provision of treatment prevents, rather than delays, onset of disorder. The results of this trial are forthcoming. The cognitively oriented psychological treatment that has been developed and evaluated at PACE has been described fully elsewhere (Phillips & Francey, 2004).

An open-label trial of low-dose lithium has also been underway at PACE for the last few years. Lithium is thought to have neurotrophic or neuroprotective effects at low doses (Manji, Moore & Chen, 2000) which, it is hoped, will translate to a preventive effect in the ARMS cohort. As this trial has not yet been completed, results have yet to be published.

A large international, multicenter trial will commence in 2008/2009 comparing the efficacy of cognitive therapy, case management, essential fatty acids and quetiapine treatment for young people who meet UHR criteria. Conducting the trial at a number of sites will ensure that a large sample can be recruited.

The UK Early Detection and Intervention Team

In Salford (UK), following the successful EDIE trial, the local health commissioners invested in a clinical service for young people experiencing psychosis. The Early Detection and Intervention Team was established and offers rapid assessment using the Comprehensive Assessment of At-Risk Mental States (Yung *et al.*, 2005) to determine whether a patient is at risk of developing psychosis. A person meeting the UHR criteria is accepted into the service and offered a range of choices regarding treatment options including individual cognitive therapy, monthly monitoring of their mental state and family intervention. In addition, a large multi-centre trial of cognitive therapy for the prevention of psychosis (EDIE-2) has been funded by the UK Medical Research Council and will evaluate the effectiveness of cognitive therapy in preventing or delaying the onset of psychosis over a 2-year follow-up period. The trial aims to recruit 320 patients across five sites and will report results in 2010.

Cologne Early Recognition and Intervention Centre for mental crisis

A different approach to identifying individuals at risk of psychosis is applied at the FETZ Clinic in Cologne, Germany. This approach is based on the concept of two distinct periods of heightened risk (Häfner *et al.*, 2004; Ruhrmann, Schultze-Lutter & Klosterkötter, 2003). The early initial prodromal state is defined by the presence of subjectively experienced abnormalities of cognition, perception, attention and movement ('basic symptoms': Huber & Gross, 1989), which predicted psychosis in 70% of individuals who experience them (Klosterkötter *et al.*, 2001). The late initial prodromal state is defined similarly to the ARMS criteria developed at PACE (Yung *et al.*, 2005). At FETZ, a psychological treatment is being evaluated with the early initial prodromal state cohort and the atypical antipsychotic amilsulpride is being trialled in the late group.

Underlying strategies of the psychological intervention developed at FETZ include improving coping resources and stress management (Bechdolf *et al.*, 2006). This intervention draws strongly from cognitive therapy strategies for working with people with psychosis (Chadwick, Birchwood & Trower, 1996; Fowler,

Garety & Kuipers, 1995; Kingdon & Turkington, 1994) and is offered in individual and group formats. A trial is currently being conducted with participants to receive either a comprehensive CBT intervention plus case management or 21 sessions of case management alone over a 12-month period. Preliminary results suggest that the CBT group experience greater improvements in depression and global functioning than the case-management group, and lower transition to full-blown psychosis (Bechdolf *et al.*, 2006).

Case study

Conor was a 17 year old who lived with his father, stepmother and younger half-siblings. He stopped attending school 6 months prior to his first appointment because he was finding that the work was increasingly difficult and he was being teased by other pupils for his poor academic achievement. He had not been able to find any employment since leaving school and was spending most of his day at home. He often used cannabis and this caused friction between him and his father and stepmother.

Conor's father became concerned when Conor revealed to him that he was having difficulty focusing his thoughts at times and that he was worried that his thoughts might be read by others at times. After discussion with his primary care physician, Conor was referred to the local child and adolescent mental health clinic for assessment. At this meeting, Conor indicated that the experiences of thought broadcasting did not happen very frequently – about three times a month over the past 3 months – but that they were scary when they happened. He said that although they did not always occur when he was 'stoned', he was concerned about his level of cannabis use but did not feel he could cut down or cease using. It was felt that Conor met ARMS criteria and he was referred to an ARMS team for monitoring and treatment.

Conor agreed to regular appointments with a psychologist at the ARMS clinic. He identified three broad treatment objectives:

- initially to reduce cannabis use but eventually to stop using altogether
- to improve the relationship with his parents
- to make a decision about future employment or education and to start working towards this goal.

In the first session, Conor and his psychologist discussed at length his recent experiences and the changes that had occurred in his life. They developed a formulation suggesting that the anxiety associated with poor school performance and subsequently being teased by other students had led to negative cognitions about himself. These negative cognitions echoed what he thought others were thinking about him ('I am dumb', 'I'm a failure'). This led to withdrawal from school and from all friends, apart from those who had also left school and were unemployed. Together they started smoking cannabis because it gave them something to do during the day. Conor said that smoking did not stop him from thinking negatively about himself but stopped him from becoming upset when he did. His experience of thinking that others could hear his thoughts first occurred when he was at home with his friends smoking in his room and he began thinking about how they were all 'failures' who would not achieve much with their lives. At the same time one of his friends expressed a similar thought and Conor was concerned that his friend knew what he had been thinking. Conor was particularly concerned that his friend would think that he thought negatively about his friends and for a short time was worried about his thoughts being heard. He had similar worries at other times when he thought negatively about someone else, and he tried to control the content of his thoughts – particularly when he was around his friends. The psychologist did not dismiss the influence of smoking cannabis on Conor's experiences, although Conor was less convinced of this. Ongoing conflict within the family and anxiety about the future was likely to be influencing the ongoing nature of his symptoms.

Conor's next two sessions with his psychologist were spent exploring his cannabis use to determine factors that led to his motivation to reduce use and eventually to stop, as well as factors that promoted increased use, within a motivational interviewing framework (Miller & Rollnick, 1991). Conor indicated that factors that promoted ongoing cannabis use were that smoking used up some of his spare time, assisted with sleep and helped him to relax. He acknowledged that his cannabis use also caused conflict at home and contributed towards his low mood and poor motivation. Further, he recognized that his use of cannabis was not assisting with being able to think clearly about the future and to plan for future employment or education. He said that he was not really enjoying how he was spending his days at the current time and regretted the impact his cannabis use had on his relationship with his parents – particularly his father.

Conor's father and stepmother attended the next appointment and the formulation was discussed with them as well as Conor's decision to reduce his cannabis use. Conor's father indicated his concern about Conor's future and was relieved to hear that Conor was willing to think about future employment or education. They agreed to try to make an appointment with the careers teacher at Conor's former school to determine what options might be available to him.

Conor attended the next appointment feeling much more positive about the future. He had seen the careers teacher and had obtained information about apprenticeships, which he was considering. He had managed to reduce his cannabis use and although he was experiencing some difficulty in sleeping was feeling much better overall as a result. His relationship with his family had improved also. Together with the psychologist, he began exploring beliefs about himself and challenging negative beliefs.

Conor's psychotic-like symptoms began reducing in frequency and intensity as he reduced his cannabis use and developed other things to do with his time. He was also able to 'reality test' his belief that friends could hear his thoughts by purposefully thinking something and asking his friends to tell him what he was thinking. His belief in the possibility of mind-reading reduced over time.

The remainder of his sessions was focused on reducing and ceasing his cannabis use, addressing his self-esteem and assisting him to develop the capacity to monitor his mood and cognitions so that he would seek assistance if the feelings of anxiety or beliefs about mind reading returned in the future. When he was discharged he had commenced a pre-apprenticeship programme and hoped to eventually become a plumber. He was free of symptoms when discharged from the clinic 6 months after initial referral.

Conclusions and recommendations

Clearly there are several promising approaches that may help young people who are at risk of developing psychosis. These range from adopting a watching brief, with regular assessments of mental state in order to engage a young person with services and reduce duration of untreated psychosis should transition occur, through to more active strategies that target the problems that ARMS patients experience. There are some ethical issues to consider when selecting specific treatment options and the potential risks of treatment have to be balanced against the potential benefits. Recent guidelines, produced by the International Early Psychosis Association Writing Group (2005), based on consideration of best clinical practice by 29 international consultants and subsequent ratification by the Executive Committee of the Association suggest that

Box 7.1. Core components of a normalizing rationale guiding psychoeducation provided to young people at risk of psychosis

Provide evidence that psychotic symptoms 'merge' with normal experiences and are points on a continuum of experience (Fowler *et al.*, 1995)

Provide evidence that psychotic symptoms can be experienced by 'normal' individuals (i.e. Johns & Van Os, 2001)

Explore whether psychotic experiences that have been reported are culturally relevant

Explore the difference between thoughts and actions and emphasize to client that at times of stress this division can become blurred

Explore the relationship between psychotic experiences and level of stress (Kingdon & Turkington, 1994)

Discuss the proposition that psychotic experiences are not necessarily dangerous or threatening

young people who meet UHR criteria and are help-seeking should be engaged and offered the following:

- regular monitoring
- treatments (including CBT) that target their presenting problems, such as anxiety, depression and relationship difficulties
- family support and education
- education about mental health, psychosis and coping strategies.

It is recommended that these interventions occur within low-stigma and non-restrictive settings. We would agree with these recommendations and, given the current evidence base plus a consideration of the risks and benefits, believe that cognitive therapy targeting psychotic experiences could be added to this list of 'front-line' interventions, reserving the offer of medication for those individuals who specifically request it or those who do not respond to the initial treatment approaches. Additionally, given the ubiquitous concerns of this client group regarding 'going mad', it is important that any psychoeducation offered utilizes a normalizing rationale (Box 7.1) to 'decatastrophize' any symptoms that are experienced. It is clear that more research in this area is required, but it is reasonable to expect that we may have a much stronger evidence base upon which to base treatment recommendations within the next few years.

REFERENCES

Addington, J. & Addington, D. (2005). Clinical trials during the prodromal stage of schizophrenia. [Letter to the editor.] *American Journal of Psychiatry*, **162**, 1387.

Addington, J. & Burnett, P. (2004). Working with families in the early stages of psychosis. In J. F. M. Gleeson & P. D. McGorry (eds.), *Psychological Interventions in Early Psychosis*. Chichester, UK: John Wiley, pp. 99–116.

Addington, J., Francey, S. M. & Morrison, A. P. (2006). *Working With People at High Risk of Developing Psychosis: A Treatment Handbook*. Chichester, UK: John Wiley.

Agerbo, E., Byrne, M., Eaton, W. W. & Mortensen, P. B. (2003). Schizophrenia, marital status and employment: a forty year study. *Schizophrenia Research*, **60**(Suppl 1), 32.

Andreasen, N. C. (1987). Creativity and mental illness: prevalence rates in writers and their first-degree relatives. *American Journal of Psychiatry*, **144**, 1288–92.

APA (1994). *Diagnostic and Statistical Manual of Mental Disorders*, 4th edn. Washington, DC: American Psychiatric Press.

Barrowclough, C., Haddock, G., Tarrier, N. *et al.* (2001). Randomized controlled trial of motivational interviewing, cognitive behaviour therapy, and family intervention for patients with comorbid schizophrenia and substance use disorders. *American Journal of Psychiatry*, **158**, 1706–13.

Bechdolf, A., Phillips, L. J., Francey, S. *et al.* (2006). Recent approaches to psychological interventions for people at risk of psychosis. *European Archives of Psychiatry and Neuroscience*, **256**, 159–73.

Beck, A. T. (1976). *Cognitive Therapy and the Emotional Disorders*. New York: International Universities Press.

Beck, A. T., Rush, A. J., Shaw, B. F. & Emery, G. (1979). *Cognitive Therapy of Depression*. New York: Guilford Press.

Bentall, R. P. & Morrison, A. P. (2002). More harm than good: the case against using antipsychotic drugs to prevent severe mental illness. *Journal of Mental Health*, **11**, 351–6.

Bernstein, D. A. & Borkovec, T. D. (1973). *Progressive Relaxation Training: A Manual for the Health Professionals*. Campaign, IL: Research Press.

Broome, M. R., Woolley, J. B., Johns, L. C. *et al.* (2005). Outreach and support in south London (OASIS): implementation of a clinical service for prodromal psychosis and the at risk mental state. *European Psychiatry*, **20**, 372–8.

Cadenhead, K. (2002). Vulnerability markers in the schizophrenia spectrum: implications for phenomenology, genetics and the identification of the schizophrenia prodrome. *Psychiatric Clinics of North America*, **25**, 837–53.

Carbone, S., Harrigan, S., McGorry, P. D., Curry, C. & Elkins, K. (1999). Duration of untreated psychosis and 12 month outcome in first-episode psychosis: the impact of treatment approach. *Acta Psychiatrica Scandinavica*, **100**, 96–104.

Caroff, S. N., Mann, S. C., Campbell, E. C. & Sullivan, K. A. (2002). Movement disorders associated with atypical antipsychotic drugs. *Journal of Clinical Psychiatry*, **63**(Suppl 4), 12–19.

Chadwick, P., Birchwood, M. & Trower, P. (1996). *Cognitive Therapy for Delusions, Voices and Paranoia*. Chichester, UK: John Wiley.

Corcoran, C., Malaspina, D. & Hercher, L. (2005). Prodromal interventions for schizophrenia vulnerability: the risks of being 'at risk'. *Schizophrenia Research*, **73**, 173–84.

Cornblatt, B. A., Lencz, T. & Kane, J. M. (2001). Treatment of the schizophrenia prodrome: is it presently ethical? *Schizophrenia Research*, 51, 31–8.

Deegan, P. E. (1988). Recovery: the lived experience of rehabilitation. *Psychosocial Rehabilitation Journal*, **11**, 11–19.

Deffenbacher, J. L. & McKay, M. (2000). *Overcoming Situational and General Anger: A Protocol for the Treatment of Anger Based on Relaxation, Cognitive Restructuring, and Coping Skills Training*. Oakland, CA: New Harbinger.

Eder-Ischia, U., Ebenbichler, C. & Fleischhacker, W. W. (2005). Olanzapine-induced weight gain and disturbances of lipid and glucose metabolism. *Essential Psychopharmacology*, **6**, 112–17.

Elkins, K., Hinton, M. & Edwards, J. (2004). Cannabis and psychosis: a psychological intervention. In J. F. M. Gleeson & P. D. McGorry (eds.), *Psychological Interventions in Early Psychosis*. Chichester, UK: John Wiley, pp. 137–56.

Falzer, P. R., Stayner, D. A. & Davidson, L. (2004). Principles and strategies for developing psychosocial treatments for negative symptoms in early course psychosis. In J. F. M. Gleeson & P. D. McGorry (eds.), *Psychological Interventions in Early Psychosis*. Chichester, UK: John Wiley, pp. 229–43.

Fowler, D., Garety, P. & Kuipers, E. (1995). *Cognitive Behaviour Therapy for Psychosis: Theory and Practice*. Chichester, UK: John Wiley.

French, P. & Morrison, A. P. (2004). *Early Detection and Cognitive Therapy for People at High Risk of Developing Psychosis: A Treatment Approach*. New York: John Wiley.

Germer, C. K., (2005). Anxiety disorders: befriending fear. In C. K. Germer, R. D. Siegel & P. R. Fulton (eds.), *Mindfulness and Psychotherapy*. New York: Guilford Press, pp. 152–72.

Häfner, H., Nowotny, B., Löffler, W., van der Heiden, W. & Maurer, K. (1995a). When and how does schizophrenia produce social deficits? *European Archives of Psychiatry and Clinical Neuroscience*, **246**, 17–28.

Häfner, H., Maurer, W., Löffler, B. *et al.* (1995b). Onset and early course of schizophrenia. In H. Häfner & W. F. Gattaz. (eds.), *Causes of Schizophrenia*, vol. III. New York: Springer, pp. 43–66.

Häfner, H., Maurer, K., Ruhrmann, S. *et al.* (2004). Are early detection and secondary prevention feasible? Facts and visions. *European Archives of Psychiatry and Clinical Neuroscience*, **254**, 117–28.

Haroun, N., Dunn, L., Haroun, A. & Cadenhead, K. S. (2006). Risk and protection in prodromal schizophrenia: ethical implications for clinical practice and future research. *Schizophrenia Bulletin*, **32**, 166–78.

Harrigan, S. M., McGorry, P. D. & Krstev, H. (2003). Does treatment delay in first-episode psychosis really matter? *Psychological Medicine*, **33**, 97–110.

Harris, M. G., Henry, L. P., Harrigan, S. M. *et al.* (2005). The relationship between duration of untreated psychosis and outcome: an eight-year prospective study. *Schizophrenia Research*, **79**, 85–93.

Hawkins, K. A., McGlashan, T. H., Quinlan, D. *et al.* (2004). Factorial structure of the Scale of Prodromal Symptoms. *Schizophrenia Research*, **68**, 339–47.

Huber, G. & Gross, G. (1989). The concept of basic symptoms in schizophrenic and schizoaffective psychoses. *Recent Progress in Medicine*, **80**, 646–52.

International Early Psychosis Association Writing Group (2005). International clinical practice guidelines for early psychosis. *British Journal of Psychiatry*, **187**(Suppl 48), s120–4.

Jablensky, A. & Eaton, W. W. (1995). Schizophrenia. In A. Jablensky (eds.), *Epidemiological Psychiatry*. London: Baillière Tindall, pp. 283–306.

Jablensky, A. Sartorius, N., Ernberg, G. *et al.* (1992). Schizophrenia: manifestations, incidence and course in different cultures. A World Health Organization ten-country study. *Psychological Medicine – Monograph Supplement*, **20**, 1–97.

Jayaram, M. B., Hosalli, P. & Stroup, S. (2006). Risperidone versus olanzapine for schizophrenia. *Cochrane Database of Systematic Reviews*, **2**, CD005237.

Johns, L. C. & van Os, J. (2001). The continuity of psychotic experiences in the general population. *Clinical Psychology Review*, **21**, 1125–41.

Kane, J. M. (2004). Tardive dyskinesia rates with atypical antipsychotics in adults: prevalence and incidence. *Journal of Clinical Psychiatry*, **65**(Suppl 9), 16–20.

Kay, S. R., Fiszbein, A. & Opler, L. A. (1987). The Positive and Negative Syndrome Scale (PANSS) for schizophrenia. *Schizophrenia Bulletin*, **13**, 261–9.

Kingdon, D. & Turkington, D. (1994). *Cognitive–Behavioural Therapy for Schizophrenia.* Hove, England: Lawrence Erlbaum.

Kinon, B. J., Kaiser, C. J., Ahmed, S., Rotelli, M. D. & Kollack-Walker, S. (2005). Association between early and rapid weight gain and change in weight over one year of olanzapine therapy in patients with schizophrenia and related disorders. *Journal of Clinical Psychopharmacology*, **25**, 255–8.

Klosterkötter, J., Hellmich, M., Steinmeyer, E. M. & Schultze-Lutter, F. (2001). Diagnosing schizophrenia in the initial prodromal phase. *Archives of General Psychiatry*, **58**, 158–64.

Larsen, T. K. (2002). The transition from the premorbid period to psychosis: how can it be described? *Acta Psychiatrica Scandinavica*, **106**(Suppl 413), S10–11.

Lencz, T., Smith, C. W., Auther, A., Correll, C. U. & Cornblatt, B. A. (2003). The assessment of 'prodromal schizophrenia': unresolved issues and future directions. *Schizophrenia Bulletin*, **29**, 717–28.

Lieberman, J. A., Tollefson, G. D., Schulz, C. *et al.* For the HGDH Study Group (2005). Antipsychotic drug effects on brain morphology in first-episode psychosis. *Archives of General Psychiatry*, **62**, 361–70.

Manji, H. K., Moore, G. J. & Chen, G. (2000). Clinical and preclinical evidence for the neurotrophic effects of mood stabilizers: implications for the pathophysiology and treatment of manic–depressive illness. *Biological Psychiatry*, **48**, 740–54.

Margolese, H. C., Chouinard, G., Kolivakis, T. T. *et al.* (2005). Tardive dyskinesia in the era of typical and atypical antipsychotics. Part 2: incidence and management strategies in patients with schizophrenia. *Canadian Journal of Psychiatry*, **50**, 703–14.

Mason, O., Startup, M., Halpin, S. *et al.* (2004). Risk factors for transition to first episode psychosis among individuals with 'at-risk mental states'. *Schizophrenia Research*, **71**, 227–37.

McFarlane, W. R., Dixon, L., Lukens, E. & Lucksted, A. (2003). Family psychoeducation and schizophrenia: a review of the literature. *Journal of Marital and Family Therapy*, **29**, 223–45.

McGlashan, T. H. (2001). Psychosis treatment prior to psychosis onset: ethical issues. *Schizophrenia Research*, **51**, 47–54.

McGlashan, T. H., Zipursky, R. B., Perkins, D. *et al.* (2003). The PRIME North America randomized double-blind clinical trial of olanzapine versus placebo in patients at risk of being prodromally symptomatic for psychosis: I. Study rationale and design. *Schizophrenia Research*, **61**, 7–18.

McGlashan, T. H., Zipursky, R. B., Perkins, D. *et al.* (2006). Randomized, double-blind trial of olanzapine versus placebo in patients prodromally symptomatic for psychosis. *American Journal of Psychiatry*, **163**, 790–9.

McGorry, P. D. (2005). Early intervention in psychotic disorders: beyond debate to solving problems. *British Journal of Psychiatry*, **187**(Suppl 48), s108–10.

McGorry, P. D., Yung, A. R. & Phillips, L. J. (2001). Ethics and early intervention in psychosis: keeping up the pace and staying in step. *Schizophrenia Research*, **51**, 17–29.

McGorry, P. D., Yung, A. R., Phillips, L. J. *et al.* (2002). Randomized controlled trial of interventions designed to reduce the risk of progression to first-episode psychosis in a clinical sample with subthreshold symptoms. *Archives of General Psychiatry*, **59**, 921–8.

Meichenbaum, D. H. (1975). Self-instructional methods. In F. H. Kanfer & Goldstein, A. P. (eds.), *Helping People Change: A Textbook of Methods.* New York: Pergamon, pp. 357–91.

Meyer, S. E., Bearden, C. E., Lux, S. R., *et al.* (2005). The psychosis prodrome in adolescent patients viewed through the lens of DSM-IV. *Journal of Child and Adolescent Psychopharmacology*, **15**, 434–51.

Miller, L. J., O'Connor, E. & DiPasquale, T. (1993). Patients' attitudes toward hallucinations. *American Journal of Psychiatry*, **150**, 584–8.

Miller, T. J., McGlashan, T. H., Rosen, J. L. *et al.* (2002). Prospective diagnosis of the initial prodrome for schizophrenia based on the Structured Interview for Prodromal Syndromes: preliminary evidence of interrater reliability and predictive validity. *American Journal of Psychiatry*, **159**, 863–5.

Miller, T. J., Zipursky, R. B., Perkins, D. *et al.* (2003a). The PRIME North America randomized double-blind clinical trial of olanzapine versus placebo in patients at risk of being prodromally symptomatic for psychosis. II Baseline characteristics of the 'prodromal' sample. *Schizophrenia Research*, **61**, 19–30.

Miller, T. J., McGlashan, T. H., Rosen, J. L. *et al.* (2003b). Prodromal assessment with the Structured Interview for Prodromal Syndromes and the Scale of Prodromal Symptoms: predictive validity, interrater reliability, and training to reliability. *Schizophrenia Bulletin*, **29**, 703–15. [Erratum in *Schizophrenia Bulletin* (2004) **30**, 217f.]

Miller, W. R. & Rollnick, S. (1991). *Motivational Interviewing: Preparing People to Change Addictive Behaviour.* New York: Guilford Press.

Morrison, A. P. (2001). The interpretation of intrusions in psychosis: an integrative cognitive approach to hallucinations and delusions. *Behavioural and Cognitive Psychotherapy*, **29**, 257–76.

Morrison, A. P., French, P., Walford, L. *et al.* (2004). Cognitive therapy for the prevention of psychosis in people at ultra-high risk. *British Journal of Psychiatry*, **185**, 291-7.

Morrison, A. P., Gumley, A. I., Schwannauer, M. *et al.* (2005). The beliefs about paranoia scale: preliminary validation of a metacognitive approach to conceptualising paranoia. *Behavioural and Cognitive Psychotherapy*, **33**, 153-64.

Morrison, A. P., French, P., Parker, S. *et al.* (2007). Three year follow-up of a randomised controlled trial of cognitive therapy for the prevention of psychosis in people at ultra-high risk. *Schizophrenia Bulletin*, **33**, 682-7.

Nemeroff, C. B. (2005). Use of atypical antipsychotics in refractory depression and anxiety. *Journal of Clinical Psychiatry*, **66**, 13-21.

Newcomer, J. W. (2005). Second-generation (atypical) antipsychotics and metabolic effects: a comprehensive literature review. *CNS Drugs*, **19**(Suppl 1), 1-93.

Norman, R. M. G., Lewis, S. W. & Marshall, M. (2005). Duration of untreated psychosis and its relationship to clinical outcome. *British Journal of Psychiatry*, **187**(Suppl 48), s19-23.

O'Reilly, T., Dunbar, R. & Bentall, R. (2001). Schizotypy and creativity: an evolutionary connection? *Personality and Individual Differences*, **31**, 1067-78.

Ost, L. G. (1987). Applied relaxation: description of a coping technique and review of controlled studies. *Behaviour Research and Therapy*, **25**, 397-410.

Phillips, L. J. & Francey, S. M. (2004). Changing PACE: psychological interventions in the pre-psychotic phase. In J. F. M Gleeson & P. D. McGorry (eds.), *Psychological Interventions in Early Psychosis: A Practical Treatment Handbook*. Chichester, UK: John Wiley, pp. 23-40.

Phillips, L. J., McGorry, P. D., Yuen, H. P. *et al.* (2007). Medium term follow-up of a randomized controlled trial of interventions for young people at ultra high risk of psychosis. *Schizophrenia Research*, **96**, 25-33.

Post, S. G. (2001). Preventing schizophrenia and Alzheimer disease: comparative ethics. *Schizophrenia Research*, **51**, 103-8.

Ramel, W., Goldin, P. R., Carmona, P. E. & McQuaid, J. R. (2004). The effects of mindfulness meditation on cognitive processes and affect in patients with past depression. *Cognitive Therapy and Research*, **28**, 433-55.

Read, J. & Harre, N. (2001). The role of biological and genetic causal beliefs in the stigmatisation of 'mental patients'. *Journal of Mental Health*, **10**, 223-35.

Read, J. & Haslam, H. (2004). Public opinion: bad things happen and can drive you crazy. In J. Read, L. R. Mosher & R. P. Bentall (eds.), *Models of Madness: Psychological, Social and Biological Approaches to Schizophrenia*. Hove, UK: Brunner-Routledge, pp. 133-45.

Roemer, L. & Orsillo, S. M. (2002). Expanding our conceptualization of and treatment for generalized anxiety disorder: integrating mindfulness/acceptance-based approaches with existing cognitive-behavioral models. *Clinical Psychology: Science and Practice*, **9**, 54-68.

Ruhrmann, S., Schultze-Lutter, F. & Klosterkötter, J. (2003). Early detection and intervention in the initial prodromal phase of schizophrenia. *Pharmacopsychiatry*, **36**(Suppl 3), S162-7.

Ryle, A. & Kerr, I. B. (2002). *Introducing Cognitive Analytic Therapy: Principles and Practice*, Chichester, UK: John Wiley.

Sachdev, P. S. (2005). Neuroleptic-induced movement disorders: an overview. *Psychiatric Clinics of North America*, **28**, 255-74.

Siddle, R. & Haddock, G. (2004). Cognitive-behavioural therapy for acute and recent-onset psychosis. In J. F. M. Gleeson & P. D. McGorry (eds.), *Psychological Interventions in Early Psychosis*. Chichester, UK: John Wiley, pp. 41-62.

Stathis, S., Martin, G. & McKenna, J. G. (2005). A preliminary case series on the use of quetiapine for posttraumatic stress disorder in juveniles within a youth detention center. *Journal of Clinical Psychopharmacology*, **25**, 539-44.

Sullivan, H. S. (1927; reprinted 1994). The onset of schizophrenia. *American Journal of Psychiatry*, **151**, 135-9.

Svirkis, T., Korkeila, J., Heinimaa, M. *et al.* (2005). Axis I disorders and vulnerability to psychosis. *Schizophrenia Research*, **75**, 439-46.

Tarrier, N., Harwood, S., Yusopoff, L., Beckett, R. & Baker, S. (1990). Coping strategy enhancement (CSE): a method of treating residual schizophrenic symptoms. *Behavioural Psychotherapy*, **18**, 283-93.

Valmaggia, L. R., van der Gaag, M., Tarrier, N., Pijnenborg, M. & Slooff, C. J. (2005). Cognitive-behavioural therapy for refractory psychotic symptoms of schizophrenia resistant to atypical antipsychotic medication. Randomised controlled trial. *British Journal of Psychiatry*, **186**, 324-30.

Warner, R. (1985). *Recovery from Schizophrenia: Psychiatry and Political Economy*. New York: Routledge & Kegan Paul.

Warner, R. (2003). How much of the burden of schizophrenia is alleviated by treatment? *British Journal of Psychiatry*, **183**, 375-6.

Warner, R. (2005). Problems with early and very early intervention in psychosis. *British Journal of Psychiatry*, **187**(Suppl 48), s104-7.

Woods, S., Zipursky, R., Perkins, D. *et al.* (2002). Olanzapine vs. placebo for prodromal symptoms. *Acta Psychiatrica Scandinavica*, **106**(Suppl 413), 43.

Woods, S. W., Breier, A., Zipursky, R. B. *et al.* (2003). Randomized trial of olanzapine versus placebo in the symptomatic acute treatment of the schizophrenic pro-drome. *Biological Psychiatry*, **54**, 453–64.

Wykes, T. & van der Gaaz, M. (2001). Is it time to develop a new cognitive therapy for psychosis: cognitive remediation therapy (CRT). *Clinical Psychology Review*, **21**, 1227–56.

Yung, A. R. & McGorry, P. D. (1996). The prodromal phase of first-episode psychosis: past and current conceptualizations. *Schizophrenia Bulletin*, **22**, 353–70.

Yung, A. R. & McGorry, P. D. (2003). Keeping an open mind: investigating options for treatment options of the pre-psychotic phase. *Journal of Mental Health*, **12**, 341–3.

Yung, A. R., Phillips, L. J. & McGorry, P. D. (2004). *Treating Schizophrenia in the Prodromal Phase*. London: Taylor & Francis.

Yung, A. R., Phillips, L. J., Yuen, H. P. *et al.* (2003). Psychosis prediction: 12 month follow-up of a high risk ('prodromal') group. *Schizophrenia Research*, **60**, 21–32.

Yung, A. R., Yuen, H. P., McGorry, P. D. *et al.* (2005). Mapping the onset of psychosis: the Comprehensive Assessment of At Risk Mental States (CAARMS). *Australian and New Zealand Journal of Psychiatry*, **39**, 964–71.

Zimmermann, G., Favrod, J., Trieu, V. H. & Pomini, V. (2005). The effect of cognitive behavioral treatment on the positive symptoms of schizophrenia-spectrum disorders: a meta-analysis. *Schizophrenia Research*, **77**, 1–9.

Zubin, J. & Spring, B. (1977). Vulnerability: a new view of schizophrenia. *Journal of Abnormal Psychology*, **86**,103–26.

Access and reducing delay to treatment: reducing the duration of untreated psychosis

Duration of untreated psychosis: definition, measurement and association with outcome

Max Marshall, Susy Harrigan and Shon Lewis

Introduction

The course of schizophrenia and other psychotic disorders shows substantial individual variation, suggesting that perhaps something can be done to improve outcome (Wiersma *et al.*, 1998). However, most of the established predictors of outcome, such as gender, age of onset and premorbid adjustment (Harrigan, McGorry & Krstev, 2003), cannot be easily changed. In this respect, duration of untreated psychosis (DUP) is exceptional, because it is potentially modifiable. This raises the exciting possibility that outcome could be improved through early detection programmes aimed at reducing DUP. In this chapter, we will systematically assess the strength and robustness of the association between DUP and outcome; however, as an essential preliminary, we will first consider the difficulties of defining and assessing DUP.

Variability of findings in duration of untreated psychosis: what reason?

There is much potential for measurement error in a concept as rarefied as DUP, and it is not reassuring that there is such a wide variability in estimates of DUP across studies (Norman & Malla, 2001; Perkins *et al.*, 2005). This variability might be attributed to heterogeneity amongst different psychotic disorders (Keshavan & Schooler, 1992) or to differences between societies and health services. However, it could equally be accounted for by measurement error. We will consider some of the most likely sources of measurement

error below. In summary, these are (1) difficulties in defining the onset and offset of untreated psychosis, (2) the problems of retrospective assessment, (3) discrepancies between the accounts of patients and carers, (4) sample bias, and (5) failure to use standardized assessment instruments.

Defining the onset and offset of untreated psychosis

The majority of studies construe DUP as a continuous period of psychosis that covers the time interval from the onset of psychosis until the initiation of treatment (Norman & Malla, 2001). However, in real life, the course of untreated psychosis can be quite variable, with some people experiencing continual symptoms and others experiencing symptoms of a more intermittent nature (Norman, Townsend & Malla, 2001). It is not known whether it is the cumulative experience of active psychosis or simply the period of time since the onset of psychotic symptoms that is most detrimental to outcome. The Early Treatment and Intervention in Psychosis study appears to have established that people presenting with an intermittent course of untreated symptoms are quite rare (Melle *et al.*, 2004). Hopefully, therefore, the fact that few studies have assessed the cumulative period of untreated psychosis is not a major problem for the DUP literature. However, even if we assume that DUP tends to be limited to a single continuous episode, there are considerable difficulties in operationalizing the beginning and endpoints of this episode.

Several authors have noted the lack of consistency in the definition of onset between studies (Keshavan &

The Recognition and Management of Early Psychosis: A Preventive Approach, ed. Henry J. Jackson and Patrick D. McGorry.
Published by Cambridge University Press. © Cambridge University Press 2009.

Schooler, 1992; Norman & Malla, 2001), which arises because no specific marker of emergent psychosis has yet been identified (Perkins *et al.*, 2005). Some studies advocate the emergence of the first psychotic symptom, even if fleeting, as the beginning point of DUP (e.g. Perkins *et al.*, 2000; Singh *et al.*, 2005; Verdoux *et al.*, 1998, 2001), whereas other studies specify that the psychotic symptom must be sustained for a defined period of time, for example, lasting '... throughout the day for several days or several times a week, not being limited to a few brief moments' (Kay, Fiszbein & Opler, 1987). Addington, van Mastrigt & Addington (2004, p. 279) and Larsen *et al.* (2003, p. 3) have both used this latter definition. The use of severity indices in the definition of onset has also been advocated (Keshavan & Schooler, 1992; Larsen, McGlashan & Moe, 1996), with the recommendation that the onset of a psychotic episode should be ascertained by a rating of at least 'moderate' on scales such as the Brief Psychiatric Rating Scale or the Positive and Negative Syndrome Scale. This contrasts with a number of earlier studies that sometimes blurred the distinction between prodromal and psychotic symptoms (e.g. Beiser *et al.*, 1993). Yet, in practice, there is often a fine and potentially arbitrary distinction to be made between judging whether an individual's behaviour or experience falls within the realm of psychosis or whether it is merely eccentric or unusual (Norman & Malla, 2001).

Studies also tend to be inconsistent in the types of symptom used to define psychosis (Norman & Malla, 2001). Although hallucinations and delusions are commonly used, many studies also include thought disorder and disorganized, bizarre or catatonic behaviour (e.g. Ho *et al.*, 2000; Keshavan *et al.*, 2003). It is debatable whether patients presenting with these last symptoms in the absence of positive symptoms (i.e. hallucinations and delusions) can be regarded as psychotic.

Determining the endpoint of DUP is also more complex than it appears at first sight. The endpoint is commonly regarded as the point at which antipsychotic medication is administered (Norman & Malla, 2001), but this begs the question of whether there is a minimum duration of treatment that is critical in determining the prospects of recovery (Perkins *et al.*, 2005). Some studies define the endpoint as the commencement of

any level of antipsychotic medication, whereas others use more stringent criteria for adequacy (Larsen *et al.*, 1996; Norman & Malla, 2001) based on duration or dose of medication. For instance, Larsen *et al.* (2000, p. 3) defined adequate treatment as '... giving an antipsychotic drug given in sufficient time and amount so that it would lead to clinical response in the average non-chronic schizophrenic patient (e.g. haldol 5 mg a day for 3 weeks)'. Others have considered that up to 12 weeks of prior treatment with antipsychotic drugs is within the limits of acceptability for determining eligibility for participation in their first-episode psychosis study (Loebel *et al.*, 1992; Robinson *et al.*, 1999a,b). The patient's adherence to their prescribed medication is usually not taken into account in applying the initiation of antipsychotic medication criteria, although it is occasionally considered (e.g. Wunderink *et al.*, 2006). This last scenario, in which any delay of actual antipsychotic treatment after the first contact (owing to compliance problems) is added to the length of the DUP period, is potentially problematic and raises issues regarding what constitutes adequate treatment for the purposes of determining the endpoint of DUP.

There are a number of alternatives to defining the endpoint of DUP as the administration of antipsychotic medication. These include admission to a psychiatric hospital (Bottlender *et al.*, 2003; Craig *et al.*, 2000; Larsen *et al.*, 2000; Ucok *et al.*, 2004; Verdoux *et al.*, 1998), entry into treatment (Browne *et al.*, 2000; McGorry, Copolov & Singh, 1990a), time until treatment response, end of a defined period of time subsequent to administration of medication (Malla *et al.*, 2002) and time until the establishment of a definitive diagnosis (Chong *et al.*, 2005).

It would seem desirable to come up with a common definition of adequate treatment, since this defines the endpoint of DUP, but is it sufficient to define treatment simply in terms of psychiatric hospitalization or the administration of an antipsychotic drug? It has been proposed that the endpoint should be 'time until exposure to evidence-based treatment for first-episode psychosis' (P. D. McGorry, personal communication, 2006). This endpoint would need a precise operational definition, but it could include such components as (1) exposure and adherence to antipsychotic medication,

(2) exposure to psychosocial treatment and (3) tenure in care and other treatment variables. In fact, there are some who argue that if the patient does not receive psychosocial treatment then they have not received proper treatment, since the early implementation of psychosocial intervention aimed at improving self-esteem, social functioning and disease management could be an important factor in long-term outcome over and above the effects of medication administration, which commonly defines the endpoint of DUP (de Haan *et al.*, 2003).

The period of *treated* psychosis is defined as the time interval from the initiation of treatment until the remission of psychotic symptoms. If long DUP has a negative effect on outcome, then it seems plausible that a long duration of treated psychosis might also have an adverse effect. Hence this variable should perhaps be considered in studies assessing the relationship between DUP and outcome. Unfortunately, this is not entirely straightforward, since the time until the resolution of treated psychotic symptoms is likely to be highly correlated with the DUP. There is another important distinction to consider in the duration of treated psychosis, and that is the concept of early treatment resistance which should only be applied when a patient has definitely received potentially effective treatment but has failed to respond. This is a different scenario from the situation where a patient has failed to engage or adhere and has not received evidence-based care as yet. True treatment resistance could be viewed as an outcome variable for studying DUP and should not be confused with treated psychosis. Furthermore, it has been suggested that individuals who fail to be exposed to a genuine first pass at evidence-based care for first-episode psychosis can be viewed as still 'clocking up' their DUP, albeit within rather than outside the health system (P. D. McGorry, personal communication, 2006).

The problems of retrospective assessment

Dating the onset of psychosis is inevitably difficult since one must rely on retrospective data (Keshavan & Schooler, 1992; Maurer & Häfner, 1995). Moreover, the onset is often insidious (Ho *et al.*, 2000) and the

definition of the actual tipping point from prodrome to psychosis is arbitrary. Presumably, the more remote the tipping point, the more arbitrary this judgement becomes. Maurer and Häfner (1995) found that, as the time grows between the tipping point and the interview, reliable ratings are only made possible by a considerable reduction in the precision of measurement. They suggested that methods for the improvement in reliability via the reduction of sources of error should include:

- specific measurement techniques such as the use of a standardized procedure
- the use of anchor events in the assessment
- the parallel collection of information from different sources
- the change from point estimation to interval assessment (although this suggestion will necessarily result in a reduction in the precision of measurement, particularly for lower estimates of DUP).

Another issue compounding the retrospective recall of the onset of psychosis is the illness status of the individual when onset information is collected (Keshavan & Schooler, 1992; Norman & Malla, 2001). If the individual is floridly psychotic as well as cognitively impaired, the accuracy of recall may be adversely affected. For these reasons, it is recommended that information should be collected when patients are symptomatically stable and that self-report should be supplemented by corroborative information from families (Keshavan & Schooler, 1992). Corroborative information from family members and other informants in relation to the onset, evolution and duration of symptomatology is essential to piece together the mosaic of the illness episode and to date its onset accurately. Nevertheless, it has been noted that observers' recall will be affected by a number of factors, including their perceptiveness, possible denial, tolerance for eccentricity and the extent to which the onset is accompanied by bizarre symptoms (Norman & Malla, 2001).

Discrepancies between the accounts of patients and carers

Reliance on retrospective data is not the only threat to accurate dating of the onset of psychosis. Psychotic symptoms are subjective phenomena whose presence is not necessarily obvious to observers (Browne *et al.*, 2000). This could mean that patients will tend to date onset earlier than relatives (Norman & Malla, 2001). This has been confirmed in a study which showed that psychotic symptoms were first noticed by relatives 12 months later than first perceived by patients (Häfner *et al.*, 1993). In the light of these findings, it has been proposed that behavioural symptoms are best identified by the family, and that subjective symptoms such as hallucinations and delusions are more reliably reported by the patient (McGorry *et al.*, 1990).

Sample bias

Most first-episode studies identify subjects at first hospitalization and, therefore, individuals with milder symptoms who do not require inpatient treatment may not be included (Perkins *et al.*, 2005). Clearly, it is important to include in DUP studies those individuals whose symptoms qualify them as psychotic, but at a less acute level, so that the full spectrum of illness severity and its relationship to outcome can be examined. Related to this point is the fact that most studies have narrow diagnostic inclusion criteria, thus excluding patients with affective psychoses. Focusing only on schizophrenia-spectrum disorders limits the generalizability of the study findings to a subgroup of patients within the broader diagnostic spectrum of psychosis, although some might argue that the inclusion of affective psychosis is a self-fulfilling prophesy, since affective psychoses are known to be characterized by a shorter duration of psychotic symptoms and a better prognosis. Examples of the few studies that have included affective psychotic disorders in their assessment of the relationship between DUP and outcome include those reported by McGorry *et al.* (1996), Craig *et al.* (2000) and Harrigan *et al.* (2003). Finally, another point to bear in mind is the thorny issue regarding bias introduced by study refusal. On the one hand, a study has found that the DUP for subjects who refused to participate in a follow-up study was significantly longer than for those subjects who agreed to participate (Friis *et al.*, 2004). On the other hand, other research has found that DUP in the participant group was

similar to that in a non-consenting group (Harrigan *et al.*, 2003).

Failure to use standardized assessment instruments

It seems intuitive that DUP should be assessed directly by standardized interview with patients and relatives, but it would be convenient if a reasonable estimate of DUP could be obtained from clinical records. As a precursor to another study, an assessment was made of how reliably DUP could be estimated from patient file notes compared with ratings derived from a 'gold-standard' interview with the patient and their family (unpublished data). The 'gold-standard' interview was based on the Royal Park Multidiagnostic Instrument for Psychosis (RP-MIP), which is a comprehensive semi-structured interview that features meticulous measurement of DUP and prodromal phases of illness according to carefully operationalized criteria (McGorry *et al.*, 1990a). The RP-MIP has demonstrated very good to excellent inter-rater reliability for specific components, including a DSM-IIIR diagnosis of schizophrenia (kappa = 0.92) and the onset and duration of symptoms (mean kappa = 0.79) (McGorry *et al.*, 1990b). Multiple sources of information were obtained by interviewing 50 patients and close relatives and the information was then merged to produce an accurate record of the onset, evolution and duration of the illness. The onset of DUP was assessed as the date of the emergence of the first sustained psychotic symptom of any type at threshold level, and it was dated as precisely as possible to the nearest day, week or month. The offset of psychosis was defined as initiation of treatment. An independent rater assessed the same variables using clinical file records, with no other sources of information used. The DUP for two patients was unable to be ascertained from the file notes, leaving 48 subjects. DUP estimates derived from the clinical records were highly unreliable when compared with the DUP ratings from the RP-MIP (interclass correlation, 0.22). There was perfect agreement on DUP for just 3 of the 48 cases, and only 10 of the sample (21%) were estimated to lie within 7 days either side of the gold-standard DUP. The clinical file method, over- or underestimated DUP by more than 1 year for eight subjects (17%). Even when the point estimation was changed to a interval assessment as a way of increasing the accuracy of onset identification, as suggested by Maurer and Häfner (1995), the magnitude of error remained unsatisfactory, with a kappa rating of 0.39, which is only fair (unpublished data). The magnitude of the discrepancies indicates that for the majority of patients, the file rating method fails to provide a reasonable estimate of DUP.

In summary, it is inevitable that there will be substantial measurement error between and within studies as a consequence of the inconsistencies in defining and measuring DUP, as described above. This error could be minimized by calibrating and standardizing operational criteria relating to the onset and offset of psychosis.

Duration of untreated psychosis and outcome

Having expressed these reservations about the difficulties of measuring DUP, we will now consider the findings of those studies that have attempted to explore the association between DUP and outcome. There has been intense interest in this association because of the proposal that psychosis is somehow neurologically or psychologically toxic (Sheitman & Lieberman, 1998). If this is true, then delay in treating people with psychosis could impair prognosis, while reducing delay could improve it (Wyatt & Henter, 2001). There are now well-established early intervention services in America, Australia and Europe, all of which are attempting to reduce DUP (Department of Health, 2000; Edwards & McGorry, 2002).

However, despite the blossoming of early intervention services, there is continuing disagreement over whether there is a real association between DUP and outcome. For example, of three recent non-systematic reviews, one concluded that the evidence for an association was conflicting (Ho & Andreasen, 2001), another that it was convincing for positive symptoms only (Norman & Malla, 2001) and a third that it was convincing across a range of outcomes (Lincoln & McGorry, 1999). These differing conclusions reflect the complex nature of the evidence that has been derived from four different types of study.

Type 1. Comparisons of cohorts from before and after the emergence of neuroleptic treatment (Wyatt, 1991). Such studies compare the outcome for service users who became ill before neuroleptic drugs were available, with that for a group who became ill after such drugs were available. These studies provide evidence of limited value because they rely on retrospectively collected data, and have difficulty controlling for inter-generational confounders, such as improved nutrition or social conditions (Norman & Malla, 2001).

Type 2. Trials of patients with acute psychoses where neuroleptic treatment was withheld. Such studies examine the long-term outcome for participants in trials where neuroleptic treatment was withheld or withdrawn in one of the trial arms, thus extending the duration of untreated psychosis for participants in that arm. These studies have the advantage of randomization and prospective data collection, but they are rare and the available data are sparse (Norman & Malla, 2001). Further data are unlikely to become available as such trials would now be considered unethical (McGlashan, 1998).

Type 3. Trials attempting to reduce DUP through early detection. Such trials could potentially provide conclusive evidence of a casual relationship between DUP and outcome. However, there is currently only one such trial (non-randomized), which has not yet been reported (Larsen *et al.*, 2000).

Type 4. Follow-up studies of cohorts of first-episode patients at first presentation and in the years following treatment. Such studies can be used to establish if there is an association between DUP and outcome, but they cannot establish if this association is causative.

The systematic review presented below is concerned only with type 4 studies because at present they are the best available source of evidence for or against a link between DUP and outcome. The review aimed to apply systematic techniques of data ascertainment, quality assessment, data extraction and synthesis to first-episode follow-up studies to determine if an association between DUP and outcome was present. However, because the review is based on data from type 4 studies, even if it were to show an association between DUP and outcome, this would not prove that longer DUP caused worse outcome, as the observed association could be because DUP and outcome were both correlated with an unknown third variable. The most likely candidate for such a 'third variable' is generally thought to be premorbid adjustment, on the assumption that people with poor premorbid adjustment are less likely to seek psychiatric help and more likely to have a poor prognosis (Verdoux *et al.*, 2001). A secondary aim of the review was, therefore, to determine how far premorbid adjustment might explain any observed association between DUP and outcome.

Review of published type 4 studies

Methods

Search strategy

A list of relevant papers was generated from the personal databases of the reviewers. A search strategy was then developed based on the indexing of these papers (Fig. 8.1). This strategy was run on CINAHL (January 1982–May 2004), the Cochrane Schizophrenia Group Register (Issue 1, 2004), EMBASE (January 1980–May 2004), MEDLINE (January 1966–May 2004) and PsycLIT (January 1967–May 2004). A sensitive rather than specific strategy was used because follow-up studies (unlike clinical trials) are not well indexed. Sensitivity was examined by scrutinizing the reference lists of relevant papers detected by the search.

Study selection

Eligible studies were those that examined prospectively the relationship between DUP and outcome in patients presenting with their first-episode of psychosis. Restriction to first-episode studies was considered essential as they were more likely to provide a representative sample of patients, and an accurate estimation of DUP (Browne, Larkin & O'Callaghan, 1999). Studies were excluded if they only reported data on

brain morphology or cognitive functioning, excluded patients with schizophrenia, were restricted to the under 16s or over 60s, or had a follow-up rate of less than 50%. Abstracts were initially screened by one reviewer and copies of potentially relevant papers were requested. Potentially relevant papers were screened by two reviewers who achieved substantial agreement on which cohorts should be included (kappa 0.9; 95% confidence interval (CI), 0.75–1.04). Disagreements between reviewers were resolved by discussion.

Methods of measuring duration of untreated psychosis

There is no universally accepted method for measuring the onset of psychosis and the early course of illness, although several instruments are available that attempt to provide a standardized approach. The instruments identified by our review are listed below:

The Nottingham Onset Schedule (Singh *et al.*, 2005). This is described as a standardized and reliable way of identifying key time points in an emerging psychosis. The claimed advantages are brevity, reliability and ease of use. Onset is broken down into three stages: (1) a prodrome of two parts, a period of 'unease' followed by 'non-diagnostic' symptoms; (2) appearance of psychotic symptoms; and (3) a build-up of diagnostic symptoms leading to a definite diagnosis (Singh *et al.*, 2005, p. 117). Information is gathered from a variety of sources including evidence from informants and case notes.

The Symptom Onset in Schizophrenia inventory (Perkins *et al.*, 2000). This dates the onset of 16 symptoms including general prodromal symptoms, and positive, negative and disorganizational symptoms. Global ratings of the onset of illness are made by the patient, their family and the clinician. The onset of psychosis is defined as the emergence of the first psychotic symptom. The inventory is claimed to be reliable, easy to administer and brief.

The Interview for the Retrospective Assessment of the Onset of Schizophrenia (Häfner *et al.*, 1992). This is administered as a semi-structured interview with both patient and key informant, and

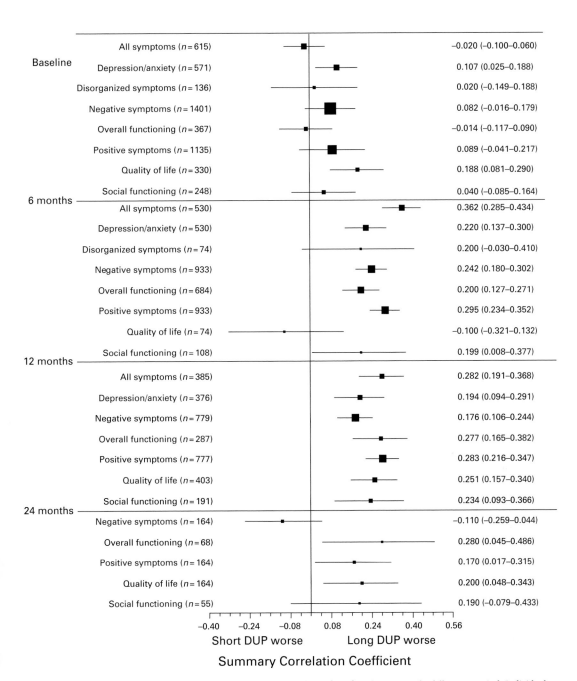

Fig. 8.1. Summary correlations between duration of untreated psychosis (DUP) and outcomes by follow-up period. Individual mean summary correlation coefficients are given with confidence intervals.

supplemented with case note information. The interview focuses on dating the onset of 66 signs and symptoms. Although it is not brief, this instrument is considered comprehensive and reliable.

The Royal Park Multidiagnostic Instrument for Psychosis (McGorry *et al.*, 1990a). This comprehensive assessment and diagnostic tool is intended for first-episode psychosis. Onset of psychosis is defined as the emergence of the first sustained psychotic symptom and is dated as precisely as possible. The RP-MIP includes detailed rating guidelines and operational criteria for onset. Multiple information sources are used to record evolution and duration of the illness. The RP-MIP is not brief, although it is comprehensive and reliable.

Despite the high reliability generally demonstrated by standardized instruments such as these, the comparability of DUP estimates derived from these different methods is unknown (Norman & Malla, 2001), with '... no agreed definition of DUP and no standardised way of measuring it' (Singh *et al.*, 2005, p. 118). It would seem that the development of a consistent and reliable measure of DUP is a major challenge in DUP research (Norman & Malla, 2001; Singh *et al.*, 2005).

Types of outcome

Outcomes were divided a priori into primary and secondary categories according to their presumed proximity to the core disease process in schizophrenia. This division was made on the assumption that if untreated psychosis is neurologically or psychologically toxic then DUP should show the strongest correlation with impairments (such as symptoms) that are closely tied to the disease process, as opposed to handicaps (such as reduced quality of life) or process variables (such as time to relapse) that arise from the interaction of impairments with social processes. Consequently, the primary outcome variables were measures of symptoms (all symptoms, positive, negative, depression/anxiety, disorganized), overall functioning and measures of remission based on symptoms. Secondary outcome variables were quality of life, social functioning and measures of relapse. Data on duration of hospital

stay or time to readmission were excluded as they were likely to be strongly related to hospital admission and discharge practices. Data were also excluded if collected using unpublished scales (Marshall *et al.*, 2000) or concerned with brain morphology or cognitive functioning.

Validity assessment

There are no broadly accepted quality criteria for follow-up studies in general, or for studies of DUP in particular. However, reasonable quality criteria appear to be restriction of participants to those with schizophrenia-like disorders, outcome assessed blind to DUP status, a follow-up rate of 80% and the use of a standardized method to assess DUP. A sensitivity analysis was performed based on these criteria. The definition of standardized method used was that either a specific instrument had been used or a precise description of the method was given in the paper describing the study.

Data extraction

Data were extracted independently by two raters, entered on a database and cross-checked for agreement. Disagreements were resolved by discussion. Nine methods were identified for analysing the association between DUP and outcome. These methods may be classified according to whether the DUP was treated dichotomously (i.e. divided into groups of long and short DUP) or continuously and whether the outcome was treated dichotomously or continuously. Data derived from each method of analysis were included in the review.

To examine the effects of premorbid adjustment as a confounding variable, data were extracted from included studies where the effect of DUP on a primary outcome had been assessed after controlling for premorbid adjustment using hierarchical multivariate analysis (Cox, stepwise logistic regression, stepwise multiple regression), partial correlation or analysis of covariance. A record was kept of the number of times when inclusion of premorbid adjustment as a covariate had led to the effect of DUP on an outcome becoming non-significant. On each occasion where this had occurred, the quality of the analysis was assessed according to two criteria. First, was there adjustment for multiple testing (because the commonest scale for measuring premorbid adjustment provides four possible summary scores: for childhood, early adolescence, late adolescence and adulthood; Cannon-Spoor, Potkin & Wyatt, 1982)? Second, were steps taken to ensure that premorbid adjustment was assessed before the onset of the psychotic phase of the disorder?

Study characteristics

Characteristics of participants and studies (including quality criteria) were recorded in tables. Most cohorts were described in more than one paper. In this chapter, for reasons of space, each cohort is referenced and identified by the earliest paper in which it was described. In Table 8.1, the date in parentheses after the cohort identifier is the date of commencement of recruitment to the cohort. Where year of recruitment was not reported, it was estimated by subtracting the length of follow-up plus an estimated delay of 2 years between study completion and publication.

Quantitative data synthesis

Data were analysed using the computer programme Comprehensive Meta-Analysis (Biostat, 2004), which permits meta-analysis and graphical presentation of rate differences, mean differences and correlations. Tests of heterogeneity were applied and where these were statistically significant the data were reanalysed using a random effects model. Data derived from survival analyses in the original paper were presented in tabular form.

A problem was presented by studies that dichotomized participants into long and short DUP groups as there is no agreed cutoff point separating 'long DUP' from 'short DUP'. Consequently, the data from such studies were presented in order of ascending length of cutoff point, to permit a visual assessment of any trends related to choice of cut-point.

Analyses based on treating DUP as a continuous variable were also problematic as the correlation coefficient can be calculated by parametric or non-parametric methods, or by parametric methods on log transformed data. Since DUP is positively skewed, the last two methods are preferable. Therefore, for each meta-analysis based on correlational data a sensitivity analysis was performed excluding data derived from a parametric correlation of untransformed data. Confidence intervals for both parametric and non-parametric correlation coefficients were calculated using Fisher's exact transformation.

Results

Cohort characteristics

After deletion of duplicates there was an initial sample of 11 458 abstracts, from which 26 included cohorts were identified (Addington et al., 2004; Barnes et al., 2000; Black et al., 2001; Bottlender, Strauss & Moller, 2000; Bottlender et al., 2002; Browne et al., 2000; Carbone et al., 1999; Craig et al., 2000; Drake et al., 2000; Fresan et al., 2003; Fuchs & Steinert 2004; Haas & Sweeney, 1992; Ho et al., 2000; Huber, Gross & Schuttler, 1975; Kalla et al., 2002 (contains two cohorts); Keshavan et al., 2003; Larsen et al., 2000; Loebel et al., 1992; Malla et al., 2002; Melle et al., 2004; Szymanski et al., 1996; Tirupati, Rangaswamy & Raman, 2004; Ucok et al., 2004; Verdoux et al., 1999; Wiersma et al., 1998). Fourteen cohorts were from Europe ($n = 2844$); nine were from the US or Canada ($n = 943$); and three were from elsewhere (Australia 1, Mexico 1, India 1; $n = 703$). The mean age of participants was 27.8 years. Women made up 39% of the sample. The mean DUP was 124 weeks, although this reduced to 103 weeks after the exclusion of an outlier (Tirupati et al., 2004).

Twenty studies were restricted to participants with schizophrenia or schizophrenia-like disorders; two reported data separately for schizophrenia and other psychoses, and four reported combined data for all psychoses (Table 8.1). All but one cohort used standardized diagnostic criteria, but only two reported that the researchers who assessed outcome were blind to DUP status at baseline. Fifteen studies had a follow-up rate of 80% or greater; two had a rate of between 70% and 80% and three a rate of between 50% and 70%. In

Table 8.1. Description of included cohorts

Study[a]	Country	Cohort size	Eligibility[b]	Diagnostic method	Definition of DUP	DUP scale[c]	Follow-up (months)[d]	Rater blind	DUP (weeks (median))	Follow-up rate (%)
Barnes et al., 2000 (1998)	UK	136	Schizophreniform	DSM-IV	1st psychotic symptom to neuroleptic treatment	SM	1.5	Unclear	59	90.6
Drake et al., 2000 (1997)	UK	248	Schizophrenia spectrum	DSM-IV	1st psychotic symptom to admission	No	2.5	No	36 (12)	86.7
Bottlender et al., 2000 (1980)	Germany	998	Schizophrenia spectrum	ICD9	1st symptom to admission	No	1.9	Unclear	–	100
Bottlender et al., 2002 (1995)	Germany	196	Schizophrenia spectrum	ICD10	1st psychotic symptom to admission	No	6.0[e]	Unclear	–	100
Fuchs & Steinert, 2004 (1999)	Germany	50	Schizophreniform	ICD10	1st psychotic symptom to admission	IRAOS	12	Unclear	68 (8)	60.0
Browne et al., 2000 (1995)	Ireland	78	Schizophrenia	DSM-IV/SCID	1st psychotic symptom to neuroleptic treatment	SM	0.0	Unclear	28.6	n/a
Wiersma et al., 1998 (1978)	Netherlands	82	Schizophrenia spectrum	ICD9/PSE	1st psychotic symptom to contact	No	180.0	Unclear	10.3	80.5
Huber et al., 1975 (1945)	Germany	502	Schizophrenia	Unclear	Unclear	No	268.8	Unclear	–	Unclear
Kalla et al., 2002 (1992)	Finland	49	Schizophrenia spectrum	DSM-IIIR	1st psychotic symptom to admission	No	0.0	Unclear	16	n/a
Larsen et al., 2000 (1993)	Norway	43	Schizophrenia spectrum	DSM-IIIR/SCID	1st psychotic symptom to admission	SM	12.0	Unclear	114 (26)	100
Melle et al., 2004 (1997)	Scandinavia	281	Schizophrenia spectrum	DSM-IV/SCID	1st psychotic symptom to neuroleptic treatment	SM	3.0	Unclear	49.4 (10)	100
Kalla et al., 2002 (1997)	Madrid	37	Schizophrenia spectrum	DSM-IIIR/SCID	1st psychotic symptom to admission	No	0.0	Unclear	39.6	n/a
Verdoux et al., 1999 (1996)	France	65	All psychoses	DSM-IV	1st psychotic symptom to admission	SM	24.0	Unclear	103 (12.8)	90.8
Ucok et al., 2004 (1996)	Turkey	79	Schizophrenia	DSM-IV/SCID	1st psychotic symptom to admission	No	6.0[e]	Unclear	– (26)	100
Addington et al., 2004 (1999)	Canada	278	Schizophrenia spectrum	DSM-IV/SCID	1st psychotic symptom to neuroleptic treatment	IRAOS	24	Yes	84.2 (28)	59

Study	Country	N	Diagnostic group	Diagnostic criteria	DUP definition	Instrument				
Black et al., 2001 (1998)	Canada	19	Schizophrenia spectrum	DSM-IV	1st psychotic symptom to neuroleptic treatment	IRAOS	6.0	Unclear	83.1	100
Malla et al., 2002 (1999)	Canada	88	All psychoses	DSM-IV/SCID	1st psychotic symptom to neuroleptic treatment	IRAOS	12	Unclear	68.1 (3.9)	79
Haas & Sweeney, 1992 (1989)	USA	71	Schizophrenia spectrum	DSM-IIIR/SCID	1st psychotic symptom to admission	No	0.0	Unclear	156	100
Loebel et al., 1992 (1986)	USA	118	Schizophrenia spectrum	RDC	1st psychotic symptom to neuroleptic treatment	No	Unclear	Yes	71	88.1
Ho et al., 2000 (1988)	USA	74	Schizophrenia	DSM-IV/CASH	1st psychotic symptom to neuroleptic treatment	No	6.0	No	60.8	Unclear
Szymanski et al., 1996 (1992)	USA	36	Schizophreniform	DSM-IIIR/SCID	unclear	No	6.0	Unclear	166.4	100
Craig et al., 2000 (1989)	USA	155	Both	DSM-IIIR/SCID	1st psychotic symptom to admission	No	24.0	No	(14)	96.1
Keshavan et al., 2003 (2000)	USA	104	All psychoses	DSM-IV/SCID	1st psychotic symptom to admission	SM	24.0	No	95.7 (34.1)	65.4
Fresan et al., 2003 (1997)	Mexico	63	All psychoses	DSM-IIIR/SCAN	1st psychotic symptom to admission	SM	0.0	Unclear	59.5	n/a
Carbone et al., 1999 (1989)	Australia	565	Both	DSM-IIIR/RPMIP	1st psychotic symptom to neuroleptic treatment	RP-MIP	12.0	Unclear	25.9 (7.1)	74.8
Tirupati et al., 2004 (1985)	India	75	Schizophrenia	ICD9/PSE	1st psychotic symptom to neuroleptic treatment	No	12.0	Unclear	796.0	100

n/a, not available; DUP, duration of untreated psychosis; IRAOS, Interview for the Retrospective Assessment for the Onset of Schizophrenia; RP-MIP, Royal Park Multidiagnostic Instrument for Psychosis; DSM, DSM, *Diagnostic and Statistical Manual of Mental Disorders*; ICD, World Health Organization *International Classification of Diseases*; SCID, Structured Clinical Interview for DSM; PSE, Present State Examination; CASH, Comprehensive Assessment of Symptoms and History; SCAN, Schedule for Clinical Assessment in Neuropsychiatry; RDC, Research Diagnostic Criteria.

[a] The date in parentheses is the date when recruiting of the cohort began, or an estimate of that date if not reported in the paper.

[b] Schizophrenia indicates the study included only schizophrenia; schizophreniform indicates the study also included schizophreniform disorders; schizophrenia spectrum indicates the study also included schizoaffective disorders; all psychoses indicates the study also included affective psychosis; both indicates data were available separately for affective and non-affective psychoses.

[c] SM indicates used a systematic method such as applying the Positive and Negative Syndrome Scale retrospectively but did not use a specifically developed standardized interview.

[d] Follow-up of 0 months indicates data available only at presentation

[e] Follow-up was at discharge from hospital, estimated to be about 6 months on average.

two studies the follow-up rate was unclear, and in four only data from first presentation were reported. Twelve studies reported the use of a systematic method to assess DUP.

Effect of duration of untreated psychosis on outcome

Summary correlations between DUP and primary or secondary outcomes at first presentation, 6, 12 and 24 month follow-up, are shown in Fig. 8.1. These summary correlations shift towards the right of the figure as the duration of follow-up increases, indicating an increasingly strong association between DUP and a range of outcomes. Thus, at first presentation, only two of eight outcomes show significant correlations with DUP (depression/anxiety and quality of life), but by follow-up at 6 months, six of eight outcomes show significant correlations, and by 12 months all outcomes are correlated. In all cases, the correlations are positive, indicating that a longer DUP is associated with a worse outcome. At follow-up at 24 months, data are substantially reduced, as only two studies have followed participants for this length of time (Addington et al., 2004; Keshavan et al., 2003), yet there are still significant correlations for three of five outcomes.

Data based on comparisons between long and short DUP groups are presented in Fig. 8.2. These data are derived from a smaller number of participants than the correlational data but display a similar pattern. At first presentation, the only significant differences between long and short DUP groups were on negative symptoms and quality of life, but by 6 months there were significant differences between all symptoms, overall functioning, positive symptoms and quality of life, though not depression/anxiety (for which data were limited to 19 subjects) or negative symptoms. No data were available at 12 months; there are some limited data from one study at 24 months (Craig et al., 2000) and another at 15 years (Bottlender et al., 2000). These data showed no significant differences between long and short DUP groups at 24 months, but at 15 years the long DUP group was significantly worse on depression/anxiety, overall functioning and positive symptoms, but not for negative symptoms.

A change over time is also seen in the extent of heterogeneity between study estimates of effect size. For example, at the time of first presentation, there was statistically significant heterogeneity between the estimates for the first-episode cohorts of the correlation between DUP and negative symptoms, and DUP and positive symptoms. However, there was no significant heterogeneity between these estimates at later follow-up points. Significant heterogeneity suggests that estimates of the strength of the correlation between DUP and an outcome vary more widely between studies than would be expected by chance alone. Therefore, there would appear to be some systematic differences in study methodology at first presentation that were leading to varying estimates of effect size.

The number of participants in remission in long and short DUP groups was reported by seven studies, with data available at follow-up at 6, 12 and 24 months (Black et al., 2001; Bottlender et al., 2002; Craig et al., 2000; Huber et al., 1975; Malla et al., 2002; Tirupati et al., 2004; Verdoux et al., 1999). Participants in the long DUP group were significantly less likely to be in remission at all follow-up points where data were available (Fig. 8.3). Despite varying definitions of 'remission', tests of heterogeneity were not significant. Two studies compared the length of DUP between participants in remission versus those not in remission and found that DUP was significantly longer in those not in remission ($n = 270$; standardized difference 0.517; 95% CI, 0.121–0.915; $p = 0.011$; heterogeneity not significant) (Carbone et al., 1999; Larsen et al., 2000). Two studies measured the time to remission and found that it was longer amongst participants with long DUP (Loebel et al., 1992; Wiersma et al., 1998). Another study found that the likelihood of remission was reduced in participants with a DUP of greater than 1 year, but it did not find that the risk of relapse was increased (Loebel et al., 1992).

Effect of premorbid adjustment

Sixteen multiple regression analyses (from nine studies) were identified that had examined the effect of controlling for premorbid adjustment when a significant association was present between DUP and one or

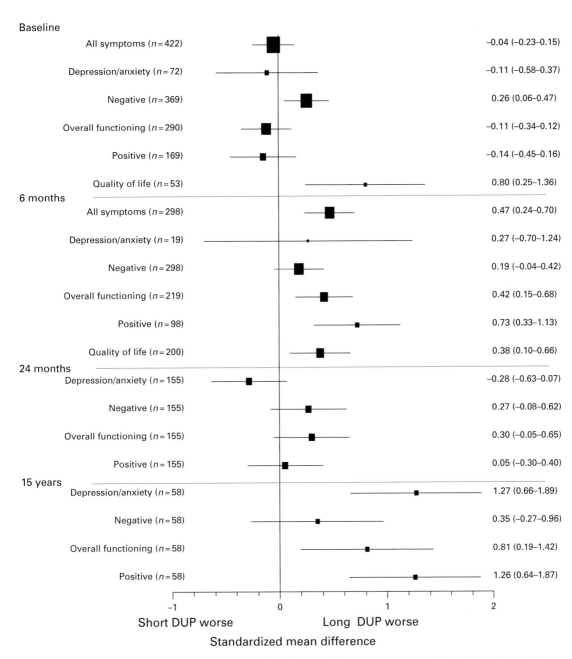

Fig. 8.2. Long versus short duration of untreated psychosis (DUP): mean differences on outcomes (with confidence intervals) by follow-up period.

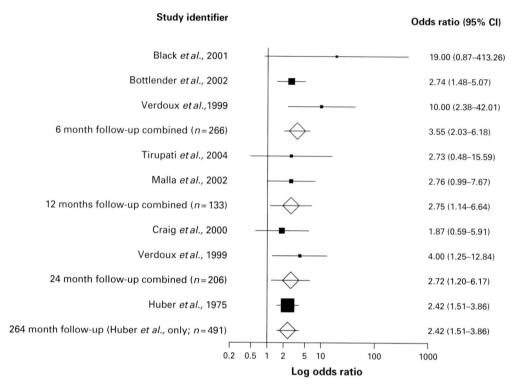

Fig. 8.3. Odds of no remission in long versus short duration of untreated psychosis groups. An odds ratio > 1 indicates that subjects in the long duration group were more likely not to be in remission at the follow-up point. Definitions of remission: no positive symptoms scoring >3 on the Positive and Negative Syndrome Scale (Black *et al.*, 2001), Global Assessment of Functioning score >62 (Bottlender *et al.*, 2002), variants of the World Health Organization Life Chart method (Craig *et al.*, 2000; Tirupati *et al.*, 2004; Verdoux *et al.*, 1999), all global items < 2 on the Scale for the Assessment of Positive Symptoms (Malla *et al.*, 2002), and no symptoms at interview (Huber *et al.*, 1975). CI, confidence interval.

more of the primary or secondary outcome variables (Table 8.2). After controlling for premorbid adjustment, the association between DUP and outcome was no longer significant in only 4 of the 16 analyses. However, three of these four analyses were suboptimal according to our predetermined quality criteria (either because they did not control for multiple testing or because they did not make it clear that premorbid adjustment was assessed before the onset of the disorder). In the other 12 analyses the association between DUP and the outcome variable stayed significant. There appeared to be a particularly robust association between DUP and positive symptoms, where four multiple regressions failed to show any effect of controlling for premorbid adjustment.

Sensitivity analysis

Sensitivity analyses on the primary outcome variables at baseline, 6 and 12 months are summarized in Table 8.3. The analyses excluded studies that included participants with affective psychoses, used Pearson's method without log transformation (correlational data only), did not use a standardized method for assessing DUP, or had a follow-up of less than 80%. The sensitivity analyses did not differ substantially from the main findings for any of the primary outcome variables. No sensitivity analyses were conducted on blinded studies as there were only two. Of these, one reported significant correlations between DUP and positive symptoms and quality of life at 0, 12 and 24 months'

Table 8.2. Effect of controlling for premorbid adjustment in the presence of a significant association between duration of untreated psychosis and outcome

Outcome	Study[a]	Method	Premorbid scale	No.	Multiple testing corrected[b]	Truly premorbid	Outcome
Negative	Larsen et al., 2000	Mult reg	PAS	43	No	No	DUP NS
	Carbone et al., 1999	Mult reg	PAS	202	Yes	Yes	No change
Positive	Malla et al., 2002	Mult reg	PAS	88	No	No	No change
	Larsen et al., 2000	Mult reg	PAS	43	No	No	No change
	Addington et al., 2004	Mult reg	PAS	200	Yes	Yes	No change
	Carbone et al., 1999	Mult reg	PAS	202	Yes	Yes	No change
All symptoms	Melle et al., 2004	Mult reg	PAS	281	Yes	Unclear	No change
	Ucok et al., 2004[c]	Mult reg	PAS	79	Yes	Unclear	DUP NS
Overall function	Craig et al., 2000	Mult reg	PAS	202	No	No	DUP NS
	Larsen et al., 2000	Mult reg	PAS	43	No	No	No change
	Bottlender et al., 2002	Log reg	Phillips scale	196	Not applicable	Unclear	No change
Remission	Loebel et al., 1992	Mult reg	PAS	70	No	No	No change
	Malla et al., 2002	Mult reg	PAS	88	No	No	No change
Quality of life	Carbone et al., 1999	Mult reg	PAS	202	Yes	Yes	No change
	Addington et al., 2004	Mult reg	PAS	200	Yes	Yes	No change
Social function	Malla et al., 2002.	Mult reg	PAS	66	Yes	Yes	DUP NS

DUP NS, association between outcome and duration of untreated psychosis no longer significant after controlling for premorbid adjustment; Mult reg, multiple regression; Log reg, logarithmic regression; PAS, Premorbid Adjustment Scale.
[a] Each cohort is identified by a reference to a single paper describing the cohort; to save space, not all references for each cohort are included. The multiple regression analyses on the cohort are not necessarily described in the cited reference; full references for each cohort are available from the authors.
[b] Yes indicates that there was a correction for the fact that there are four ways of measuring premorbid adjustment using the PAS
[c] Analysis based on baseline data only.

follow-up (Addington et al., 2004), while the other found a significant association between DUP and level of functioning (Loebel et al., 1992).

Discussion

The main finding of this systematic review was convincing evidence of a moderately strong association between DUP and a range of outcomes at 6 and 12 months of follow-up. The association was not usually obvious at the time of first presentation but emerged after the patient had received treatment. At 6 and 12 months' follow-up, only four of 21 comparisons in Figs. 8.1 and 8.2 were not statistically significant (and three of the four negative comparisons were based on very small amounts of data). At 24 months' follow-up, the evidence of an association between DUP and outcome was weaker (though only limited amounts of data were available); however, data from a single study at follow-up after 15 years continued to provide support for an association between DUP and affective symptoms, overall functioning and positive symptoms. The review also found an association between DUP and the odds of remission at 6, 12, 24 and even 269 months' follow-up. The strength of the association between DUP and outcome, based on data from correlational analyses, was only moderately strong, approximately 13% of the variance in outcome. Yet long DUP seemed

Table 8.3. Summary of sensitivity analyses (with 95% confidence intervals) for primary outcomes

Follow-up point	Outcome	All data	Data excluded by sensitivity analysis			
			Subjects include affective psychoses	Correlation derived by simple Pearson's	Measure of DUP not standardized	Study follow-up rate <80%
Correlational data						
0 months	All symptoms	0.01 (−0.2 to 0.22)[a]	0.01 (−0.2 to 0.22)[a]	0.01 (−0.2 to 0.22)[a]	0.08 (−0.02 to 0.19)	Not applicable
	Positive symptoms	0.08 (−0.04 to 0.21)[a]	**0.12 (0.00 to 0.24)**[a]	0.12 (−0.02 to 0.26)[a]	0.04 (−0.13 to 0.22)[a]	Not applicable
	Negative symptoms	0.08 (−0.01 to 0.17)[a]	0.08 (−0.01 to 0.17)[a]	0.05 (−0.00 to 0.12)	0.06 (−0.01 to 0.13)	Not applicable
	Overall functioning	0.23 (−0.28 to 0.65)[a]	0.23 (−0.28 to 0.65)[a]	0.23 (−0.28 to 0.65)[a]	**−0.15 (−0.26 to 0.03)**	Not applicable
	Depression/anxiety	**0.10 (0.02–0.18)**	**0.10 (0.02–0.18)**	**0.10 (0.02–0.19)**	0.084 (−0.02–0.19)	Not applicable
6 months	All symptoms	**0.36 (0.28–0.43)**	**0.36 (0.28–0.43)**	**0.36 (0.28–0.43)**	**0.39 (0.29–0.48)**	**0.36 (0.29–0.44)**
	Positive symptoms	**0.29 (0.23–0.35)**	**0.29 (0.23–0.35)**	**0.33 (0.26–0.40)**	**0.38 (0.28–0.47)**	**0.31 (0.18–0.42)**[a]
	Negative symptoms	**0.24 (0.18–0.30)**	**0.24 (0.18–0.30)**	**0.18 (0.10–0.26)**	**0.20 (0.10–0.31)**	**0.26 (0.20–0.32)**
	Overall functioning	**0.20 (0.12–0.27)**	**0.20 (0.12–0.27)**	**0.25 (0.15–0.35)**	**0.30 (0.18–0.40)**	**0.22 (0.02–0.40)**[a]
	Depression/anxiety	**0.22 (0.13–0.30)**	**0.22 (0.13–0.30)**	**0.22 (0.13–0.30)**	**0.22 (0.11–0.32)**	**0.21 (0.13–0.30)**
12 months	All symptoms	**0.28 (0.18–0.37)**	**0.28 (0.18–0.37)**	**0.28 (0.18–0.37)**	**0.32 (0.17–0.45)**	**0.25 (0.12–0.37)**
	Positive symptoms	**0.28 (0.21–0.34)**	**0.27 (0.20–0.34)**	**0.27 (0.20–0.33)**	**0.29 (0.21–0.37)**	**0.28 (0.17–0.39)**
	Negative symptoms	**0.17 (0.10–0.24)**	**0.18 (0.10–0.25)**	**0.16 (0.09–0.23)**	**0.18 (0.10–0.26)**	**0.18 (0.06–0.30)**
	Overall functioning	**0.27 (0.16–0.38)**	**0.35 (0.22–0.47)**	**0.23 (0.11–0.35)**	**0.27 (0.16–0.38)**	**0.50 (0.23–0.69)**
	Depression/anxiety	**0.19 (0.09–0.29)**	**0.22 (0.10–0.33)**	**0.18 (0.07–0.28)**	**0.23 (0.08–0.38)**	**0.18 (0.06–0.29)**
24 months	All symptoms	No data	No data	No data	No data	No data
	Positive symptoms	**0.17 (0.01–0.31)**	**0.17 (0.01–0.31)**	**0.17 (0.01–0.31)**	**0.17 (0.01–0.31)**	No data
	Negative symptoms	−0.11 (−0.25 to 0.04)	−0.11 (−0.25 to 0.04)	−0.11 (−0.25 to 0.04)	−0.11 (−0.25 to 0.04)	No data
	Overall functioning	**0.28 (0.04–0.48)**	**No data**	**0.28 (0.04–0.48)**	**0.28 (0.04–0.48)**	No data
	Depression/anxiety	No data	No data	No data	No data	No data
Data from long versus short DUP group comparisons						
0 months	All symptoms	−0.04 (−0.23 to 0.14)	0.01 (−0.25 to 0.28)	0.01 (−0.25 to 0.28)	−0.02 (−0.26 to 0.21)	Not applicable
	Positive symptoms	−0.14 (−0.44 to 0.16)	−0.14 (−0.44 to 0.16)	Not applicable	0.41 (−0.55 to 1.38)	Not applicable
	Negative symptoms	**0.26 (0.05 to 0.46)**	0.29 (0.00–0.58)	Not applicable	**0.30 (0.04–0.57)**	Not applicable
	Overall functioning	−0.11 (−0.34 to 0.11)	−0.33 (−0.75 to 0.09)	Not applicable	0.00 (−0.27 to 0.25)	Not applicable
	Depression/anxiety	−0.10 (−0.57 to 0.36)	−0.10 (−0.57 to 0.36)	Not applicable	−0.10 (−0.57 to 0.36)	Not applicable

6 months	All symptoms	0.47 (0.24–0.69)	**0.81 (0.41–1.21)**	Not applicable	**0.32 (0.05–0.58)**	**0.81 (0.41–1.21)**
	Positive symptoms	**0.72 (0.32–1.12)**	**0.72 (0.32–1.12)**	Not applicable	**1.08 (0.11–2.05)**	**0.72 (0.32–1.12)**
	Negative symptoms	0.18 (−0.04–0.41)	0.19 (−0.20 to 0.59)	Not applicable	0.20 (−0.05 to 0.47)	0.19 (−0.20 to 0.59)
	Overall functioning	**0.41 (0.15–0.68)**	**1.00 (0.03–1.96)**	Not applicable	**0.41 (0.15–0.68)**	**1.00 (0.03–1.96)**
	Depression/anxiety	0.27 (−0.69–1.24)	0.27 (−0.69 to 1.24)	Not applicable	0.27 (−0.69 to 1.24)	0.27 (−0.69 to 1.24)
24 months	All symptoms	No data	No data	Not applicable	No data	No data
	Positive symptoms	0.05 (−0.29 to 0.40)	0.05 (−0.29 to 0.40)	Not applicable	No data	0.05 (−0.29 to 0.40)
	Negative symptoms	0.27 (−0.07 to 0.62)	0.27 (−0.07 to 0.62)	Not applicable	No data	0.27 (−0.07 to 0.62)
	Overall functioning	0.29 (−0.05 to 0.64)	0.29 (−0.05 to 0.64)	Not applicable	No data	0.29 (−0.05 to 0.64)
	Depression/anxiety	−0.28 (−0.63 to 0.06)	−0.28 (−0.63 to 0.06)	Not applicable	No data	−0.28 (−0.63 to 0.06)

[a] DUP, duration of untreated psychosis. Test for heterogeneity significant; effect size and confidence intervals derived by random effects model. A negative value for the effect size indicates that shorter DUP is correlated with a worse outcome. Effect sizes in bold are statistically significant at $p < 0.05$. No data are available at 12 months for long versus short DUP comparison.

to account for approximately 1 in 3 to 1 in 4 of those who did not achieve remission.

Notwithstanding the consistency of the association seen in this meta-analysis, some of the included studies reached the conclusion that there was no association. These include three important American studies that are often cited as proving that there is no association between DUP and outcome (Craig *et al.*, 2000; Ho *et al.*, 2000; Loebel *et al.*, 1992). However, on closer scrutiny, the findings of all three studies are actually consistent with the findings of this review. In the Iowa prospective study (Ho *et al.*, 2000), a small sample size meant that, although the correlations obtained for positive symptoms and overall functioning were not significant, the 95% CI values overlapped the estimate of the pooled correlation obtained by this review. They might also have done so for negative symptoms, had not 'disorganized' symptoms been reported separately. In the Hillside study (Loebel *et al.*, 1992), a preliminary report found a significant association between DUP and level of remission, but a later report, using hazard ratios, found that DUP was not a predictor of first relapse. However, because so many analyses were conducted on the dataset, the later report used 99% CI values to determine significance and was consequently underpowered. The Suffolk County study (Craig *et al.*, 2000) found no significant difference between long and short DUP groups at 24 months of follow-up, but it did find that fewer patients with long DUP were in remission at 24 months. Although this effect was not significant within the study, it was of a similar size to that found at 24 months by the only other study examining this outcome at the same time point (Verdoux *et al.*, 1999) and the cumulative results from the two studies are significant (Fig. 8.3).

The main methodological limitation of a review based on follow-up studies is that it cannot exclude the possibility that any observed association between DUP and outcome is a consequence of both being correlated with an unknown third variable. Premorbid adjustment is generally considered the best candidate for the role of the 'third variable' on the grounds that people with poor premorbid adjustment are known to have a poor outcome and could be reluctant or less able to make contact with psychiatric services. However, we found little evidence to support this hypothesis in our scrutiny of multiple regressions that had included premorbid adjustment as a predictor variable.

A further limitation of this review is that there were insufficient data to justify a formal analysis of publication bias for any outcome. However, the consistency of results across outcomes and methods of analysis (DUP treated as continuous or categorical) and the inclusion of several large studies suggest that publication bias is an unlikely explanation for the findings. The fact that only two studies used raters who were blind to DUP status is also a limitation, since it means that we cannot exclude the possibility that ratings of outcome may have been biased by awareness of participants' DUP. Future studies of first-episode cohorts should ensure that raters are blind to DUP status.

In the course of the review, we uncovered two incidental findings that may be related and that could shed some light on the nature of the relationship between DUP and outcome. Our first finding was that the size of the difference in outcome between long and short DUP groups bore no relationship to the cutoff point used to define 'long' DUP. In other words, the difference in outcome between long and short DUP groups was much the same regardless of whether long DUP was defined as 6 months or 12 months. Our second finding was that there was heterogeneity in effect size between studies at first presentation but this was absent at follow-up. These observations are compatible with the hypothesis that the long-term harm caused by psychosis occurs principally in the first few months or even weeks following onset (Drake *et al.*, 2000). This hypothesis explains the first observation because only the choice of a cutoff point very close to the onset of psychosis would have a noticeable influence on the size of the difference in outcome between long and short DUP groups. It also explains the second observation because people with short duration of psychosis, who tend to respond quickly to treatment, would also make the predominant contribution to any observed correlation between DUP and outcome. Therefore, studies where the 'baseline' assessment began before treatment was started would find no relationship between DUP and outcome, but those that delayed assessment until a few days after treatment would find a substantial difference.

If baseline data were derived from a mixture of studies using both of these approaches, then the result would be substantial heterogeneity between studies at baseline, which would disappear at subsequent follow-up points, as observed by this review.

Despite the promising findings of this review, it would be foolish at this stage to predict that reducing DUP will improve outcome. However, the Early Treatment and Intervention in Psychosis project has already demonstrated that DUP can be shortened by a meticulous early detection programme (Larsen *et al.*, 2001). The next big challenge for researchers around the world examining early intervention is to carry out the definitive clinical trial that will establish beyond doubt whether the link between DUP and outcome is causative. Whether or not such trials are successful, at the very least it seems likely that controlled attempts to manipulate DUP will substantially increase our understanding of psychosis.

REFERENCES

Addington, J., van Mastrigt, S. & Addington, D. (2004). Duration of untreated psychosis: impact on 2-year outcome. *Psychological Medicine*, **34**, 277–84.

Barnes, T., Hutton, S. B., Chapman, M. J. *et al.* (2000). West London first-episode study of schizophrenia. Clinical correlates of duration of untreated psychosis. *British Journal of Psychiatry*, **177**, 207–11.

Beiser, M., Erickson, D., Fleming, J. A. E. & Iacono, W. G. (1993). Establishing the onset of psychotic illness. *American Journal of Psychiatry*, **150**, 1349–54.

Biostat. Comprehensive Meta-Analysis Version 1.0.23. Englewood, NJ: Biostat. http//www.Meta-Analysis.com (accessed 13 February 2004).

Black, K., Peters, L., Rui, Q. *et al.* (2001). Duration of untreated psychosis predicts treatment outcome in an early psychosis program. *Schizophrenia Research*, **47**, 215–22.

Bottlender, R., Strauss, A. & Moller, H. (2000). Impact of duration of symptoms prior to first hospitalization on acute outcome in 998 schizophrenic patients. *Schizophrenia Research*, **44**, 145–50.

Bottlender, R., Sato, T., Jager, M. *et al.* (2002). The impact of duration of untreated psychosis and premorbid functioning on outcome of first inpatient treatment in schizophrenic and schizoaffective patients. *European Archives of Psychiatry and Clinical Neuroscience*, **252**, 226–31.

Bottlender, R., Sato, T., Jager, M. *et al.* (2003). The impact of the duration of untreated psychosis prior to first psychiatric admission on the 15-year outcome in schizophrenia. *Schizophrenia Research*, **62**, 37–44.

Browne, S., Larkin, C. & O'Callaghan, E. (1999). Outcome studies in schizophrenia. *Irish Journal of Psychological Medicine*, **16**, 140–4.

Browne, S., Clarke, M., Gervin, M. *et al.* (2000). Determinants of quality of life at first presentation with schizophrenia. *British Journal of Psychiatry*, **176**, 173–6.

Cannon-Spoor, H. E., Potkin, S. G. & Wyatt, R. J. (1982). Measurement of premorbid adjustment in chronic schizophrenia. *Schizophrenia Bulletin*, **8**, 470–84.

Carbone, S., Harrigan, S., McGorry, P., Curry, C. & Elkins, K. (1999). Duration of untreated psychosis and 12-month outcome in first-episode psychosis: the impact of treatment approach. *Acta Psychiatrica Scandinavica*, **100**, 96–104.

Chong, S., Mythily, Lum, A., Chan, Y. H. & McGorry, P. (2005). Determinants of duration of untreated psychosis and the pathway to care in Singapore. *International Journal of Social Psychiatry*, **51**, 55–62.

Craig, T., Bromet, E. J., Fennig, S., Tanenberg-Karant, M., Lavelle, J. & Galambos, N. (2000). Is there an association between duration of untreated psychosis and 24-month clinical outcome in a first-admission series? *American Journal of Psychiatry*, **157**, 60–6.

de Haan, L., Linszen, D. H., Lenior, M. E., de Win, E. D. & Gorsira, R. (2003). Duration of untreated psychosis and outcome of schizophrenia: delay in intensive psychosocial treatment versus delay in treatment with antipsychotic medication. *Schizophrenia Bulletin*, **29**, 341–8.

Department of Health (2000). *The NHS Plan. A Plan For Investment, A Plan For Reform*. London: Department of Health.

Drake, R. J., Haley, C. J., Akhtar, S. & Lewis, S. W. (2000). Causes and consequences of duration of untreated psychosis in schizophrenia. *British Journal of Psychiatry*, **177**, 511–15.

Edwards, J. & McGorry, P. D. (2002). Multi-component early intervention: models of good practice. In J. Edwards & P. D. McGorry (eds.), *Implementing Early Intervention in Psychosis*. London: Martin Dunitz, pp. 63–84.

Fresan, A., Apiquian, R., Ulloa, R. E. *et al.* (2003). Premorbid functioning by gender and its relationship with duration of untreated psychosis in first psychotic episode. *Actas Españolas de Psiquiatría*, **31**, 53–8.

Friis, S., Melle, I., Larsen, T. K. *et al.* (2004). Does duration of untreated psychosis bias study samples of first-episode psychosis? *Acta Psychiatrica Scandinavica*, **110**, 286–91.

Fuchs, J. & Steinert, T. (2004). Duration of untreated psychosis (DUP): a useful predictor of outcome in schizophrenia? *Fortschritte der Neurologie-Psychiatrie*, **72**, 79–87.

Haas, G. & Sweeney, J. A. (1992). Premorbid and onset features of first-episode schizophrenia. *Schizophrenia Bulletin*, **18**, 373–86.

Häfner, H., Riecher-Rossler, A., Hambrecht, M. *et al.* (1992). IRAOS: an instrument for the assessment of onset and early course of schizophrenia. *Schizophrenia Research*, **6**, 209–23.

Häfner, H., Maurer, K., Loffler, W. & Riecher-Rossler, A. (1993). The influence of age and sex on the onset and early course of schizophrenia. *British Journal of Psychiatry*, **162**, 80–6.

Harrigan, S. M., McGorry, P. D. & Krstev, H. (2003). Does treatment delay in first-episode psychosis really matter? *Psychological Medicine*, **33**, 97–110.

Ho, B. & Andreasen, N. C. (2001). Long delays in seeking treatment for schizophrenia. *Lancet*, **357**, 898–9.

Ho, B., Andreasen, N. C., Flaum, M., Nopoulos, P. & Miller, D. (2000). Untreated initial psychosis: its relation to quality of life and symptom remission in first-episode schizophrenia. *American Journal of Psychiatry*, **157**, 808–15.

Huber, G., Gross, G. & Schuttler, R. (1975). A long-term follow-up study of schizophrenia: psychiatric course of illness and prognosis. *Acta Psychiatrica Scandinavica*, **52**, 49–57.

Kalla, O., Aaltonen, J., Wahlstrom, J. *et al.* (2002). Duration of untreated psychosis and its correlates in first-episode psychosis in Finland and Spain. *Acta Psychiatrica Scandinavica*, **106**, 265–75.

Kay, S. R., Fiszbein, A. & Opler, L. A. (1987). The Positive and Negative Syndrome Scale (PANSS) for schizophrenia. *Schizophrenia Bulletin*, **13**, 261–76.

Keshavan, K. S. & Schooler, N. R. (1992). First-episode studies in schizophrenia: criteria and characterization. *Schizophrenia Bulletin*, **18**, 491–513.

Keshavan, M. S., Haas, G., Miewald, J. *et al.* (2003). Prolonged untreated illness duration from prodromal onset predicts outcome in first episode psychoses. *Schizophrenia Bulletin*, **29**, 757–69.

Larsen, T. K., McGlashan, T. J. & Moe, L. C. (1996). First-episode schizophrenia: I. Early course parameters. *Schizophrenia Bulletin*, **22**, 241–56.

Larsen, T. K., Moe, L. C., Vibe-Hansen, L. & Johannessen, J. O. (2000). Premorbid functioning versus duration of untreated psychosis in 1 year outcome in first-episode psychosis. *Schizophrenia Research*, **45**, 1–9.

Larsen, T. K., McGlashan, T. H., Johannessen, J. O. *et al.* (2001). Shortened duration of untreated first episode of psychosis:

changes in patient characteristics at treatment. *American Journal of Psychiatry*, **158**, 1917–19.

Lincoln, C. & McGorry, P. D. (1999). Pathways to care in early psychosis: clinical and consumer perspectives. In P. D. McGorry & H. J. Jackson (eds.), *The Recognition and Management of Early Psychosis: A Preventive Approach.* Cambridge, UK: Cambridge University Press, pp. 51–79.

Loebel, A. D., Lieberman, J. A., Alvir, J. M. *et al.* (1992). Duration of psychosis and outcome in first-episode schizophrenia. *American Journal of Psychiatry*, **149**, 1183–8.

Malla, A. K., Norman, R. M. G., Manchanda, R. *et al.* (2002). One year outcome in first episode psychosis: influence of DUP and other predictors. *Schizophrenia Research*, **54**, 231–42.

Marshall, M., Lockwood, L., Bradley, C. *et al.* (2000). Unpublished rating scales: a major source of bias in randomised controlled trials of treatments for schizophrenia? *British Journal of Psychiatry*, **176**, 249–53.

Maurer, K. & Häfner, H. (1995). Methodological aspects of onset assessment in schizophrenia. *Schizophrenia Research*, **15**, 265–76.

McGlashan, T. H. (1998). Early detection and intervention of schizophrenia: rationale and research. *British Journal of Psychiatry*, **172**, 3–6.

McGorry, P., Copolov, D. & Singh, B. (1990a). Royal Park Multidiagnostic Instrument for Psychosis: Part 1. Rationale and review. *Schizophrenia Bulletin*, **16**, 501–15.

McGorry, P. D., Dossetor, C. R., Kaplan, I. *et al.* (1990). *The Royal Park Multidiagnostic Instrument for Psychosis: Glossary and Guidelines for Administration.* Melbourne, Australia: Royal Park Hospital. Available from Professor P. D. McGorry, Department of Psychiatry, University of Melbourne.

McGorry, P. D., Edwards, J., Mihalopoulos, C., Harrigan, S. M. & Jackson, H. J. (1996). EPPIC: an evolving system of early detection and optimal management. *Schizophrenia Bulletin*, **22**, 305–26.

McGorry, P. D., Singh, B. S., Copolov, D. L. *et al.* (1990b). The Royal Park Multidiagnostic Instrument for Psychosis: Part II. Development, reliability and validity. *Schizophrenia Bulletin*, **16**, 517–36.

Melle, I., Larsen, T. K., Haahr, U. *et al.* (2004). Reducing the duration of untreated first-episode psychosis: effects on clinical presentation. *Archives of General Psychiatry*, **61**, 143–50.

Norman, R. & Malla, A. K. (2001). Duration of untreated psychosis: a critical examination of the concept and its importance. *Psychological Medicine*, **31**, 381–400.

Norman, R., Townsend, L. & Malla, A. (2001). Duration of untreated psychosis and cognitive functioning in first-episode patients. *British Journal of Psychiatry*, **179**, 340–5.

Perkins, D. O., Leserman, J., Jarskog, L. F. *et al.* (2000). Characterizing and dating the onset of symptoms in psychotic illness: the Symptom Onset in Schizophrenia (SOS) inventory. *Schizophrenia Research*, **44**, 1–10.

Perkins, D. O., Gu, H., Boteva, K. & Lieberman, J. A. (2005). Relationship between duration of untreated psychosis and outcome in first-episode schizophrenia: a critical review and meta-analysis. *American Journal of Psychiatry*, **162**, 1785–804.

Robinson, D. G., Woerner, M. G., Alvir, J. A. J. *et al.* (1999a). Predictors of relapse following response from a first-episode of schizophrenia or schizoaffective disorder. *Archives of General Psychiatry*, **56**, 241–7.

Robinson, D. G., Woerner, M. G., Alvir, J. A. J. *et al.* (1999b). Predictors of treatment response from a first-episode of schizophrenia or schizoaffective disorder. *American Journal of Psychiatry*, **156**, 544–9.

Sheitman, B. & Lieberman, J. A. (1998). The natural history and pathophysiology of treatment resistant schizophrenia. *Journal of Psychiatric Research*, **32**, 143–50.

Singh, S. P., Cooper, J. E., Fisher, H. L. *et al.* (2005). Determining the chronology and components of psychosis onset: the Nottingham Onset Schedule (NOS). *Schizophrenia Research*, **80**, 117–30.

Szymanski, S., Cannon, T. D., Gallacher, F., Erwin, R. J. & Gur, R. E. (1996). Course of treatment response in first-episode and chronic schizophrenia. *American Journal of Psychiatry*, **153**, 519–25.

Tirupati, N. S., Rangaswamy, T. & Raman, P. (2004). Duration of untreated psychosis and treatment outcome in schizophrenia patients untreated for many years. *Australian and New Zealand Journal of Psychiatry*, **38**, 339–43.

Ucok, A., Polat, A., Genc, A., Cakir, S. & Turan, N. (2004). Duration of untreated psychosis may predict acute treatment response in first-episode schizophrenia. *Journal of Psychiatric Research*, **38**, 163–8.

Verdoux, H., Bergey, C., Assens, F. *et al.* (1998). Prediction of duration of psychosis before first admission. *European Psychiatry*, **13**, 346–52.

Verdoux, H., Liraud, F., Gonzales, B. *et al.* (1999). Short-term outcome in first admission for psychosis. *Encephale*, **25**, 213–20.

Verdoux, H., Liraud, F., Bergey, C. *et al.* (2001). Is the association between duration of untreated psychosis and outcome confounded? A two year follow-up study of first-admitted patients. *Schizophrenia Research*, **49**, 231–41.

Wiersma, D., Nienhuis, F., Slooff, C. J. & Giel, R. (1998). Natural course of schizophrenic disorders: a 15-year follow up of a Dutch incidence cohort. *Schizophrenia Bulletin*, **24**, 75–85.

Wunderink, A., Nienhuis, F. J., Sytema, S. & Wiersma, D. (2006). Treatment delay and response rate in first episode psychosis. *Acta Psychiatrica Scandinavica*, **113**, 332–9.

Wyatt, R. (1991). Early intervention with neuroleptics may decrease the long-term morbidity of schizophrenia. *Schizophrenia Research*, **5**, 201–2.

Wyatt, R. & Henter, I. (2001). Rationale for the study of early intervention. *Schizophrenia Research*, **51**, 69–76.

9

Improving the community's mental health literacy as a means of facilitating early intervention

Anthony F. Jorm and Annemarie Wright

Role of mental health literacy in pathways to care

There can be long delays between the initial appearance of psychotic symptoms and the initiation of appropriate treatment (Marshall *et al.*, 2005). This duration of untreated psychosis (DUP) causes unnecessary suffering in both the patient and family and has consequences for the maintenance of social networks and for the achievement of educational and occupational goals (Harris *et al.*, 2005). Some have argued that earlier treatment may also improve long-term prognosis, but this remains to be firmly established (Marshall *et al.*, 2005). Whether or not early intervention affects prognosis, there are clear reasons for trying to reduce DUP.

A number of authors have pointed out that there are two components to DUP: (1) the period between onset of psychotic symptoms and professional contact, and (2) the period between first contact and the initiation of appropriate treatment (Lincoln, Harrigan & McGorry, 1998; Norman *et al.*, 2004). It is also possible to extend the first component back even further from the onset of the first prodromal changes, which may themselves warrant intervention. In the case of schizophrenia, the most frequent initial symptom is depressed mood, often followed by negative symptoms and functional impairment, with positive symptoms occurring some years after the first prodromal changes (Häfner *et al.*, 2005). Reducing each of these components of DUP involves different kinds of action. The period from onset to professional contact requires better recognition and help-seeking by the person who is affected, their social network and health service gatekeepers

such as teachers and welfare workers, whereas the period from contact to adequate treatment requires better skills in health professionals. It has been proposed that reducing the first component of DUP would require greater community awareness of psychotic disorders and the appropriate types of help available (Addington *et al.*, 2002; Bertolote & McGorry, 2005). This is an aspect of mental health literacy that has been defined as: 'knowledge and beliefs about mental disorders which aid their recognition, management or prevention' (Jorm *et al.*, 1997a, p. 182). The present chapter examines the role that the community's mental health literacy might play in DUP, in particular with the first component from onset to professional contact. It also reviews evidence on interventions to improve mental health literacy and whether these have any benefits for earlier recognition and treatment.

Public knowledge about psychotic disorders

Public knowledge has many aspects, but here we review those aspects of greatest relevance to reducing DUP: recognition of psychosis, first aid skills and beliefs about the effectiveness of health professionals and treatments.

Recognition of psychosis

Contacts with services are typically initiated by patients and families. Delays in making contact occur because patients, families and other gatekeepers to care may recognize that changes are occurring but do not

The Recognition and Management of Early Psychosis: A Preventive Approach, ed. Henry J. Jackson and Patrick D. McGorry.
Published by Cambridge University Press. © Cambridge University Press 2009.

identify these as symptoms of a psychotic disorder (de Haan *et al.*, 2004; Perkins *et al.*, 1999). For example, a study of mothers of psychotic patients found that the initial psychotic symptoms were frequently seen as being the result of drug use or another mental disorder such as depression (de Haan *et al.*, 2004).

Given the importance of better community recognition for reducing DUP, community surveys in a number of developed countries have assessed the ability of the public to label a psychotic disorder correctly. One methodology has been to present a case vignette of a person with schizophrenia or psychosis and ask the respondent what they think is wrong with this person. Such surveys have been carried out with Australian adults (Jorm *et al.*, 1997a, 2005a) and youth (Wright *et al.*, 2005), Italian adults (Magliano *et al.*, 2004), and Japanese adults (Jorm *et al.*, 2005a). Box 9.1 shows a

---

Box 9.1 Vignette of a person with schizophrenia/psychosis

John is 24 and lives at home with his parents. He has had a few temporary jobs since finishing school but is now unemployed. Over the last 6 months he has stopped seeing his friends and has begun locking himself in his bedroom and refusing to eat with the family or to have a bath. His parents also hear him walking about his bedroom at night while they are in bed. Even though they know he is alone, they have heard him shouting and arguing as if someone else is there. When they try to encourage him to do more things, he whispers that he won't leave home because he is being spied upon by the neighbour. They realize he is not taking drugs because he never sees anyone or goes anywhere.

From Jorm *et al.* (1997a).

---

typical vignette used in these studies and Table 9.1 summarizes the findings. The consistent finding has been that only a minority of respondents give the correct psychiatric label, although most recognize a mental health problem of some kind, often of a less serious type than psychosis (e.g. depression). Another approach has been to ask about understanding of the term *schizophrenia*. As summarized in Table 9.2, studies of university students and adults in several countries have found that many people wrongly associate the term with *split personality* (Angermeyer & Matschinger, 1999; Furnham & Chan, 2004; Lauber *et al.*, 2005a), which is likely to affect correct recognition.

Because psychosis may often present as depression in the prodromal phase, public recognition of depression may also assist earlier help-seeking. Surveys assessing recognition of depression find that this is better than for psychosis (65% versus 41% in Australian adults; 49% versus 25% in Australian youth; and 23% versus 17% in Japanese adults) (Jorm *et al.*, 2005a; Wright *et al.*, 2005). However, many members of the public still label depression with less-serious terms such as *stress* or *crisis* (Jorm *et al.*, 1997a; Lauber *et al.*, 2003).

The results of community surveys showing low recognition give support to the view that lack of public knowledge could contribute to DUP. However, there has been no research directly testing whether DUP is shorter where patients, families and other gate-keepers have greater knowledge about psychosis.

First aid skills

When families are faced with a loved one developing psychotic symptoms, they will often try to deal with

---

Table 9.1. Correct recognition of schizophrenia/psychosis in vignettes by members of the public

Study	Country	Age group surveyed (years)	Labelling vignette correctly (%)	Recognizing some sort of mental health problem (%)
Jorm *et al.*, 1997a	Australia	18–74	27	84
Jorm *et al.*, 2005a	Australia	18+	41	Not reported
Jorm *et al.*, 2005a	Japan	20+	17	Not reported
Magliano *et al.*, 2004	Italy	18–70	21	Not reported
Wright *et al.*, 2005	Australia	12–25	25	70

Table 9.2. Association of the term 'schizophrenia' with 'split personality' in surveys of the public

Study	Country	Group surveyed	Associating term with split personality (%)
Angermeyer & Matschinger, 1999	Germany	Adults	29
Angermeyer & Matschinger, 1999	Germany	Medical students before exposure to psychiatric knowledge	'Two-thirds'
Furnham & Chan, 2004	England and Hong Kong	Convenience sample mainly of university students	28
Lauber *et al.*, 2005a	Switzerland	University students	64

these themselves (Perkins *et al.*, 1999). They will also be important gateways to professional help-seeking. This role will be more effective if the family member possesses good first aid skills. This is an aspect of mental health literacy that has not been greatly researched. However, a recent Australian survey investigated first aid skills of the public ($n = 997$) by presenting a vignette of a young person developing schizophrenia (see Box 9.1) and then asking what the respondent would do if this was someone they knew and cared about (Jorm *et al.*, 2005b). Seventy per cent said they would talk/listen/support the person, but only 58% said they would encourage professional help-seeking. The health professionals most often mentioned in this regard were primary care physician (general practitioner, GP)/doctor unspecified (27%), counsellor (8%), psychiatrist (6%) and psychologist (2%). More sophisticated approaches to encouraging help-seeking were uncommon: only 10% said they would accompany the person to the professional helper, and 13% would contact a health professional on their behalf. Other uncommon first aid responses were to listen/talk/support family (8%), assess the problem or risk of harm (10%), give or seek information (9%) and encourage self-help (12%).

Beliefs about mental health professionals

The first port of call for professional help will depend in part on the type of health system operating in a country. For those countries with a widespread system of GPs, they are often the first point of professional contact for people with psychotic disorders (Addington *et al.*, 2002;

Lincoln *et al.*, 1998; Norman *et al.*, 2004). However, whether a particular profession is seen as likely to be helpful for a person with psychosis may be an important influence. Table 9.3 summarizes the findings from surveys in a number of countries on beliefs about various types of professional help. Surveys of the public from Australia (Jorm *et al.* 2005a; Wright *et al.*, 2005), Switzerland (Lauber, Nordt & Rössler, 2005b) and Germany (Riedel-Heller, Matschinger & Angermeyer, 2005) show that GPs are frequently seen as a suitable source of help. By contrast, in Japan, GPs are not seen as likely to be helpful and they do not take a major role in mental healthcare (Jorm *et al.*, 2005a). In Austria too, GPs are not so often seen as a source of help for people with schizophrenia (Jorm, Angermeyer & Katschnig, 2000).

When the public are asked about other health professionals, psychiatrists generally rank highly as a potential source of help for people with schizophrenia (Jorm *et al.*, 2005a; Lauber *et al.*, 2005b; Riedel-Heller *et al.*, 2005; Wright *et al.*, 2005). However, in both Australia and Japan, counsellors rank even higher than psychiatrists amongst adults (Jorm *et al.*, 2005a) while amongst Australian youth, counsellors/psychologists are also more often seen as providing better help than psychiatrists (Wright *et al.*, 2005). In Germany, psychotherapists are amongst the highest rated professions for helping individuals with schizophrenia (Riedel-Heller *et al.*, 2005). The high preference for counsellors and psychotherapists suggests that schizophrenia is being seen by some members of the public in terms of life problems or crises rather than as a medical problem.

Table 9.3. Beliefs about the helpfulness of various professionals for psychosis/schizophrenia

Study	Country	Age group surveyed (years)	Method of assessing beliefs	Favouring each profession (%)
Jorm et al., 2000	Austria	15+	Respondents asked what they would do if family member suffered from problem in a vignette	GP 15% Psychiatrist 38% Psychologist 18%
Jorm et al., 2005a	Australia	18+	Respondents asked if professional likely to be helpful for person in vignette	GP 77% Psychiatrist 80% Psychologist 74% Counsellor 85%
Jorm et al., 2005a	Japan	20+	Respondents asked if professional likely to be helpful for person in vignette	GP 19% Psychiatrist 73% Psychologist 56% Counsellor 87%
Lauber et al., 2005b	Switzerland	16–76	Respondents asked if professional likely to be helpful (score of 1) or harmful (score of –1) for person in vignette	GP mean score, 0.46 Psychiatrist mean score, 0.54 Psychologist mean score, 0.66
Riedel-Heller et al., 2005	Germany	18+	Respondents asked to choose preferred source of help from a list for person in vignette	Family physician 17% Psychiatrist 35% Psychotherapist 25%
Wright et al., 2005	Australia	12–25	Respondents asked if professional likely to be helpful for person in vignette	Family doctor/GP 70% Psychiatrist 84% Counsellor/psychologist 80%

GP, general practitioner (primary care physician).

Beliefs about treatments

While antipsychotic medication is a cornerstone of treatment, public beliefs across a number of developed countries tend to be negative about all psychotropic medication, including antipsychotic drugs (Jorm et al., 2000; 2005a; Lauber et al., 2005b; Magliano et al. 2004; Wright et al., 2005; see Table 9.4). Reasons for these negative attitudes include concern about side effects and the belief that medication only deals with the symptoms and not the causes (Angermeyer, Däumer & Matschinger, 1993, Fischer et al., 1999).

By contrast, public beliefs about psychological treatments and counselling are generally much more favourable (Table 9.4). In both Australia and Japan, seeing a counsellor is one of the most favourably viewed interventions, and both telephone counselling and psychotherapy are rated much higher than medication (Jorm et al., 2005a). Australian youth also rate

counselling/psychotherapy very highly for psychosis (Wright et al., 2005). Similarly, in Germany, psychotherapy was the top choice of treatment when members of the public were asked to choose from a list (Riedel-Heller et al., 2005), while in Austria a large majority believed that psychosis responded 'exclusively' or 'mainly' to psychotherapy (Jorm et al., 2000).

While inpatient admission is often a component of psychosis management, this is regarded very unfavourably by the public in a range of countries, with many people seeing it as harmful (Table 9.4; Jorm et al., 2005a; Lauber et al., 2005b; Magliano et al., 2004).

In summary, the public tend to favour psychological treatments and be negative about medication and admission to hospital. Whether these beliefs affect DUP is not known, but it seems likely that they will affect patients' and families' willingness to accept some standard interventions.

Table 9.4. Beliefs about the helpfulness of medications, psychological treatments and hospital admission for psychosis/schizophrenia

Study	Country	Age group surveyed (years)	Method of assessing beliefs	Favouring each intervention (% or mean)
Jorm *et al.*, 2000	Austria	15+	Respondents asked whether problem in a vignette responds exclusively or mainly to intervention	Medication 35% Psychotherapy 65%
Jorm *et al.*, 2005a	Australia	18+	Respondents asked if intervention likely to be helpful for person in vignette	Antipsychotic drugs 4% Phone counselling 57% Psychotherapy 59% Hospital admission 32%
Jorm *et al.*, 2005a	Japan	20+	Respondents asked if intervention likely to be helpful for person in vignette	Antipsychotic drugs 5% Phone counselling 36% Psychotherapy 54% Hospital admission 22%
Lauber *et al.*, 2005b	Switzerland	16–76	Respondents asked if intervention likely to be helpful (score of 1) or harmful (score of –1) for person in vignette	Antipsychotic drugs mean, –0.12 Phone counselling mean, 0.08 Hospital admission mean, 0.18
Magliano *et al.*, 2004	Italy		Respondents asked if intervention useful for person in vignette and rate as 'completely true'	Drugs 25% 'Other interventions' 58% 'Asylum' admission 2%
Riedel-Heller *et al.*, 2005	Germany	18+	Respondents asked to choose preferred source of help from a list for person in vignette	Psychotropic drugs 15% Psychotherapy 65%
Wright *et al.*, 2005	Australia	12–25	Respondents asked if intervention likely to be helpful for person in vignette	Antipsychotic drugs 40% Counselling/psychotherapy 92%

Contrast between public and professional beliefs

It will be apparent that some beliefs held commonly by members of the public are at variance with the consensus of mental health professionals. The contrast between public and professional beliefs has been specifically investigated in Australia, where a modified version of a questionnaire for the public was administered to GPs, psychiatrists, clinical psychologists and mental health nurses (Caldwell & Jorm, 2000; Jorm *et al.*, 1997b). For schizophrenia, there was consensus across the professions that it would be helpful to see a GP, clinical psychologist or psychiatrist, receive antipsychotic medication and be admitted to a psychiatric ward. While these views are similar to those of the public in some areas (e.g. the helpfulness of GPs and

counselling), there are major discrepancies in others. In particular, the professionals were much more positive about the helpfulness of antipsychotic drugs and admission to a psychiatric ward for schizophrenia (Jorm *et al.*, 1997b). Conversely, the public tended to be much more favourably disposed to vitamins, special diets and reading self-help books for schizophrenia. Table 9.5 summarizes the relevant data.

A similar study was conducted in Switzerland (Lauber *et al.*, 2005b), where the public were compared with psychiatrists, psychologists, nurses and other mental health professionals. For schizophrenia, psychiatrists and psychologists most strongly recommended psychiatrists, antipsychotic drugs and psychiatric hospital, whereas nurses and other professionals recommended psychiatrists, psychiatric hospital and GPs. The public's top recommendations were psychologists, psychiatrists,

Table 9.5. Most favoured interventions for psychosis/schizophrenia by public compared with professionals

Study	Country	Group surveyed (No.)	Most highly rated interventions (mean rating)[a]
Jorm et al., 1997b; Caldwell & Jorm, 2000	Australia	Public (1021)	Physical activity (0.85) Getting out more (0.85) Counsellor (0.84) Courses on relaxation (0.79) GP (0.77)
		Psychiatrists (1128)	Psychiatrist (0.99) Antipsychotic drugs (0.99) GP (0.98) Hospital admission (0.98) Clinical psychologist (0.67)
		Clinical psychologists (454)	Psychiatrist (0.97) Clinical psychologist (0.95) Antipsychotic drugs (0.93) Hospital admission (0.91) GP (0.86)
		GPs (872)	GP (1.00) Psychiatrist (0.99) Antipsychotic drugs (0.96) Hospital admission (0.88) Clinical psychologist (0.76)
		Mental health nurses (673)	Psychiatrist (0.99) Antipsychotic drugs (0.97) Hospital admission (0.82) GP (0.80) Clinical psychologist (0.79)
Lauber et al., 2005b	Switzerland	Public (98)	Psychologist (0.66) Psychiatrist (0.54) GP (0.46) Fresh air (0.45) Psychotherapy (0.42)
		Psychiatrists and psychologists (94)	Psychiatrist (0.93) Antipsychotic drugs (0.82) Psychiatric hospital (0.71) GP (0.62) Psychologist (0.29)
		Nurses, social workers, vocational workers (289)	Psychiatrist (0.90) Psychiatric hospital (0.70) GP (0.61) Antipsychotic drugs (0.54) Psychologist (0.40)

GP, general practitioner (primary care physician).
[a] Rating on a scale from 1 (helpful) to –1 (harmful).

GPs, fresh air and psychotherapy, with neither psychiatric hospital nor antipsychotic drugs seen favourably. Again, the main findings are summarized in Table 9.5.

Historical improvements in mental health literacy for psychotic disorders

While there are some major discrepancies between public and professional beliefs, there are signs that this may be changing, at least in some countries. In Australia between 1995 and 2003–4, correct recognition of a schizophrenia vignette increased from 27% to 42%. There were also major changes in beliefs about professionals and treatments. For example, belief in the helpfulness of psychiatrists increased from 71% to 82%, in antipsychotic drugs from 23% to 34%, and in admission to a psychiatric ward from 18% to 33% (Jorm, Christensen & Griffiths, 2006). A similar change has been found in Germany between 1990 and 2001 (Angermeyer & Matschinger, 2004, 2005). For example, agreement with the statement: 'The benefit brought about by drug treatment far outweighs the risk associated with it' increased from 22% to 30% in the western part of Germany and from 14% to 23% in the east. Positive changes have also been observed in beliefs about psychiatrists and psychotherapists for schizophrenia and for willingness to recommend therapy in general. However, despite these improvements, substantial gaps remain between public and professional beliefs.

Interventions to improve mental health literacy for psychotic disorders

Although some countries have seen some significant improvements in mental health literacy over quite short historical periods, the causes of these changes are unknown. Nevertheless, there are a number of specific interventions that have been quite well evaluated and it is likely that programmes like these have been contributors. Interventions to improve mental health literacy can be implemented in a variety of settings. Here we group these as community campaigns, school-based programmes and individual training

---

Box 9.2 The Early Treatment and Intervention in Psychosis campaign

Information was conveyed in a variety of ways, including a brochure distributed to households, mass media advertisements, postcards, car stickers, T-shirts and public meetings. All elements of the campaign used the slogan 'Seek help as early as possible and you have the best chance to recover' and a standard list of symptoms of psychosis. Newspaper advertisements were a major focus of the campaign and their message design was phrased to address a range of attitudinal and knowledge areas. These included messages showing the myths (images from the movie *One Flew Over the Cuckoo's Nest*) and reality (images of treating teams, patient–clinician interactions, etc.) of psychiatric treatment, images such as a line of dominoes to illustrate how symptoms gradually develop, and the use of cognitive dissonance techniques to challenge the notion that it is difficult to get help for psychosis.

From Johannessen *et al.* (2001).

---

programmes. Many of these interventions are not specific to psychosis, which is quite appropriate given that the prodromal changes typically involve non-psychotic symptoms.

Community campaigns

In a number of countries, community awareness campaigns have been developed to improve mental health literacy and/or reduce DUP. Those that have been rigorously evaluated are reviewed here.

In Norway, the Early Treatment and Intervention in Psychosis (TIPS) programme has been implemented in Rogaland county with the aim of reducing DUP (Johannessen *et al.*, 2001). This programme involves early detection teams and an information programme about early psychosis targeting the general population, schools and health professionals. The information campaign (Box 9.2) aims to increase the community's knowledge of mental disorders in general and the early signs of serious disorders in particular. It tries to increase earlier help-seeking by giving information about available help, positive outcomes from help and by reducing stigma around disorders and services.

To evaluate the TIPS programme, a comparison was carried out of DUP in the intervention region with two comparison regions having similar early psychosis services – one in Norway and one in Denmark (Melle *et al.*, 2004). It was found that the median DUP was significantly shorter in the TIPS region (5 weeks) compared with the comparison region (16 weeks). Symptom levels were also lower at intake in the TIPS region (e.g. $d = 0.59$ for symptoms on the Global Assessment of Functioning) and the difference sustained 3 months later ($d = 0.42$), supporting the effectiveness of the campaign. However, it was unclear at what point the reduction in DUP occurred, whether through greater patient, family or GP awareness, or as a result of the establishment of the early detection teams in the mental health service. Furthermore, baseline measures of DUP and symptom levels were not reported, so the differences observed may be naturalistic rather than a result of the intervention itself.

In Australia, the Compass Strategy was a mental health literacy community awareness campaign targeting young people aged 12–25 years and their supporters (Wright et al, 2006). The programme ran in the western part of Melbourne and the adjacent regional/rural area of Barwon between 2001 and 2003. Southeastern metropolitan Melbourne and the adjacent regional/rural area of Mornington Peninsula/southeast Gippsland served as a control for evaluation purposes. The Precede–Proceed Model (Green & Kreuter, 1999) guided the population assessment, campaign strategy development and evaluation. The campaign messages were based on findings from the population assessment and the Health Belief Model (Janz & Becker, 1984), and were pre-tested in focus groups to facilitate their refinement. Box 9.3 outlines the campaign.

An evaluation of the programme through repeated community surveys of mental health literacy found a number of significant changes in the intervention region compared with the control region (Figure 9.1), including greater awareness of mental health campaigns, greater knowledge of prevalence and suicide risk associated with the disorders, more self-identified depression in young people, a reduction in perceived barriers to help-seeking, and greater help sought for depression in the previous year. Given that the

---

Box 9.3 The Compass Strategy campaign

The major message of the programme was that there are benefits of early recognition and help-seeking for depression and psychosis. This translated into the core slogan 'Get on top of it before it gets on top of you'. Other key messages were that young people are particularly susceptible, that symptoms should be taken seriously, the core symptoms to look for, getting help early is a key to successful treatment, and sources of further information. These messages were conveyed through a variety of media including vibrant and youthful advertisements in cinemas, newspapers and magazines; posters, brochures and postcards; a website; and an information phone line. They were supported by regular liaison with relevant community service providers. Below are some examples of campaign elements.

Newspaper advertisement text

Spinning out
Or is it a sign of something else?
1 in 4 young people will experience a mental health problem, such as psychosis.
Signs include:

- Finding it more difficult than usual to cope with work or study
- Difficulty relating to family and friends
- Seeing and hearing things that others can't
- Strange or unusual ideas that aren't based on reality

Getting help early is a key to successful treatment

To find out how you can help someone get on top of psychosis, call 1300 … … or visit www.getontop.org.

The message used a lead word or phrase such as 'spinning out', 'moody', 'confused', which are lay terms commonly used by young people to describe the experience of depression or psychosis. This was used to get the readers' attention and followed by a question to urge them to take it more seriously. The '1in 4' statistic was used to highlight susceptibility of young people, and a short list of core symptoms was provided to ensure that the message was simple enough to be retained. The benefits of early treatment were highlighted and, as with all campaign elements, finished with recommended action.

Cinema advertisement script

Every year 1 in 4 young Australians experience a mental health problem. And like any health problem ignore it and it can get out of hand. But help is available – and getting help from the start can get you back on track. For more information about depression and psychosis visit our website or call 1300 … … … and get on top of it before it gets on top of you.

This was a 30 second advertisement with a focus on raising general awareness and promoting the website and information line.

Website components

- Detailed information about signs and symptoms of psychosis, depression and bipolar disorder
- Recommended forms of treatments available
- Recommended sources of professional help and how they operate
- A search engine for sources of help in a person's local town or suburb
- Tips on how to assist a person in getting the help they need
- Personal stories and feedback.

evaluation was carried out after only 14 months of a moderate intensity campaign, these findings are impressive.

In Canada, an Early Case Identification Programme has been set up, but with different results (Malla *et al.*, 2005). The programme was implemented in two phases in London, Ontario. In the first phase, a new service was established for first-episode psychosis and made known to referring agencies. The service took referrals from any source, including self-referrals. In the second phase, the Early Case Identification Programme was launched. Materials were distributed community wide describing early psychosis and the advantages of early treatment. The materials included posters, bookmarks, calendars, pamphlets, a film clip, cinema advertisements and talks to referring agencies. However, a comparison of median DUP from 2 years before the programme was implemented until 2 years after showed no improvement (21.9 and 24.3 weeks, respectively). A possible reason for the lack of effect was that the programme needed to run longer to have a detectable effect. There was no assessment of mental health literacy, so it is unclear if the programme succeeded even at increasing knowledge. However, the authors suggested that an alternative approach, targeted at training referring agencies in early identification of cases, might be more productive.

More positive results were found for a similar nationwide programme in Singapore: the Early Psychosis Intervention Programme (Chong, Mythily & Verma,

2005). An awareness programme targeted the general public and primary health professionals. The public campaign involved public forums on psychosis; advertising on radio, newspapers and free postcards using corporate sponsorship; articles on TV and other media; art exhibitions with a psychosis theme; and an easy-to-read book for patients and carers. With the primary care professionals, information was distributed to GPs, student counsellors and counsellors with non-government organizations. A comparison of the median DUP from before until after the programme showed a large improvement (at 12 months and 4 months, respectively). A possible reason for the more favourable results than in Canada was that the median DUP before the programme was much longer, allowing considerable scope for improvement. Again, there was no assessment of whether mental health literacy was a mediator of this improvement and, similarly to the TIPS programme, it is unclear whether the reduction in DUP occurred through community awareness initiatives or primary health service enhancement.

Taken together, there is evidence that programmes to enhance awareness in the community and with referral sources can increase help-seeking and reduce DUP, particularly where the median DUP is long to start with. Whether enhanced mental health literacy underlies the change is unclear, because only the Compass Strategy in Australia has reported on changes in knowledge.

School-based programmes

Schools have often been used as a setting for mental health education. Much of this work has been aimed at reducing stigma, rather than promoting knowledge or behaviour conducive to earlier help-seeking. Furthermore, little of it has been formally evaluated. Here, we review those studies with some relevance to increasing help-seeking, particularly for psychosis, and where there has been some evaluation of impact.

In the USA, Battaglia, Coverdale and Bushong (1990) evaluated a mental illness awareness week in several high schools, which involved professionals working in psychiatry (residents) giving talks to students ($n = 1380$). The talks were not standardized, but they covered topics such as psychiatry, drugs and alcohol, suicide and

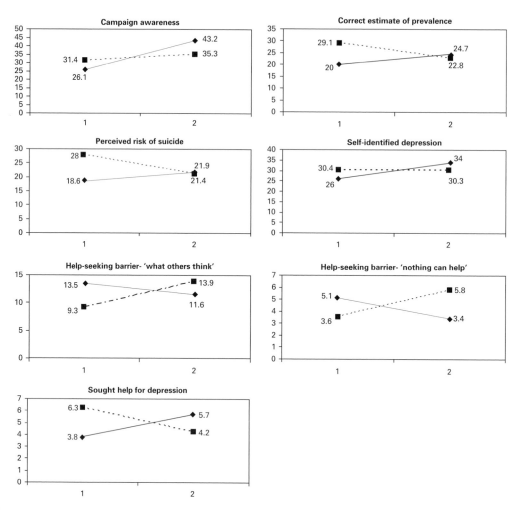

Fig. 9.1. Percentage change in outcome variables for the experimental (—) and control (- - -) regions before (1) and after (2) the Compass Strategy campaign.

depression. The aim was to change attitudes towards seeking help and to psychiatrists. It was found that there were differences in attitudes at the end of the week compared with a non-randomly assigned comparison group. For example, the intervention group said that they were more likely to seek help from a psychiatrist (10% versus 6%), counsellor (10% versus 4%) and less likely to tell family (16% versus 22%). However, there was no longer-term evaluation of effects on attitudes or actual help-seeking.

In the UK, Pinfold *et al.* (2003) implemented a programme in five secondary schools (472 students) to increase mental health literacy and reduce stigma. The programme involved two lectures, one of which included a video of people living with depression and schizophrenia, and the other which challenged stereotypes and labelling and was supported by a person living with a mental disorder. There were gains in mental health literacy and stigma reduction that were maintained over 6 months. While the programme was not specifically designed to promote earlier help-seeking, there were changes in relevant knowledge about the prevalence of mental disorders (from 35% correct at baseline to 61% at follow-up), the chances of recovery (from 68% to 83%) and understanding of the term schizophrenia (from 10% to 29%).

In Australia, there is a programme of mental illness education in high schools in which a person with personal experience of a mental disorder gives an interactive presentation. An evaluation of this programme on knowledge and attitudes, from before until immediately after the presentation, has been carried out with 457 students. This evaluation showed a strong impact on knowledge (partial $\eta^2 = 18\%$), a modest one on stigma (7%) and a weak one on help-seeking intentions (3%) (Rickwood *et al.*, 2004). Longer-term effects and impact on actual help-seeking were not evaluated.

The conclusion to be drawn from this body of work is that while schools are a promising setting for promoting early intervention, efforts have been piecemeal and there has been no evaluation of longer-term impact on beliefs or actual help-seeking.

Individual training programmes

Individual training programmes lasting for a day or more have been developed to facilitate early intervention and help-seeking in the community. These programmes are not specific to psychosis but train participants in skills that promote earlier intervention with psychotic disorders. They are potentially applicable across a range of settings. Here we review two programmes that have had published evaluations.

Family, friends and providers of social services can be an important gateway to professional help. However, as reviewed above, many members of the public lack basic knowledge and first aid skills. To overcome this lack, a mental health first aid course has been developed, following the model successfully applied to conventional first aid (Kitchener & Jorm, 2002a; see Box 9.4 for details). Several trials have been carried out to evaluate the effects of the course. The first trial was an uncontrolled study with 210 members of the public, who were assessed at the beginning and end of the course and at a follow-up 6 months later (Kitchener & Jorm, 2002b). The

---

Box 9.4 Mental health first aid training

Mental health first aid is a 12-hour training course, usually delivered as four 3-hour sessions. The course is designed to train members of the public in how to assist someone developing a mental disorder or in a mental health crisis situation. The mental disorders covered include depression, anxiety and psychosis. The comorbidity of these disorders with substance misuse is also discussed. The crisis situations covered include suicidal thoughts and behaviour, acute stress reaction, panic attacks and acute psychotic behaviour. First aiders are taught an action plan consisting of five basic steps.

1. Assess risk of suicide or harm
2. Listen non-judgmentally
3. Give reassurance and information
4. Encourage person to get appropriate professional help
5. Encourage self-help strategies.

First aiders do the course for three main reasons: they work in a human services job that gives them increased contact with people experiencing mental health problems; they have a relative or friend who is affected; or they see it as their duty as a citizen. The course is being run in a number of countries. Further information can be found at the Mental Health First Aid website: http://www.mhfa.com.au/.

---

training was found to produce several significant changes: better recognition of schizophrenia from a case vignette (from 57% correct before to 76% after), beliefs about treatment of schizophrenia that were more like those of mental health professionals (from 74% agreement before to 88% after), reduced social distance from the person in the schizophrenia vignette ($d = 0.22$), greater confidence in providing help to others (from 62% confident before to 83% after) and an increase in the number actually providing help (from 54% providing help to 62%). Two subsequent trials involved randomized comparison with wait-list controls, evaluating change from before the course until 5 months afterwards (Kitchener & Jorm, 2006). The first trial was in a workplace setting and involved 301 employees of government departments (Kitchener & Jorm, 2004). This was an efficacy trial under ideal conditions, with the originator of the course doing the training and the participants doing the course during work time. The second trial involved 753 members of the public from a large rural area (Jorm *et al.*, 2004). This was an effectiveness trial under realistic conditions, with staff from the local health service running the training for members of the public, who undertook the course in their own time. Both trials used similar measures to the uncontrolled trial and found similar benefits.

Another individual training programme, the Suicide Intervention Project, used a peer education approach with university students to encourage early intervention and prevention (Pearce, Rickwood & Beaton, 2003). Although nominally about suicide intervention, the programme was actually much broader. Students ($n = 42$) were trained how to recognize mental disorders in others and to feel comfortable talking about them with other students, and were given information about mental health support services available to students. There were significant changes from before to after training in mental health literacy (from 68% to 76%), confidence ($d = 1.05$) and intention to talk to other students about mental health problems ($d = 0.91$). However, there was only a brief 2-week follow-up to measure behavioural change and, not surprisingly, little was found. As with school-based programmes, these more-intensive individual training programmes show promise, but a link to reduced DUP remains to be investigated.

Conclusions

People developing psychotic disorders, their family and friends and key community members can play an important role in recognizing the presence of a serious mental disorder and seeking help earlier. However, community surveys from a range of developed countries show that knowledge of psychotic disorders is deficient and that attitudes to some standard psychiatric treatments are frequently negative. Nevertheless, there are encouraging signs that change is occurring. Historical comparisons in Australia and Germany show that mental health literacy and attitudes are improving. There is also evidence that specific interventions can improve mental health literacy and reduce the delay to treatment. However, research in this area is still in its infancy. The biggest remaining challenge is to

investigate whether increasing mental health literacy has benefits to the uptake of appropriate treatments and ultimately to the mental health of the community.

REFERENCES

Addington, J., van Mastrigt, S., Hutchinson, J. & Addington, D. (2002). Pathways to care: help seeking behaviour in first episode psychosis. *Acta Psychiatrica Scandinavica*, **106**, 358–64.

Angermeyer, M. C. & Matschinger, H. (1999). Social representations of mental illness among the public. In J. Guimon, W. Fischer & N. Sartorius (eds.), *The Image of Madness: The Public Facing Mental Illness and Psychiatric Treatment*. Basel: Karger, pp. 20–8.

Angermeyer, M. C. & Matschinger, H. (2004). Public attitudes towards psychotropic drugs: have there been any changes in recent years? *Pharmacopsychiatry*, **37**, 152–6.

Angermeyer, M. C. & Matschinger, H. (2005). Have there been any changes in the public's attitudes towards psychiatric treatment? Results from representative population surveys in Germany in the years 1990 and 2001. *Acta Psychiatrica Scandinavica*, **111**, 68–73.

Angermeyer, M. C., Däumer, R. & Matschinger, H. (1993). Benefits and risks of psychotropic medication in the eyes of the general public: results of a survey in the Federal Republic of Germany. *Pharmacopsychiatry*, **26**, 114–20.

Battaglia, J., Coverdale, J. H. & Bushong, C. P. (1990). Evaluation of a mental illness awareness week program in public schools. *American Journal of Psychiatry*, **147**, 324–9.

Bertolote, J. & McGorry, P. D. (2005). Early intervention and recovery for young people with early psychosis: consensus statement. *British Journal of Psychiatry*, **187**(Suppl), s116–19.

Caldwell, T. M. & Jorm, A. F. (2000). Mental health nurses' beliefs about interventions for schizophrenia and depression: a comparison with psychiatrists and the public. *Australian and New Zealand Journal of Psychiatry*, **34**, 602–11.

Chong, S. A., Mythily, S. & Verma, S. (2005). Reducing the duration of untreated psychosis and changing help-seeking behaviour in Singapore. *Social Psychiatry and Psychiatric Epidemiology*, **40**, 619–21.

de Haan, L., Welborn, K., Krikke, M. & Linszen, D. H. (2004). Opinions of mothers on the first psychotic episode and the start of treatment of their child. *European Psychiatry*, **19**, 226–9.

Fischer, W., Goerg, D., Zbinden, E. & Guimon, J. (1999). Determining factors and the effects of attitudes towards psychotropic medication. In J. Guimon, W. Fischer &

N. Sartorius (eds.), *The Image of Madness: The Public Facing Mental Illness and Psychiatric Treatment*. Basel: Karger, pp. 162–86.

Furnham, A. & Chan, E. (2004). Lay theories of schizophrenia: a cross-cultural comparison of British and Hong Kong Chinese attitudes, attributions and beliefs. *Social Psychiatry and Psychiatric Epidemiology*, **39**, 543–52.

Green, L. W. & Kreuter, M. W. (1999). *Health Promotion Planning: An Educational and Ecological Approach*, 3rd edn. Mountain View, CA: Mayfield.

Häfner, H., Maurer, K., Trendler, G. *et al.* (2005). Schizophrenia and depression: challenging the paradigm of two separate diseases: a controlled study of schizophrenia, depression and healthy controls. *Schizophrenia Research*, **77**, 11–24.

Harris, M. G., Henry, L. P., Harrigan, S. M. *et al.* (2005). The relationship between duration of untreated psychosis and outcome: an eight-year prospective study. *Schizophrenia Research*, **79**, 85–93.

Janz, N. K. & Becker, M. H. (1984). The health belief model: a decade later. *Health Education Quarterly*, **11**, 1–47.

Johannessen, J. O., McGlashan, T. H., Larsen, T. K. *et al.* (2001). Early detection strategies for untreated first-episode psychosis. *Schizophrenia Research*, **51**, 39–46.

Jorm, A. F., Korten, A. E., Jacomb, P. A. *et al.* (1997a). 'Mental health literacy': a survey of the public's ability to recognize mental disorders and their beliefs about the effectiveness of treatment. *Medical Journal of Australia*, **166**, 182–6.

Jorm, A. F., Korten, A. E., Jacomb, P. A. *et al.* (1997b). Helpfulness of interventions for mental disorders: beliefs of health professionals compared to the general public. *British Journal of Psychiatry*, **171**, 233–7.

Jorm, A. F., Angermeyer, M. C. & Katschnig, H. (2000). Public knowledge of and attitudes to mental disorders: a limiting factor in the optimal use of treatment services. In G. Andrews & S. Henderson (eds.), *Unmet Need in Psychiatry: Problems, Resources, Responses.* Cambridge, UK: Cambridge University Press, pp. 399–413.

Jorm, A. F., Kitchener, B. A., O'Kearney, R. & Dear, K. B. G. (2004). Mental health first aid training of the public in a rural area: a cluster randomized trial. *BMC Psychiatry*, **4**, 33.

Jorm, A. F., Nakane, Y., Christensen, H. *et al.* (2005a). Public beliefs about treatment and outcome of mental disorders: a comparison of Australia and Japan. *BMC Medicine*, **3**, 12.

Jorm, A. F., Blewitt, K. A., Griffiths, K. M., Kitchener, B. A. & Parslow, R. A. (2005b). Mental health first aid responses of the public: results from an Australian national survey. *BMC Psychiatry*, **5**, 9.

Jorm, A. F., Christensen, H. & Griffiths, K. M. (2006). The public's ability to recognize mental disorders and their beliefs about

treatment: changes in Australia over 8 years. *Australian and New Zealand Journal of Psychiatry*, **40**, 36–41.

Kitchener, B. A. & Jorm, A. F. (2002a). *Mental Health First Aid Manual.* Canberra: Centre for Mental Health Research.

Kitchener, B. A. & Jorm, A. F. (2002b). Mental health first aid training for the public: evaluation of effects on knowledge, attitudes and helping behavior. *BMC Psychiatry*, **2**, 10.

Kitchener, B. A. & Jorm, A. F. (2004). Mental health first aid training in a workplace setting: a randomized controlled trial. *BMC Psychiatry*, **4**, 23.

Kitchener, B. A. & Jorm, A. F. (2006). Mental health first aid training: review of evaluation studies. *Australian and New Zealand Journal of Psychiatry*, **40**, 6–8.

Lauber, C., Nordt, C., Falcato, L. & Rössler, W. (2003). Do people recognize mental illness? Factors influencing mental health literacy. *European Archives of Psychiatry and Clinical Neuroscience*, **253**, 248–51.

Lauber, C., Ajdacic-Gross, V., Fritschi, N., Stulz, N. & Rossler, W. (2005a). Mental health literacy in an educational elite: an online survey among university students. *BMC Public Health*, **5**, 44.

Lauber, C., Nordt, C. & Rössler, W. (2005b). Recommendations of mental health professionals and the general population on how to treat mental disorders. *Social Psychiatry and Psychiatric Epidemiology*, **40**, 835–43.

Lincoln, C., Harrigan, S. & McGorry, P. D. (1998). Understanding the topography of the early psychosis pathways: an opportunity to reduce delays in treatment. *British Journal of Psychiatry*, **172**(Suppl), S21–5.

Magliano, L., Fiorillo, A., De Rosa, C., Malangone, C. & Maj, M. (2004). Beliefs about schizophrenia in Italy: a comparative nationwide survey of the general public, mental health professionals, and patients' relatives. *Canadian Journal of Psychiatry*, **49**, 322–30.

Malla, A., Norman, R., Scholten, D., Manchanda, R. & McLean, T. (2005). A community intervention for early identification of first episode psychosis: impact of duration of untreated psychosis (DUP) and patient characteristics. *Social Psychiatry and Psychiatric Epidemiology*, **40**, 337–44.

Marshall, M., Lewis, S., Lockwood, A. *et al.* (2005). Association between duration of untreated psychosis and outcome in cohorts of first-episode patients: a systematic review. *Archives of General Psychiatry*, **62**, 975–83.

Melle, I., Larsen, T. K., Haahr, U. *et al.* (2004). Reducing the duration of untreated first-episode psychosis: effects on clinical presentation. *Archives of General Psychiatry*, **61**, 143–50.

Norman, R. M. G., Malla, A. K., Verdi, M. B., Hassall, L. D. & Fazekas, C. (2004). Understanding delay in treatment for first-episode psychosis. *Psychological Medicine*, **34**, 255–66.

Pearce, K., Rickwood, D. & Beaton, S. (2003). Preliminary evaluation of a university-based suicide intervention project: impact on participants. *Australian e-Journal for the Advancement of Mental Health*, **2**. www.auseinet.com/journal/vol2iss1/Pearce.pdf.

Perkins, D. O., Nieri, J. M., Bell, K. & Lieberman, J. A. (1999). Factors that contribute to delay in the initial treatment of psychosis. *Schizophrenia Research*, **36**, 52.

Pinfold, V., Toulmin, H., Thornicroft, G. *et al.* (2003). Reducing psychiatric stigma and discrimination: evaluation of educational interventions in UK secondary schools. *British Journal of Psychiatry*, **182**, 342–6.

Rickwood, D., Cavanagh, S., Curtis, L. & Sakrouge, R. (2004). Educating young people about mental health and illness: evaluating a school-based programme. *International Journal of Health Promotion*, **6**, 23–32.

Riedel-Heller, S. G., Matschinger, H. & Angermeyer, M. C. (2005). Mental disorders: who and what might help? Help-seeking and treatment preferences of the lay public. *Social Psychiatry and Psychiatric Epidemiology*, **40**, 167–74.

Wright, A., Harris, M. G., Wiggers, J. H. *et al.* (2005). Recognition of depression and psychosis by young Australians and their beliefs about treatment. *Medical Journal of Australia*, **183**, 18–23.

Wright, A., McGorry, P. D., Harris, M. G., Jorm, A. F. & Pennell, K. (2006). Development and evaluation of a youth mental health community awareness campaign: the Compass Strategy, *BMC Public Health*, **6**, 215–28.

10

Pathways to care and reducing treatment delay in early psychosis

Ross M. G. Norman and Ashok K. Malla

Introduction

Interest in the potential benefits of early intervention for psychotic disorders has stimulated extensive research on duration of untreated illness as a predictor of treatment outcome. Recent reviews of the relevant literature suggest that a longer period of untreated psychosis predicts aspects of treatment outcome, at least over the first few years (Marshall *et al.*, 2005; Norman & Malla, 2001; Norman, Lewis & Marshall, 2005a; Perkins *et al.*, 2005). Such findings have provided impetus to the early intervention movement because they suggest that by reducing the delay between onset of psychosis and initiation of effective treatment we may be able to bring about better outcomes for those suffering from these very serious disorders (Malla, Norman & Voruganti, 1999; McGorry, Krstev & Harrigan, 2000). In addition, it is important to reduce the unnecessary suffering that is an intrinsic part of treatment delay (Ho & Andreasen, 2001; Lieberman & Fenton, 2000).

It might be supposed that the delay in providing treatment for psychotic disorders would be comparatively short because of the severity of psychotic symptoms. Estimates of mean delays from onset of frank psychotic symptoms to treatment vary widely but are often in the range of 1 to 2 years, with median values around 4 to 6 months (Compton, Kaslow & Walker, 2004; Gundez-Bruce *et al.*, 2005; Marshall *et al.*, 2005; McGlashan, 1999; Norman & Malla, 2001; Norman *et al.*, 2004). Internationally, the distribution of the period of untreated psychosis is found to be positively skewed, and often includes delays of 15 years or longer.

While such delays are not as long as sometimes reported for other forms of psychopathology, such as anxiety and affective disorders (e.g. Christiana *et al.*, 2000; Jenike, 2004; Kessler *et al.*, 1999; Thompson, Hunt & Issakidis, 2004), they still provide cause for concern given the likely associated disruption in social circumstances and/or vocational/educational pursuits. Moreover, there are hypotheses that untreated psychosis may have lasting 'neurotoxic' effects (Wyatt, 1991) and that delays of even a few weeks may have a major impact on the extent of recovery possible once treatment is started (Drake *et al.*, 2000; Harrigan, McGorry & Krstev, 2003).

In order to understand and perhaps reduce treatment delay, it may be important to identify its separable components. For instance, we think that there are compelling reasons for distinguishing between the period between onset of symptoms and initial contact with a professional service provider, and the period between that first contact and initiation and acceptance of appropriate treatment (Fuchs & Steinart, 2004; Gater & Goldberg, 1991; Johnstone *et al.*, 1986; Lincoln, Harrigan & McGorry, 1998; Norman *et al.*, 2004). Reducing each of these components of delay might require somewhat different approaches. Reducing the first component is likely to require education of the public concerning symptoms of psychosis and the importance of seeking help quickly. Interventions with service providers to help them to identify signs of psychosis and appreciate the need for prompt treatment are likely to be more relevant to the second component of delay. Most research on treatment delay does not separate these components, and we realize that the importance of this differentiation can be

The Recognition and Management of Early Psychosis: A Preventive Approach, ed. Henry J. Jackson and Patrick D. McGorry. Published by Cambridge University Press. © Cambridge University Press 2009.

overstated as there are some processes that can have a profound impact across phases of treatment delay. For instance, a strong aversion to accepting that a serious psychiatric disorder is occurring can delay help-seeking, impede willingness to accept referral to an appropriate service provider and interfere with engagement in treatment even when it is readily available.

We have organized the existing research about pathways to care in psychotic disorders around three issues: (1) what is known about the nature and determinants of the major milestones in seeking help, (2) the factors which predict the amount of time that it takes to progress along the relevant pathways, and (3) the interventions that have been evaluated for effectiveness in reducing treatment delay.

Milestones in help-seeking

The relevant literature suggests the following observations about initial help-seeking.

Help is often sought before the definite onset of psychosis

Many individuals who develop psychotic disorders have actually sought mental health treatment before the onset of psychosis. Preda *et al.* (2002) found that 90% of a small sample of individuals meeting criteria for a prodromal state (Miller *et al.*, 1999) had previously received psychotropic medication and/or had been seen by a mental health service provider. The subjects in this study may not be representative of all individuals with prodromal symptoms because they had all initiated treatment seeking or been referred for evaluation. This may well have resulted in an overestimate of previous help-seeking. A different perspective is provided by two Canadian studies. Addington *et al.* (2002) and Norman *et al.* (2004) independently found that just under 40% of patients admitted to different Canadian early intervention programmes for psychosis had previously sought help for mental health concerns such as depression,

disruption of functioning, anxiety or stress prior to the onset of psychosis. Lincoln *et al.* (1998), in examining pathways to care in an Australian sample, commented that 50% of their sample initiated help-seeking prior to the onset of psychosis. Norman *et al.* (2004) found that those who sought help in the prodromal period may be at particular risk of extended delay to treatment once the onset of psychosis occurred. This is a somewhat counterintuitive finding and, if replicated, could suggest that there may be a delay in responding when psychosis occurs in patients who have an established mental health record for other concerns, such as depression and anxiety disorders, and/or prodromal states of psychosis (Norman *et al.*, 2004; Preda *et al.*, 2002).

Help-seeking is often initiated for reasons other than psychotic symptoms

Understandably, one might assume that once psychosis is present, the initiation of help-seeking would be prompted primarily by the severity of the defining symptoms, such as bizarre behaviour, hallucinations and delusions. The evidence, however, is that those suffering from such disorders often do not recognize a need for treatment, or, if they do, their reasons for seeking treatment often concern non-specific symptoms such as dysphoric mood, anxiety, somatic concerns or concerns about decline in functioning (Addington *et al.*, 2002; de Haan *et al.*, 2002; Norman *et al.*, 2004). Several studies that have examined reasons for seeking help suggest that even when psychotic symptoms are clearly identified as a precipitator of help-seeking this may occur in the context of psychotic symptoms which have been experienced over an extended period of time – perhaps intermittently – and that help-seeking does not occur immediately upon awareness of their presence. In many cases, these symptoms are responded to only when they become perceived as dangerous, disruptive or embarrassing, or the coping resources of family or social supports have been exhausted (e.g. Compton *et al.*, 2004; de Haan *et al.*, 2004; Yamazawa *et al.*, 2004).

Help-seeking is often prompted by the actions of family or other members of the ill-person's social network

The onset of a psychotic disorder often occurs in late adolescence or early adulthood, and those afflicted often do not believe that what they are experiencing is an illness requiring treatment (Amador *et al.*, 1991; de Haan *et al.*, 2002). It is not surprising, therefore, that family members, usually parents, can play a crucial role in help-seeking (Helgason, 1990; Johnstone *et al.*, 1986). de Haan *et al.* (2002) found that 80% of a sample of 56 patients with recent-onset schizophrenia acknowledged that family members were critical in initiating help-seeking, and non-family contacts such as teachers and police were important for a further 10% (although others such as Addington *et al.* (2002) and Lincoln *et al.* (1998) reported lower levels of family involvement). While family members and others may eventually be more aware of the need for treatment than the ill-person, it is essential to recognize that there may be a significant delay between the onset of positive symptoms and awareness by friends and acquaintances (de Haan *et al.*, 2002). Furthermore, close relatives, especially parents, can underestimate the seriousness of what they are seeing. Even if they are aware of psychotic symptoms, family members may cultivate the hope that what they are observing is a reflection of temporary mood states, stress, relational problems or other circumstances that would justify waiting for the situation to resolve on its own (Compton *et al.*, 2004; de Haan *et al.*, 2004). In addition, given the relatively high rate of substance use in those at risk, it would not be surprising if family observers assume that habit change rather than psychiatric treatment is most needed. de Haan *et al.* (2002) found no significant relationship between the involvement of family in seeking care and the length of treatment delay.

Primary healthcare providers such as family physicians are often the first points of contact in accessing treatment

It is unfortunate that we know little about the patterns of consultation and help-seeking that occurs with friends,

Table 10.1. Frequency of general practitioner (primary care physician) as first point of contact when seeking help for psychotic disorder

Study	Country	First contact with GP (%)
Balestrieri *et al.*, 1994	Italy	43
Cole *et al.*, 1995	England	39.8
Cougnard *et al.*, 2004a	France	36.8
Lincoln *et al.*, 1998	Australia	35.5
Norman *et al.*, 2004	Canada	39

extended family members and co-workers (Lincoln & McGorry, 1995; Lincoln *et al.*, 1998). Perhaps such consultations are most likely to occur at earlier stages of the pathways to care. To the extent that interventions to reduce treatment delay could address such informal components, they would presumably be in the context of education of the general public (improving mental health literacy, as discussed in Ch. 9). Most attempts to map points of contact in help-seeking have focused on contacts with 'professional helpers', especially those working in health settings – although those in educational, social service, law enforcement and religious settings are sometimes included in such enquiries. Given the variation in the methods used, types of contact enquired about and how the data are reported, it is a difficult literature to summarize. To the extent that there is a consistency, it is with respect to the important role of primary care providers such as general practitioners/family physicians. Table 10.1 provides information on the first point of contact for individuals seeking help at some stage of a psychotic illness. As the table shows, figures from studies in Australia, the UK, Canada and Italy are remarkably similar in indicating that 35% to 45% of first contacts when looking for professional help for a psychotic disorder involved a general practitioner (GP; primary care physician) (Balestrieri *et al.*, 1994; Cole *et al.*, 1995; Cougnard *et al.*, 2004a; Lincoln *et al.*, 1998; Norman *et al.*, 2004). When treatment is being sought after the onset of frank psychosis, emergency rooms also become an important first point of contact (Addington *et al.*, 2002; Norman *et al.*, 2004). The involvement of GPs *at some point* in the pathway to care is reported for at least 50% of patients presenting with recent-onset psychosis (Cole *et al.*, 1995; Johnstone *et al.*, 1986; Lincoln *et al.*, 1998; Norman *et al.*, 2004). The most noteworthy exception to these findings is a report from Fuchs and Steinert (2004) in Germany, who found that less than 30% of patients had initially consulted a GP. Although these authors attributed the difference to the fact that in Germany a GP's referral was not required for accessing appropriate psychiatric care, this was also true of at least some of the settings reporting higher levels of GP involvement (Addington *et al.*, 2002; Balestrieri *et al.*, 1994; Cougnard et al, 2004a; Norman *et al.*, 2004).

Not only are GPs frequently involved in pathways to care, but there is also evidence that their involvement may be associated with shorter delays in accessing appropriate treatment and reduced likelihood of having to use compulsory methods (Burnett *et al.*, 1999; Cole *et al.*, 1995; Fuchs & Steinert, 2004; Skeate *et al.*, 2002).

Some barriers to help-seeking are potentially modifiable

Some barriers to help-seeking are probably related to intrinsic aspects of the illness. These could include the social withdrawal that can characterize the early stages of psychotic disorders, and thereby interfere with the recognition of problems by others. In addition, the rather non-specific nature of some initial symptoms can make it easy to attribute any anomalies to other causes (Compton *et al.*, 2004; Larsen, Johannessen & Opjordsmoen, 1998; McGorry, 2000). Qualitative interviews suggest that there is often a substantial period of uncertainty about what is happening and how to respond (Compton *et al.*, 2004; Etheridge, Yarrow & Peet, 2004), and this may be particularly likely to occur if the illness onset is gradual (Chen *et al.*, 2005; Kalla *et al.*, 2002; Larsen *et al.*, 1998). Such potentially modifiable psychological factors such as lack of information about early signs and who to approach, anticipated effectiveness of treatment and embarrassment related to the stigma of mental illness are likely to increase the likelihood of denial or otherwise encourage inertia in responding (Compton *et al.*, 2004; Etheridge, Yarrow & Peet, 2004; Larsen *et al.*, 1998;

McGorry, 2000; Phillips *et al.*, 1999). While structural factors such as availability and cost of services may be important barriers in some countries (Compton *et al.*, 2004; Wells *et al.*, 1994), lengthy delays in help-seeking occur in contexts where free and appropriate services are readily available (de Haan *et al.*, 2002; Norman *et al.*, 2004). There is evidence that, in seeking help for mental health problems generally, knowledge and attitudes may be the most important sources of delay (Christiana *et al.*, 2000; Thompson *et al.*, 2004).

Once help is sought, there is considerable variation in how readily it is provided

After an approach has been made to a professional helper, then that individual and any other helpers subsequently recruited into the process can serve as facilitators or hindrances in the pathway to care. Some investigations of pathways to care have attempted to assess the number and/or variety of contacts that occur between the initial professional consultation and accessing appropriate care. As noted above, comparisons between the results of studies in pathways to care are hindered by differences in methodology, including inclusion criteria, the types of contact recorded, whether the contacts are related to the period before or after the onset of psychosis (which is often not specified) and how the contacts are classified and summarized. It is clear from all relevant studies that the range of contacts with helping professionals before accessing treatment is wide: Johnstone *et al.* (1986) reported a range from 1 to 33, Lincoln *et al.* (1998) from 1 to 17, Cougnard *et al.* (2004a) up to 7, and Addington *et al.* (2002) up to 4 in the pre-psychosis period and up to 6 after the onset of psychosis. The estimated mean number of contacts prior to treatment varied between 4.9 (Johnstone *et al.*, 1986; Lincoln *et al.*, 1998) and 2.3 (extrapolated from data reported in Addington *et al.*, 2002). It is tempting to assume that a larger number of contacts would represent a longer delay, but there are no published data assessing whether such a relationship holds. Recent unpublished data from the Prevention and Early Intervention Programme for Psychoses in Montreal did find a number of contacts to correlate positively with treatment delay. In addition, most studies do not report the extent to which multiple contacts are with the same or different help providers. A quick succession of multiple different contacts that result in an appropriate referral could sometimes be more efficient than a comparable number or even fewer contacts with a single provider who fails to recognize psychosis and facilitate appropriate treatment. Several studies reported that patients and/or families often report difficulty in accessing a professional who will correctly assess the nature of the problem (de Haan *et al.*, 2004; Etheridge *et al.*, 2004; Johnstone *et al.*, 1986; Perkins *et al.*, 1999). As noted above, Norman *et al.* (2004) provided evidence that those who are actually being seen on an ongoing basis by a mental health service provider prior to the onset of psychosis are at particular risk of delay in being correctly diagnosed and treated.

There is wide variation in who facilitates the final connection to appropriate services

Lincoln *et al.* (1998) have commented that in seeking help for psychotic disorders some people find themselves diverted into 'dead-ends' by dealing with helpers who really do not provide the help needed or do not refer on to those who can, and this unnecessarily lengthens delay in treatment. So, in addition to the first point of contact and number of contacts that are made in seeking help, it could also be helpful to know which contacts are most likely to lead to appropriate interventions. Unfortunately, there has been relatively little investigation of this issue. Addington *et al.* (2002), in Calgary, Canada, found that the most common final referral source for appropriate treatment was an emergency department (48%) followed by family physicians and psychiatrists (18% each). In Singapore, where patients can directly access specialist services, 21% of referrals to a facility for treatment of first-episode psychosis came from GPs and 32% of admissions involved police in the final stage (Chong *et al.*, 2005a). These may be roughly comparable findings given that emergency room psychiatric consultations can often involve the police. As noted above, Fuchs and Steinert (2004) found less frequent use of GPs in pathways to care for psychosis in Germany, and in that context only 10% of admissions to the psychiatric service had their penultimate contact with GPs.

By comparison, Burnett *et al.* (1999), in a London, UK sample, found that 46% of referrals for admission or psychiatric care were made by GPs. The last finding is consistent with findings that GPs are often the primary source of referral to a range of mental health services (e.g. Amaddeo *et al.*, 2001; Balestrieri *et al.*, 1994). It appears, however, that in the case of psychotic disorders hospital-based emergency services and police also become prominent final points of referral for psychiatric treatment as the symptoms become more severe (Chong *et al.*, 2005a; Garety & Rigg, 2001; Norman *et al.*, 2004). While there are some reports of a relationship between longer treatment delay and increased likelihood of the use of compulsory admission, Cougnard *et al.* (2004b) and Kelly *et al.* (2004) did not replicate this finding.

Accessing the right service does not automatically mean immediate treatment

There is considerable variation in the endpoint used in studies of pathways to care or treatment delay for psychotic disorder, including entry into a mental health service or hospital (Balestrieri *et al.*, 1994; Compton *et al.*, 2004; Kalla *et al.*, 2002; Verdoux *et al.*, 2001), initial prescription of an antipsychotic drug (Chen *et al.*, 2005; de Haan *et al.*, 2004; Yamazawa *et al.*, 2004), receiving an antipsychotic drug for a specified period (Fuchs & Steinert, 2004; Larsen *et al.*, 1998; Norman *et al.*, 2004), prescription of any psychotropic drug (Cougnard *et al.*, 2004a), and time to definitive diagnosis (Chong *et al.*, 2005a) or an unspecified endpoint (Drake *et al.*, 2000; Haley *et al.*, 2003; Peralta *et al.*, 2005). Common clinical experience suggests that a psychotic disorder can go untreated for some time following diagnosis and availability of treatment, particularly if the individual's circumstances do not justify compulsory treatment. Although some researchers have made the effort to separate delay in help-seeking from delay in reaching the appropriate source of help, it may be of benefit also to assess the extent to which treatment delay reflects a delay in the patient engaging in treatment once it is available. Our own data from the Prevention and Early Intervention Programme for Psychoses (PEPP) in London, Canada, suggests that, on average, this delay in patients accepting antipsychotic treatment once it is prescribed represents less than 5% of total treatment delay from onset of psychosis. Nevertheless, in some cases, this delay in engagement can be quite lengthy – over 3 months for about 5% of patients.

What predicts treatment delay?

There are now several research reports that have examined predictors of treatment delay or duration of untreated psychosis (DUP). The findings are of interest for two primary reasons. First, if reliable predictors can be detected they might allow us to target interventions better to reduce treatment delay. Second, examination of predictors of treatment delay could also be important in assessing the extent to which the relationship between DUP and treatment outcome represent the influence of confounding variables such as gender and premorbid adjustment (McGlashan, 1999; Norman & Malla, 2001; Norman et al., 2005a).

Demographic and personal circumstances

A US study by Loebel et al. (1992) of DUP in first-episode schizophrenia is often cited as evidence that men have a longer treatment delay than women. Larsen and colleagues reported a similar difference among patients with a non-affective psychotic disorder admitted to a Norwegian programme (Larsen, McGlashan & Moe, 1996; Melle et al., 2004), although this difference was less apparent when the sample was restricted to those with a diagnosis of schizophrenia (Larsen et al., 1998). Most studies across several different countries, however, have not found that treatment delay once psychosis occurs is significantly related to gender (Black et al., 2001; Chen et al., 2005; Cohen, Gotowiec & Seeman, 2000; de Haan et al., 2002; Drake et al., 2000; Fuchs & Steinert, 2004; Kalla et al., 2002; Norman et al., 2004). Of particular interest are recent studies in Singapore and Japan that found longer delays for women than men (Chong et al., 2005a; Yamazawa et al., 2004), the former examining non-affective psychosis and the latter restricted to schizophrenia. The authors of these two papers suggested that their findings may be at least partly

attributable to the high stigmatization of mental illness in Asian cultures.

Verdoux et al. (1998), in a study in Bordeaux, and Melle et al. (2004), in a Scandinavian population, found lower level of education to be associated with longer treatment delay, whereas Chong et al. (2005a), in Singapore, found the opposite: those with post-secondary education had longer treatment delays. Several other studies have found no relationship between education level and delay (e.g. Black et al., 2001; Cougnard et al., 2004a; de Haan et al., 2002; Fuchs & Steinert, 2004).

There have been several studies examining whether ethnic minority groups within a country show longer treatment delays. Although there has been some evidence that ethnic minorities, in general, may be less likely to use mental health services (e.g. Gallo, Ford & Anthony, 1995), there is inconsistent evidence concerning whether longer treatment delays are systematically influenced by ethnicity (Bhugra et al., 1999; Burnett et al., 1999; Chong et al., 2005a; Cole et al., 1995; Drake et al., 2000). Moreover, findings from two UK studies on treatment delay in first-episode patients (Bhugra et al., 1999; Cole et al., 1995) do not support the hypothesis that when admissions occur they are more likely to be compulsory for ethnic minorities. Ethnic minority status can be related to socioeconomic status but the predictive role of this more general construct has not been widely investigated. In a Canadian study Norman et al. (2004) did not find that parental socioeconomic status predicted treatment delay, whereas using the same measure in a Spanish study, Peralta et al. (2005) found lower parental socioeconomic status to be related to longer DUP.

Perhaps the aspect of personal circumstance that has been most widely investigated in relation to treatment delay is the nature and extent of the affected individual's social network. Given that many individuals in the initial stages of psychosis do not readily recognize they need help, one might predict, on the one hand, that having a stronger network of social connections would facilitate the detection of problems and encourage help-seeking. On the other hand, under some circumstances strong social support might help to reduce the impact of illness and allow someone to function for longer periods without seeking treatment. Several studies have found the presence of fewer social contacts around the time of illness onset to be associated with longer treatment delay (Drake *et al.*, 2000; Kalla *et al.*, 2002; Larsen *et al.*, 1998; Malla *et al.*, 2004; Melle *et al.*, 2004). While Chen *et al.* (2005) found some suggestive evidence that belonging to a single member household was associated with longer treatment delay, other researchers have not (e.g. Fuchs & Steinert, 2004; Yamazawa *et al.*, 2004); it may be that being single is a more critical predictor of delay than living alone (Chong *et al.*, 2005a; Cole *et al.*, 1995; Cougnard *et al.*, 2004a). Peralta *et al.* (2005) found that a high level of diffuse social contact through work and school was related to shorter delay, but more intimate contacts such as the presence of confidants and close family did not predict delay.

The role of social networks in treatment delay is of particular interest for two reasons. First, to the extent that good social network support predicts shorter treatment delay, it could be a confounding factor in the relationship between treatment delay and outcome. This is because social support can be a significant predictor of prognosis (Erikson, Beiser & Iacono 1998; Erikson *et al.*, 1989; Norman *et al.*, 2005b). A second possibility is that the extent of an individual's social network at the time of onset of psychosis may be at least partly related to aspects of early clinical presentation, such as premorbid functioning and social withdrawal.

Aspects of illness onset

The previous section suggests that very few aspects of the social circumstances of an individual reliably predict length of time between onset of a psychotic disorder and obtaining treatment. Perhaps more robust predictors will be identified if the characteristics of the onset of the disorder are examined.

It is not surprising that many authors have speculated that the more precipitous the onset of a psychotic disorder the more likely it is to be noticed by the person's acquaintances and family and responded to (e.g. Lincoln & McGorry, 1995; Moller, 2001). Research related to the mode of onset can be identified by the measurement of constructs such as 'premorbid adjustment', 'level of functioning' and 'insidious versus acute onset'. The

definition of these constructs and their measures are likely to overlap substantially and so we shall not endeavour to distinguish between them for current purposes.

Perhaps one of the most provocative findings in this respect is that of Verdoux *et al.* (2001), whose data indicate that a higher peak level of functioning in the period prior to hospital admission is associated with shorter treatment delay and that controlling for prior level of functioning greatly reduced the importance of DUP in predicting subsequent course of illness. These findings suggest the possibility that the relationship between treatment delay and treatment outcome might simply be the result of the relationship between premorbid functioning and long-term course, or that the relationship between premorbid functioning and outcome may be mediated by treatment delay. Larsen *et al.* (1998) found that premorbid adjustment with reference to early life was not related to DUP, but that greater deterioration of functioning in adolescence and early adulthood and more active social avoidance predicted longer treatment delay. Results consistent with this pattern of longer delay being associated with poorer social and vocational functioning prior to, or around, the onset of frank psychosis and/or a gradual mode of onset have also been reported by others (Chen *et al.*, 2005; Cole *et al.*, 1995; Johannessen, Larsen & McGlashan, 1999; Kalla *et al.*, 2002; Melle *et al.*, 2004; Moller, 2000). One might expect severity of negative symptoms to be related to some of these premorbid characteristics, and Melle *et al.* (2004) have found a slight but significant trend for longer DUP to be related to more severe negative symptoms at presentation, but others have not (e.g. Barnes *et al.*, 2000; Drake *et al.*, 2000; Kalla *et al.*, 2002). The relationship between negative symptoms and treatment delay may depend on the specific symptoms. Malla *et al.* (2002) found that treatment delay was greater for those showing more apathy and social anhedonia, but was unrelated to affective flattening and alogia. The finding with respect to social anhedonia and apathy are likely to be conceptually related to the relationship discussed earlier between the extent of social contacts and treatment delay. Perhaps related to the role of gradual versus acute onset are the findings that those who meet diagnostic criteria for schizophrenia-spectrum disorders may have a longer treatment delay than those with affective disorders with psychotic features (e.g. Beiser *et al.*, 1993; Melle *et al.*, 2004; Verdoux *et al.*, 1998).

Although the role of premorbid functioning and acuity of onset appear to be among the more robust predictors of treatment delay, the relationships may turn out to be more complex upon closer examination. Drake *et al.* (2000) derived two indices from the Social Functioning Scale (Birchwood *et al.*, 1990): one to assess social relationships and one to assess daily living competence. They found that maintenance of social relationships was associated with shorter DUP (consistent with the above reports) but preserved ability to cope with the challenges of daily living correlated with longer delay.

Another contextual factor that might influence the speed with which the onset of psychosis is recognized and responded to is whether there is a family history of psychotic disorder (Cohen *et al.*, 2000). Hambrecht (1995) noted that one could hypothesize that having a family history of psychotic disorder could result either in more rapid recognition of what is happening when onset occurs or denial or tolerance of signs of illness. After interviewing the relatives of 30 patients with recent-onset schizophrenia-spectrum disorders in Germany, he concluded that when there is a positive family history relatives are more able to detect the presence of hallucinations and delusions, but they are less sensitive to non-specific early signs as possible harbingers of psychosis. The latter could result in delay to treatment given that such non-specific signs may not only precede the onset of psychosis but may also be the only external signs for some time after the onset. Chen *et al.* (2005) reported that longer delay was associated with a family history of psychosis, but others have failed to find such a relationship (de Haan *et al.*, 2002; Norman *et al.*, 2004, 2007). Verdoux *et al.* (1998) reported a longer delay in getting treatment when a family member had previously been hospitalized for any psychiatric disorder, but delay was not associated specifically with a family history of psychotic disorder.

We noted earlier that some individuals report a delay in seeking treatment because they assume that symptoms are a result of substance abuse. One might, therefore, expect that the occurrence of substance abuse at around the time of onset of psychosis would be associated with longer treatment delay. While there are some reports consistent with such a prediction (e.g. Chong *et al.*, 2005a; Cougnard *et al.*, 2004a), several studies have not found the presence of substance abuse to be related to treatment delay (e.g. Cohen *et al.*, 2000; de Haan *et al.*, 2002; Drake *et al.*, 2000; Fuchs & Steinert, 2004; Norman & Malla, 2002).

Interventions to reduce treatment delay for psychotic disorders

An essential aspect of any efforts to reduce delay in treatment for psychotic disorders is the presence of appropriate specialized assessment and consultation and treatment programmes that can be readily accessed. Programmes staffed by professionals able to diagnose psychotic disorders quickly and accurately, and provide coordinated, comprehensive treatment, are a sine qua non of any effort to reduce treatment delay and improve outcome (Malla & Norman, 2001, 2002). However, the presence of such programmes does not ensure reduction in treatment delay. Based on the above findings of descriptive and correlational investigations of pathways to care for psychotic disorders, it is clear that reducing treatment delay poses many additional challenges. Two of the most reliable findings appear to be that the presence of psychosis is often not detected by the affected person and/or others – particularly if there is a gradual onset accompanied by social withdrawal and restricted social contacts – and that primary care providers such as family physicians or GPs (as well as school counsellors, community therapists, youth workers, etc.) are often important points of contact in pathways to care for those with psychosis – even when referral from such professionals are not required for prompt access to appropriate specialized services.

Attempts to evaluate systematically the impact of community efforts to reduce treatment delay have typically been carried out in settings where the required specialized treatment facilities are readily available. Consistent with the above reasoning, these community interventions have typically emphasized two components. The first is widespread public education about the early signs of psychosis, the importance of early treatment and how to access appropriate treatment readily. Literature relevant to this approach is reviewed in Ch. 9. Another approach is to target primary health-care and social service providers. The objective would be to increase the likelihood of such professionals considering whether a psychotic disorder is responsible for the presenting problems of their patients and clients. In addition, such targeted interventions could reinforce the importance of early treatment and provide information on how to access appropriate facilities.

There are four noteworthy quasi-experimental studies reported which include education of helping professions in an effort to reduce treatment delay for psychotic disorders. These are The Early Psychosis Prevention and Intervention Centre (EPPIC) in Melbourne, Australia (Krstev et al., 2004; McGorry et al., 1996); the PEPP in London, Canada (Malla et al., 2005); the Treatment and Intervention in Psychosis Study (TIPS) in Scandinavia (Friis et al., 2005; Johannessen et al., 2001; Larsen et al., 2001; Melle et al., 2004); and the Early Psychosis Intervention Programme (EPIP) in Singapore (Chong, Mythily & Verma, 2005b). Each of these studies included a public education campaign as well as interventions targeted at professionals who are likely to be consulted by those seeking help for psychotic disorders. The latter interventions generally included education about the early signs of psychosis and the advantages of early intervention, as well as information on how to obtain prompt assessment and consultation for patients with specialist teams. In EPPIC, the interventions targeted at helping professionals included the establishment of working groups involving relevant service providers, visits to relevant work settings such as GPs' practices to provide information, holding special education workshops, mail-outs of information and videos. In PEPP, service providers were targeted through a peripatetic consultation programme initiated with the secondary schools and the local college and university through the relevant guidance, counselling and health services, as well as provision of information directly to family physicians through multiple means. Neither the EPPIC nor the PEPP interventions resulted in a decrease in treatment delay. In both programmes there was some evidence of changes in the distributions of treatment delay in the years immediately after the early detection

initiatives (Krstev et al., 2004; Malla et al., 2005). One interpretation of these findings is that the interventions may have had two main effects: reduction in delay for those with recent-onset psychosis plus detection of those with long-standing illness who may otherwise have not been identified (see also McGorry et al., 1996).

Perhaps the most ambitious study of reducing treatment delay is the TIPS, which involves four Scandinavian health sectors. Two of the sectors (in Rogaland County, Norway) carried out extensive interventions to reduce treatment delay while two sectors (one in Oslo County, Norway and one in Roskilde County, Denmark) served as controls. The nature of and accessibility to treatment, which was publicly funded, remained comparable in all four sectors. The early detection programmes in the intervention sectors consisted of extensive public information campaigns using newspapers, radio and cinema advertising. In addition, there were targeted campaigns to service providers such as GPs, school health services and social workers, and the establishment of special early detection teams with the mandate to carry out assessments of patients with potential psychosis within 24 hours wherever convenient to the affected person and/or the referring person.

The design of the TIPS project allowed two comparisons of relevance to the effectiveness of the early detection initiative. The first is a historical comparison of DUP in the intervention sectors before and after the initiation of the early detection programme, and the second is a comparison of treatment delay between the intervention and control sectors. While there is evidence that the campaigns resulted in a reduction in treatment delay (Johannessen et al., 2001; Larsen et al., 2001), it is not possible to determine the relative importance of public education, targeted interventions with service providers and/or the establishment of early detection teams in bringing about such a change.

Data from EPIP in Singapore also suggest that combined public and professional education programmes can bring about a reduction in treatment delay. One of the objectives of EPIP was to raise awareness of psychosis among the general public as well as among primary healthcare workers such as GPs, polyclinic doctors and counsellors. In addition to a public education campaign, networks were established with GPs, students and other community counsellors. Bimonthly newsletters and forums for primary service providers were provided, and it was ensured that telephone consultations were readily available. The impact was evaluated by a before and after comparison of patients seen at the Institute of Mental Health in Singapore in the 1 year prior to EPIP and the 2 years after its establishment. This comparison showed a significant decrease in the DUP from a median of 12 months to 4 months, with an increase in the proportion of self or family referrals and decrease in police referrals (Chong *et al.*, 2005b).

It is difficult to assess why the TIPS project and EPIP appear to have had greater success in reducing treatment delay than the Australian or Canadian initiatives. The greater success of the TIPS programme may have resulted from differences in intensity or duration of interventions or from the differential use of mobile early detection teams as part of the intervention – the latter apparently allowing greater access to services on an outpatient basis. Data concerning the extent to which reduced treatment delay was specifically associated with cases seen by these teams would be helpful. However, the successful EPIP intervention does not appear to have included any changes in availability or circumstances of patient access. It is also important to acknowledge that the designs used in evaluating the effectiveness of interventions to reduce treatment delay often do not include blinds to reduce risk of assessment bias.

Conclusions: what have we learned?

Unfortunately few reports have presented information relevant to the reliability of measures of pathways to care or treatment delay (Norman *et al.*, 2004, 2007), and there is certainly a need for the development of more standardized instruments in the field (Singh & Grange, 2006). Nevertheless, there are three reasonably reliable findings from the existing literature on pathways to care for psychotic disorders. The first is that help-seeking in the presence of psychosis is most likely to be delayed when the presentation is an insidious one accompanied by a gradual reduction in functioning and social withdrawal. The second is that help-seeking is often initiated by families or others in contact with the affected individual, rather than the person himself or herself. The third is that primary service providers are often involved as important contacts for those seeking help even in settings where access to specialized services are readily available without an intermediary referral source.

The first two observations are relevant to the challenges of identifying the presence of psychosis and initiating help-seeking, and support the importance of continuing to include public education about possible signs of early psychosis. Many of the early signs of psychosis are non-specific and can frequently occur, especially in young people, without indicating risk of psychosis. Even when frank psychosis is present, it may be obscured by social withdrawal or represent an imperceptible increase in eccentricity over time to which the ill-person and those who interact with him or her may have adapted. It seems important, therefore, that education of the public emphasizes not only what may be the signs of psychosis but also that initial consultation is readily available for purposes of assessing whether there is reason to suspect psychosis. The extent to which the public takes advantage of such services will undoubtedly be influenced by how quickly and conveniently they can be provided. Descriptive research suggests that the early course of psychosis is often one of intermittent periods of worrisome signs. What causes concern today may seem bearable tomorrow, and a process of increasing demand for adaptation may go on for a long time before a definitive crisis occurs (Compton *et al.*, 2004; de Haan *et al.*, 2002, 2004; Etheridge *et al.*, 2004; Larsen *et al.*, 1998; Moller, 2001). Under such circumstances, the availability of a very prompt skilled consultation, in a convenient, non-stigmatizing setting, might well make a great difference in both the likelihood of early help-seeking and its effectiveness. As noted above, the presence of early detection teams in the TIPS may be one of the critical factors in determining the effectiveness of the programme in reducing treatment delay.

The challenges in identifying early signs of psychosis apply not only to ill-persons and their informal social contacts but also to the care providers who are often consulted. Although GPs are among those primary healthcare providers often cited in this respect, they are by no means the only ones. Depending on the circumstances and preferences of the individuals involved, these contacts can include school or college counsellors or health service providers, community-based therapists, clergy and social and youth workers. Given the nature of their training and experience, they are unlikely to have particular expertise in identification of psychosis. Their importance to pathways to care is not through their expertise but rather through the frequency with which they are an early contact for those seeking help. In many ways, the challenges they have in identifying early psychosis parallels that of the general public. The findings that those who have sought help for mental health problems prior to the onset of psychosis may be at particular risk of delay in getting adequate treatment (Norman *et al.*, 2004) suggests that clinicians can sometimes develop a cognitive set about the nature of their patient's problems which interferes with the detection of a psychotic disorder at onset. Primary care providers may hope for a readily accessible consultation for their patient or client not only for the ill-person's sake but also for themselves in deciding whether or how to pursue the possibility of a psychotic disorder being present. While knowledge of the possible signs of psychosis and the benefits of early identification is important, knowledge of the ease and promptness with which a consultation with experts is available may be crucial. There may well be parallels between the reactions of a service provider and those of other members of the ill-person's social network. It has also been our experience that primary service providers sometimes do not respond to psychosis in those who consult with them because of concerns about the person's or family's response to such a stigmatizing suggestion. This concern plus scepticism about the likelihood of recovery sometimes result in those in primary care taking a 'wait and see' approach rather than facilitating prompt referral. As with the individual's social network, these hesitancies on the part of service providers can allow a gradual exacerbation of the course of the disorder until a crisis occurs. When such crises do occur, police and emergency health services are more likely to become involved (Addington *et al.*, 2002; Chong *et al.*, 2005b; Norman *et al.*, 2004).

In general, the literature reviewed in this chapter suggests that public education and education chiefly aimed at primary service providers are likely to be important for early identification and treatment of psychotic disorders, particularly when the onset is not abrupt or dramatic. In addition, making access to excellent consultation, assessment and treatment services as easy and quick as possible is clearly essential. It is important to note that most efforts to facilitate early intervention for psychosis have, up to this point, been carried out in areas characterized by at least moderate population density. As the interest in early intervention expands, there is likely to be increasing interest in how to expand such efforts into rural areas. This will undoubtedly present an additional set of challenges. It has been our experience that both the establishment of websites and development of electronically aided virtual family-support groups can be of considerable help to those dealing with early psychosis in comparatively isolated areas. Unfortunately, while such assistance is of value, it often highlights the paucity of appropriate clinical services outside urban areas. The challenges of reducing treatment delay are many – not just in shortening the pathway to care but also in ensuring the usefulness of what is found at its end.

REFERENCES

Addington, J., van Mastrigt, S., Hutchinson, J. & Addington, D. (2002). Pathways to care: help seeking behaviour in first-episode psychosis. *Acta Psychiatrica Scandinavica*, **106**, 358–64.

Amaddeo, F., Zambello, F., Tansella, M. & Thornicroft, G. (2001). Accessibility and pathways to psychiatric care in a community-based mental health system. *Social Psychiatry and Psychiatric Epidemiology*, **36**, 500–7.

Amador, X. F., Strauss, D. H., Yale, S. A. & Gorman, J. M. (1991). Awareness of illness in schizophrenia. *Schizophrenia Bulletin*, **17**, 113–32.

Balestrieri, M., Bon, M. G., Rodriguez-Sacristan, A. & Tansella, M. (1994). Pathways to psychiatric care in South-Verona, Italy. *British Journal of Psychiatry*, **24**, 641–9.

Barnes, T. R., Hutton, S. B., Chapman, M. J. *et al.* (2000). West London first episode study of schizophrenia: clinical correlates of duration of untreated psychosis. *British Journal of Psychiatry*, **177**, 207–11.

Beiser, M., Erickson, D., Fleming, J. A. E. & Iacono, W. G. (1993). Establishing the onset of psychotic illness. *American Journal of Psychiatry*, **150**, 1349–54.

Bhugra, D., Corridan, B., Rudge, S., Leff, J. & Mallett, R. (1999). Early manifestations, personality traits and pathways to care for Asian and white first-onset cases of schizophrenia. *Social Psychiatry and Psychiatric Epidemiology*. **34**, 595–9.

Birchwood, M., Smith, J., Cochrane, R., Wetton, S. & Copestake, S. (1990). The Social Functioning Scale. The development and validation of a new scale of social development for use in family intervention programmes with schizophrenic patients. *British Journal of Psychiatry*, **157**, 853–9.

Black, K., Peters, L., Rui, Q. *et al.* (2001). Duration of untreated psychosis predicts treatment outcome in an early psychosis program. *Schizophrenia Research*, **47**, 215–22.

Burnett, R., Mallett, R., Bhugra, D. *et al.* (1999). The first contact of patients with schizophrenia with psychiatric services: social factors and pathways to care in a multi-ethnic population. *Psychological Medicine*, **29**, 475–83.

Chen, E. Y-H., Dunn, E. L-W., Miao, M. Y-K. *et al.* (2005). The impact of family experience on the duration of untreated psychosis (DUP) in Hong Kong. *Social Psychiatry and Psychiatric Epidemiology*, **40**, 350–6.

Chong, S-A., Mythily, S., Lum, A., Chan, Y. H. & McGorry, P. D. (2005a). Determinants of duration of untreated psychosis and the pathway to care in Singapore. *International Journal of Social Psychiatry*, **51**, 55–62.

Chong, S-A., Mythily, S. & Verma, S. (2005b). Reducing the duration of untreated psychosis and changing help-seeking behaviour in Singapore. *Social Psychiatry and Psychiatric Epidemiology*, **40**, 619–21.

Christiana, J. M., Gilman, S. E., Guardino, M. *et al.* (2000). Duration between onset and time of obtaining initial treatment among people with anxiety and mood disorders: an international survey of members of mental health patient advocate groups. *Psychological Medicine*, **30**, 693–703.

Cohen, R. Z., Gotowiec, A. & Seeman, M. V. (2000). Duration of pretreatment phases in schizophrenia: women and men. *Canadian Journal of Psychiatry*, **45**, 544–7.

Cole, E., Leavey, G., King, M., Johnson-Sabine, E. & Hoar, A. (1995). Pathways to care for patients with a first episode of psychosis: a comparison of ethnic groups. *British Journal of Psychiatry*, **167**, 770–6.

Compton, M. T., Kaslow, N. J. & Walker, E. F. (2004). Observations on parent/family factors that may influence the duration of untreated psychosis among African American first-episode schizophrenia patients. *Schizophrenia Research*, **68**, 373–85.

Cougnard, A., Kalmi, E., Desage, A. *et al.* (2004a). Pathways to care of first-admitted subjects with psychosis in South-Western France. *Psychological Medicine*, **34**, 267–76.

Cougnard, A., Kalmi, E., Desage, A. *et al.* (2004b). Factors influencing compulsory admission in first episode subjects with psychosis. *Social Psychiatry and Psychiatric Epidemiology*, **39**, 804–9.

de Haan, L., Peters, B., Dingemans, P., Wouters, L. & Linszen, D. (2002). Attitudes of patients toward the first psychotic episode and the start of treatment. *Schizophrenia Bulletin*, **28**, 431–42.

de Haan, L., Welborn, K., Krikke, M. & Linszen, D. (2004). Opinions of mothers on the first psychotic episode and the start of treatment of their child. *European Psychiatry*, **19**, 226–9.

Drake, R. J., Haley, C. J., Akhtar, S. & Lewis, S. W. (2000). Causes and consequences of duration of untreated psychosis in schizophrenia. *British Journal of Psychiatry*, **177**, 511–15.

Erikson, D. H., Beiser, M., Iacono, W. G., Fleming, J. A. & Lin, T. (1989). The role of social relationships in the course of first-episode schizophrenia and affective psychosis. *American Journal of Psychiatry*, **146**, 1456–61.

Erikson, D. H., Beiser, M. & Iacono, W. G. (1998). Social support predicts 5-year outcome in first-episode schizophrenia. *Journal of Abnormal Psychology*, **107**, 681–5.

Etheridge, K., Yarrow, L. & Peet, M. (2004). Pathways to care in first episode psychosis. *Journal of Psychiatric and Mental Health Nursing*, **11**, 125–8.

Friis, S., Vaglum, P., Haahr, U. *et al.* (2005). Effect of an early detection programme on duration of untreated psychosis: part of the Scandinavian TIPS study. *British Journal of Psychiatry*, **187**(Suppl 48), s29–32.

Fuchs, J. & Steinert, T. (2004). Patients with a first episode of schizophrenia spectrum psychosis and their pathways to psychiatric hospital care in South Germany. *Social Psychiatry and Psychiatric Epidemiology*, **39**, 375–80.

Gallo, J. J., Ford, S. M. & Anthony, J. C. (1995). Filters on the pathway to mental healthcare, II. Sociodemographic factors. *Psychological Medicine*, **25**, 1149–60.

Garety, P. A. & Rigg, A. (2001). Early psychosis in the inner city: a survey to inform service planning. *Social Psychiatry and Psychiatric Epidemiology*, **36**, 537–44.

Gater, R. & Goldberg, D. (1991). Pathways to psychiatric care in Manchester. *British Journal of Psychiatry*, **159**, 90–6.

Gundez-Bruce, H., McMeniman, M., Robinson, D. G. *et al.* (2005). Duration of untreated psychosis and time to treatment response for delusions and hallucinations. *American Journal of Psychiatry*, **162**, 1966–9.

Haley, C. J., Drake, R. J., Bentall, R. P. & Lewis, S. W. (2003). Health beliefs link to duration of untreated psychosis and attitudes to later treatment in early psychosis. *Social Psychiatry and Psychiatric Epidemiology*, **38**, 311–16.

Hambrecht, M. (1995). A second case of schizophrenia in the family: is it observed differently? *European Archives of Psychiatry and Clinical Neuroscience*, **245**, 267–9.

Harrigan, S. M., McGorry, P. D. & Krstev, H. (2003). Does treatment delay in first-episode psychosis really matter? *Psychological Medicine*, **33**, 97–110.

Helgason, L. (1990). Twenty years follow-up of first psychiatric presentation for schizophrenia: what could have been prevented? *Acta Psychiatrica Scandinavica*, **81**, 231–5.

Ho, B-C. & Andreasen, N. C. (2001). Long delays in seeking treatment for schizophrenia. *Lancet*, **157**, 898–900.

Jenike, M. A. (2004). Obsessive – compulsive disorder. *New England Journal of Medicine*, **350**, 259–65.

Johannessen, J. O., Larsen, T. K. & McGlashan, T. (1999). Duration of untreated psychosis: an important target for intervention in schizophrenia? *Nordic Journal of Psychiatry*, **53**, 275–83.

Johannessen, J. O., McGlashan, T. H., Larsen, T. K. *et al.* (2001). Early detection strategies for untreated first-episode psychosis. *Schizophrenia Research*, **51**, 39–46.

Johnstone, E. C., Crow, T. C., Johnson, A. L. & MacMillan, J. F. (1986). The Northwick Park study of first episodes of schizophrenia. I. Presentation of the illness and problems related to admission. *British Journal of Psychiatry*, **148**, 115–20.

Kalla, O., Aaltonen, J., Wahlstrom, J. *et al.* (2002). Duration of untreated psychosis and its correlates in first episode psychosis in Finland and Spain. *Acta Psychiatrica Scandinavica*, **106**, 265–75.

Kelly, B. D., Clark, M., Browne, S. *et al.* (2004). Clinical predictors of admission status in first-episode schizophrenia. *European Psychiatry*, **19**, 67–71.

Kessler, D., Lloyd, K., Lewis, G. & Gray, D. P. (1999). Cross sectional study of symptom attribution and recognition of depression and anxiety in primary care. *British Medical Journal*, **318**, 136–40.

Krstev, H., Carbone, S., Harrigan, S. M. *et al.* (2004). Early intervention in first-episode psychosis: the impact of a community development campaign. *Social Psychiatry and Psychiatric Epidemiology*, **39**, 711–19.

Larsen, T. K., McGlashan, T. H. & Moe, L. C. (1996). First episode schizophrenia: I. Early course parameters. *Schizophrenia Bulletin*, **22**, 241–56.

Larsen, T. K., Johannessen, J. O. & Opjordsmoen, S. (1998). First episode schizophrenia with long duration of untreated psychosis: pathways to care. *British Journal of Psychiatry*, **172**(Suppl 3), s45–52.

Larsen, T. K., McGlashan, T. H., Johannessen, J. O. *et al.* (2001). Shortened duration of untreated first episode of psychosis: change in patient characteristics at treatment. *American Journal of Psychiatry*, **158**, 1917–19.

Lieberman, J. A. & Fenton, W. S. (2000). Delayed detection of psychosis: causes, consequences, and effect on public health. *American Journal of Psychiatry*, **157**, 1727–30.

Lincoln, C. V. & McGorry, P. D. (1995). Who cares? Pathways to psychiatric care for young people experiencing a first episode of psychosis. *Psychiatric Services*, **46**, 1166–71.

Lincoln, C. V., Harrigan, S. & McGorry, P. D. (1998). Understanding the topography of the early psychosis pathway. *British Journal of Psychiatry*, **172**(Suppl 33), s21–5.

Loebel, A. D., Lieberman, J. A., Alvir, J. M. J. *et al.* (1992). Duration of psychosis and outcome in first-episode schizophrenia. *American Journal of Psychiatry*, **149**, 1183–8.

Malla, A. K. & Norman, R. M. G. (2001). Treating psychosis: is there more to early intervention than intervening early? *Canadian Journal of Psychiatry*, **46**, 645–8.

Malla, A. K. & Norman, R. M. G. (2002). Early intervention in schizophrenia and related disorders: advantages and pitfalls. *Current Opinion in Psychiatry*, **15**, 17–23.

Malla, A. K., Norman, R. M. G. & Voruganti, L. P. (1999). Improving outcome in schizophrenia: the case for early intervention. *Canadian Medical Association Journal*, **160**, 843–6.

Malla, A. K., Takhar, J. J., Norman, R. M. G. *et al.* (2002). Negative symptoms in first episode non-affective psychosis. *Acta Psychiatrica Scandinavica*, **105**, 431–9.

Malla, A. K., Norman, R. M. G., McLean, T. S. *et al.* (2004). Determinants of quality of life in first episode psychosis. *Acta Psychiatrica Scandinavica*, **109**, 46–54.

Malla, A. K., Norman, R. M. G., Scholten, D., Manchanda, R. & McLean, T. (2005). A community intervention for early identification of first-episode psychosis: impact on duration of untreated psychosis (DUP) and patient characteristics. *Social Psychiatry and Psychiatric Epidemiology*, **40**, 337–44.

Marshall, M., Lewis, S., Lockwood, A. *et al.* (2005). Association between duration of untreated psychosis and outcome in cohorts of first-episode patients. *Archives of General Psychiatry*, **62**, 975–83.

McGlashan, T. H. (1999). Duration of untreated psychosis in first episode schizophrenia: marker or determinant of course? *Biological Psychiatry*, **46**, 899–907.

McGorry, P. D. (2000). Evaluating the importance of reducing the duration of untreated psychosis. *Australian and New Zealand Journal of Psychiatry*, **34**(Suppl), s145–9.

McGorry, P. D., Edwards, J., Mihalopoulos, C., Harrigan, S. M. & Jackson, H. J. (1996). EPPIC: an evolving system of early detection and optimal management. *Schizophrenia Bulletin*, **22**, 305–26.

McGorry, P. D., Krstev, H. & Harrigan, S. (2000). Early detection and treatment delay: implications for outcomes in early psychosis. *Current Opinion in Psychiatry*, **13**, 37–43.

Melle, I., Larsen, T. K., Haahr, U. *et al.* (2004). Reducing the duration of untreated first-episode psychosis: effects on clinical presentation. *Archives of General Psychiatry*, **61**, 143–50.

Miller, T. J., McGlashan, T. H., Woods, S. W. *et al.* (1999). Symptom assessment in schizophrenia prodromal states. *Psychiatric Quarterly*, **70**, 273–87.

Moller, P. (2000). First-episode schizophrenia: do grandiosity, disorganization, and acute initial development reduce duration of untreated psychosis? An exploratory naturalistic case study. *Comprehensive Psychiatry*, **41**, 184–90.

Moller, P. (2001). Duration of untreated psychosis: are we ignoring the model of initial development? *Psychopathology*, **34**, 8–14.

Norman, R. M. G. & Malla, A. K. (2001). Duration of untreated psychosis: a critical examination of the concept and its importance. *Psychological Medicine*, **31**, 381–400.

Norman, R. M. G. & Malla, A. K. (2002). Examining adherence to medication and substance abuse as possible confounds of duration of untreated psychosis. *Journal of Nervous and Mental Disease*, **190**, 331–4.

Norman, R. M. G., Malla, A. K., Verdi, M. B., Hassall, L. D. & Fazekas, C. (2004). Understanding delay in treatment for first-episode psychosis. *Psychological Medicine*, **34**, 255–66.

Norman, R. M. G., Lewis, S. W. & Marshall, M. (2005a). Duration of untreated psychosis and its relationship to clinical outcome. *British Journal of Psychiatry*, **187**(Suppl 48), s19–23.

Norman, R. M. G., Malla, A. K., Manchanda, R. *et al.* (2005b). Social support and three-year symptom and admission outcomes for first episode psychosis. *Schizophrenia Research*, **80**, 227–34.

Norman, R. M. G., Malla, A. K., Manchanda, R., Harricharan, R. & Northcott, S. (2007). Delay in treatment for psychosis: its relation to family history. *Social Psychiatry and Psychiatric Epidemiology*, **42**, 507–12.

Peralta, V., Cuesta, M. J., Matinez-Larrea, A., Serrano, J. E. & Langarica, M. (2005). Duration of untreated psychotic illness: the role of premorbid social support networks. *Social Psychiatry and Psychiatric Epidemiology*, **40**, 345–9.

Perkins, D. O., Nieri, J. M., Bell, K. & Lieberman, J. A. (1999). Factors that contribute to delay in the initial treatment of psychosis. *Schizophrenia Research*, **36**, 52.

Perkins, D. O., Gu, H., Boteva, K. & Lieberman, J. A. (2005). Relationship between duration of untreated psychosis and outcome in first-episode schizophrenia: a critical review and meta-analysis. *American Journal of Psychiatry*, **162**, 1785–804.

Phillips, L., Yung, A. R., Hearn, N. *et al.* (1999). Preventive mental healthcare: accessing the target population. *Australian and New Zealand Journal of Psychiatry*, **33**, 912–17.

Preda, A., Miller, T. J., Rosen, J. L. *et al.* (2002). Treatment histories of patients with a syndrome putatively prodromal to schizophrenia. *Psychiatric Services*, **53**, 342–4.

Singh, S. P. & Grange, T. (2006). Measuring pathways to care in first episode psychosis: a systematic review. *Schizophrenia Research*, **81**, 75–82.

Skeate, A., Jackson, C., Birchwood, M. & Jones, C. (2002). Duration of untreated psychosis and pathways to care in first episode psychosis: investigation of help-seeking behaviour in primary care. *British Journal of Psychiatry*, **181**(Suppl 43), s73–7.

Thompson, A., Hunt, C. & Issakidis, C. (2004). Why wait? Reasons for delay and prompts to seek help for mental health problems in an Australian clinical sample. *Social Psychiatry and Psychiatric Epidemiology*, **39**, 810–17.

Verdoux, H., Bergey, C., Assens, F. *et al.* (1998). Prediction of duration of psychosis before first admission. *European Psychiatry*, **13**, 346–52.

Verdoux, H., Liraud, F., Bergey, C. *et al.* (2001). Is the association between duration of untreated psychosis and outcome confounded? A two year follow-up study of first-admitted patients. *Schizophrenia Research*, **49**, 231–41.

Wells, J. E., Robins, L. N., Bushnell, J. A. *et al.* (1994). Perceived barriers to care in St. Louis (USA) and Christchurch (NZ): reason for not seeking help for psychological distress. *Social Psychiatry and Psychiatric Epidemiology*, **29**, 155–64.

Wyatt, R. J. (1991). Neuroleptics and the natural course of schizophrenia. *Schizophrenia Bulletin*, **17**, 325–51.

Yamazawa, R., Mizuno, M., Nemoto, T. *et al.* (2004). Duration of untreated psychosis and pathways to psychiatric services in first-episode schizophrenia. *Psychiatry and Clinical Neurosciences*, **58**, 76–81.

SECTION 5

The first episode

Initial assessment and initial pharmacological treatment in the acute phase

Martin Lambert

Introduction

Treatment of patients with first-episode psychosis (FEP) is a challenging task. The early detection of illness and the pursuit of integrative treatment in specialized services give patients and their families hope for a better course and outcome. The combination of pharmacotherapy and psychosocial interventions markedly increases the chance of remission and subsequent long-lasting recovery (Petersen *et al.*, 2005). However, the complex psychosocial problems of these patients may still result in incomplete remission and recovery – at least for a proportion of people.

Initially, engagement and comprehensive assessments of FEP patients are fundamental to developing a positive therapeutic alliance and initial formulation of the person's condition, which provides the foundation for later successful treatment. The initial pharmacotherapy of these patients rests on some important principles, which should guide clinicians in the way they use antipsychotic and other psychotropic medications. Optimizing the initial pharmacological management is not only vital to maximizing the chance of remission and recovery, but also crucial in minimizing the potential for future relapses, morbidity and mortality.

This chapter, which mainly covers the first 3 months of treatment, provides an overview about engagement, initial assessment and the initial psychopharmacological treatment in FEP. It is chiefly based on several recently published guidelines for schizophrenia-spectrum disorders (e.g. APA, 2004a; NICE, 2002; Royal Australian and New Zealand College of Psychiatrists, 2005), for bipolar disorder (e.g. APA, 2004b; Royal Australian and New Zealand College of Psychiatrists, 2004), for major depressive disorder (e.g. APA, 2004c) and on articles focusing on the initial pharmacological treatment in this early phase.

Aims of acute treatment in first-episode psychosis

Engagement and development of a therapeutic alliance

The quality of relationships with clinicians during the initial contacts and the subsequent development of a trustworthy therapeutic alliance appears to be an important determinant of a patient's attitude toward treatment, adherence to medication and engagement (Day *et al.*, 2005; Power & McGorry, 1999); all these factors are known to decrease the likelihood of relapse and to improve long-term symptomatic and functional outcome as well as quality of life (Coldham, Addington & Addington, 2002; Gray, Wykes & Gournay, 2002; Schimmelmann *et al.*, 2006). However, the initial engagement process could be aggravated by a variety of factors, such as negative attitudes towards psychiatry, the present mental state of the patient, including behavioural disturbances, fears, suspiciousness, unawareness of the illness, cognitive problems in processing information; and concerns of the family and carers. The family and carers may have already made several unsuccessful attempts at obtaining help and at encouraging the patient to attend a psychiatric assessment (de Haan *et al.*, 2004; Power & McGorry, 1999). Unfortunately,

The Recognition and Management of Early Psychosis: A Preventive Approach, ed. Henry J. Jackson and Patrick D. McGorry.
Published by Cambridge University Press. © Cambridge University Press 2009.

most patients fulfil at least one of these complicating factors by the time of initial presentation. This implies that the first contact with the service is often critical, and that engagement, initial assessment and (early) treatment need to occur as parallel processes. Usually, this process is more successful if it occurs as early as possible prior to any major crises and if the initial treating clinician continues with the care of the patient.

Planning of the initial contact is also important. All sources of information should be gathered before arranging the first assessment. This information will assist in choosing the most appropriate setting with the highest chance of engagement, safety and successful initiation of treatment. The main goal of the first contact(s) with a new patient and the family is developing a trustworthy therapeutic alliance. The principles of this goal include, first, well-trained and experienced staff; second, an individually adapted interview situation (calm, friendly, safe and sufficient time); and, third, an appropriate interview technique (listening carefully, taking patient's concerns seriously, dispelling patient's fears, establishing trust, attempting to understand the personal context in which the person's psychosis has developed; see Power & McGorry, 1999).

Recognition of psychosis and understanding its personal context

The recognition of psychosis and understanding its personal context becomes the foundation upon which a treatment plan can be formed. However, confirmation of psychosis, especially in the early stages, could be hampered by a variety of clinical factors, including (1) slowly evolving, fluctuating and subtle symptoms, which may mimic behavioural changes related to puberty or non-psychotic disorders commonly seen in adolescents; and (2) difficult clinical constellations such as non-bizarre delusions, a primary deficit syndrome with exclusively negative symptoms, or the existence of certain comorbid disorders, especially substance-use disorders, schizotypal or borderline personality disorder, obsessive–compulsive disorder or mental retardation (Jarbin, Ott & von Knorring, 2003; Poyurovsky, Fuchs & Weizman, 1999; Sim *et al.*, 2004). Therefore, assured recognition of psychosis, recognition of the *form of*

psychosis and subsequent diagnostic formulation is often a longitudinal process, which is based on detailed psychosocial and biological investigations (see below). However, there is a common belief that a diagnostic categorization is necessary before initiation of treatment. This view, which can hinder an appropriate treatment, fails to take into account knowledge about diagnostic instability and the known difficulty in initially differentiating between diagnostic entities in FEP (Schimmelmann *et al.*, 2005a).

Understanding the personal context of the patient's psychosis is another goal of initial and subsequent psychotherapeutic treatment. This process involves a number of issues, including assessment of (1) the individual biological and psychosocial predictors of psychosis (e.g. family history, early developmental delays, schizotypal personality traits, traumatic events); (2) the consequences of the psychotic illness on the lives of the patient and his or her relatives (e.g. delayed personality development, initiation of drug use, disruption of functional development, duration of symptoms, stressors and traumatic events, development of comorbid disorders); and (3) the personal resources of the patient (e.g. premorbid personality, task-coping skills, social strengths and resources, family support). This information should be gathered in an optimistic and supportive atmosphere and constitutes the content of the integrated treatment plan (see below).

Treatment of behavioural disturbances

In the acute phase, a third and important treatment goal is to prevent and control acutely disturbed behaviours such as agitation, hostility, violence/aggression, pathological excitement or suicidal ideation in a way that does not traumatize the patient and their family. Of course, behavioural disturbances in psychosis could be caused by a variety of reasons. The most common reasons for behavioural disturbances are disorganization, suspiciousness/delusions, dysphoric and/or manic syndromes, antisocial personality traits, catatonic excitement, drug intoxication or command hallucinations (Allen *et al.*, 2001). Prevention, early detection and rapid consequent treatment of psychiatric emergencies related to a FEP are needed to prevent harm and to reduce traumatizing experiences, which can destroy all efforts to establish and maintain a trustworthy alliance.

Symptomatic and functional remission, adequate quality of life

Many patients with a FEP initially present with complex psychosocial problems. These problems include a variety of psychotic and other symptoms at initial presentation (e.g. positive, negative, cognitive, depressive, manic, anxiety), often with impaired functioning (e.g. unemployment, no or interrupted occupation, inability to live independently and impaired social contacts) and a low quality of life (e.g. Law *et al.*, 2005). These three outcome domains are only weakly interrelated with each other (Drake *et al.*, 2006) and, as such, different integrated interventions are needed to promote different outcome domains (Lambert *et al.*, 2007). Patients with FEP can achieve symptomatic and functional remission as well as adequate quality of life within the first 3 months of treatment (Lambert *et al.*, 2006, 2007; Malla *et al.*, 2006). However, early response within the first 12 weeks of treatment has been found to be predictive of mid- and long-term outcome (Lambert *et al.*, 2006, 2007). In other words, patients who do not achieve a good outcome in the short term are at risk for poor overall outcome in the long term. This finding, that the course of the disorder depends on early outcome, points toward a critical 'window of opportunity' in the initial treatment of FEP. Therefore, a high quality of early treatment and early detection of incomplete remission and subsequent treatment adaptations are mandatory in the initial treatment of these patients (Lambert *et al.*, 2006, 2007).

Formulation of an integrated treatment plan

The fifth goal of the acute treatment is the formulation of an individual phase- and stage-specific integrated treatment plan in cooperation with patients, relatives and treatment providers. All interventions and necessary treatment steps should be repeatedly explained and actively discussed in a shared-decision process with the patient and their family (Hamann, Leucht & Kissling, 2003; Hamann *et al.*, 2005).

Once the presence of psychosis (in general and whether it is non-affective or affective) has been confirmed, and the personal context of the psychosis explored, an acute treatment plan should be developed. However, at the time such a plan is developed, there is often only limited information about the complexity and acuteness of a patient's problems. Consequently, this plan should be actively discussed with other experienced clinicians before implementation and it should be frequently reviewed, particularly in the first days and weeks after initial presentation. If safety and intensive support are addressed, many patients with FEP, who were formerly hospitalized, could receive 'home-based' treatment and may not require hospitalization at all. This requires a multiprofessional, flexible and easily accessible care team with sufficient experience in acute interventions (Edwards & McGorry, 2002). Once the patient has accepted and initiated treatment, time is needed to strengthen further the therapeutic alliance and gather information from a number of sources. This is required in order to improve the understanding of the personal context of the patient's psychosis and the life circumstances in which it developed. In this process, it is helpful to involve the patient's relatives as early as possible.

Also important for the formulation of short- and long-term treatment plans is the assessment of risk factors for inadequate (antipsychotic) response and poor outcome (e.g. long duration of untreated psychosis (DUP), poor premorbid functioning, insufficient early response in the first 4 weeks, existence of (untreated) comorbid psychiatric disorders or non-adherence; e.g. Flyckt *et al.*, 2006; Lambert *et al.*, 2007; Perkins *et al.* 2004). All of these issues, insofar still treatable, have to be included in the treatment plan as core targets of therapeutic interventions. Once the patient begins to recover, the goals of treatment and thereby the therapeutic strategies shift towards a more intense psychotherapeutic approach, with the goals of complete remission of symptoms, improvement in social functioning and achievement of an adequate quality of life. The vulnerability-stress-coping model provides a framework for integrating the different therapeutic strategies and adapting interventions to the patient's functioning level. Such integrated treatment, according to the patient's needs and adapted according to the patient's functioning, was repeatedly found to be superior compared with treatment as usual, with significantly lower symptoms at follow-up, less comorbid substance use, better adherence to treatment and higher satisfaction with treatment (Petersen *et al.*, 2005; Thorup *et al.*, 2005). This integrative treatment is best accomplished through designation of a treatment team consisting of a case manager and a psychiatrist (Edwards & McGorry, 2002).

Comprehensive psychobiological assessments

Clinical and personal history

Assessment of the clinical and personal history of people with a psychotic disorder should include a detailed biography and developmental and past psychiatric history, which must be obtained as early as possible. Nevertheless, as misinformation or misinterpretation may occur in the acute phase, this information should be verified and complemented by reports from significant others and re-evaluated when the patient has stabilized. Because the biography of the patient and his/her developmental and past psychiatric history are often closely related, the assessment should be performed chronologically. However, because many patients in the acute phase are easily stressed and disturbed in such interviews, the assessments should be adapted according to the patient's actual mental state, which may require the assessment to be conducted over several sessions. Furthermore, clinicians should explain why they are asking specific questions and the links between the lines of questioning and the patient's actual situation. Table 11.1 gives an overview about the most important contents of this initial assessment.

Important information about predictors of psychosis and actual psychosocial problems may be revealed by assessment of the family history (up to second-degree relatives); perinatal history; birth complications; developmental history (early), including delayed neuromotor and cognitive development; signs of schizotypal personality traits, including a reduced social confidence with a high degree of social anxiety; and traumatic events or cannabis use in adolescence (Jones *et al.*, 1994; Maki *et al.*, 2005; Mueser & McGurk, 2004). Furthermore, the premorbid functioning should be explored in three domains: academic functioning, ability to live independently and social contacts. These domains reflect certain behavioural precursors that may predict subsequent illness manifestations. Clinically, the level of premorbid functioning, especially in the year before initial presentation and whether it *suddenly* decreased, is of particular importance (Larsen *et al.*, 2004). However, its assessment is often confounded by unrecognized early prodromal states or the fact that some patients have a lower functioning level throughout their whole life.

The assessment should further include a systematic history of evolving prodromal symptoms and primary and secondary symptoms of psychosis, including onset, duration, the patient's responses and behavioural disturbances such as risk of violence, suicide and risk-taking behaviour (e.g. drug and alcohol use, criminal activity). Furthermore, the factors influencing the transition from prodrome to psychosis should be explored (Olsen & Rosenbaum, 2006a,b).

The duration of untreated illness including the untreated prodromal psychosis phase and the untreated psychotic phase (DUP) should be carefully assessed together with patients *and* relatives. This is of great importance as these phases, particularly DUP, along with other predictors, have been found to predict independently antipsychotic response and overall outcome (Lambert *et al.*, 2005a; Marshall *et al.*, 2005; Perkins *et al.*, 2004; see Ch. 8). However, retrospective assessment of these variables is often crucial, especially in patients with long prodromal and untreated phases.

Furthermore, the psychiatric assessment should include a detailed forensic history, previous and recent psychosocial stressors and the state of personality development. As many patients with FEP have a subjectively diminished quality of life, this important outcome aspect should also be assessed at baseline and follow-up (Bechdolf *et al.*, 2005; Lambert & Naber, 2004a).

A valuable source for collateral information comes from families and relevant others (e.g. family doctors, teachers, friends) and they should be explored as soon as possible. In particular, information about family history

Table 11.1. Overview of the most important psychiatric assessment domains in first-episode psychosis

Assessment	Content
Clinical history	Psychiatric history of family (e.g. psychiatric disorders in relatives, expressed emotion, genetic risk)
	Pregnancy and obstetric complications (e.g. intrauterine infection, hypoxia, premature birth)
	Early developmental events (e.g. delayed speaking and walking)
	Functional problems during early childhood (e.g. in kindergarten or elementary school)
	Premorbid functioning and intelligence
	Trauma in early childhood or youth
	Schizotypal personality traits
	Psychosocial stressors
	Prodromal symptoms (including brief limited initial psychotic symptoms, attenuated psychotic symptoms, reduced functioning level in the last 12 months, duration of prodrome, time point of ongoing positive symptom manifestation)
	DUP, including symptoms and symptomatic development
	Consequences of DUP (e.g. functioning and social)
	Comorbid psychiatric disorder (premorbid, during prodrome, during DUP, and at initial presentation)
	If comorbid substance-use disorder, previous drug-induced psychosis
	Forensic history
	Pathways to care
	Psychodynamic context
Biography	Details include developmental milestones, school/work status and functioning, peer relationships
Mental state examination	Positive symptoms (e.g. hallucinations, systematized delusions)
	Negative symptoms (e.g. primary deficit syndrome, secondary negative symptoms)
	Disorganization, thought disorder
	Manic or depressive syndromes, anxiety
	Cognitive dysfunctions (neuropsychological tests)
	Insight
Comorbid psychiatric disorder	Substance-use disorder (e.g. type, abuse or dependency, onset, actual use, reasons for use, previous treatment, insight)
	Major depression (e.g. onset, course, previous treatment, actual severity)
	Anxiety disorder (e.g. onset, course, previous treatment, actual severity; especially social phobia and post-traumatic stress disorder)
	Obsessive–compulsive disorder (e.g. onset, course, previous treatment, actual severity)
	Personality disorder/traits (e.g. onset, course, previous treatment, actual severity; especially antisocial and avoidant personality disorder)
	Mental retardation and/or learning disability
	Attention deficit hyperactivity disorder
Risk assessment	Suicidal risk (e.g. actual thoughts or plans, past suicide attempts, actual depression, delusion-related anxiety, actual substance use, command hallucinations, tragic loss)
	Violent/aggressive behaviour (e.g. previous violent behaviour, agitation, disorganization, suspiciousness/delusions, dysphoric and/or manic symptoms, antisocial personality, catatonic excitement, drug intoxication)
	Risk of victimization by others (e.g. disorganization, manic–psychotic mental state)
	Risk of treatment non-adherence (e.g. insufficient therapeutic alliance, persistent comorbid substance-use disorder, lack of insight, negative attitude towards medication, negative subjective well-being under antipsychotic drugs, lack of social support)
	Risk of service disengagement and unauthorized absconding from hospital (e.g. young age, male, persistent substance-use disorder, antisocial personality, lack of insight)
Social assessment	Actual situation and problems at school or work
	Living situation
	Financial situation, debts
	Family situation

DUP, duration of untreated psychosis.

of psychiatric, neurological and other somatic disorders; perinatal and birth complications; early developmental problems; and premorbid functioning must be obtained from these sources and thereby reconfirmed.

Mental state examination

A patient's mental state can vary considerably in response to different interview settings, different staff members and over time. A full overview about a patient's symptoms and understanding their context is based on repeated interviews and a trustworthy relationship. However, patients have the ability to learn not to reveal information about psychotic phenomena if this can have negative consequences such as prolonged hospital stays or an increase of medication. For these various reasons, serial clinical assessments of a patient's psychopathology, undertaken by different clinicians, are very useful (McGorry, Copolov & Singh, 1990a; McGorry *et al.*, 1990b).

The mental state examination should focus on all symptoms, signs and behavioural disturbances related to non-affective and affective psychosis, and different comorbid psychiatric disorders. During the acute phase, it is difficult to differentiate between non-affective and affective psychosis, because manic or depressive symptoms can also exist in patients with non-affective psychosis and because first-rank schizophrenia symptoms also exist in affective psychosis (Conus *et al.*, 2004). Furthermore, during the acute state, it is also difficult to decide whether a symptom belongs to the psychosis itself or to different comorbid psychiatric disorders. An additional problem is that some symptoms (e.g. negative symptoms) can be 'masked' by other psychopathological symptoms (e.g. positive symptoms). Finally, the degree of functional disability related to symptoms, especially related to negative symptoms, comorbid social phobia or schizotypal personality traits, is often difficult to assess when a patient is hospitalized. For these various reasons, the mental state examination should take into account the development of symptoms prior to and at initial presentation, after reduction or remission of positive symptoms, and in relation to the patient's situation in his/her own environment.

Several mental state areas/symptoms are of special importance. First, the cognitive deficits of a patient require serial assessments, especially in the stabilization and the early recovery phase (see below) because they are predictive of (functional) outcome (Carlsson *et al.*, 2006). Second, patients presenting with more prolonged episodes of untreated psychosis often have developed systematized delusions. Prior to these delusions, many of these patients have had prolonged periods of depression. As such, there is a high risk of suicidal behaviour when these patients recover from psychosis and when depression emerges again. Third, a patient's level and quality of insight is of particular importance as it is linked to non-adherence to medication or service disengagement and other important clinical variables (McEvoy *et al.*, 2006; Schimmelmann *et al.*, 2006). However, insight is a complex construct; therefore, individual circumstances have to be explored carefully.

Assessment of comorbid disorders

Special attention should be paid to previous episodes of psychiatric disorders. Many FEP patients suffer from a comorbid psychiatric disorder (Lambert *et al.*, 2005a; Sim *et al.* 2004; Wade *et al.*, 2006), which may already be evident in the premorbid or prodromal phase (Kim-Cohen *et al.*, 2003; Lencz *et al.*, 2004; Rosen *et al.*, 2006). However, as assessment often occurs retrospectively, these disorders are sometimes difficult to differentiate from symptoms of the prodromal or the early psychotic states. Confirmation of these diagnoses could be reached by contacting previous attending physicians, obtaining information from significant others or undertaking a formal diagnostic interview, as most of these disorders are still evident at initial presentation.

In particular, these diagnoses include major depression; anxiety disorders, including social phobia and post-traumatic stress disorders; obsessive–compulsive disorder; attention deficit hyperactivity disorder; conduct and/or oppositional defiant disorder; personality traits/disorders mainly involving schizotypal and antisocial personality traits; and mental retardation (Kim-Cohen *et al.*, 2003; Lencz *et al.*, 2004; Poyurovsky *et al.*, 1999; Sim *et al.* 2004). These comorbid disorders could be linked to a poor overall outcome and poor quality of life, especially if they are untreated (Sim *et al.*, 2006); therefore, it is important that they are assessed in detail.

Special attention should be paid to comorbid substance-use disorders as diagnostic criteria for such disorders are fulfilled in 30–70% of FEP patients (see Lambert *et al.*, 2005a; Wade *et al.*, 2006). This is of great importance as substance misuse has been found to be one of the major predictors and outcome confounders in psychosis. For example, cannabis use before the age of 15 years was found to be a risk factor for psychosis (Arseneault *et al.*, 2002) and therefore, possibly related to an earlier onset of psychosis (Barnes *et al.*, 2006). Furthermore, persistent substance use was linked to an increased risk of inpatient admissions, relapse and shorter times to relapse (Wade *et al.*, 2006), symptomatic non-remission, service disengagement and non-adherence (Lambert *et al.*, 2005a). Many patients concurrently fulfil diagnostic criteria for two or more substance-use disorders and there is a subgroup of patients with a so-called multiple-substance-use disorder. This subgroup comprises high-risk patients for persistent substance use as most of them are dependent on three or more different drugs (Lambert *et al.*, 2005a).

Beside psychiatric disorders, many patients with psychosis suffer from long-standing medical disorders. Comorbid medical disorders mainly are coronary heart disease, metabolic syndrome, diabetes mellitus, cancer and infection with the human immunodeficiency virus and/or the hepatitis viruses (see below), all of which are associated with several indices of harmful dysfunction, decrements in functional outcomes, increased utilization of medical services and poor quality of life (e.g. McIntyre *et al.*, 2006).

Risk assessment

A major goal of the first assessment is to minimize the risks for the patient and others (Table 11.1). The risk assessment covers (1) risk of suicidal attempt or completed suicide, (2) risk of neglect or death, (3) risk of violence and aggression, (4) risk of victimization by others, (5) risk of non-adherence to treatment and service disengagement, and (6) risk of absconding

from hospital. There are some general recommendations with regard to all risks. The first is that all patients, especially new and unknown FEP patients, should be assessed initially and regularly. Second, all single risk conditions and their most important predictors should be recorded on the general assessment form of the respective service and the staff should be made aware of them. Third, the staff should have specific and systematic treatment procedures to manage and treat the identified risk(s).

The importance of assessing *suicide risk* cannot be underestimated, given that FEP patients are a high-risk group (Ch. 15). Approximately 15% of patients have already attempted suicide before initial presentation, and another 5–10% will attempt suicide during the first 18 months of treatment. Despite this risk, patients are infrequently asked about suicidal ideation and staff may be insufficiently educated about the most important predictors. Factors with robust evidence of increased risk of suicide are previous depressive disorders, previous suicide attempts, drug misuse, agitation or motor restlessness, fear of mental disintegration, poor adherence to treatment and recent tragic loss. As such, prevention of suicide is likely to result from treatment of affective symptoms, improving adherence to treatment and maintaining special vigilance of patients with risk factors (Hawton *et al.*, 2005).

Apart from the suicidal risk, the *assessment and prediction of violence* and other behavioural disturbances is vital in FEP. The characteristics of a high-risk patient include being a young male; being recently admitted with a drug misuse history; possibly with comorbid (antisocial) personality traits/disorder; a diagnosis of schizophrenia or acute dysphoric or mixed mania; or being hostile, agitated, disorganized and suspicious (e.g. Allen *et al.*, 2001).

Victimization by others is another major risk for FEP patients, especially females (Gearon & Bellack, 1999), which is largely underestimated and under researched. Cognitive and social competency deficits exacerbated by the effects of substance use or the psychosis itself may make females with psychosis particularly vulnerable. Information-processing deficits may impair the ability to identify risk situations, and make it difficult to remember and hence avoid situations, people or places previously proven dangerous. Social competency deficits interfere with the ability to form lasting relationships, negotiate out of dangerous situations, refuse unreasonable requests and problem solve effectively.

Assessment of the risk of non-adherence and service disengagement is another part of the risk assessment. In FEP, the risk of non-adherence with medication is likely to be substantially greater than in patients with multiple episodes. However, an important determinant of a patient's attitude toward treatment and adherence to medication appears to be the quality of relationships with clinicians during acute admission (Day *et al.*, 2005). Risk factors that contribute to predicting service disengagement include a lower severity of illness at baseline, living without family during treatment and persistent substance use during treatment (Schimmelmann *et al.*, 2006).

Biomedical evaluation

Additionally, a full biomedical assessment should be undertaken (Table 11.2). These examinations are important to detect already evident medical comorbid disorders and risk factors for future medical diseases, especially for cardiovascular disease, and include obesity, smoking, hypertension, dyslipidaemia and type 2 diabetes. Furthermore, the medical assessment gives information about any organic cause of psychosis and any risk factors for incomplete remission or treatment resistance (e.g. wide ventricles seen by magnetic resonance spectroscopy). They also establish a baseline against which possible future side effects and complications of pharmacological treatment can be measured.

Neuropsychological assessment

Many FEP patients (approximately 75%) display cognitive dysfunctions in a wide variety of domains at initial presentation (Bilder *et al.*, 2000; Joyce *et al.*, 2005), particularly in the domains of verbal learning and memory, psychomotor speed and attention. However, in comparison with patients with a longer illness history, they demonstrate significantly superior performance. In longitudinal studies, cognitive functioning generally remains static, suggesting limited change in

Table 11.2. Recommendations for physical, laboratory and medical assessments in first-episode psychosis

Examinations and tests	Assessments indicated
Physical status	Medical history
	Physical examination (including waist circumference)
	Neurological examination
Vital signs	Blood pressure, pulse, temperature
Laboratory tests	Hematology
	Liver function tests
	Renal function tests (blood urea nitrogen/ creatinine ratio)
	Thyroid function tests (basal thyroid-stimulating hormone, total and free trilodothyronine/thyroxine)
	Electrolytes
	Serum calcium and phosphates
	Fasting blood lipids (including triglycerides, total cholesterol and high and low density lipoprotein cholesterol)
	Blood sugar (fasting test optional; include one blood sugar daily profile before initiating treatment)
	Metabolic syndrome (if indication)[a]
	Blood coagulation (if indication)
	Urine illicit drug screen (if indication)
	Prolactin test (always drawn at same time, morning)
Other tests	Electrocardiology
	Electroencephalography
	Computed tomography or magnetic resonance imaging
	Lumbar puncture (if indication)
	Pregnancy test (if indication)
	Body weight (kg; assessing for ≥ 7% increase; body mass index)
	Neuropsychological testing (including attention span, concentration, memory)

[a] Risk factors for metabolic syndrome are detailed in the text; the syndrome is evident if three or more of these risk factors are fulfilled

performance over the first several years of the illness (Townsend & Norman, 2004).

Cognitive assessment is important because empirical evidence has shown that cognitive deficits are determinants of functional outcome. Furthermore, they are linked to other clinical variables such as insight or the ability to take medication as prescribed (Green *et al.*, 2000; Joyce *et al.*, 2005). Moreover, undisturbed cognitive abilities are important for patients to benefit successfully from psychotherapeutic interventions. As such, it is useful to conduct a formal neuropsychological assessment when the patient is not floridly psychotic and has stabilized. In most cases, a repeat neuropsychological assessment is recommended about 6 months after the first.

Diagnostic evaluation

An integrated short- and long-term treatment plan is based on an accurate diagnostic evaluation. However, early diagnostic identification of psychotic and comorbid disorders in FEP is hampered by several factors, such as the existence of several diagnostic entities within the term 'psychosis' and diagnostic instability (e.g. Schimmelmann *et al.*, 2005a; Schwartz *et al.*, 2000), the large range of differential diagnoses (Table 11.3) and a high rate of patients with comorbid psychiatric disorders.

Diagnostic stability in psychotic patients at first admission varies depending on psychosis subtype and the diagnostic system used. Schizophrenia, especially since the introduction of the 6-month duration criterion with the American Psychiatric Association's *Diagnostic and Statistical Manual* (DSM-III; APA, 1980), is reported to be the most stable diagnosis (about 90%) over a period of 6 months to 40 years (Schwartz *et al.*, 2000). Conversely, with diagnostic shifts varying from 10 to 50%, other psychotic disorders such as schizophreniform or schizoaffective disorder are reported to be less stable. Furthermore, recent studies suggest that many patients with initial substance-induced psychosis are subsequently diagnosed with a schizophrenia-spectrum disorder (Arendt *et al.*, 2005). Important reasons for a diagnostic shift include (1) a change of the clinical picture within the follow-up period, (2) additional information on past symptomatic evolution, and/or (3) an initially unreliable assessment.

These findings support the need for a longitudinally based diagnostic process in FEP. The main psychosis diagnosis as well as comorbid psychiatric disorders could be additionally assessed using standardized diagnostic interviews, e.g. the Royal Park Multidiagnostic Instrument for Psychosis (McGorry *et al.*, 1990a,b) or the Structured Clinical Interview for DSM-IV (APA, 1994; Ventura *et al.*, 1998). These interviews should be performed when the patient is stabilized and repeated 12–24 months after the initial presentation. Nevertheless, as new information becomes available, the patient's diagnosis should be reassessed, and the treatment plan subsequently modified.

Pharmacological interventions

Principles of pharmacotherapy in first-episode psychosis

Patients with FEP are a special patient population. Treatment should not only be based on general treatment principles but also must consider aspects specific to this population (Lambert *et al.*, 2003a; Remington, 2005; Robinson *et al.*, 2005). Optimal administration of pharmacotherapy must take into account that the first experience of psychotropic medication has considerable influence on subsequent engagement and adherence to treatment. The following guidelines are important (see also International Early Psychosis Association Writing Group, 2005).

Reduction of treatment delay improves antipsychotic response

Prolonged DUP, especially in combination with other non-response risk factors, seems to be predictive of decreased antipsychotic response (Flyckt *et al.*, 2006; Perkins *et al.*, 2004; Robinson *et al.*, 1999a) and also of a reduced satisfaction with care (Mattsson *et al.*, 2005). The time to response for delusions seems to be specifically associated with DUP (Gunduz-Bruce *et al.*, 2005). Consequently, early detection and optimal integrated treatment could improve response to (antipsychotic) treatment.

Table 11.3. Differential diagnosis of first-episode psychosis according to ICD-10 or DSM-IV; most important diagnoses are given in bold

ICD-10/DSM-IV	Differential diagnosis
F0/290, 293, 294 organic, including symptomatic mental disorders	Encephalitis (e.g. herpes encephalitis, HIV encephalitis, Creutzfeldt–Jakob disease, neurosyphilis)
	Traumatic cerebral injury
	Cerebral tumours
	Epilepsy
	Hormonal disorders (e.g. Cushing syndrome, hyperthyroidism)
	Neurodegenerative disorders (e.g. dementia, Friedreich ataxia, Huntington chorea, Parkinson's disease)
	Endocrine disorders (e.g. acute intermittent porphyria, Wilson's disease, uraemia, vitamin B_{12} insufficiency, zinc insufficiency)
	Rheumatic disorders (e.g. lupus erythematosus)
	Multiple sclerosis
	Others (e.g. narcolepsy, pregnancy, heart disorders, endocrinopathies, postoperative states)
F1/291–305 mental and behavioural disorders due to psychotropic substances	**Drug-induced psychotic disorder**
	Intoxications
	Withdrawal syndrome with or without delirium
F2/293–298 schizophrenia spectrum disorders	**Brief psychotic episode**
	Schizophreniform disorder (ICD-10: ≤ 1 months; DSM-IV: ≤ 6 months)
	Schizoaffective disorder (manic, mixed and depressive type)
	Delusional disorder
	Drug-induced psychotic disorder (for subtype see F1 or 291–305)
	Psychotic disorder not otherwise specified
	Schizotypal disorder
	Acute transient delusional disorder
	Induced delusional disorder
F3/293–296 affective disorders	**Bipolar (affective) disorder** (manic, mixed and depressive type)
	Severe depressive episode with psychotic symptoms
	Recurrent depressive disorder, presently severe depressive episode, with psychotic symptoms
F4 neurotic, stress and somatoform disorders	Dissociative stupor
	Depersonalization and derealization syndrome
F6 personality and behavioural disorders	Paranoid personality disorder
	Schizoid personality disorder
	Emotional-instable personality disorder (borderline type)
	Artificial disorders
F8 development disorders	Asperger syndrome
	Autistic spectrum disorders

ICD-10, *International Classification of Diseases*, 10th edn (WHO, 1992); DSM-IV, *Diagnostic and Statistical Manual of Mental Disorders*, 4th edn (APA, 1994), reproduced with permission.

Integrated treatment is a prerequisite for antipsychotic response

Studies on incomplete remission and treatment resistance, which were mainly conducted in schizophrenia, have shown that insufficient psychological interventions are a risk factor for poor outcome (Lambert & Naber, 2004a,b). Psychosocial interventions complement pharmacological interventions and often serve as a prerequisite for the effectiveness of pharmacotherapy. Repeated individualized education (both in verbal and written format) about psychosis and its (pharmacological) treatment is of particular importance, as the knowledge base within patients, families and other relevant people in the patient's circle is often found to be limited and their attitude towards pharmacological treatment is often negative (de Haan *et al.*, 2004).

Non-affective and affective psychoses should receive separate approaches to initial pharmacotherapy

An epidemiological cohort of FEP patients with rather short DUP has been shown to be made up of those with non-affective psychosis (about 40% with schizophreniform disorder and 25% with schizophrenia), and those with affective psychosis (about 15% with bipolar I disorder, 10% with schizoaffective disorder and 5% with major depression with psychotic features) (Lambert *et al.*, 2005a). However, at initial presentation it is often difficult to differentiate between these diagnostic entities (see above). Therefore, a pragmatic approach in which initial pharmacotherapy is applied broadly according to a 'non-affective' or an 'affective' psychotic syndrome is recommended (see below).

Patients and relatives should participate in treatment planning

Patients' participation in treatment planning is being increasingly advocated in mental health. The model of 'shared decision making' is proposed as a promising method of engaging patients and their families in medical decisions. This is of special importance in FEP as negative attitudes toward medical treatment and younger age are associated with less willingness to engage in treatment (Hamann *et al.*, 2005).

Initial low-dose antipsychotic treatment is recommended

Patients with FEP are more responsive to treatment and more sensitive to antipsychotic drug side effects than are patients who have experienced multiple episodes (reviewed by Lambert *et al.*, 2003a). To date, there are approximately 20 studies that have assessed the efficacy/effectiveness and tolerability of conventional and atypical antipsychotic drugs in patients with mainly non-affective FEP (Tables 11.4 and 11.5). They have shown that the majority of patients respond to a lower antipsychotic dose than is recommended for patients who have had multiple episodes (a 'minimal effective dose'). These results are in line with recent positron emission tomographic studies on occupancy rates for dopamine D_2 receptors (reviewed by Remington, 2005). Nevertheless, studies have also shown that approximately 10–30% of patients do not respond fully to initial low-dose treatment, especially patients with an initial diagnosis of schizophrenia (Lambert *et al.*, 2005b,c).

Medication side effects should be avoided or treated early to promote response and future adherence

All side effects of antipsychotic drugs can cause major subjective distress, which clinicians may overlook if they only judge the severity of side effects objectively (Schimmelmann *et al.*, 2005b). Therefore, clinicians need to discuss with patients the severity of, and distress with, the side effects in order to encourage future adherence. Furthermore, as many antipsychotic side effects (e.g. extrapyramidal motor symptoms (EPMS), weight gain, sexual dysfunctions) are dose dependent and often caused by rapid titration, low-dose treatment and a slow titrating process are recommended. Early detection of side effects and early treatment adaptation is also important, for example binge eating in the first week after initiation of antipsychotic treatment, with the risk of subsequent weight gain and possible consequences of metabolic syndrome, type 2 diabetes or cardiovascular disease.

Table 11.4. Studies in first-episode non-affective psychosis giving information about used average antipsychotic dose, and dose equivalents for different antipsychotic drugs based on dopamine D_2 occupancy[a]

Source	Study design	Antipsychotic agent	Dosage (mg/day)
McEvoy, Hogarty & Steingard, 1991	CT	Haloperidol	2.1
Zhang-Wong et al., 1999	CT	Haloperidol	2.0
Oosthuizen et al., 2001	CT	Haloperidol	1.8
Sanger et al., 1999	RCT	Olanzapine	11.2
Lambert et al., 2003b	CT	Olanzapine	15.1
Lieberman et al., 2003	RCT	Olanzapine	10.2
		Haloperidol	4.8
Keefe et al., 2004	RCT	Olanzapine	11.3
		Haloperidol	4.9
Emsley, 1999	CT	Risperidone	6.1
		Haloperidol	5.6
McGorry, 1999	CT	Risperidone	2.5
Yap et al., 2001	CT	Risperidone	2.7
Merlo et al., 2002	CT	Risperidone	2.0
Zalsman et al., 2003 (adolescent)	CT	Risperidone	3.1
Huq, 2004	CT	Risperidone	3.5–3.8
Malla et al., 2004	CT	Risperidone	2.5
		Olanzapine	10.0
Lambert et al., 2005b	File review	Risperidone	2.8
		Olanzapine	10.5
Schooler et al., 2005	RCT	Risperidone	3.3
		Haloperidol	2.9
Kopala et al., 2006	CT	Quetiapine	600

CT, controlled study; RCT, randomized controlled trial. There are many discrepancies between studies, especially with regard to assessed population, duration of treatment, and primary study aims. To the author's knowledge, there are so far no published studies for ziprasidone, amisulpride or aripiprazole.

Untreated comorbid psychiatric disorders can reduce response

At initial presentation, approximately 80–90% of FEP patients fulfil diagnostic criteria for at least one comorbid psychiatric disorder, including substance-use disorders

Table 11.5. Theoretical average dosages for different antipsychotic drugs and dose equivalents based on dopamine D_2 receptor occupancy

Drug	Dosage
Theoretical average daily dosage	
Haloperidol	3.4
Risperidone	3.4
Olanzapine	11.4
Quetiapine	600
Dose equivalents based on D_2 occupancy	
Haloperidol	2
Olanzapine	10
Risperidone	2.5–3.0
Ziprasidone	80

Dose equivalents according to Remington (2005).

(Lambert et al., 2005a). Untreated and persistent comorbid disorders could be a risk factor for incomplete remission, misdiagnosis (social phobia or major depression as negative symptoms), or suicidal ideation and completed suicide (major depression). As such, these comorbid disorders should be treated as early as possible. Second-generation antipsychotic drugs are increasingly used as add-on therapy for various non-psychotic disorders, which is an argument for their first-line use in psychotic disorders (Fountoulakis et al., 2004).

Adherence to pharmacological treatment should be monitored regularly

Patients with FEP are a major risk group for early medication non-adherence (Robinson et al., 1999b, 2002). Reasons for this behaviour as well as its negative clinical consequences are manifold (Lacro et al., 2002). As such, a preventive approach should be implemented. For example, using compliance therapy even in patients without risk factors of non-adherence may be useful.

Adaptation of pharmacotherapy according to diagnostic shift is needed

In FEP, diagnoses are often unstable in the beginning and some patients fulfil diagnostic criteria for another psychotic disorder after initial assessment (Schimmelmann *et al.*, 2005a). In this instance, the adaptations of pharmacological (and psychological) interventions are important in order to prevent incomplete remission.

Patients with an unfavourable outcome should be identified early

All patients with FEP are at risk for delayed response and remission, incomplete remission or even treatment resistance (Emsley, Rabinowitz & Medori, 2006; Malla *et al.*, 2006; Manchanda *et al.*, 2005). There is evidence that incomplete initial response within the first 4 weeks of treatment predicts non-response in the first 3 months (Lambert *et al.*, 2007) and that non-response in the first 3 months predicts incomplete remission in the first 24 months of treatment (Lambert *et al.*, 2006). Furthermore, there seem to be certain risk factor combinations that predict poor outcome when added together (e.g. low premorbid functioning in the year before initial assessment, poor school performance or limited social contact; Flyckt *et al.*, 2006). To initiate adequate interventions, it is crucial to identify patients experiencing FEP who are likely to have an unfavourable outcome. The predictive rating scale developed by Flyckt *et al.* (2006) is a feasible tool for early detection of these patients.

Some patients need a longer time to achieve treatment response and remission

For many years it has been customary to carry out trials of an antipsychotic drug over 6–8 weeks in order to establish response (Remington, 2005). However, Emsley and colleagues (2006) have reported that the time to antipsychotic response varies widely, with approximately 10–15% of FEP patients needing longer than 8 weeks. This finding is supported by studies showing that some patients need longer periods to achieve full symptomatic remission (e.g. 7 to 10 weeks in non-affective psychosis; Lambert *et al.*, 2005b; Malla *et al.*, 2006). This implies that in some patients a 'sufficient' response should be reached during the first 6–8 weeks, but not necessarily 'full' remission of symptoms. These patients should be kept on the first medication

and a longer treatment trial should be applied. Criteria such as a total score reduction of ≥ 20% on the Positive and Negative Syndrome Scale or a reduction of ≥ 2 on the Clinical Global Impression Severity scale have been applied to measure a 'sufficient' response and thereby predict later remission. However, newer studies have suggested that a certain increase of subjective well-being in the first 4 weeks (defined as ≥ 20% increase in the Subjective Well-being Under Neuroleptic Treatment Scale; Lambert *et al.* 2006, 2007) has the best predictive power for subsequent remission of symptoms, functioning and quality of life (Lambert *et al.*, 2007).

Pharmacotherapy of acute first-episode non-affective psychosis

Pharmacotherapy of FEP begins with the assessment of the psychopathological syndrome(s), the differentiation between non-affective and affective psychosis and the severity of the clinical presentation. In those with acute disturbed behaviour and/or aggression/hostility, treatment should first follow the recommendations for psychiatric emergencies (see below).

Antipsychotic treatment of patients with non-affective disorders should start with a low dose of an atypical antipsychotic drug (APA, 2004a; International Early Psychosis Association Writing Group, 2005; NICE, 2002; Fig. 11.1). Because a low dose will not have a rapid effect on distress, insomnia and behavioural disturbances, a safe and supportive environment, skilled staff and regular and liberal doses of benzodiazepines are essential interim components. If a patient responds to the initial dose by 1–3 weeks (Fig. 11.1), but their response remains incomplete, the dose should be slowly increased. If there is still an inadequate response despite dose increase after 6–8 weeks, a crossover switch to another antipsychotic drug is recommended. Where the use of conventional antipsychotic drugs is indicated, they should be started on very low dosage (e.g. haloperidol 1–2 mg/day) and titrated slowly according to EPMS and other side effects. The maximum dosage should not exceed 4–6 mg/day haloperidol equivalents for the majority of patients. Non-adherence with antipsychotic treatment is a major confounding factor for the success of all therapeutic

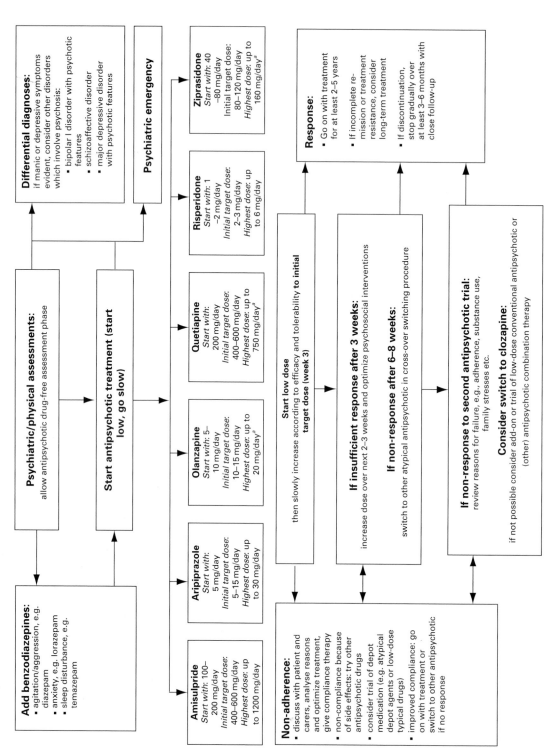

Fig. 11.1. Pharmacotherapy of first-episode non-affective psychosis. These are general guidelines. The individual needs of each patient must be considered. [a]Positive experiences with higher dosages exist, but mainly in patients who have had multiple episodes.

interventions. If non-adherence is confirmed, putative reasons should be explored and discussed with the patient and relatives. If side effects (e.g. EPMS) have impaired the patient's adherence, one possibility is to switch to another oral atypical antipsychotic drug with a lower EPMS risk. In the case of confirmed non-adherence, a (temporary) switch to an atypical depot medication could be tried (e.g. injectable risperidone).

Pharmacotherapy of acute first-episode affective psychosis

There are some special recommendations for the pharmacological treatment of affective psychosis. First, it is important that the pharmacotherapy must rapidly and securely control manic/depressive *and* psychotic symptoms, and it should possess acute and long-term mood stabilizing properties. Second, it should have minimal potential for induction of side effects that could be misinterpreted as symptoms of the disorder (e.g. akinesia as depression or akathisia as agitation). Finally, it should have the lowest possible risk for EPMS and tardive dyskinesia, as patients with affective psychosis are even more vulnerable than patients with non-affective psychosis.

Figure 11.2 gives an overview of pharmacological treatment options in patients with affective FEP and a severe manic or mixed psychotic syndrome should begin treatment with a combination of a mood stabilizer and an (atypical) antipsychotic drug (Perlis, 2005). In most cases, short-term adjunctive therapy with benzodiazepines is recommended. With regards to mood stabilizing, lithium carbonate (preferable for euphoric mania) and sodium valproate (preferable for rapid cycling and acute psychotic mania) are recommended as first-line treatments. Previously prescribed antidepressants should be discontinued immediately. In the case of inadequate manic control or mixed symptom control with first-line treatment, the mood stabilizer should be switched to an alternative mood stabilizer; electroconvulsive therapy should also be considered. If psychotic symptoms persist, the next step entails switching to another (atypical) antipsychotic drug and continuing with mood-stabilizing treatment. There are

differential pharmacological long-term treatment recommendations for bipolar I or schizoaffective disorders, which differ in various guidelines (APA 2004a,b,c). In summary, most patients with schizoaffective disorder require a long-term combination of mood stabilizer and antipsychotic drug. Patients with bipolar I disorder should be initially treated with mood stabilizer alone. Alternatively, (atypical) antipsychotic drugs can be tried as monotherapy or in combination with mood stabilizer. Intermittent and sometimes long-term add-on antidepressant therapy is also often needed.

For patients with psychotic symptoms in the context of a major depression, a combination therapy of a selective serotonin-reuptake inhibitor (SSRI) with an add-on low-dose (atypical) antipsychotic drug is recommended as first-line treatment, especially with a non-sedative (atypical) antipsychotic drug in a low- to mid-range dosage (APA, 2004c). For patients with a bipolar depression, the first step is to optimize or start a mood stabilizer in combination with low-dose (atypical) antipsychotic treatment, and, second, to add an antidepressant, preferably a SSRI (e.g. Goodwin *et al.*, 2003). With regard to the choice of mood-stabilizing compound, lithium has shown antidepressant effects alone and in combination with antidepressants (Perlis, 2005). Antidepressant monotherapy is not recommended in most cases (Perlis, 2005). When evaluating treatment effectiveness, it is important to consider that the antidepressive effect may take significantly longer to manifest (2 weeks or longer) and it is possible that psychotic symptoms may remit while depressive symptoms remain. With a biphasic course of illness or family history of bipolar disorder, early combination treatment of an antidepressant with mood stabilizer is recommended. For further treatment steps and long-term recommendations, see the APA guidelines (2004b,c). Further information on the treatment of first-episode mania is also covered in detail in Ch. 13.

Pharmacotherapy in psychiatric emergencies

During an acute psychotic episode, some patients become behaviourally disturbed and may need

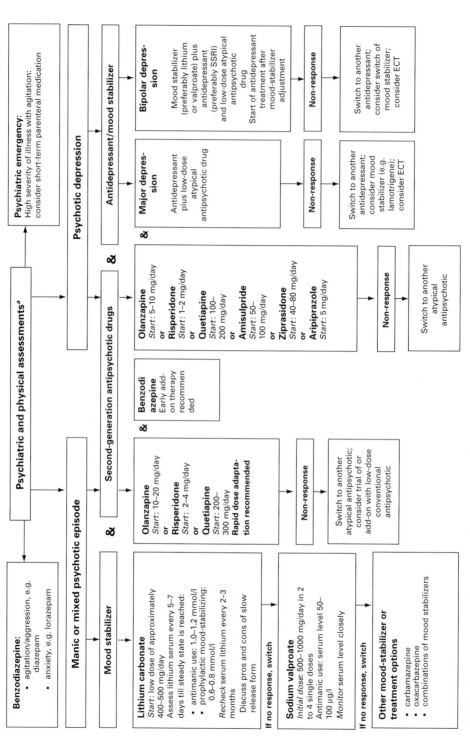

Fig. 11.2. Pharmacotherapy of first-episode affective psychosis. These are general guidelines and the individual needs of each patient must be considered. [a]There are differential pharmacological long-term treatment recommendations for bipolar I disorder, schizoaffective disorder or major depressive disorder. SSRI, selective-serotonin reuptake inhibitor; ECT, electroconvulsive therapy.

emergency pharmacological (and psychological) interventions. To decrease the incidence and severity of psychiatric emergencies, it is necessary to ensure that the environment is prepared and that staff are well trained. The goal of emergency management is to assure safety for patients and staff alike and to resolve the situation without harm and traumatic experiences (NICE, 2002).

In a psychiatric emergency, the clinical team should first undertake an assessment of the underlying causes. It is recommended that the clinicians avoid unprepared confrontations, defuse escalating tensions, establish the patient's concerns, attempt to resolve conflict and only if necessary encourage the patient to be admitted into an intensive care area.

The first pharmacological step is to try oral therapy with benzodiazepines (dissolvable tablets) in combination with a preferably sedative antipsychotic drug (dissolvable tablets or syrup). In most patients, this step is sufficient to resolve the crisis. If the patient refuses medication, or a rapid response is needed owing to violent behaviour or other behavioural disturbances, parenteral medication will be necessary. In this situation, the team members must all ensure that they clearly communicate the necessity of parenteral medication and calmly explain this to the patient. Here, it is necessary to understand that agitation usually results from psychotic anxiety, and measures taken against the will of the patient can exacerbate this anxiety and lead to traumatization. Therefore, such a decision should be taken after all alternatives have been considered and a psychiatrist consulted.

Recommended preparations for use in rapid tranquillization are intramuscular preparations of lorazepam (if not available, intramuscular clonazepam or midazolam, with appropriate caution) or olanzapine. A well-established option to avoid repeated intramuscular injections is the use of short-life depot medications (e.g. zuclopenthixol acetate (Accuphase), 50–100 mg for FEP). A disadvantage of this short-acting depot medication is the delayed onset of action (2–8 hours), although patients may respond after 30–45 minutes. Zuclopenthixol acetate is effective for 24–36 hours; repeated zuclopenthixol injections within 24 hours of a previous dose are mostly not required.

After parenteral tranquillization, vital parameters should be monitored, including temperature, pulse, blood pressure and respiratory rate every 10 minutes for 1 hour, then half-hourly to hourly according to the half-life of the medication. Caution is required because of the risk of reduced respiratory rate, irregular or slow pulse, a fall in blood pressure, acute dystonia and unconsciousness. If available, electrocardiographic monitoring is also recommended. Once the acute situation is resolving, growing awareness and traumatic reactions in patients, staff, family members or other caregivers may make a 'debriefing process' necessary. All emergency steps including the debriefing process should be documented.

Management of adverse events and medical disorders

A variety of adverse event risks are associated with pharmacological treatment of psychotic disorders, including EPMS, tardive dyskinesia, elevated prolactin levels, sexual dysfunctions, somnolence, weight gain, hyperlipidaemia, hypothyroidism, hepatic toxicity and impaired memory (Newcomer, 2006). These adverse events occur in different frequencies with different psychotropic drugs and can be separated into tolerability and safety issues. Tolerability refers to non-lethal, time-limited adverse events, whereas safety culminates in treatment-related life-threatening side effects. This is of particular importance in FEP because adverse events can start as a tolerability problem (e.g. weight gain) and then subsequently cause a safety problem (e.g. metabolic syndrome or type 2 diabetes).

Of particular concern for treatment of FEP patients are the metabolic side effects with antipsychotic drugs because they occur rapidly, are very distressful and have long-term medical consequences. Consequently, there are many preventive strategies, including preventive education, lifestyle changes, early treatment adaptations and early treatment of adverse events, all intended to decrease the risk of long-term medical disorders. In this process it is important to be honest about potential adverse effects of each medication, to discuss alternative treatment options and to monitor the

Table 11.6. Comparison of atypical antipsychotic drugs in terms of potential side effects

Atypical antipsychotic	Severe side effects	Commonly reported side effects[a]	EPMS liability	Most common EPMS reported
Amisulpride	Elevated prolactin levels; can cause EPMS at higher dosage	Insomnia, anxiety	Low (at low dosage)	Akathisia
Aripiprazole	Can cause EPMS at higher dosage	Restlessness, sleep disturbance, anxiety	Low (at low dosage)	Tremor, akathisia
Clozapine	Weight gain; metabolic syndrome with possible diabetic complications; agranulocytosis; cardiovascular/respiratory arrest	Hypersalivation, sedation, cognitive deficits	Extremely low	Bradykinesia, akathisia
Olanzapine	Weight gain; metabolic syndrome with possible diabetic complications	Cognitive deficits, insomnia, anxiety	Very low	Tremor, subjective akathisia
Quetiapine	Moderate weight gain	Somnolence, dizziness, orthostatic hypotension (mostly in elderly)	Extremely low	Tremor, akathisia
Risperidone	Elevated prolactin levels; can cause EPMS at higher dosage; moderate weight gain	Headaches, insomnia, anxiety	Low (= 4 mg/day)	Acute dystonia, parkinsonism, few cases of tardive dyskinesia
Ziprasidone	Prolongs QT interval	Somnolence, dizziness	Very low	Tremor, akathisia
Zotepine	Can cause electrocardiographic changes; moderate weight gain	Nausea, somnolence, dizziness	Low (at low dosage)	Acute dystonia, parkinsonism

EPMS, extrapyramidal motor symptoms.

[a] All antipsychotic drugs are associated with hyperglycaemia and possible diabetes mellitus.

patient's early side effects closely (Table 11.6 lists the side effects of atypical antipsychotic drugs). The most important antipsychotic side effects for FEP patients are described in detail below.

Extrapyramidal motor symptoms and tardive dyskinesia

Antipsychotic drugs have the potential to produce short-term reversible EPMS and long-term, mostly irreversible, movement disorders such as tardive dyskinesia. Treatment with conventional antipsychotic drugs is associated with a high risk of acute and long-term motor side effects (Correll, Leucht & Kane, 2004; Lambert *et al.*, 2003a). As there is little difference in threshold between the dose required for efficacy and the dose required for EPMS, the latter are often an

inevitable accompaniment of treatment with conventional agents (see Remington, 2005). Atypical antipsychotic drugs generally have a lower, but also dose-dependent, propensity to induce EPMS and tardive dyskinesia (Correll *et al.*, 2004; Leucht *et al.*, 1999). However, in the therapeutic dose range, the risk of EPMS remains relatively low. Acute EPMS can lead to several consequences, such as reduction of subjective well-being/quality of life, diminished cognitive functioning, a higher risk of developing tardive dyskinesia, medication non-adherence, impaired acute antipsychotic response and a variety of social consequences, especially stigmatization (see Lambert & Naber, 2004b). Clinical recommendations include weekly assessments of acute EPMS and akathisia until the medication dose has been stabilized, and assessment of tardive dyskinesia every 6 months when taking conventional, and every 12 months when taking atypical, antipsychotic drugs (Marder *et al.*, 2004). The best treatment is prevention.

Weight gain and obesity

Weight gain and subsequent obesity can have serious consequences for the health of patients with psychotic disorders (Marder *et al.*, 2004; Newcomer, 2006). These health problems include cardiovascular disease, type 2 diabetes, hypertension, osteoarthritis, stroke and some types of cancer. Consequences are usually seen on both the somatic level, as medication adherence, self-esteem, somatic discomfort, and in well-being, such as social functioning and quality of life. Almost all antipsychotic drugs can cause weight gain and obesity, although prevalence and extent varies from drug to drug. It has been estimated that it affects 30–60% of patients sufficiently to cause increases that exceed ideal body weight by 20% or greater (Newcomer, 2006), with clozapine and olanzapine showing the greatest risk (Allison *et al.*, 1999). For prevention and management, it is important to inform patients about the risks and about suggestions for behaviour to counteract these effects. It is also important to monitor the patient's weight and eating behaviour regularly. Patients with an initial body mass index of >25 should be treated with weight-sparing antipsychotic drugs. As subsequent weight loss is very difficult, early assessment within the first 3–7 days of increase in appetite, loss of feeling full or satiated, as well as eating binges, has to be observed. If these risk factors are evident, an early switch of antipsychotic treatment should be considered. Detailed management recommendations are discussed by Faulkner, Soundy & Lloyd (2003) and Marder *et al.* (2004).

Metabolic syndrome and diabetes

The metabolic syndrome comprises the following clinical variables: (1) abdominal obesity (waist circumference >102 cm in males and >88 cm in females), (2) triglycerides ≥150 mg/dl (1.5 g/l), (3) high density lipoprotein cholesterol increases (>40 mg/dl (400 mg/l) in males, >50 mg/dl (500 mg/l) in females), (4) blood pressure ≥130/85 mmHg, and (5) fasting blood glucose ≥110 mg/dl (1.1 g/l); the syndrome is evident if three or more of these risks factors are fulfilled (Newcomer, 2006). In the long-term, 40–50% of patients with schizophrenia are diagnosed with metabolic syndrome (McEvoy *et al.*, 2005) and 15% with type 2 diabetes (Newcomer, 2006); both are risk factors for cardiovascular disease. This knowledge has increased the concerns about the causal relationship between treatment with atypical antipsychotic drugs and these medical disorders. A number of recommendations can be made. Clinicians should be aware that patients with psychosis are more prone to diabetes than the general population for various reasons, including unhealthy lifestyle, antipsychotic drug-induced reduction of basal metabolic output, weight gain, cognitive deficits resulting in difficulties in detecting early warning signs of diabetes, and a higher rate of family history of diabetes compared with the general population. Patients who are starting treatment with antipsychotic agents should be evaluated with a fasting plasma glucose test or haemoglobin A_{1c} level. In the absence of clinical signs for diabetes and significant weight gain and/or risk factors for diabetes (family history, body mass index ≥25, waist size ≥88 cm in women and ≥100 cm in men), patients should be monitored for symptoms of diabetes 4 months later and then yearly. Fasting serum glucose ≥126 mg/dl (1.26 g/l), random serum glucose >200 mg/dl (2.0 g/l), or haemoglobin A_{1c} >6.1% suggest increased risk. Levels of fasting glucose between 100 and 125 mg/dl (1.0–1.25 g/l) are indicative of pre-diabetes. Furthermore, clinicians should educate patients about early warning signs (such as excessive thirst or hunger, polyuria or other physical symptoms) and weight control (e.g. diet, eating habits, exercise). If there are preexisting risk factors, an antipsychotic drug with the lowest risk of weight gain should be chosen.

Endocrine and sexual side effects

Although sexuality and sexual disorders receive little attention in clinical practice, they are important issues to be addressed in FEP. It is estimated that the prevalence of hormonal and sexual dysfunctions in antipsychotic drug-treated patients is 30–60% (see Lambert *et al.*, 2003a) including galactorrhaea, gynaecomastia, breast enlargement, amenorrhaea, anovulation, decreased libido, hypogonadism among men, impotence, anorgasmia, infertility and possibly increases in the risk of breast cancer (Marder *et al.*, 2004). Hyperprolactinaemia, which is considered of central importance in the aetiology of sexual dysfunctions, is a common side effect of conventional antipsychotic drugs, especially with amisulpuride and risperidone and antipsychotic combination therapy (Lambert *et al.*, 2003a). Clozapine, olanzapine, quetiapine, ziprasidone and aripiprazole have a minimal risk. If sexual dysfunction occurs, a differentiation between antipsychotic causation and other causes is necessary. If it is clearly caused by the drug treatment, a dose reduction should be tried if the clinical picture allows it (but is unlikely to resolve the problem). If dose reduction does not lead to a change, a switch to an antipsychotic drug with less potential for hyperprolactinaemia should follow.

Conclusions

The first contact of adolescents and young adults with a psychiatric service, especially if confused by psychotic symptoms, is often accompanied by fears, negative attitudes towards such institutions and their treatments and (self-) stigmatization. Consequently, the first contact – often called the 'initial assessment' – has a major impact on a patient's attitude towards staff members, the respective psychiatric service and even psychiatry in general. If the initial engagement fails, it is difficult to re-engage the patient. This implies that all efforts should be made to build a positive and trustworthy therapeutic alliance from the very first contact.

The initial assessment(s) are a central part of the engagement and alliance process; the way they are accomplished and the resultant quality of information and understanding contribute to the success of psychosocial interventions. Consequently, engagement, initial assessments and treatment occur as parallel processes. The pharmacological interventions should support this process by eliminating disturbing symptoms. However, from the patient's perspective, the action of antipsychotic drugs is best characterized by a detachment

from symptoms rather than an eradication or elimination of symptoms. This result, a so-called 'dampening of the salience of psychotic symptoms', is not concordant with the patient's expectations prior to antipsychotic exposure. At this point many patients start to weigh the pros and cons of psychotropic drugs, which can result in medication non-adherence. However, as many FEP patients are in need of longer pharmacological relapse prevention, a positive therapeutic alliance can help to encourage the patient to continue the medication. The inclusion of significant others in this process is often very important. A low-dose antipsychotic treatment with a low side effect profile and no or minimal cognitive–emotional disturbances can help to promote adherence. Nevertheless, treatment with some antipsychotic drugs is accompanied by very distressful, life-threatening medical consequences. As such, the initial pharmacological management is vital not only to maximize the chance of remission and recovery but also to minimize the potential for future relapses, morbidity and mortality.

REFERENCES

Allen, M. H., Currier, G. W., Hughes, D. H., Reyes-Harde, M. & Docherty, J. P. (2001). The Expert Consensus Guideline Series. Treatment of behavioral emergencies. *Postgraduate Medicine*, 1–88.

Allison, D. B., Mentore, J. L., Heo, M. *et al.* (1999). Antipsychotic-induced weight gain: a comprehensive research synthesis. *American Journal of Psychiatry*, **156**, 1686–96.

APA. (1980). *Diagnostic and Statistical Manual of Mental Disorders*, 3rd edn. Washington, DC: American Psychiatric Press.

APA. (1994). *Diagnostic and Statistical Manual of Mental Disorders*, 4th edn. Washington, DC: American Psychiatric Press.

APA. (2004a). Practice guideline for the treatment of patients with schizophrenia (second edition). In *American Psychiatric Association, Practice Guidelines for the Treatment of Psychiatric Disorders. Compendium 2004*, Washington, DC: American Psychiatric Press, pp. 249–440.

APA. (2004b) Practice guideline for the treatment of patients with bipolar disorder (second edition). In *American*

Psychiatric Association, Practice Guidelines for the Treatment of Psychiatric Disorders. Compendium 2004, Washington, DC: American Psychiatric Press, pp. 525–612.

APA. (2004c). Practice guideline for the treatment of patients with major depressive disorder (second edition). In *American Psychiatric Association, Practice Guidelines for the Treatment of Psychiatric Disorders. Compendium 2004*, Washington, DC: American Psychiatric Press, pp. 440–524.

Arendt, M., Rosenberg, R., Foldager, L., Perto, G. & Munk-Jorgensen, P. (2005). Cannabis-induced psychosis and subsequent schizophrenia-spectrum disorders: follow-up study of 535 incident cases. *British Journal of Psychiatry*, **187**, 510–15.

Arseneault, L., Cannon, M., Poulton, R. *et al.* (2002). Cannabis use in adolescence and risk for adult psychosis: longitudinal prospective study. *British Medical Journal*, **325**, 1212–13.

Barnes, T. R., Mutsatsa, S. H., Hutton, S. B., Watt, H. C. & Joyce, E. M. (2006). Comorbid substance use and age at onset of schizophrenia. *British Journal of Psychiatry*, **188**, 237–42.

Bechdolf, A., Pukrop, R., Kohn, D. *et al.* (2005). Subjective quality of life in subjects at risk for a first episode of psychosis: a comparison with first episode schizophrenia patients and healthy controls. *Schizophrenia Research*, **79**, 137–43.

Bilder, R. M., Goldman, R. S., Robinson, D. *et al.* (2000). Neuropsychology of first-episode schizophrenia: initial characterization and clinical correlates. *American Journal of Psychiatry*, **157**, 549–59.

Carlsson, R., Nyman, H., Ganse, G. & Cullberg, J. (2006) Neuropsychological functions predict 1- and 3-year outcome in first-episode psychosis. *Acta Psychiatrica Scandinavica*, **113**, 102–11.

Coldham, E. L., Addington, J. & Addington, D. (2002). Medication adherence of individuals with a first episode of psychosis. *Acta Psychiatrica Scandinavica*, **106**, 286–90.

Conus, P., Abdel-Baki, A., Harrigan, S., Lambert, M. & McGorry, P. D. (2004). Schneiderian first rank symptoms predict poor outcome within first episode manic psychosis. *Journal of Affective Disorders*, **81**, 259–68.

Correll, C. U., Leucht, S. & Kane, J. M. (2004). Lower risk for tardive dyskinesia associated with second-generation antipsychotics: a systematic review of 1-year studies. *American Journal of Psychiatry*, **161**, 414–25.

Day, J. C., Bentall, R. P., Roberts, C. *et al.* (2005). Attitudes toward antipsychotic medication: the impact of clinical variables and relationships with health professionals. *Archives of General Psychiatry*, **62**, 717–24.

de Haan, L., Welborn, K., Krikke, M. & Linszen, D. H. (2004). Opinions of mothers on the first psychotic episode and the start of treatment of their child. *European Psychiatry*, **19**, 226–9.

Drake, R. E., McHugo, G. J., Xie, H. *et al.* (2006). Ten-year recovery outcomes for clients with co-occurring schizophrenia and substance use disorders. *Schizophrenia Bulletin*, **32**, 464–73.

Edwards, J. & McGorry, P. (2002). *Implementing Early Intervention in Psychosis*. London: Martin Dunitz.

Emsley, R. A. (1999). Risperidone in the treatment of first-episode psychotic patients: a double-blind multicenter study. Risperidone Working Group. *Schizophrenia Bulletin*, **25**, 721–9.

Emsley, R. A., Rabinowitz, J. & Medori, R. (2006). Time course for antipsychotic treatment response in first-episode schizophrenia. *American Journal of Psychiatry*, **163**, 743–5.

Faulkner, G., Soundy, A. A. & Lloyd, K. (2003). Schizophrenia and weight management: a systematic review of interventions to control weight. *Acta Psychiatrica Scandinavica*, **108**, 324–32.

Flyckt, L., Mattsson, M., Edman, G., Carlsson, R. & Cullberg, J. (2006). Predicting 5-year outcome in first-episode psychosis: construction of a prognostic rating scale. *Journal of Clinical Psychiatry*, **67**, 916–24.

Fountoulakis, K. N., Nimatoudis, I., Iacovides, A. & Kaprinis, G. (2004). Off-label indications for atypical antipsychotics: a systematic review. *Annual General Hospital Psychiatry*, **3**, 1–10.

Gearon, J. S. & Bellack, A. S. (1999). Women with schizophrenia and co-occurring substance use disorders: an increased risk for violent victimization and HIV. *Community Mental Health Journal*, **35**, 401–19.

Goodwin, G. M. for the Consensus Group of the British Association of Psychopharmacology (2003). Evidence-based guidelines for treating bipolar disorder: recommendations from the British Association for Psychopharmacology. *Journal of Psychopharmacology*, **17**, 149–73.

Gray, R., Wykes, T. & Gournay, K. (2002). From compliance to concordance: a review of the literature on interventions to enhance compliance with antipsychotic medication. *Journal of Psychiatry and Mental Health Nursing*, **9**, 277–84.

Green, M. F., Kern, R. S, Braff, D. L. & Mintz J. (2000). Neurocognitive deficits and functional outcome in schizophrenia: are we measuring the 'right stuff'? *Schizophrenia Bulletin*, **26**, 119–36.

Gunduz-Bruce, H., McMeniman, M., Robinson, D. G. *et al.* (2005). Duration of untreated psychosis and time to treatment response for delusions and hallucinations. *American Journal of Psychiatry*, **162**, 1966–9.

Hamann, J., Leucht, S. & Kissling W. (2003). Shared decision making in psychiatry. *Acta Psychiatrica Scandinavica*, **107**, 403–9.

Hamann, J., Cohen, R., Leucht, S., Busch, R. & Kissling W. (2005). Do patients with schizophrenia wish to be involved in decisions about their medical treatment? *American Journal of Psychiatry*, **162**, 2382–4.

Hawton, K., Sutton, L., Haw, C., Sinclair, J. & Deeks, J. J. (2005). Schizophrenia and suicide: systematic review of risk factors. *British Journal of Psychiatry*, **187**, 9–20.

Huq, Z. U. For the RIS-GBR-32 Investigators (2004). A trial of low doses of risperidone in the treatment of patients with first-episode schizophrenia, schizophreniform disorder, or schizoaffective disorder. *Journal of Clinical Psychopharmacology*, **24**, 220–4.

International Early Psychosis Association Writing Group (2005). International clinical practice guidelines for early psychosis. *British Journal of Psychiatry*, **187**(Suppl 48), s120–4.

Jarbin, H., Ott, Y. & von Knorring, A. L. (2003). Adult outcome of social function in adolescent-onset schizophrenia and affective psychosis. *Journal of the American Academy of Child and Adolescent Psychiatry*, **42**, 176–83.

Jones, P., Rodgers, B., Murray, R. & Marmot, M. (1994). Child development risk factors for adult schizophrenia in the British 1946 birth cohort. *Lancet*, **19**, 1398–402.

Joyce, E. M., Hutton, S. B., Mutsatsa, S. H. & Barnes, T. R. (2005). Cognitive heterogeneity in first-episode schizophrenia. *British Journal of Psychiatry*, **187**, 516–22.

Keefe, R. S., Seidman, L. J., Christensen, B. K. *et al.* (2004). Comparative effect of atypical and conventional antipsychotic drugs on neurocognition in first-episode psychosis: a randomized, double-blind trial of olanzapine versus low doses of haloperidol. *American Journal of Psychiatry*, **161**, 985–95.

Kim-Cohen, J., Caspi, A., Moffitt, T. E. *et al.* (2003). Prior juvenile diagnoses in adults with mental disorder: developmental follow-back of a prospective-longitudinal cohort. *Archives of General Psychiatry*, **60**, 709–17.

Kopala, L. C., Good, K. P., Milliken, H. *et al.* (2006). Treatment of a first episode of psychotic illness with quetiapine: an analysis of 2 year outcomes. *Schizophrenia Research*, **81**, 29–39.

Lacro, J. P., Dunn, L. B., Dolder, C. R., Leckband, S. G. & Jeste, D. V. (2002). Prevalence of and risk factors for medication non-adherence in patients with schizophrenia: a comprehensive review of recent literature. *Journal of Clinical Psychiatry*, **63**, 892–909.

Lambert, M. & Naber, D. (2004a). Current issues in schizophrenia: overview of patient acceptability, functioning capacity and quality of life. *CNS Drugs*, **18**(Suppl 2), 5–17.

Lambert, M. & Naber, D. (2004b). *Current Schizophrenia*. London: Science Press.

Lambert, M., Conus, P., Lambert, T. & McGorry, P. D. (2003a). Pharmacotherapy of first-episode schizophrenia. *Expert Opinion on Pharmacotherapy*, **4**, 717–51.

Lambert, M., Holzbach, R., Moritz, S. *et al.* (2003b). Objective and subjective efficacy as well as tolerability of olanzapine in the acute treatment of 120 patients with schizophrenia spectrum disorders. *International Clinical Psychopharmacology*, **18**, 251–60.

Lambert, M., Conus, P., Lubman, D. I. *et al.* (2005a). The impact of substance use disorders on clinical outcome in 643 patients with first-episode psychosis. *Acta Psychiatrica Scandinavica*, **112**, 141–8.

Lambert, M., Conus, P., Schimmelmann, B. *et al.* (2005b). Comparison of olanzapine and risperidone in 367 first-episode patients with non-affective or affective psychosis: results of an open retrospective medical record study. *Pharmacopsychiatry*, **38**, 206–13.

Lambert, M., Conus, P., Schimmelmann, B., Naber, D. & McGorry, P. D. (2005c). Olanzapine in patients with a first-episode psychosis non-responsive, intolerant or non-compliant to a first-line trial of risperidone. *International Journal of Psychiatry in Clinical Practice*, **9**, 244–50.

Lambert, M., Schimmelmann, B., Naber, D. *et al.* (2006). Prediction of remission as a combination of symptomatic and functional remission and adequate subjective well-being in 2960 patients with schizophrenia. *Journal of Clinical Psychiatry*, **67**, 1690–7.

Lambert, M., Naber, D., Eich, F. X. *et al.* (2007). Remission of severely impaired subjective well-being in 727 patients with schizophrenia treated with amisulpride. *Acta Psychiatrica Scandinavica* **115**, 106–13.

Larsen, T. K., Friis, S., Haahr, U. *et al.* (2004). Premorbid adjustment in first-episode non-affective psychosis: distinct patterns of pre-onset course. *British Journal of Psychiatry*, **185**, 108–15.

Law, C. W., Chen, E. Y., Cheung, E. F. *et al.* (2005). Impact of untreated psychosis on quality of life in patients with first-episode schizophrenia. *Quality of Life Research*, **14**, 1803–11.

Lencz, T., Smith, C. W., Auther, A., Correll, C. U. & Cornblatt, B. (2004). Nonspecific and attenuated negative symptoms in patients at clinical high-risk for schizophrenia. *Schizophrenia Research*, **68**, 37–48.

Leucht, S., Pitschel-Walz, G., Abraham, D. & Kissling, W. (1999). Efficacy and extrapyramidal side effects of the new antipsychotics olanzapine, quetiapine, risperidone, and sertindole compared to conventional antipsychotics and placebo. A meta-analysis of randomized controlled trials. *Schizophrenia Research*, **35**, 51–68.

Lieberman, J. A., Tollefson, G., Tohen, M. *et al.* For the HGDH Study Group (2003). Comparative efficacy and safety of atypical and conventional antipsychotic drugs in first-episode psychosis: a randomized, double-blind trial of olanzapine versus haloperidol. *American Journal of Psychiatry*, **160**, 1396–404.

Maki, P., Veijola, J., Jones, P. B. *et al.* (2005). Predictors of schizophrenia: a review. *British Medical Bulletin*, **73–74**, 1–15.

Malla, A., Norman, R., Scholten, D. *et al.* (2004). A comparison of two novel antipsychotics in first episode non-affective psychosis: one-year outcome on symptoms, motor side effects and cognition. *Psychiatry Research*, **129**, 159–69.

Malla, A., Norman, R., Schmitz, N. *et al.* (2006). Predictors of rate and time to remission in first-episode psychosis: a two-year outcome study. *Psychological Medicine*, **36**, 649–58.

Manchanda, R., Norman, R. M., Malla, A. K., Harricharan, R. & Northcott, S. (2005). Persistent psychoses in first episode patients. *Schizophrenia Research*, **80**, 113–16.

Marder, S. R., Essock, S. M., Miller, A. L. *et al.* (2004). Physical health monitoring of patients with schizophrenia. *American Journal of Psychiatry*, **161**, 1334–49.

Marshall, M., Lewis, S., Lockwood, A. *et al.* (2005). Association between duration of untreated psychosis and outcome in cohorts of first-episode patients: a systematic review. *Archives of General Psychiatry*, **62**, 975–83.

Mattsson, M., Lawoko, S., Cullberg, J. *et al.* (2005). Background factors as determinants of satisfaction with care among first-episode psychosis patients. *Social Psychiatry and Psychiatric Epidemiology*, **40**, 749–54.

McEvoy, J. P., Hogarty, G. E. & Steingard, S. (1991). Optimal dose of neuroleptic in acute schizophrenia. A controlled study of the neuroleptic threshold and higher haloperidol dose. *Archives of General Psychiatry*, **48**, 7397–45.

McEvoy, J. P., Meyer, J. M., Goff, D. C. *et al.* (2005). Prevalence of the metabolic syndrome in patients with schizophrenia: baseline results from the Clinical Antipsychotic Trials of Intervention Effectiveness (CATIE) schizophrenia trial and comparison with national estimates from NHANES III. *Schizophrenia Research*, **80**, 19–32.

McEvoy, J. P., Johnson, J., Perkins, D. *et al.* (2006). Insight in first-episode psychosis. *Psychological Medicine*, **36**, 1385–93.

McGorry, P. D. (1999). Recommended haloperidol and risperidone doses in first-episode psychosis. *Journal of Clinical Psychiatry*, **60**, 794–5.

McGorry, P. D., Copolov, D. L. & Singh, B. S. (1990a). Royal Park Multidiagnostic Instrument for Psychosis: Part I. Rationale and review. *Schizophrenia Bulletin*, **16**, 501–15.

McGorry, P. D., Singh, B. S., Copolov, D. L. *et al.* (1990b). Royal Park Multidiagnostic Instrument for Psychosis: Part II. Development, reliability, and validity. *Schizophrenia Bulletin*, **16**, 517–36.

McIntyre, R. S., Konarski, J. Z., Soczynska, J. K. *et al.* (2006). Medical comorbidity in bipolar disorder: implications for functional outcomes and health service utilization. *Psychiatric Services*, **57**, 1140–4.

Merlo, M. C., Hofer, H., Gekle, W. *et al.* (2002). Risperidone, 2 mg/d vs. 4 mg/d, in first-episode, acutely psychotic patients: treatment efficacy and effects on fine motor functioning. *Journal of Clinical Psychiatry*, **63**, 885–91.

Mueser, K. T. & McGurk, S. R. (2004). Schizophrenia. *Lancet*, **363**, 2063–72.

NICE. (2002). *Schizophrenia. Core Interventions in the Treatment and Management of Schizophrenia in Primary and Secondary Care. Clinical Guideline 1*. London: National Collaborating Centre for Mental Health.

Newcomer J W. (2006). Medical risk in patients with bipolar disorder and schizophrenia. *Journal of Clinical Psychiatry*, **67**(Suppl 9), 25–30.

Olsen, K. A. & Rosenbaum, B. (2006a). Prospective investigations of the prodromal state of schizophrenia: assessment instruments. *Acta Psychiatrica Scandinavica*, **113**, 273–82.

Olsen, K. A. & Rosenbaum, B. (2006b). Prospective investigations of the prodromal state of schizophrenia: review of studies. *Acta Psychiatrica Scandinavica*, **113**, 247–72.

Oosthuizen, P., Emsley, R. A., Turner, J. & Keyter, N. (2001). Determining the optimal dose of haloperidol in first-episode psychosis. *Journal of Psychopharmacology*, **15**, 251–5.

Perkins, D., Lieberman, J., Gu, H. *et al.* For the HGDH Research Group (2004). Predictors of antipsychotic treatment response in patients with first-episode schizophrenia, schizoaffective and schizophreniform disorders. *British Journal of Psychiatry*, **185**, 18–24.

Perlis, R. H. (2005). The role of pharmacologic treatment guidelines for bipolar disorder. *Journal of Clinical Psychiatry*, **66**(Suppl 3), 37–47.

Petersen, L., Jeppesen, P., Thorup, A. *et al.* (2005). A randomised multicentre trial of integrated versus standard treatment for patients with a first episode of psychotic illness. *British Medical Journal*, **331**, 602–10.

Power, P. & McGorry, P. D. (1999). Initial assessment in first-episode psychosis. In P. D. McGorry & H. J. Jackson (eds.), *The Recognition and Management of Early Psychosis. A Preventive Approach*. Cambridge, UK: Cambridge University Press, pp. 155–84.

Poyurovsky, M., Fuchs, C. & Weizman, A. (1999). Obsessive-compulsive disorder in patients with first-episode schizophrenia. *American Journal of Psychiatry*, **156**, 1998–2000.

Remington, G. (2005). Rational pharmacotherapy in early psychosis. *British Journal of Psychiatry*, **48**(Suppl), s77–84.

Robinson, D. G., Woerner, M. G., Alvir, J. M. *et al.* (1999a). Predictors of treatment response from a first episode of schizophrenia or schizoaffective disorder. *American Journal of Psychiatry*, **156**, 544–9.

Robinson, D. G., Woerner, M. G., Alvir, J. M. *et al.* (1999b). Predictors of relapse following response from a first episode of schizophrenia or schizoaffective disorder. *Archives of General Psychiatry*, **56**, 241–7.

Robinson, D. G., Woerner, M. G., Alvir, J. M. *et al.* (2002). Predictors of medication discontinuation by patients with first-episode schizophrenia and schizoaffective disorder. *Schizophrenia Research*, **57**, 209–19.

Robinson, D. G., Woerner, M. G., Delman, H. M. & Kane, J. M. (2005). Pharmacological treatments for first-episode schizophrenia. *Schizophrenia Bulletin*, **31**, 705–22.

Rosen, J. L., Miller, T. J., D'Andrea, J. T., McGlashan, T. H. & Woods, S. W. (2006). Comorbid diagnoses in patients meeting criteria for the schizophrenia prodrome. *Schizophrenia Research*, **85**, 124–31.

Royal Australian and New Zealand College of Psychiatrists (2004). Australian and New Zealand clinical practice guidelines for the treatment of bipolar disorder. *Australian and New Zealand Journal of Psychiatry*, **38**, 280–305.

Royal Australian and New Zealand College of Psychiatrists (2005). Royal Australian and New Zealand College of Psychiatrists clinical practice guidelines for the treatment of schizophrenia and related disorders. *Australian and New Zealand Journal of Psychiatry*, **39**, 1–30.

Sanger, T. M., Lieberman, J. A., Tohen, M. *et al.* (1999). Olanzapine versus haloperidol treatment in first-episode psychosis. *American Journal of Psychiatry*, **156**, 79–87.

Schimmelmann, B., Conus, P., Edwards, J., McGorry, P. D. & Lambert, M. (2005a). Diagnostic stability 18-month after a first diagnosis of psychosis. *Journal of Clinical Psychiatry*, **66**, 1239–46.

Schimmelmann, B., Paulus, S., Tilgner, C. *et al.* (2005b). Side effects, subjective distress and subjective well-being in first admitted adolescents with early onset psychosis treated with atypical antipsychotics. *Journal of Child and Adolescent Psychopharmacology*, **15**, 249–58.

Schimmelmann, B., Conus, P., Schacht, M., McGorry, P. D. & Lambert, M. (2006). Predictors of service disengagement in first admitted adolescents with psychosis. *Journal of the American Academy of Child and Adolescent Psychiatry*, **45**, 990–9.

Schooler, N., Rabinowitz, J., Davidson, M. *et al.* For the Early Psychosis Global Working Group (2005). Risperidone and haloperidol in first-episode psychosis: a long-term randomized trial. *American Journal of Psychiatry*, **162**, 947–53.

Schwartz, J. E., Fennig, S., Tanenberg-Karant, M. *et al.* (2000). Congruence of diagnoses 2 years after a first-admission diagnosis of psychosis. *Archives of General Psychiatry*, **57**, 593–600.

Sim, K., Swapna, V., Mythily, S. *et al.* (2004). Psychiatric comorbidity in first episode psychosis: the Early Psychosis Intervention Programme (EPIP) experience. *Acta Psychiatrica Scandinavica*, **109**, 23–9.

Sim, K., Chua, T. H., Chan, Y. H., Mahendran, R. & Chong, S. A. (2006). Psychiatric comorbidity in first episode schizophrenia: a 2 year, longitudinal outcome study. *Journal of Psychiatry Research*, **40**, 656–63.

Thorup, A., Petersen, L., Jeppesen, P. *et al.* (2005). Integrated treatment ameliorates negative symptoms in first episode psychosis: results from the Danish OPUS trial. *Schizophrenia Research*, **79**, 95–105.

Townsend, L. A. & Norman, R. M. (2004). Course of cognitive functioning in first episode schizophrenia spectrum disorders. *Expert Review of Neurotherapeutics*, **4**, 61–8.

Ventura, J., Liberman, R. P., Green, M. F., Shaner, A. & Mintz, J. (1998). Training and quality assurance with the Structured Clinical Interview for DSM-IV (SCID-I/P). *Psychiatry Research*, **15**, 163–73.

Wade, D., Harrigan, S., Edwards, J. *et al.* (2006). Substance misuse in first-episode psychosis: 15-month prospective follow-up study. *British Journal of Psychiatry*, **189**, 229–34.

WHO (1992). *International Classification of Diseases*, 10th edn. Geneva: World Health Organization.

Yap, H. L., Mahendran, R., Lim, D. *et al.* (2001). Risperidone in the treatment of first-episode psychosis. *Singapore Medical Journal*, **42**, 170–3.

Zalsman, G., Carmon, E., Martin, A. *et al.* (2003). Effectiveness, safety, and tolerability of risperidone in adolescents with schizophrenia: an open-label study. *Journal of Children and Adolescent Psychopharmacology*, **13**, 319–27.

Zhang-Wong, J., Zipursky, R. B., Beiser, M. & Bean G. (1999). Optimal haloperidol dosage in first-episode psychosis. *Canadian Journal of Psychiatry*, **44**, 164–7.

12

Complete and incomplete recovery from first-episode psychosis

Jean Addington, Tim Lambert and Peter Burnett

Introduction

The overall aims of early intervention are to offer prompt and effective intervention for young people experiencing psychosis. Specialized and potentially effective early intervention programmes are being developed worldwide. Offering intervention promptly implies reducing the duration of untreated psychosis and starting effective treatments as soon as possible and certainly prior to the development of a crisis (Jackson & Birchwood, 1996, p. 487): 'The first two or three years following a first episode of psychosis is a crucial period for high-quality psychosocial and biological interventions and a time slot which may influence recovery and long-term outcome'.

Expectations are high and successful recoveries are reported. Early intervention with optimal pharmacological and psychosocial interventions may have a substantial influence on recovery and long-term outcome (Jackson & Birchwood, 1996; Lincoln & McGorry, 1995). In fact, the initial course of the illness may be a particularly strong predictor of longer-term disability and functional outcomes (Harrison et al., 1996). These findings support the notion that intervention as early as possible with optimum treatments may set longer-term stability at a higher functional level. It is, of course, a concern when not all patients with first-episode psychosis make a full recovery. Nevertheless, one possible advantage of early intervention and specialized care may be that it has the potential to address the recovery process of those who do not achieve remission of symptoms or recover adequately from their first episode of psychosis (Edwards, Harris & Bapat, 2005).

In schizophrenia research, there is a lack of agreement on the criteria that define outcome of treatment. Recovery and remission are not the same thing; recovery is a 'higher hurdle and long-term goal' (van Os et al., 2006, p. 92). Traditionally, recovery was considered to be an outcome that occurred after an illness, at a specific time when an individual returned to a normal, healthy status. Complete recovery implies that the individual has the ability to function in the community, socially and vocationally and has no signs of psychopathology. Anthony (2000) offered a broader redefinition of recovery for mental health in which recovery is not a discrete event but rather a process that actually incorporates a belief that, even for those with the most severe form of illness, there is hope for an improved future. This includes hope 'to participate in meaningful activities, exercise self-determination and live in a society without stigma and discrimination' (Resnick et al., 2005, p. 120).

Clearly, recovery is a long-term and probably a far more demanding phenomenon than remission (Andreasen et al., 2005). Recently two working groups, one in the USA and one in Europe, have attempted to develop a consensus definition of remission in schizophrenia (Andreasen et al., 2005; van Os et al., 2006). The US working group (Andreasen et al., 2005, p. 442) defined remission as 'a necessary but not sufficient step towards recovery … and a state in which patients have experienced an improvement in core signs and symptoms to the extent that any remaining symptoms are of such low intensity that they no longer interfere significantly with behaviour and are below the threshold typically utilized in justifying an initial diagnosis of

The Recognition and Management of Early Psychosis: A Preventive Approach, ed. Henry J. Jackson and Patrick D. McGorry. Published by Cambridge University Press. © Cambridge University Press 2009.

schizophrenia'. Thus, remission is not limited only to positive symptoms but also includes negative symptoms. These two working groups proposed remission criteria as three or less on the following items from the Positive and Negative Syndrome Scale (PANSS): delusions (P1), unusual thought content (G9), hallucinatory behaviour (P3), conceptual disorganization (P2), posturing/mannerisms (G5), blunted affect (N1), passive/apathetic social withdrawal (N4) and lack of spontaneity and flow of conversation (N6) (van Os et al., 2006).

For recovery, we can add a more clinically based approach and consider recovery in a number of domains. These might include positive, negative, cognitive, affective and aggressive symptoms or syndromes, as well psychosocial function, behaviour and occupational activity.

Despite our best treatments and attempts to intervene early, there are, unfortunately, individuals who are described as not 'responding well to pharmacological interventions' and who continue to experience positive and negative symptoms. The reported rates of 1- and 2-year incomplete recovery (variously defined) range from 9% to 30% (Edwards et al., 1998; Lieberman et al., 1993; Manchanda et al., 2005). Correspondingly, good prognosis rates seem comparable with reports that at 5 years only 9–14% are in full remission (Robinson et al., 2005; Svedberg, Mesterton & Cullberg, 2001) and at 15 years 8% have good outcomes (Ropcke & Eggers, 2005).

These individuals have been labelled as 'treatment resistant' with the term implying that they have not responded to medication and continue to experience positive symptoms. Since the term 'resistant' implies both that there is little if anything that can be done to improve schizophrenia symptoms and that the patients themselves are actually resisting treatment rather than the illness itself being resistant to treatment, 'incomplete recovery' has been suggested as a preferred term (Pantelis & Lambert, 2003).

The purpose of this chapter is to examine the recovery phase following a first-episode of psychosis. Since the majority of first-episode patients generally meet criteria for schizophrenia or schizophreniform psychosis (Addington, Chaves & Addington, 2006; M. Lambert et al., 2003a), this group will be the principal focus of this chapter. We first describe the early recovery phase and the kinds of treatment that can be offered. We consider early recovery to be anywhere from a few weeks after initial treatment up to 3 months, although this will vary from one individual to another. The initial pharmacological treatment in the acute phase is dealt with in Ch. 11. Both Chs. 11 and 12 should be read in conjunction. Next, we offer a description of an incomplete recovery: what does this look like in an individual compared with someone who appears to be doing well prognostically? The third focus is on the factors contributing to and maintaining an incomplete recovery. Finally, we offer potential treatment strategies for those with a poorer recovery.

Early recovery phase: pharmacological treatments

The vast majority of patients entering the recovery phase have received pharmacotherapy in the acute phase. Indeed, pharmacotherapy has been described as the cornerstone of the treatment of psychosis, and it forms the platform upon which psychosocial interventions may have their greatest effect. Before starting treatment, the target symptoms should be clearly defined. The potential risks and benefits of the proposed intervention require discussion with the young person and their family – a discussion that should include a review of current treatment experiences in both adult and child psychiatry. The treatment is designed such that both response and side effects can be adequately monitored. Initial assessment and pharmacological intervention in the acute phase is the focus of Ch. 11.

The essential tasks of pharmacotherapy in the recovery phase are to (1) ensure adequate adherence to therapy; (2) adjust dosage for optimal efficacy; (3) monitor and minimize side effects (e.g. autonomic, neurological, metabolic, cognitive, sexual); (4) offer psychoeducation that addresses the illness, the treatment, the rationale for the use of a particular drug, the positive effects of medication, the potential side effects and its long-term effectiveness; and (5) work towards maintaining a positive therapeutic relationship and effective treatment for at least 12 months. The young person's first experience of psychotropic medication may have considerable influence on subsequent engagement and treatment (Zipursky, 2001).

At the beginning of the recovery phase, the patient's progress is continually reviewed. Numerous studies have shown that the treatment of choice for first-episode psychosis is low-dose second-generation antipsychotic drugs (SGAs) (Power *et al.*, 1998) and, where available, SGAs should be the first, second and third line of antipsychotic treatment (Royal Australian and New Zealand College of Psychiatrists, 2005). If SGAs are not available, then very low-dose first-generation antipsychotic drugs (FGAs) could be used with enhanced monitoring of the risks and benefits (Schooler *et al.*, 2005).

Poor efficacy

In our experience, about 60% of first-episode patients respond to low-dose antipsychotic drugs in the first 6 weeks following a first episode (Addington, Leriger & Addington, 2003a). In cases where the clinician feels there are no problems with tolerability or adherence, the patient may require either a higher dose or a different class of drug. Psychosocial interventions may, to some degree, obviate the need to alter core pharmacological management (Canadian Psychiatric Association, 2005; Lehman *et al.*, 2004).

Poor tolerability

It is the role of the treatment team to review difficulties with medication, such as side effects, that may directly or indirectly impair adherence or control of the psychosis (Ch. 11). An active enquiry regarding the presence or absence of key side effects, such as sexual side effects, should be undertaken by the team at least every 3 months, or more frequently if there is any change to the medication regimen or if there are complaints from patients, carers or other staff. A validated self-report instrument of the side effects of antipsychotic drugs, such as the Liverpool University Neuroleptic Side-Effect Rating Scale, is effective in this respect

(T. J. Lambert *et al.*, 2003b). Uncontrolled akathisia, for example, can worsen psychosis and even promote suicidal urges. A rapid increase in weight, especially in the sensitive adolescent, is an unacceptable cost of treatment. The control of unwanted side effects, combined with psychoeducation involving motivational interviewing, may help to avoid unnecessary increases in dose or changes in medication.

Ensuring frequent reviews

If the patient is showing a good response, frequent progress reviews should be undertaken to ensure continuing adherence. Taking a preventive stance will balance the benefits and costs of the treatment in a dynamic manner. Although maintenance therapy may result in long periods of fixed-dose therapy, minor perturbations in mental state, difficulties with life events and the vagaries of existence may require short-term interventions with various adjunctive treatments (both physical and psychosocial). A regular appraisal of long-term effects such as those associated with the metabolic syndrome and tardive dyskinesia should be standard practice in this phase (Lambert & Chapman, 2004).

Switching treatments

When the previous interventions have not ameliorated the target symptoms within 6–10 weeks and there are adverse effects, then changing to a different class of SGA may be warranted, or if receiving an FGA, switching to an SGA. Most antipsychotic medications have optimal dose–response curves, with maximum efficacy versus adverse effects occurring within a prescribed range. Doses higher than recommended have not usually been shown to improve outcome (Little, Gay & Vore, 1989).

Long-acting novel antipsychotic drugs

Where there is strong evidence for covert or overt non-adherence that is not remediable following attempts at treatment optimization, the use of a long-acting intra-muscular injection may be necessary. At the time of writing, the only such preparation available is for risperidone (Consta; Lambert, 2006). Depot forms of FGAs may also be an option where long-acting SGAs are unavailable, but the perception of some mental health workers of increases in inherent toxicity, and evidence of long-term motor disorders, suggests that they require frequent risk–benefit monitoring (T. J. Lambert *et al.*, 2003c; Lambert & Castle, 2003).

Relapse

Linzsen and colleagues (1994) defined three kinds of relapse: remission followed by relapse, partial remission followed by exacerbation, and persisting symptoms followed by significant exacerbation. Relapse factors are identifiable antecedents to the relapse, which is often, but not exclusively, related to poor adherence. Examples of relapse factors are substance abuse or stressful life events.

Early recovery phase: psychosocial treatments

When young people develop a psychosis, they often fall out of step with their peers, become socially isolated, have an altered self-perception and are unable to complete their education or training. As a result, the potential for achievements is reduced and, as the gap between themselves and their peers widens, catching up becomes more difficult. Thus, failure or difficulty in accomplishing these developmental tasks, along with any experiences of stigma, could potentially have a major impact on the young person over and above the psychotic illness itself (Corrigan & Watson, 2002; McGorry, 2002).

Functional recovery (e.g. social, vocational, interpersonal) remains a major challenge and is one of the principal domains in multidimensional approaches to incomplete recovery. The illness can remain disabling and problematic for patients and their families since symptom improvement is not always matched with functional improvement (Addington, Young & Addington, 2003b; Tohen *et al.*, 2000). Consequently, it is critical that we develop treatment approaches to complement

pharmacotherapy in order to improve outcome. Furthermore, such treatment needs to focus on limiting psychosocial damage by offering sustained treatment during this critical early period when vulnerability is at its peak and 'we have the best opportunity to provide a degree of damage control' (McGorry, 2002, p. 156). A range of psychosocial interventions is available to help in recovery from a first episode. They include psychoeducation, individual cognitive–behaviour therapy (CBT), phase-specific groups, interventions focusing on vocation, and family work. The goals of a psychosocial treatment encompass not only the symptoms of the illness but also the impact of the illness on an individual. This includes isolation from families and friends, damage to social and working relationships, depression and demoralization, and an increased risk of self-harm, aggression and substance abuse. Persistent symptoms that remain after the early recovery phase are an additional problem and add to the already disrupted developmental trajectory. These will be discussed later in this chapter.

Psychoeducation

Through psychoeducation – a clinical technique that can increase understanding and change behaviour – we can offer information about symptoms, aetiology, and treatment of psychosis. These young people do have the right to be fully informed about the nature of their illness so that they can gain knowledge that helps them to understand and integrate their experiences of themselves and their world. Knowledge can be empowering if it helps clients to take an active role in the management of their illness (Rosenberg, 1984).

Psychoeducation offered individually or in a group format is particularly important in early psychosis since the patients and their families probably have little experience with or knowledge about psychosis. Psychoeducation can include a wide range of topics such as symptoms and diagnoses, models and theories of psychosis, impact of substance use, medications, warning signs, how to avoid relapse and the agencies and personnel involved in treatment. The origins of, and factors influencing, the illness are presented in terms of a stress – vulnerability model (Addington & Addington, 2006).

Cognitive–behaviour therapy

Use of CBT is gaining recognition as a potentially effective treatment for improving outcome among patients with schizophrenia, with several randomized controlled trials demonstrating effectiveness of CBT for individuals with a more chronic course of illness (Tarrier & Wykes, 2004). In those RCTs that compared CBT with varied forms of supportive therapy, the positive impact of CBT was inconsistently diminished relative to the supportive therapy, although *never outperformed* (Tarrier & Wykes, 2004).

Very few CBT trials have focused on first-episode populations. The SoCRATES trial (Lewis *et al.*, 2002) used a large representative sample ($n = 315$; 83% with first-episode psychosis) to compare a 5-week treatment package of (1) CBT plus routine care, (2) supportive therapy plus routine care and (3) routine care alone during the acute phase of the psychotic illness. At 70 days, there were trends towards faster improvement of positive symptoms in the CBT group compared with the other two groups (Lewis *et al.*, 2002). At 18-months follow-up, CBT demonstrated significant advantages in outcome over routine care and some advantages over supportive therapy (Tarrier *et al.*, 2004). Importantly, there are significant limitations to this study. The CBT was delivered over a time period that was probably insufficient to make a longer-term impact (5 weeks). A high recovery rate in the acute phase under routine care is to be expected since we know that up to 85% of patients recover from a first episode under a standardized drug regimen. In this context, there is little room for CBT to impact on positive symptoms at the acute phase. Unfortunately, this is disappointing as SoCRATES was clearly a step in the right direction.

In the Active Cognitive Therapy for Early Psychosis study in Melbourne, active cognitive therapy outperformed a supportive therapy (befriending) in reducing negative symptoms and in improving functioning in the first 6.5 weeks of treatment. There were, however, no significant differences at 1-year follow-up, nor in terms of hospital admissions. These results again suggest that CBT promotes early recovery (Jackson *et al.*, 2008, Killackey, Jackson & McGorry, 2008).

The goal of the COPE strategy (cognitively orientated psychotherapy for early psychosis; Jackson *et al.*, 1999) was to facilitate adjustment after a first episode of psychosis. McGlashan, Docherty & Siris (1976) noted that patients deal differently with the experience of having a first psychosis. Some do not want to know about it, denying its impact (i.e. 'sealing over'), while others express a desire and interest to understand the process and give it some personal significance (i.e. 'integration'). In an open trial, those receiving COPE demonstrated improved illness adaptation as assessed by an integration and sealing-over scale (McGlashan, Wadeson & Carpenter, 1977) compared with those who had not participated (Jackson *et al.*, 2001). It has been demonstrated (Thompson, McGorry & Harrigan, 2003) that sealing over/integration is an important factor related to recovery, which is malleable over time. The results from clinical trials of CBT for psychosis and the need to develop psychosocial interventions for first-episode patients make CBT a compelling treatment to consider as an integral part of early psychosis services. However, more research is clearly warranted.

We have proposed and described elsewhere a modular approach to CBT for first-episode psychosis (Addington & Gleeson, 2005). The modules include engagement, education, addressing adaptation, treating coexisting anxiety or depression, coping strategies, relapse prevention and treating positive and negative symptoms. These modules have been guided by a wide range of texts and manuals of empirically supported treatment models that offer both unique and complementary perspectives of CBT for psychosis.[1] An advantage of this approach is that there is a range of interventions to meet the needs of first-episode clients. It is recommended that CBT be introduced to first-episode patients once medication, stabilization and

---

[1] Three texts offer both a theoretical basis for, and a systematic guide to, the therapy (Chadwick, Birchwood & Trower, 1996; Fowler, Garety & Kuipers, 1995; Kingdon & Turkington, 2005); Nelson (1997) has offered a detailed description of CBT for symptoms as a practice manual and others offer a range of useful case studies (Kingdon & Turkington, 2002; Morrison, 2002). Drawing from the work of several of the above texts, *Systematic Treatment of Persistent Psychosis* (*STOPP*): A *Psychological Approach to Facilitating Recovery in Young People with First-episode Psychosis* (Herrmann-Doig, Maude & Edwards, 2003) is the only manual that has a specific focus on CBT for first-episode psychosis. Relapse prevention is addressed by Gumley and Schwannauer (2006).

Box 12.1. Modular approach to cognitive-behavioural therapy

1. **Engagement, assessment and formulation phase**
   - Formation and development of the therapeutic alliance
   - Use of instruments assessing functioning and symptoms
   - Use of instruments specifically relevant to the focus of the therapy
   - Development of an individualized formulation that begins at the first session and continues through several sessions
   - Identification of problem areas
   - Development of understanding of the key elements leading to the psychotic disorder and of the factors that maintain the problem areas
   - Assessment of the background to psychosis for biological, psychological and social context
   - Presentation to client of therapist's understanding of the aetiology, development and maintenance of the problem
   - Presentation of a rationale for the intervention and length and frequency of sessions
   - Development of a consensus about treatment goals
   - Continued elaboration and refinement of the formulation

2. **Psychoeducation**
   - Offered in an individual or group format as described above

3. **Adaptation to psychosis**
   - Individual's understanding of the disorder
   - Impact of psychosis on the self
   - Ways to adapt to the psychosis

4. **Treatment of secondary morbidity**
   - Depression, anxiety and substance abuse
   - Challenging of underlying beliefs and assumptions

5. **Coping strategies**
   - For positive and negative symptoms
   - For functional and emotional problems that arise from the symptoms
   - Use distraction and focusing techniques for voices
   - Use behavioural self-monitoring, paced activity scheduling, assertiveness training and diary recording of mastery and pleasure for negative symptoms

6. **Relapse prevention**
   - Monitoring for early-warning signs of relapse
   - Cognitive restructuring of enduring self-schema associated with elevated risk of relapse

7. **Techniques to address delusions and beliefs about voices**
   - For auditory hallucinations: collaborative critical analysis of beliefs about the origin and nature of the voice(s),

use of voice diaries, reattribution of the cause of the voices and generation of possible coping strategies
   - For delusions: identifying precipitating and maintenance factors, modifying distressing appraisal of the symptoms and generating alternative hypotheses for abnormal beliefs

symptom remission has begun, in order to enhance the goal and expectation of optimum recovery, with a focus on enhancing functioning. A brief outline of the CBT modular approach is presented in Box 12.1.

In this early recovery phase, the most important areas to be addressed after the engagement and formulation phase would be psychoeducation and adaptation to psychosis.

Phase-specific group treatment

Communicating with peers who are having similar experiences of psychosis, in combination with opportunities to explore alternative explanatory models of illness, can assist with the development of a personal model of psychosis that enhances rather than hinders positive self-esteem (Albiston, Francey & Harrigan, 1998; Early Psychosis Prevention and Intervention Centre (EPPIC), 2000). Groups provide many opportunities to develop skills, improve social relationships and increase understanding of a psychotic illness, and as such should be designed to help the individual to manage different phases of illness and recovery following the first episode. A range of groups can be offered and these may be specific to the phase of recovery, including psychosis education, recovery, interpersonal skills and substance abuse. Specific details of these groups have been described elsewhere (Addington, 2003; Addington & Addington, 2006; Early Psychosis Prevention and Intervention Centre (EPPIC), 2000). In the early stages of recovery, groups that focus on education about psychosis and on recovery issues may be the most appropriate at that time.

Interventions focusing on vocation

Studies of vocational programmes in psychosis generally have demonstrated the efficacy of supported employment programmes (Drake, Becker & Bond, 2003; Killackey, 2004). There is support for its efficacy in a first-episode population (Rinaldi *et al.*, 2004; see Ch. 18).

Family treatments

The goals of working with families at the first episode is to maximize the adaptive functioning of the family; minimize disruption to family life and the risk of long-term grief, as well as stress and burden; and reduce the risk of negative outcomes for the patient (Addington & Burnett, 2004). The family must be collaborators in this process. Issues that are unique to the first episode and ways of working with these families have been well discussed in the literature (Addington & Burnett, 2004; see Ch. 17).

A recovery-stage model for families, based upon the course of recovery for a person experiencing their first psychotic episode, was initially described by Addington *et al.* (2005a). The recovery model was developed in the Calgary Early Psychosis Program and has since been expanded for use in the Toronto First Episode Psychosis Program. The model has four stages: (1) managing the crisis, (2) initial stabilization and facilitating recovery, (3) consolidating the gains, and (4) prolonged recovery; each stage has specific interventions and clearly defined goals. Briefly, in the first stage of treatment, the primary goal is crisis management, engaging the family and developing a good working relationship. Individual families are provided with support and education about psychosis. The second stage focuses on stabilizing the patient and family and facilitating recovery. Families are offered both individual and group treatment at this stage. In stage three, the family worker helps the family to integrate the information and skills learned in the previous stages into their daily life. In the final stage of treatment, families are prepared to transition into appropriate long-term treatment programmes. Note that at each phase of treatment, families identified as at high risk for difficulties are offered additional interventions and support. Lengths of the stages vary with the needs of the family and the rate of recovery for the individual. Typically, the crisis stage may last a few months, followed by a 3–12 month recovery stage and a 12-month consolidation stage.

A 3-year follow-up of a large sample of first-episode families from the Calgary Early Psychosis Program demonstrated several clinically relevant results (Addington, McCleery & Addington, 2005b). First-episode families had high levels of distress and experienced many difficulties. Notably, the level of stress was higher if the ill family member was younger or had an early age of onset. Second, distress improved significantly after 1 year, but those with more severe distress often took 2 years to recover. Finally, it was the families' appraisals of the impact and consequences of the illness that was most associated with their psychological well-being, not the severity of the illness. More than 80% of available families participated, and of those participating, 50% were still available after 3 years. These results are encouraging because they indicate that family interventions are acceptable, can be effective in real clinical situations and that it is advantageous to engage with families at the first episode. This model fits very well with determining how to work in these very early stages of recovery (Ch. 17 has a full discussion of family interventions).

Therefore, in the early stages of recovery, there is a range of both pharmacological and psychological interventions available. Many of these have been well described in the literature and it is beyond the scope of this chapter to offer more than an overview and a guide (see Chs. 14–19 for more comprehensive discussion).

Incomplete recovery 3 months after the acute episode

Both services and the existing research literature have, in the past, focused on the persistence of positive symptoms as the index of poor or incomplete recovery. However, if the philosophy of early intervention services is to be realized, incomplete recovery may be better conceptualized in a multidimensional manner (Brenner *et al.*, 1990; Pantelis & Lambert, 2003). Disability itself is more likely to occur as a result of problems in a variety of these dimensions, which include symptom domains, behaviour, function, suicidality and ability to work (among others) (see Box 1 in Pantelis & Lambert, 2003). This next section will describe the background to incomplete recovery, review the factors contributing to developing and continuing incomplete recovery and discuss relevant treatment approaches.

Background

Ongoing positive symptoms

Studies generally demonstrate that by 3 months there will be a clinically and statistically significant improvement in positive symptoms (Addington *et al.* 2003a). Tohen *et al.* (2000) demonstrated that 50% of hospitalized first-episode patients achieved recovery after 3 months, which increased to 70% by 6 months. The Iowa group (Gupta *et al.*, 1997) examined a small inpatient sample and showed that significant symptomatic improvement was observed in three dimensions at time of discharge from hospital: psychotic symptoms, disorganization and negative symptoms. Improvement was mainly accounted for by positive symptoms. Once the patients were discharged, there was no significant improvement in the subsequent months up to 1 year. Likewise, in the Hillside first-episode study Lieberman *et al.* (1993) demonstrated 83% were in remission by 1 year.

Negative symptoms

Unlike the improvement in positive symptoms, there are differing reports pertaining to changes in negative symptoms, with little change being reported over the first 12 months (Addington *et al.*, 2003a; Gupta *et al.*, 1997). In an Australian study with a large first-episode sample, Edwards *et al.* (1999) examined negative symptoms and reported that the percentage achieving caseness for enduring negative symptoms varied markedly depending on the method of assessment used.

Depression and anxiety

Depression and anxiety are not uncommon symptoms at the first-episode (Koreen *et al.*, 1993). In the Calgary study, depression increased at 3 months but significantly improved by 12 months (Addington *et al.*, 2003a). Thirty-two percent of the sample met DSM-IV

(APA, 2000) criteria for social phobia and approximately 60% of participants were experiencing elevated levels of social anxiety according to the Social Phobia and Anxiety Inventory ($M = 69.57$; $SD = 27.42$; Voges & Addington, 2005). Negative symptoms and negative self-statements, but not social anxiety, were significant predictors of social functioning. This has implications for addressing these negative cognitions in early psychosis. In the Hillside first-episode study (Lieberman *et al.*, 1993), 22% were depressed at onset and 15% experienced a post-psychotic depression (Koreen *et al.*, 1993).

Social deficits

Poor social and occupational functioning is a defining feature of psychotic illnesses, in particular of schizophrenia. A decline in social functioning may even begin before the first full-blown psychotic episode (Häfner *et al.*, 1999) with further deterioration occurring within the first 2–3 years (Birchwood, Todd & Jackson, 1998). McGorry *et al.* (1996) reported 23–25% improvement in quality of life scores 1 year after admission to EPPIC. Malla *et al.* (2001) demonstrated significant improvement in quality of life as subjectively judged by 41 first-episode subjects after 1 year of treatment in a community first-episode treatment programme. In the Calgary First Episode Program at the 1-year follow-up, there was significant improvement in quality of life using the Quality of Life Scale (Addington *et al.*, 2003b). Although these results of improvement are promising, studies have shown that first-episode patients have deficits in social functioning equivalent to those observed in individuals with a more chronic course of schizophrenia (Grant *et al.*, 2001; Priebe, Roeder-Wanner & Kise, 2000). In fact, even those first-episode patients experiencing a remission from positive symptoms had lower Quality of Life Scale scores than the non-psychiatric controls (Addington *et al.*, 2003b). These young patients often fail to attain age-appropriate social and vocational functioning (Lieberman *et al.*, 1992). They demonstrate high levels of social impairment, with many (43–60%) remaining unemployed after 1 and 2 years (Gupta *et al.*, 1997; Ho *et al.*, 1998).

Therefore, although we are seeing good symptomatic recovery with many first-episode subjects, the same may not be true for functional recovery (Tohen *et al.*, 2000). The comparison with normal controls provides a context for understanding the concepts of remission and recovery (Addington *et al.*, 2003b).

Cognitive deficits

It has been demonstrated that individuals experiencing their first-episode of schizophrenia show cognitive deficits that are often equivalent to those seen in patients with a more chronic course of illness (Addington, Brooks & Addington, 2003c). A recent study reported results from a 2-year longitudinal study examining the cognitive performance, using a comprehensive battery of tests, of 247 individuals who recently presented with a first-episode of psychosis. There were several significant improvements in cognition over the 2-year period, which were usually matched by improvements in a matched non-psychiatric control group. These results suggest that impaired cognition exists in the very early stages of a psychotic illness and that there is no decline over time (Addington, Saeedi & Addington, 2005c).

Although there is a wide range of studies offering considerable support for longitudinal associations between cognition and functional outcome in schizophrenia, little is known about this association in early psychosis (Green, Kern & Heaton, 2004). An examination of the impact of cognitive functioning on outcome demonstrated that deficits on a wide range of cognitive tasks were significantly associated with outcome as assessed by the Quality of Life Scale (Addington *et al.*, 2005c). However, positive and negative symptoms were clearly associated with functional outcome. Controlling for positive and negative symptoms revealed that cognition made a small but significant contribution (4–6%) to the model only at the 1-year follow-up, which appears contrary to other findings in the literature for a more chronic population. These results are important in attempting to understand further the crucial issue of the relationship between cognitive functioning and the longitudinal outcome in psychosis, which has a profound effect on recovery.

Summary of factors seen in incomplete recovery

Studies conducted with first-episode subjects demonstrate that these individuals do improve over time, with most positive-symptom improvement being seen in the early months and negative-symptom improvement being less and taking more time. What is striking is the appearance of negative symptoms early on in the course of the illness, an observation made by a number of research groups. This supports previous suggestions that negative symptoms may be well established prior to the point of entry into treatment and may either delay presentations or become entrenched through the lack of detection and treatment. Early identification of the group who will have enduring negative symptoms may also be assisted through examination of negative symptoms during the prodromal period prior to first psychotic symptoms (Häfner *et al.*, 1999). Of course, examination of *each* of the multidimensional domains should be carried out, for example, social and occupational functioning.

As a general principle, identification of those with incomplete recovery should be achieved as soon as possible. This may be undertaken by special subservices of more general first-episode programmes.[2] A clinical flow chart for considering how to manage such patients is shown in Fig. 12.1.

The problem of incomplete recovery can be addressed in three stages. The first stage considers the factors that may confound outcome. The second addresses impaired adherence and the third focuses on whether it is caused by 'treatment resistance'.

Stage 1: dealing with outcome confounders

The first step is to identify in which of the dimensions of the recovery process the patient has become 'stuck' and to consider relevant reasons for this. Within the context of a biopsychosocial integrated approach to treatment and care, incomplete recovery may occur as a consequence of a number of confounding factors. These may

---

[2] The Treatment Resistance and Assessment Team at EPPIC in Victoria, Australia is one example of such a programme. Screening for incomplete recovery occurs from 9 weeks onwards.

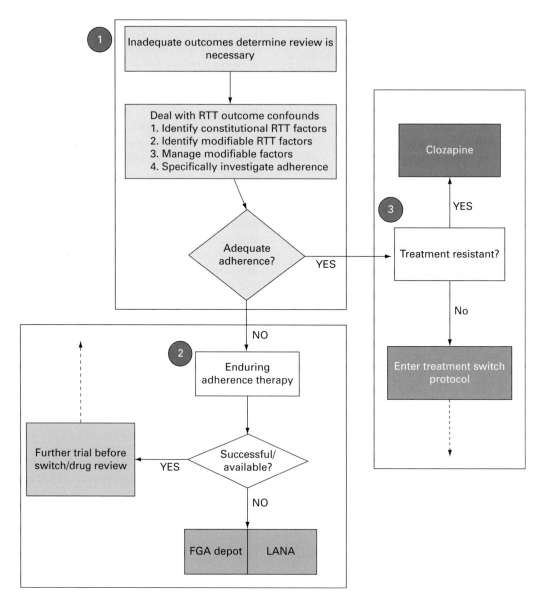

Fig. 12.1. Treatment flow chart following incomplete recovery showing three stages. RTT, resistance to treatment; FGA, first-generation antipsychotic drug; LANA, long-acting novel antipsychotic drug.

give rise to a clinical state of resistance to treatment, which should be contrasted with treatment resistant (schizophrenia). The next step is to identify both constitutional (essentially unmodifiable) and potentially modifiable confounders of recovery. A review of these is presented in Table 12.1.

At this stage, if a number of constitutional factors have been identified, such as a long duration of

Table 12.1. Factors relevant in establishing and perpetuating incomplete recovery in psychosis

Factors	Unmodifiable	Potentially modifiable
Patient	Poor prognosis factors: males, single, intellectual disability	Comorbidity: substance-use disorders, depression
	Diagnosis of schizophrenia	Psychological adjustment: sealing over versus integration recovery style
		Psychosocial milieu including family
Illness	Poor premorbid adjustment	Severity of psychopathology for each domain (see Box 12.1)
	Marked cognitive impairment	
	Early and/or insidious onset	Negative symptoms at first admission ± poor functioning
	Longer duration of prodrome, delays in treatment initiation, and/or longer duration of untreated psychosis	Unawareness of negative symptoms
	Organic factors: abnormal brain features, indicated by computed tomography, magnetic resonance imaging, baseline abnormal electroencephalograph; poor integrity of the dorsolateral prefrontal cortex	Poor cognitive function at stabilization
Treatment	Pharmacokinetics: incorrect dose, Drug–drug interactions, bioavailability problems, therapeutic windows	Impaired adherence: psychosocial treatments, medical treatments
		Inadequate rehabilitation programme or lack of services and resources
		Side effects (e.g. extrapyramidal symptoms, metabolic, cognitive, etc.)

Based in part on Pantelis and Lambert (2003).

untreated psychosis (DUP), for example, clinicians should be alerted to the potential for the patient to be at high risk in terms of achieving a poor outcome. Identifying potentially modifiable confounders is important so that appropriate interventions can be designed. A number of these factors will be briefly reviewed.

Comorbidity

First-episode patients have high rates of substance-use disorder, with lifetime rates approaching 80% in those attending specialized services (Wade *et al.*, 2005). Such patients are likely to have poorer initial and distal outcomes, compounded by an affective component, which is itself associated with poorer outcome (Edwards *et al.*, 1998; Resnick, Rosenheck & Lehman, 2004). Not surprisingly, persistent substance use is associated with non-adherence, treatment dropout and poor remission rates. Additionally, substance use may negatively impact on antipsychotic responsiveness (Green *et al.*, 2004) and lead to earlier relapse, even in those who are adherent to therapy (Hunt, Bergen & Bashir, 2002).

Effective management of psychosis within an integrated service is associated with reductions in substance-use disorder over the course of treatment, and young patients with comorbid psychosis and substance use should be offered comprehensive treatment that addresses both disorders as early as possible (Lambert *et al.*, 2005; Ch. 14).

Adequacy of psychosocial interventions

Pharmacological treatment serves mainly to provide a stable platform upon which to build critical psychosocial interventions. Psychosocial interventions as described above should be routinely available to all patients and their families. This integrated approach of psychosocial treatments and pharmacotherapy has been shown to lead to significantly better outcomes than standard outpatient care, with improvements in adherence, reduced substance abuse and greater satisfaction (Penn *et al.*, 2005; Petersen *et al.*, 2005). Vocational rehabilitation (and obtaining paid employment) can have a major effect on symptom level, social function and quality of life (Marwaha & Johnson, 2004; Ch. 18). From the perspective of incomplete recovery, a review of the services offered to the patient, whether they were appropriate and whether the patient was able to participate, may help with estimating whether further developing these modalities could enhance distal outcomes or the speed of recovery.

Psychological adjustment to psychosis

Adjustment to psychosis is an important variable in recovery. Patients respond to their first psychotic episode using either a 'sealing over' or 'integration' recovery style. Sealing over predicts low engagement in the service, and seems independent of insight (Tait, Birchwood & Trower, 2003). Those who employ sealing over have worse outcomes than those who use integration, the latter showing better functioning at 12 months. Fortunately, recovery style is not a stable trait and may be amenable to psychoeducation and other psychological interventions (Thompson *et al.*, 2003).

Further psychological intervention at this stage may also include reviewing whether the provision of CBT-based strategies for persistent symptoms would be helpful (Garety, Fowler & Kuipers, 2000). Stress, long considered a precipitant and perpetuating factor in psychological and physical illness in general, may be particularly relevant in those with psychosis in remission or in those prone to psychosis (Myin-Germeys, Delespaul & van Os, 2005). Psychological techniques to help manage stress proneness may well lead to better symptom reduction.

Adherence

As with multi-episode patients, first-episode patients are prone to non-adherence and relapse (Robinson *et al.*, 1999; Ucok *et al.*, 2006). The rates of adherence

in first-episode psychosis appear broadly similar to those in patients with a more chronic course of illness, with 39% being non-adherent, 21% partially adherent and 41% fully adherent (Coldham, Addington & Addington, 2002). Enhancing adherence in early psychosis may substantially improve the long-term course (Robinson *et al.*, 2002). However, relatively little is known about the predictors of non-adherence in first-episode patients. Likely candidates include premorbid cognitive deficits, parkinsonism or other harmful side effects, male gender, social inactivity, low positive and high overall scores on the PANSS and young age (Kampman *et al.*, 2002; Robinson *et al.*, 2002). According to Coldham *et al.* (2002), non-adherent first-episode patients demonstrate more positive symptoms, more relapses, more alcohol and cannabis use, reduced insight and poorer quality of life. They are also younger, have an earlier age of onset and are less likely to have a family member involved in treatment. Results for this group are similar to other results reported in the literature. However, several of the correlates are often the consequence of non-adherence. In any individual, however, a number of factors with weaker predictive power may, in aggregate, strongly determine non-adherence. These include characteristics inherent in the patient (age, ethnicity, gender, cognitive deficit), in the family environment and related to the level of positive symptom psychopathology and side effects (Lacro *et al.*, 2002; Perkins, 2002). From the patient's perspective, those who do not believe that they need treatment and who believe that drug treatment offers little benefit are more likely to show non-adherence for periods of more than 1 week (Perkins *et al.*, 2006). This is consistent with the health belief model, tapping into the domains of susceptibility and subsequent estimations of risk and benefit (Perkins, 1999).

A difficulty for the clinician at this stage is how actually to determine the level of adherence. In terms of attendance at therapeutic appointments, group programmes and so forth, records are easily available. For medication, estimating the rate of adherence is far more difficult (Bond & Hussar, 1991). Doctors and patients may be the least reliable sources of adherence estimations; therefore, biological means are preferred where possible. Differences in adherence may be two- or three-fold between clinical impressions and physical evidence (Cramer & Rosenheck, 1998; Velligan *et al.*, 2003). Often a number of sources have to be queried in order to arrive at a consensus. One of the key reasons for identifying early non-adherence lies in its relationship to persistence of (positive) symptoms, which may reflect some brain toxicity. Therefore, non-adherence has to be anticipated and relationships maintained with patients and families in order to allow intervention as soon as possible to minimize the consequence of non-adherence.

Duration of untreated psychosis, before and within treatment

The DUP has been associated with a range of poor outcome and delayed recovery variables. A number of lines of evidence suggest that untreated psychosis is toxic to the brain (Lieberman *et al.*, 2001), although this view has been contested (Ho *et al.*, 2003). Notwithstanding this debate, meta-analysis finds that there is a significant (if modest) association between DUP and outcome; patients with longer DUP are less likely to achieve remission (Marshall *et al.*, 2005). However, there is more consistent support for the idea that prolonged DUP may be 'psychosocially toxic' (Harrigan, McGorry & Krstev, 2003; Ch. 8).

Beyond the contribution of DUP to outcome, there potentially exists an equally concerning influence: the duration of untreated psychosis *in treatment*. This posits that the opportunity for secondary prevention may be wasted if the patient has been identified and enrolled in a first-episode treatment programme but owing to reasons mainly associated with covert or undiscovered non-adherence does not respond to treatment. Consequently, when considering the patient with incomplete recovery, the duration of effective non-adherence needs to be identified so that the duration of active psychosis can be calculated (the total duration of untreated psychosis, before detection (DUP) plus while in treatment). The longer this duration of active untreated psychosis, the greater the likelihood of a prolonged or delayed recovery.

Once an impression of adherence is obtained, the review of incomplete recovery can proceed. Where it is clear that the patient is significantly non-adherent, overtly or covertly and that this is temporally related to the poor recovery, the clinician should proceed to stage 2 (Fig. 12.1).

Stage 2: dealing with impaired adherence

Given the importance of setting up an established physical treatment platform, the issue of adherence must be dealt with as soon as possible. Where resources exist, the next step is to engage the patient in some form of adherence therapy. Strategies that have been suggested to improve adherence are related to the patient, the doctor/treating team, the social environment and the treatment itself. Nosé, Barbui & Tansella (2003) undertook a meta-analysis of clinical interventions to improve treatment non-adherence. The rank order (lesser to greater) in terms of effectiveness was prompts, education, psychotherapy, specific service policies and family therapy. However, the benefits of the adherence interventions declined with time, suggesting the need for periodic 'topping up'. An earlier review was less enthusiastic about the role of interventions in improving medication adherence, noting that only about a third of studies identified a benefit (Zygmunt *et al.*, 2002). Methods that are more likely to work include providing concrete problem-solving skills, unambiguous direct instructions and taking a motivational interviewing approach (as commonly done with patients with a comorbid subtance-use disorder). Directly addressing issues of adherence has a more powerful effect than if the approach is embedded in broader psychosocial or psychotherapeutic strategies.

If adherence therapy is undertaken, it is important to determine ahead of time what changes in outcome will signify an improvement and to be very clear as to how adherence will be monitored in this period. If the process is successful, the patient can be returned to routine clinical monitoring. If this therapy is unsuccessful (or not available), then long-acting intramuscular antipsychotic drugs are indicated. In general, FGAs are not recommended for first-episode patients and depot FGAs are similarly not recommended unless no other option exists. With the advent of the long-acting novel antipsychotic agents, there is the possibility of providing all the benefits of SGAs in combination with the certainty of adherence. Guidelines have been developed for selecting patients who are likely to be good candidates for this therapeutic option (Lambert, 2006). If after 5 or 6 months at appropriate dosage, the patient remains with persistent symptoms, adherence may not be as salient as the possibility that the patient has treatment resistance. For such a patient, or one who was determined to be sufficiently adherent to oral treatment in stage 1, the clinician should proceed to stage 3 (Fig. 12.1).

Stage 3: determining whether incomplete recovery is a result of treatment resistance

For individuals with a more chronic course of schizophrenia and experiencing multiple episodes, it has been estimated that up to 40% show only a partial response or are fully treatment resistant (Conley & Buchanan, 1997; Pantelis & Barnes, 1996). Questions remain as to the incidence and prevalence of treatment resistance in first-episode patients (Robinson *et al.*, 2005). At a minimum, it is likely to be in the order of 10% (Edwards *et al.*, 1998). The process by which an appellation of treatment resistance is conferred on the patient is beyond the scope of the present chapter.[3] However, having worked through the confounders of resistance to treatment in stage 1, and in some cases having tried a long-acting novel antipsychotic drug in stage 2, the likelihood should be readily appreciated. Although a variety of therapeutic strategies for such patients exist (Pantelis & Lambert, 2003), the evidence is perhaps most convincing for clozapine (Wahlbeck *et al.*, 1999). Given the arguments presented above, early intervention with clozapine should be considered as soon as it is indicated. There is evidence that treatment resistance may evolve with time and that the earlier the intervention in those with delayed resistance the better the response (Lieberman *et al.*, 1998; Meltzer, Lee & Cola, 1998; see also Sheitman & Lieberman, 1998). Clearly, early intervention in those developing

resistance is important and clinicians should not wait until the patient has severely worsened before considering this agent. It is noteworthy that, in comparing response rates and side effects to clozapine in first- and multi-episode patients, there appears to be no difference, although response in both groups lessens with age (Hofer *et al.*, 2003).

If the patient does not meet the resistance criteria, it may well be that he or she may respond to a different agent. At this stage, switching is appropriate, preferably combined with the integrated psychosocial strategies described above.

Treatment approaches for incomplete recovery

Outcome after a first-episode of psychosis should be considered across a number of dimensions, including positive symptoms, negative symptoms, cognitive function, affective state, suicidal risk, behaviour and psychosocial function. It is important to monitor outcome and intervene actively as early as possible in order to prevent poor outcomes becoming entrenched and difficult to treat. For example, at EPPIC in Melbourne, case managers are asked to report ongoing positive or negative symptoms 9 weeks after treatment. If these are still present at 12 weeks, the patient's treatment is reviewed by a panel of senior clinicians in the treatment resistance early assessment team.

The first step is to review the diagnosis and initial treatment. Although approximately 70% of first-episode patients suffer from schizophrenia-spectrum disorders, the remaining 30% may require different treatments, for example, mood stabilizers for bipolar patients or more psychotherapy for patients with post-traumatic stress disorder, atypical psychosis or comorbid psychosis with borderline personality disorder. Any review of previous treatment must pay particular attention to adherence to medication regimens, dosage used, presence of substance abuse and engagement with case management and any psychosocial intervention. The aim is to determine whether the poor recovery is caused by the illness being difficult to treat or the patient avoiding treatment.

---

[3] For an overview see Pantelis and Lambert (2003), the Royal Australian and New Zealand College of Psychiatrists (2005) and Ch. 20.

If it is caused by the patient avoiding treatment, then interventions are directed accordingly. Inadequate doses should be increased and the patient's response monitored for a reasonable period (6 weeks). Adequate doses for SGAs in adult patients with multiple episodes of psychosis are in the ranges of risperidone 4–6 mg, olanzapine 15–25 mg, quetiapine 250–1000 mg, amisulpride 400–1200 mg (Pantelis & Lambert, 2003); first-episode patients are likely to need doses in the lower half of these ranges, or less. Poor adherence may be addressed by psychological techniques such as adherence therapy (Kemp *et al.*, 1996) and/or by the use of long-acting (depot) medications. Substance-abuse issues may respond to psychoeducation and motivational interviewing, and engagement of specialist workers with experience in substance misuse. Factors leading to poor engagement should be explored; possible remedies include provision of transportation to attend appointments, home visits, engagement of family members to provide assistance and focusing on practical issues which may be less challenging for the patient.

Medication strategies

Positive symptoms

Incomplete recovery in schizophrenia generally has been a rather neglected area of research, perhaps because of definitional and logistic problems with this population, and reluctance of drug companies to commit to studies in an area where outcomes are uncertain (Buckley & Shendarkar, 2005). No published papers have specifically addressed this issue in a first-episode population.

Guidelines for management of incomplete recovery in schizophrenia include those of the Texas Medication Algorithm Project (Miller *et al.*, 2004) and the PORT group (Lehman *et al.*, 2004), and these have received widespread acceptance. Patients who do not respond to trials of at least two different antipsychotic drugs, one of which is a SGA, should proceed to a trial of clozapine. Clozapine has demonstrated unique efficacy in the treatment of resistant positive symptoms (Barnes & McEvedy, 1996; Peuskens, 1999). A period of at least 6 months is recommended, although responders usually show signs of response within 8 weeks of reaching their therapeutic dose (Conley, Carpenter & Taminga, 1997).

When clozapine also fails to relieve symptoms, various strategies have been suggested, including adjunctive therapy with other antipsychotic drugs (particularly potent dopamine D_2 receptor blockers), lithium, sodium valproate and benzodiazepines. Successful case reports are found but there is little systematic evidence (Pantelis & Barnes, 1996). Electroconvulsive therapy can be effective (Chanpattana *et al.*, 1999; Chanpattana & Kramer, 2004) and certainly should be considered. More esoteric suggestions with some supportive evidence include omega-3 fatty acids (Arvindakshan *et al.*, 2003).

Other domains

Although most studies have focused on positive symptoms, there are some studies of antipsychotic effects on negative symptoms and cognitive dysfunction. Several studies have demonstrated efficacy of low dose (100–300 mg) amisulpride on negative symptoms. Clozapine has also demonstrated an effect, although this may be secondary to its effect on persisting positive symptoms (Murphy *et al.*, 2006).

Most SGAs have demonstrated greater efficacy on cognitive dysfunction than the FGAs. Overall, the effect size is small (Harvey *et al.*, 2004). It is noteworthy that it may take some time before the differential effectiveness manifests, and clinicians should take a longer-term perspective on the time to recovery for these symptoms. However, for the sufferer, marginal gains may be important in many day-to-day activities.

Psychosocial treatments

Further to the above discussion on psychosocial treatments in the recovery phase, these remain an essential component of the strategies to improve incomplete recovery.

Individual therapy

As discussed above, there is a general finding of significant reduction of both positive and negative symptoms at the end of the treatment phase of CBT, with maintenance of gains into the follow-up period, when this is compared with treatment as usual and in some cases with other psychological therapies. Specific CBT for incomplete recovery in early psychosis has been developed by the Systematic Treatment of Persistent Psychosis programme at EPPIC, the essential features of which are described in the manual by Hermann-Doig and co-workers (2003). The programme has four phases: (1) developing a collaborative working relationship, (2) exploring and coping with psychosis, (3) strengthening the capacity, to relate to others, and (4) finishing and moving on. The efficacy of this approach in conjunction with clozapine for treatment of incomplete recovery in early psychosis is currently being evaluated. The dominant psychotherapeutic approach in psychosis is CBT, and there have been few published papers on other approaches, and none focusing specifically on the incomplete recovery group.

Group, vocational and family approaches

As yet, there are no specific studies of the efficacy of group approaches in those with incomplete recovery. However, given that this is a group with the greatest needs, it follows that all psychosocial treatments should be employed as much as possible for these patients.

Service level

The EPPIC programme has routinely mandated review of all patients with incomplete recovery by a panel of senior, multidisciplinary clinicians at 12 weeks after entry. This process ensures that there is a high level of awareness of the problem of incomplete recovery, and appropriate intervention.

Conclusions

The concept of recovery is very important for maintaining hope in patients with early psychosis and their families. Fortunately, most (80–90%) make a good symptomatic recovery from the first episode. We have reviewed a wide range of psychosocial and pharmacological interventions that should be made available for all first-episode patients and which may all contribute in varying degrees to the recovery of these young people after a first episode. However, it is essential to ensure that those who do not recover are identified early and are given access to all therapeutic resources available. We have discussed the key issues that relate to the identification of factors that may contribute to and perpetuate an incomplete recovery. It is likely that we have only a brief window of opportunity to intervene successfully with those experiencing a first-episode psychosis and it is important that clinicians are alerted to the need to pursue incomplete recovery vigorously.

REFERENCES

Addington, J. (2003). An integrated treatment approach to substance abuse in an early psychosis program. In H. Graham, K. Mueser, M. Birchwood & A. Copello (eds.), *Substance Misuse in Psychosis: Approaches to Treatment and Service Delivery*. Chichester, UK: John Wiley, pp. 121–35.

Addington, J. & Addington, D. (2006). Phase specific group treatment in an early psychosis program. In J. O. Johannessen, B. Martindale & J. Cullberg (eds.), *Evolving Psychosis: Different Stages Different Treatments*. London: Brunner-Routledge, pp. 124–38.

Addington, J. & Burnett, P. (2004). Working with families in the early stages of psychosis. In J. F. M. Gleeson & P. D. McGorry (eds.), *Psychological Interventions for Early Psychosis*. Chichester, UK: John Wiley, pp. 99–116.

Addington, J. & Gleeson, J. (2005). Implementing cognitive behaviour therapy for first episode psychosis, *British Journal of Psychiatry*, **187**(Suppl 48), s272–6.

Addington, J., Leriger, E. & Addington, D. (2003a). Symptom outcome one year after admission to an early psychosis program. *Canadian Journal of Psychiatry*, **48**, 204–7.

Addington, J., Young, J. & Addington, D. (2003b). Social outcome in early psychosis. *Psychological Medicine*, **33**, 1119–24.

Addington, J., Brooks, B. & Addington, D. (2003c). Cognitive functioning in first episode psychosis: initial presentation. *Schizophrenia Research*, **62**, 59–64.

Addington, J., Collins, A., McCleery, A. & Addington, D. (2005a). The role of family work in early psychosis. *Schizophrenia Research*, **79**, 77–83.

Addington, J., McCleery, A. & Addington, D. (2005b). Three year outcome of family work in an early psychosis program. *Schizophrenia Research*, **79**, 107–16.

Addington, J., Saeedi, H. & Addington, D. (2005c). The course of cognitive functioning in first episode psychosis: changes over time and impact on outcome. *Schizophrenia Research*, **78**, 35–43.

Addington, J., Chaves, A. C. & Addington, D. (2006). Diagnostic stability over one year in first episode psychosis. *Schizophrenia Research*, **86**, 71–5.

Albiston, D. J., Francey, S. M. & Harrigan, S. M. (1998). Group programmes for recovery from early psychosis. *British Journal of Psychiatry*, **172**(Suppl 33), s117–21.

APA (2000). *Diagnostic and Statistical Manual of Mental Disorders DSM-IV-TR (text revision)*, 4th edn [DSM-IV]. Washington, DC: American Psychiatric Press.

Andreasen, N. C., Carpenter, W. T., Jr, Kane, J. M., *et al.* (2005). Remission in schizophrenia: proposed criteria and rationale for consensus. *American Journal of Psychiatry*, **162**, 441–9.

Anthony, W. A. (2000). A recovery-oriented service system: setting some system level standards. *Psychiatric Rehabilitation Journal*, **24**, 159–69.

Arvindakshan, M., Ghate, M., Ranjekar, P. K., Evans, D. R. & Mahadik, S. P. (2003). Supplementation with a combination of omega-3 fatty acids and antioxidants (vitamins E and C) improves the outcome of schizophrenia. *Schizophrenia Research*, **62**, 195–204.

Barnes, T. R. E. & McEvedy, C. J. B. (1996). Pharmacological treatment strategies in the non-responsive schizophrenic patient. *International Clinical Psychopharmacology*, **11**, 67–71.

Birchwood, M., Todd, P. & Jackson, C. (1998). Early intervention in psychosis: the critical period hypothesis. *British Journal of Psychiatry*, **172**(Suppl 33), s53–9.

Bond, W. S. & Hussar, D. A. (1991). Detection methods and strategies for improving medication compliance. *American Journal of Hospital Pharmacy*, **48**, 1978–88.

Brenner, H. D., Dencker, S. J., Goldstein, M. J. *et al.* (1990). Defining treatment refractoriness in schizophrenia. *Schizophrenia Bulletin*, **16**, 551–61.

Buckley, P. F. & Shendarkar, N. (2005). Treatment-refractory schizophrenia. *Current Opinion in Psychiatry*, **18**, 165–73.

Canadian Psychiatric Association (2005). Clinical practice guidelines for schizophrenia. *Canadian Journal of Psychiatry*, **50**(Suppl 1).

Chadwick, P., Birchwood, M. & Trower, P. (1996). *Cognitive Therapy for Delusions, Voices and Paranoia*. New York: John Wiley.

Chanpattana, W. & Kramer, B. A. (2004). Acute and maintenance ECT with flupenthixol in refractory schizophrenia: sustained improvement in psychopathology, quality of life and social outcomes. *Schizophrenia Research*, **66**, 177–81.

Chanpattana, W., Chakrabhand, M. L., Kongaskon, R., Techakasem, P. & Buppanharun, W. (1999). Short-term effect of combined ECT and neuroleptic therapy in treatment-resistant schizophrenia. *Journal of ECT*, **15**, 129–39.

Coldham, E. L., Addington, J. & Addington, D. (2002). Medication adherence of individuals with a first episode of psychosis. *Acta Psychiatrica Scandinavica*, **106**, 286–90.

Conley, R. R. & Buchanan, R. W. (1997). Evaluation of treatment-resistant schizophrenia. *Schizophrenia Bulletin*, **23**, 663–74.

Conley, R. R., Carpenter, W. R. J. & Taminga, C. A. (1997). Time to response and response-dose in a 12-month clozapine trial. *American Journal of Psychiatry*, **154**, 1243–7.

Corrigan, P. W. & Watson, A. C. (2002). The paradox of self-stigma and mental illness. *Clinical Psychology, Science and Practice*, **9**, 35–53.

Cramer, J. A. & Rosenheck, R. (1998). Compliance with medication regimens for mental and physical disorders. *Psychiatric Services*, **49**, 196–201.

Drake, R., Becker, D. & Bond, G. (2003). Recent research on vocational rehabilitation for persons with severe mental illness. *Current Opinion in Psychiatry*, **16**, 451–5.

Early Psychosis Prevention and Intervention Centre (EPPIC) (2000). *Early Psychosis Manuals, 3: Working with Groups in Early Psychosis*. Melbourne, Australia: Psychiatric Services Branch, Victoria Health Service.

Edwards, J., Maude, D., McGorry, P. D., Harrigan, S. M. & Cocks, J. T. (1998). Prolonged recovery in first-episode psychosis. *British Journal of Psychiatry*, **172**(Suppl 33), s107–16.

Edwards, J., McGorry, P., Waddell, F. & Harrigan, S. (1999). Enduring negative symptoms in first-episode psychosis: comparison of six methods using follow-up data. *Schizophrenia Research*, **40**, 147–58.

Edwards, J., Harris, M. G. & Bapat, S. (2005). Developing services for first episode psychosis and the critical period. *British Journal of Psychiatry*, **187**(Suppl 48), s91–7.

Fowler, D., Garety, P. & Kuipers, E. (1995). *Cognitive Behavior Therapy for Psychosis*. Chichester, UK: John Wiley.

Garety, P. A., Fowler, D. & Kuipers, E. (2000). Cognitive-behavioral therapy for medication-resistant symptoms. *Schizophrenia Bulletin*, **26**, 73–86.

Grant, C., Addington, J., Addington, D. & Konnert, C. (2001). Social functioning in first- and multi-episode schizophrenia. *Canadian Journal of Psychiatry*, **46**, 746–9.

Green, A. I., Tohen, M. F., Hamer, R. M. *et al.* for the HGDH Research Group (2004). First episode schizophrenia-related psychosis and substance use disorders: acute response to olanzapine and haloperidol. *Schizophrenia Research*, **66**, 125–35.

Green, M. F., Kern, R. S. & Heaton, R. K. (2004). Longitudinal studies of cognition and functional outcome in schizophrenia: implications for MATRICS. *Schizophrenia Research*, **72**, 41–51.

Gumley, A. & Schwannauer, M. (2006). *Staying Well After Psychosis: A Cognitive Interpersonal Approach to Recovery and Relapse Prevention*. Chichester, UK: John Wiley.

Gupta, S., Andreasen, N. C., Arndt, S. *et al.* (1997). The Iowa longitudinal study of recent onset psychosis: one-year follow-up of first episode patients. *Schizophrenia Research*, **23**, 1–13.

Häfner, H., Loffler, W., Maurer, K., Hambrecht, M. & an der Heiden, W. (1999). Depression, negative symptoms, social stagnation and social decline in the early course of schizophrenia. *Acta Psychiatrica Scandinavica*, **100**, 105–18.

Harrigan, S. M., McGorry, P. D. & Krstev, H. (2003). Does treatment delay in first-episode psychosis really matter? *Psychological Medicine*, **33**, 97–110.

Harrison, G., Croudace, T., Mason, P., Glazebrook, C. & Medley, I. (1996). Predicting the long-term outcome of schizophrenia. *Psychological Medicine*, **26**, 697–705.

Harvey, P. D., Meltzer, H., Simpson, G. M. *et al.* (2004). Improvement in cognitive function following a switch to ziprasidone from conventional antipsychotics, olanzapine, or risperidone in outpatients with schizophrenia, *Schizophrenia Research*, **66**, 101–13.

Hermann-Doig, T., Maude, D. & Edwards, J. (2003). *Systematic Treatment of Persisting Psychosis (STOPP): A Guide for Facilitating Recovery From First Episode Psychosis*. London: Martin Dunitz.

Ho, B. C., Nopoulos, P., Flaum, M., Arndt, S. & Andreasen, N. C. (1998). Two-year outcome in first-episode schizophrenia: predictive value of symptoms for quality of life. *American Journal of Psychiatry*, **155**, 1196–201.

Ho, B. C., Alicata, D., Ward, J. *et al.* (2003). Untreated initial psychosis: relation to cognitive deficits and brain morphology in first-episode schizophrenia. *American Journal of Psychiatry*, **160**, 142–8.

Hofer, A., Hummer, M., Kemmler, G. *et al.* (2003). The safety of clozapine in the treatment of first- and multiple-episode patients with treatment-resistant schizophrenia. *International Journal of Neuropsychopharmacology*, **6**, 201–6.

Hunt, G. E., Bergen, J. & Bashir, M. (2002). Medication compliance and comorbid substance abuse in schizophrenia: impact on community survival four years after a relapse. *Schizophrenia Research*, **54**, 253–64.

Jackson, C. & Birchwood, M. (1996). Early intervention in psychosis: opportunities for secondary prevention. *British Journal of Clinical Psychology*, **35**, 487–502.

Jackson, H., Edwards, J., Hulbert, C. & McGorry, P. D. (1999). Recovery from psychosis. In P. McGorry & H. J. Jackson (eds.), *The Recognition and Management of Early Psychosis: A Preventive Approach*. Cambridge, UK: Cambridge University Press, pp. 265–307.

Jackson, H., McGorry, P., Henry, L. *et al.* (2001). Cognitively oriented psychotherapy for early psychosis (COPE): a 1 year follow-up. *British Journal of Clinical Psychology*, **40**, 57–70.

Jackson, H. J., McGorry, P. D., Killackey, E. *et al.* (2008). Acute phase and 1-year follow-up results of a randomized controlled trial of CBT versus befriending for first-episode psychosis: the ACE project. *Psychological Medicine*, **38**, 725–35.

Kampman, O., Laippala, P., Vaananen, J. *et al.* (2002). Indicators of medication compliance in first-episode psychosis. *Psychiatry Research*, **110**, 39–48.

Kemp, R., Hayward, P., Applewhaite, G., Everitt, B. & David, A. (1996). Compliance therapy in psychotic patients: randomised controlled trial. *British Medical Journal*, **312**, 345–9.

Killackey, E. (2004). Psychosocial treatment. In M. Lambert & D. Naber (eds.), *Current Schizophrenia*. London: Science Press, pp. 65–74.

Killackey, E., Jackson, H. J. & McGorry, P. D. (2008). Vocational intervention in first-episode psychosis: individual placement and support v. treatment as usual. *British Journal of Psychiatry*, **193**, 114–20.

Kingdon, D. G. & Turkington, D. (2002). *The Case Study Guide to Cognitive Behaviour Therapy of Psychosis*. Chichester, UK: John Wiley.

Kingdon, D. G. & Turkington, D. (2005). *Cognitive-Behavioral Therapy of Schizophrenia*. London: Guilford Press.

Koreen, A. R., Siris, S. G., Chakos, M. *et al.* (1993). Depression in first-episode schizophrenia. *American Journal of Psychiatry*, **150**, 1643–8.

Lacro, J. P., Dunn, L. B., Dolder, C. R., Leckband, S. G. & Jeste, D. V. (2002). Prevalence of and risk factors for medication nonadherence in patients with schizophrenia: a comprehensive review of recent literature. *Journal of Clinical Psychiatry*, **63**, 892–909.

Lambert, M., Conus, P., Lambert, T. & McGorry, P. D. (2003a). Pharmacotherapy of first-episode psychosis. *Expert Opinion in Pharmacotherapy*, **4**, 717–50.

Lambert, M., Conus, P., Lubman, D. I. *et al.* (2005). The impact of substance use disorders on clinical outcome in 643 patients with first-episode psychosis. *Acta Psychiatrica Scandinavica*, **112**, 141–8.

Lambert, T. (2006). Selecting patients for long-acting novel antipsychotic therapy. *Australasian Psychiatry*, **14**, 38–42.

Lambert, T. & Castle, D. (2003) Pharmacological approaches to the management of schizophrenia. *Medical Journal of Australia*, **178** (9 Suppl), S57–61.

Lambert, T. J., Cock, N., Alcock, S. J., Kelly, D. L. & Conley, R. R. (2003b). Measurement of antipsychotic-induced side effects: support for the validity of a self-report (LUNSERS) versus structured interview (UKU) approach to measurement. *Human Psychopharmacology*, **18**, 405–11.

Lambert, T. J., Brennan, A., Castle, D., Kelly, D. L. & Conley, R. R. (2003c) Perception of depot antipsychotics by mental health professionals. *Journal of Psychiatric Practice*, **9**, 252–60.

Lambert, T. J., Chapman, L. H. for the Consensus Working Group (2004). Diabetes, psychotic disorders and antipsychotic therapy: a consensus statement. *Medical Journal of Australia*, **181**, 544–8.

Lehman, A. F., Kreyenhuhl, J., Buchanan, R. W., *et al.* (2004). The Schizophrenia Patient Outcomes Research Team (PORT): updated treatment recommendations 2003. *Schizophrenia Bulletin*, **30**, 193–217.

Lewis, S., Tarrier, N., Haddock, G. *et al.* (2002). Randomised controlled trial of cognitive–behavioral therapy in early schizophrenia: acute-phase outcomes. *British Journal of Psychiatry*, **181**(Suppl), s91–7.

Lieberman, J., Alvir, J., Woerner, M. *et al.* (1992). Prospective study of psychobiology in first-episode schizophrenia at Hillside Hospital. *Schizophrenia Bulletin*, **18**, 351–71.

Lieberman, J., Jody, D., Geisler, S. *et al.* (1993). Time course and biologic correlates of treatment response in first-episode schizophrenia. *Archives of General Psychiatry*, **50**, 369–76.

Lieberman, J. A., Sheitman, B., Chakos, M. *et al.* (1998). The development of treatment resistance in patients with schizophrenia: a clinical and pathophysiologic perspective. *Journal of Clinical Psychopharmacology*, **18**(Suppl), S20–4.

Lieberman, J. A., Chakos, M., Wu, H. *et al.* (2001). Longitudinal study of brain morphology in first episode schizophrenia. *Biological Psychiatry*, **49**, 487–99.

Lincoln, C. V. & McGorry, P. (1995). Who cares? Pathways to psychiatric care for young people experiencing a first episode of psychosis. *Psychiatric Services*, **46**, 1166–71.

Linzsen, D. H., Dingemans, P. M., Lenior, M. E. *et al.* (1994). Relapse criteria in schizophrenic disorders: different perspectives. *Psychiatry Research*, **54**, 273–81.

Little, K. Y., Gay, T. L. & Vore, M. (1989). Predictors of response to high dose antipsychotics in chronic schizophrenics. *Psychiatry Research*, **30**, 1–9.

Malla, A. K., Norman, R. M. G., McLean, T. S. & McIntosh, E. (2001). Impact of phase-specific treatment of first episode of psychosis on Wisconsin Quality of Life Index (client version). *Acta Psychiatrica Scandinavica*, **103**, 355–61.

Manchanda, R., Norman, R. M., Malla, A. K., Harricharan, R. & Northcott, S. (2005). Persistent psychoses in first episode patients. *Schizophrenia Research*, **80**, 113–16.

Marshall, M., Lewis, S., Lockwood, A. *et al.* (2005). Association between duration of untreated psychosis and outcome in cohorts of first-episode patients: a systematic review. *Archives of General Psychiatry*, **62**, 975–83.

Marwaha, S. & Johnson, S. (2004). Schizophrenia and employment: a review. *Social Psychiatry and Psychiatric Epidemiology*, **39**, 337–49.

McGlashan, T. H., Docherty, J. P. & Siris, S. (1976). Integrative and sealing-over recoveries from schizophrenia: distinguishing case studies. *Psychiatry*, **39**, 325–38.

McGlashan, T. H., Wadeson, H. S. & Carpenter, W. T. (1977). Art and recovery style from psychosis. *Journal of Nervous and Mental Disease*, **164**, 182–90.

McGorry, P. D. (2002). The detection and optimal management of early psychosis. In J. Lieberman & R. M. Murray (eds.), *Comprehensive Care of Schizophrenia*. London: Martin Dunitz, pp. 153–66.

McGorry, P. D., Edwards, J., Mihalopoulos, C., Harrigan, S. M. & Jackson, H. J. (1996). EPPIC: an evolving system of early detection and optimal management. *Schizophrenia Bulletin*, **22**, 305–26.

Meltzer, H. Y., Lee, M. & Cola, P. (1998). The evolution of treatment resistance: biologic implications. *Journal of Clinical Psychopharmacology*, **18**(Suppl 1), S5–11.

Miller, A. L., Hall, C. S., Buchanan, R. W. *et al.* (2004). The Texas Medication Algorithm Project antipsychotic algorithm for schizophrenia: 2003 update. *Journal of Clinical Psychiatry*, **65**, 500–8.

Morrison, A. P. (ed.) (2002). *A Casebook of Cognitive Therapy For Psychosis*. New York: Taylor & Francis.

Murphy, B. P., Chung, Y. C., Park, T. W. & McGorry, P. D. (2006). Pharmacological treatment of primary negative symptoms in schizophrenia: a systematic review. *Schizophrenia Research*, **88**, 5–25.

Myin-Germeys, I., Delespaul, P. & van Os, J. (2005). Behavioural sensitization to daily life stress in psychosis. *Psychological Medicine*, **35**, 733–41.

Nelson, H. (1997). *Cognitive Behavioral Therapy with Schizophrenia*. Cheltenham, UK: Nelson Thornes.

Nosé, M., Barbui, C. & Tansella, M. (2003). How often do patients with psychosis fail to adhere to treatment programmes? A systematic review. *Psychological Medicine*, **33**, 1149–60.

Pantelis, C. & Barnes, T. R. (1996). Drug strategies and treatment-resistant schizophrenia. *Australian and New Zealand Journal of Psychiatry*, **30**, 20–37.

Pantelis, C. & Lambert, T. J. (2003). Managing patients with 'treatment-resistant' schizophrenia. *Medical Journal of Australia*, **178**(Suppl), S62–6.

Penn, D. L., Waldheter, E. J., Perkins, D. O., Mueser, K. T. & Lieberman, J. A. (2005). Psychosocial treatment for first-episode psychosis: a research update. *American Journal of Psychiatry*, **162**, 2220–32.

Perkins, D. O. (1999). Adherence to antipsychotic medications. *Journal of Clinical Psychiatry*, **60**(Suppl 21), 25–30.

Perkins, D. O. (2002). Predictors of noncompliance in patients with schizophrenia. *Journal of Clinical Psychiatry*, **63**, 1121–8.

Perkins, D. O., Johnson, J. L., Hamer, R. M. *et al.* for the HGDH Research Group (2006). Predictors of antipsychotic medication adherence in patients recovering from a first psychotic episode. *Schizophrenia Research*, **83**, 53–63.

Petersen, L., Jeppesen, P., Thorup, A. *et al.* (2005). A randomised multicentre trial of integrated versus standard treatment for patients with a first episode of psychotic illness. *British Medical Journal*, **331**, 602.

Peuskens, J. (1999). The evolving definition of treatment resistance. *Journal of Clinical Psychiatry*, **60**(Suppl 12), 4–8.

Power, P., Elkins, K., Adlard, S. *et al.* (1998). Analysis of the initial treatment phase in first-episode psychosis. *British Journal of Psychiatry*, **172**(Suppl), s71–6.

Priebe, S., Roeder-Wanner, U. & Kise, W. (2000). Quality of life in first admitted schizophrenia patients: a follow-up study. *Psychological Medicine*, **30**, 225–30.

Resnick, S. G., Rosenheck, R. A. & Lehman, A. F. (2004). An exploratory analysis of correlates of recovery. *Psychiatric Services*, **55**, 540–7.

Resnick, S. G., Fontana, A., Lehman, A. F. & Rosenheck, R. A. (2005). An empirical conceptualization of the recovery orientation. *Schizophrenia Research*, **75**, 119–28.

Rinaldi, M., McNeil, K., Firn, M. *et al.* (2004). What are the benefits of evidence-based supported employment for patients with first-episode psychosis? *Psychiatric Bulletin*, **28**, 281–4.

Robinson, D., Woerner, M. G., Alvir, J. M. *et al.* (1999). Predictors of relapse following response from a first episode of schizophrenia or schizoaffective disorder. *Archives of General Psychiatry*, **56**, 241–7.

Robinson, D. G., Woerner, M. G., Alvir, J. M. *et al.* (2002). Predictors of medication discontinuation by patients with first-episode schizophrenia and schizoaffective disorder. *Schizophrenia Research*, **57**, 209–19.

Robinson, D. G., Woerner, M. G., Delman, H. M. & Kane, J. M. (2005). Pharmacological treatments for first-episode schizophrenia. *Schizophrenia Bulletin*, **31**, 705–22.

Ropcke, B. & Eggers, C. (2005). Early-onset schizophrenia: a 15-year follow-up. *European Child and Adolescent Psychiatry*, **14**, 341–50.

Rosenberg, P. P. (1984). Support groups. *Small Group Behavior*, **15**, 173–86.

Royal Australian and New Zealand College of Psychiatrists (2005). Clinical practice guidelines for the treatment of schizophrenia and related disorders. *Australian and New Zealand Journal of Psychiatry*, **39**, 1–30.

Schooler, N., Rabinowitz, J., Davidson, M. *et al.* (2005). Risperidone and haloperidol in first-episode psychosis: a long-term randomized trial. *American Journal of Psychiatry*, **162**, 947–53.

Sheitman, B. B. & Lieberman, J. A. (1998). The natural history and pathophysiology of treatment resistant schizophrenia. *Journal of Psychiatric Research*, **32**, 143–50.

Svedberg, B., Mesterton, A. & Cullberg, J. (2001). First-episode non-affective psychosis in a total urban population: a 5-year follow-up. *Social Psychiatry and Psychiatric Epidemiology*, **36**, 332–7.

Tait, L., Birchwood, M. & Trower, P. (2003). Predicting engagement with services for psychosis: insight, symptoms and recovery style. *British Journal of Psychiatry*, **182**, 123–8.

Tarrier, N. & Wykes, T. (2004). Is there evidence that cognitive behaviour therapy is an effective treatment for schizophrenia? A cautious or cautionary tale? *Behaviour Research and Therapy*, **42**, 1377–401.

Tarrier, N., Lewis, S., Haddock, G. *et al.* (2004) Cognitive-behavioral therapy in first-episode and early schizophrenia. *British Journal of Psychiatry*, **184**, 231–9.

Thompson, K. N., McGorry, P. D. & Harrigan, S. M. (2003). Recovery style and outcome in first-episode psychosis. *Schizophrenia Research*, **62**, 31–6.

Tohen, M., Strakowski, S. M., Zarate, C. Jr *et al.* (2000). The McLean-Harvard first-episode project: 6-month symptomatic and functional outcome in affective and non-affective psychosis. *Biological Psychiatry*, **48**, 467–76.

Ucok, A., Polat, A., Cakir, S. & Genc, A. (2000). One year outcome in first episode schizophrenia: predictors of relapse. *European Archives of Psychiatry and Clinical Neuroscience*, **256**, 37–43.

van Os. J., Burns, T., Cavallaro, R. *et al.* (2006). Standardized remission criteria in schizophrenia. *Acta Psychiatrica Scandinavica*, **113**, 91–5.

Velligan, D. I., Lam, F., Ereshefsky, L. & Miller, A. L. (2003). Psychopharmacology: perspectives on medication adherence and atypical antipsychotic medications. *Psychiatric Services*, **54**, 665–7.

Voges, M. & Addington, J. (2005). The association between social anxiety and social functioning in first episode psychosis. *Schizophrenia Research*, **76**, 287–92.

Wade, D., Harrigan, S., Edwards, J. *et al.* (2005). Patterns and predictors of substance use disorders and daily tobacco use in first-episode psychosis. *Australian and New Zealand Journal of Psychiatry*, **39**, 892–8.

Wahlbeck, K., Cheine, M., Essali, A. & Adams, C. (1999). Evidence of clozapine's effectiveness in schizophrenia: a systematic review and meta-analysis of randomized trials. *American Journal of Psychiatry*, **156**, 990–9.

Zipursky, R. B. (2001). Optimal pharmacologic management of the first episode of schizophrenia. In R. B. Zipursky & S. C. Schulz (eds.), *The Early Stages of Schizophrenia*. Washington, DC: American Psychiatric Press, pp. 81–106.

Zygmunt, A., Olfson, M., Boyer, C. A. & Mechanic, D. (2002). Interventions to improve medication adherence in schizophrenia. *American Journal of Psychiatry*, **159**, 1653–64.

13

Preventive strategies in bipolar disorders: identifying targets for early intervention

Philippe Conus, Michael Berk, Nellie Lucas, José Luis Vázquez-Barquero and Craig Macneil

Introduction

Intervention in the early phases of mental disorders has become a major clinical and research focus and is one of the main challenges facing contemporary mental health. This growing interest has led to the development of new lines of enquiry as well as the implementation of new types of treatment programme and services. In this context, the early phase of psychosis has attracted considerable attention in recent years; the therapeutic strategies that have been developed as a consequence may be beginning to improve the outcome of these conditions (McGorry & Jackson, 1999). Yet, most of the attention has been directed to schizophrenia, probably in reaction to the pessimism traditionally associated with this disorder (Conus & McGorry, 2002). Bipolar disorders, usually considered with more optimism, have been relatively neglected by this movement in comparison with schizophrenia. However, while Kraepelin's (1919) initial view of mental illness was excessively pessimistic regarding schizophrenia, it was also excessively optimistic regarding manic depression, and the assumption of a generally good outcome in manic depression has now been challenged many times (Conus et al., 2006a; Coryell et al., 1993; Dion et al., 1988; Harrow et al., 1990; Tohen et al., 1990a, 2000a,b). For the many reasons given in this chapter, it is imperative that a preventive approach should also be extended to bipolar disorders. Indeed, it is likely that the key targets of early intervention in psychosis, namely early detection and optimal, intensive and sustained intervention during the early years of illness, are relevant to bipolar disorders.

Nevertheless, much remains to be explored, and certain basic concepts that are crucial to the development of early intervention need clarification in the context of bipolar disorders. In particular, while the definition of the bipolar spectrum of disorders has received extensive attention (Akiskal, 1999), much less has been achieved in characterizing the various phases leading from the onset of the initial symptoms to the full-blown disorder. Moreover, the study of prodromal manifestations and early phases of bipolar disorders is particularly complex owing to some of the characteristics of the disorder itself.

In this chapter, we review the arguments justifying the development of early intervention in bipolar disorders and then summarize knowledge gathered about the onset of bipolar disorders. We attempt to develop a concept that would facilitate research in this area and provide a basis for a new treatment approach. Importantly, it must be mentioned that 'early intervention in bipolar disorders', the focus of this chapter, is distinct from 'intervention in early-onset bipolar disorders'. The latter group form a controversial subset of bipolar disorders with onsets during childhood. They may also justify specific treatment strategies, but they will not be discussed here.

Rationale for early intervention in bipolar disorders

Until recently, it was considered that bipolar disorders were characterized not only by their cyclic nature but also by full recovery between acute episodes,

The Recognition and Management of Early Psychosis: A Preventive Approach, ed. Henry J. Jackson and Patrick D. McGorry.
Published by Cambridge University Press. © Cambridge University Press 2009.

Table 13.1. Outcome after a manic episode in multiple and first-episode mania

Source	Setting	Results
Multi-episode mania		
Tsuang *et al.*, 1979	Field follow-up of 685 patients with schizophrenia, affective disorders and non-psychiatric conditions over 30–40 years	24% failed to return to work up to 30 years after manic episode
Keck *et al.*, 1998	Outcome in 134 bipolar I patients 12 months after manic or mixed episode	48% syndromic recovery, 26% symptomatic recovery, 24% functional recovery
Dion *et al.*, 1988	Outcome in 44 patients with bipolar I 6 months after manic episode	80% resolution manic syndrome, 43% returned to professional activity, 21% returned to previous employment level
Tohen *et al.* 1990a	Outcome 4 years after manic episode	Marked discrepancy between symptomatic and functional outcome remained after 4 years
First-episode mania		
Dion *et al.*, 1988	Outcome at 6 months in 14 patients	85% symptomatic remission, 64% returned to professional activity
Tohen *et al.*, 1992	Outcome at 6 months	85% symptomatic remission, 68% returned to premorbid functional level
Strakowski *et al.*, 1998	Outcome 12 months after first hospitalization in 109 patients with an affective psychosis	56% syndromic remission, 35% symptomatic remission, 35% functional recovery
Tohen *et al.*, 2000a	Outcome at 6 months	86% syndromal remission, 33% returned to premorbid functional level
Tohen *et al.*, 2000b	Outcome at 24 months	98% syndromal remission, 40% returned to premorbid functional level
Conus *et al.*, 2006a	Outcome at 12 months	90% syndromal remission, 60% symptomatic remission, 39% functional recovery

and globally by a rather favourable outcome. Many relatively recent publications have come to challenge this assumption for an important subset of patients (Coryell *et al.*, 1993; Dion *et al.*, 1988; Harrow *et al.*, 1990; Tsuang, Woolson & Fleming, 1979; Tohen *et al.*, 1990a). Various factors have contributed to the development of a more realistic view of bipolar disorders. One of them is the development of a more critical exploration of outcome (Table 13.1). While most studies have focused on the observation of the relatively rapid disappearance of manic symptoms, Tsuang *et al.* (1979) were among the first to observe that 24% of patients failed to return to work for up to 30 years after the first manic episode. Similarly, Dion *et al.* (1988) observed 44 patients: while 35 (80%) had no manic symptoms 6 months after hospitalization for a manic episode, only 19 (43%) had a job, and

only 9 (21%) worked at their level of premorbid competence. Such a discrepancy between syndromal and functional outcome has been replicated many times since (Coryell *et al.*, 1993; Harrow *et al.*, 1990; Keck *et al.*, 1998; Strakowski *et al.*, 1998; Tohen *et al.*, 1990a, 2000a). However, it should be mentioned that most of these studies were conducted in private clinics and, therefore, in selected populations, which do not include more ill and refractory individuals. Follow-up studies in broader, more naturalistic and representative samples are needed to confirm if these findings are generally applicable.

Very few studies have explored outcome after a first manic episode. All of them outline a similar discrepancy between syndromal remission (not meeting criteria for a manic syndrome according to the *Diagnostic and Statistical Manual of Mental*

Disorders, 4th edn (DSM-IV; APA, 1994) criteria), symptomatic remission (absence of significant symptoms) and functional recovery (return to premorbid level of functioning). For example, Tohen *et al.* (2000a), in the frame of the McLean–Harvard First Episode Project, have explored outcome after a first manic episode. They found that only 33% of patients had returned to their previous functional level 6 months after a first manic episode, although 86% had recovered from the manic syndrome (Tohen *et al.*, 2000a). At 24 months after the initial manic episode, while 98% had fully recovered from the manic syndrome, only 40% met the criteria for functional recovery (Tohen *et al.*, 2000b). These data confirmed previous results (Dion *et al.*, 1988; Strakowski *et al.*, 1998; Tohen *et al.*, 1990b, 1992). A recent analysis of the outcome of bipolar patients treated for a first manic episode at the Early Psychosis Prevention and Intervention Centre (EPPIC) in Melbourne, Australia, between 1989 and 1997 showed similar results, in that 90% of patients achieved syndromal remission at 6 and 12 months but 40% did not meet symptomatic remission criteria at these points, mainly because of a host of anxiety and depressive features (Conus *et al.*, 2006a). Moreover, 66% of patients at 6 months and 61% of patients at 12 months failed to return to previous levels of functioning. Shorter duration of untreated psychosis predicted better symptomatic outcome, while younger age at intake, family history of affective disorder, illicit drug use and absence of functional recovery at 6 months predicted poorer functional outcome at 12 months (Conus *et al.*, 2006a). These results are in keeping with data from Tohen *et al.* (1990b) and Coryell *et al.* (1993), who showed that psychosocial impairment extends to all areas of functioning.

It should be mentioned, however, that various factors, such as increased prevalence of substance abuse and a possible deleterious effect of certain forms of pharmacological treatment, may have induced a deterioration in the outcome of mania over the last century (Zarate *et al.*, 2000). It appears that the prescription of antidepressants has contributed to an increase in manic relapses (Angst, 1985) and rapid cycling (Goodwin & Jamison, 1990). Additionally, excessive prescription of typical neuroleptic drugs appears to be associated with an increased rate of depressive episodes (Kukopulos *et al.*, 1980) and poorer functional outcome (Tohen *et al.*, 1990a). It is also possible that living in a more complex society, decreased social support, stigma related to mental illness and high rates of unemployment in certain countries hampers return to work. Finally, in some countries, the process of de-institutionalization, without a corresponding increase in community care, may have an additional role in reducing access to necessary ongoing care.

Nevertheless, the occurrence of such a poor outcome after a first manic episode is of significance and establishes the need for development of new treatment strategies. In 1990, Goodwin and Jamison commented that, notwithstanding difficulties in distinguishing early signs of the illness from 'normal' manifestation of adolescence, attempting to identify these signs was of paramount importance considering the potential beneficial impact of an early start of treatment on later outcome. Certain treatment principles developed in the frame of early intervention in psychotic disorders seem to have the potential to bring us a little closer to this ideal. It is, therefore, important to determine if targets identified in early psychosis are relevant to bipolar illness and can be adapted to the treatment of these disorders.

Are targets for early intervention in psychotic disorders relevant to bipolar disorders?

Early intervention in psychosis has two main objectives: (1) to decrease the delay to initiation of treatment (through early detection and engagement of new patients, and if possible detection of high-risk individuals in order to provide preventive treatment) and (2) to provide optimal and specific management for this early phase of the illness. There are some data to indicate that these objectives may have equal applicability to bipolar disorders, and that patients may benefit from treatments based on similar principles. These arguments are discussed in the following sections.

Need for early detection of new cases: treatment delay in bipolar disorders

The occurrence of a long delay between the onset of psychotic symptoms and the start of treatment in psychosis, and its implications, have been discussed in detail in Chs. 8–10. Strategies to overcome this hurdle and their efficacy have also been described in these chapters. Various studies on bipolar disorders converge to show that, on average, there is a very long delay between the onset of the illness and the time when adequate levels of care are given (Baethege *et al.*, 2003; Egeland *et al.*, 1987; Post *et al.*, 2003). For example, Post *et al.* (2003, p. 317) reported an 'average of 10 years between first symptoms meeting diagnostic threshold and first treatment', and Baethege *et al.* (2003) found an average mean latency of 9.3 years between first medical contact for the mood disorder and the commencement of treatment with a mood stabilizer.

Various factors can be responsible for such a delay in diagnosing bipolar disorders. First, the index episode of illness is depressive in the majority of patients, and, as a consequence, the most common initial diagnosis is of unipolar depression (Lish *et al.*, 1994). Second, because of the often atypical clinical presentation of mania (high rate of mixed episodes, presence of irritability and flight of ideas rather than the typical euphoria and grandiosity, high rate of psychotic symptoms and comorbidities), many professionals fail to identify mania in adolescents and young adults (Joyce, 1984). Third, hypomania is often pleasant and not associated with impairment and, therefore, not mentioned by patients (Berk *et al.*, 2006). Fourth, the presence of substance-abuse comorbidity may deflect diagnostic attention (Berk *et al.*, 2006). Finally, delay is sometimes not linked to failed diagnosis but rather to patients' reluctance to ask for mental healthcare. For example, ten Have *et al.* (2002), in the Netherlands Mental Health Survey and Incidence Study on bipolar disorders in the Dutch general population, observed that only 4 out of 10 patients with bipolar disorder had contacted mental heath services in order to receive care. Moreover, a large percentage of those who established contact with mental health services did not present complaints related to their bipolar disorder, an observation already made by Lish *et al.* (1994).

Case vignette

John was 14 when his teachers began to complain about his disruptive behaviour. He had started skipping school and smoking cannabis and his parents noticed periods of irritability when he was going out all night with his friends, and others where he withdrew and avoided contact. When he was 17, he was admitted for the first time to hospital after a week of sleepless nights where he was smoking a lot, listening to loud music and speaking to himself in his room. He was very agitated and convinced his mind was controlled by aliens who wanted him to fulfil a special mission. He was diagnosed with a first episode of psychosis, recovered quickly from his psychotic symptoms and was discharged with a neuroleptic treatment that he stopped a week after discharge. Between 17 and 21 years of age, he was admitted four times with a similar clinical presentation and was diagnosed with schizophrenia. During his sixth admission when he was 22, clinicians realized that the successive periods of irritability and withdrawal corresponded to manic and depressive phases of a bipolar disorder; a mood stabilizer was introduced, and since then John has begun to progress towards stability.

Consequences of delayed diagnosis

First, some authors have suggested that there may be a reduction in the effect of lithium with increasing delay between onset of the disorder and the instigation of medication (Post *et al.*, 2003). This issue is still debated, however, since other authors have failed to find such an association (Baethege *et al.*, 2003; Baldessarini, Tondo & Hennen, 2003). Whatever the case may be, most authors agree that delay in treatment is linked to poorer social adjustment, a higher number of hospitalizations (Goldberg & Ernst, 2002), increased risk of suicide, development of comorbidities, forensic complications and global impairment of the capacity to face developmental tasks (Conus & McGorry, 2002). Second, increasing numbers of episodes are also associated with a shortening of the frequency of the cycle (Angst, Felder & Lohmeyer, 1980; Roy-Byrne *et al.*, 1985; Zis *et al.*, 1980). This may be linked to Post's (1992) neurosensitization model, which suggests that an increasing number of relapses produces not only acute modifications but also more permanent alterations in neuronal activity, possibly transduced at the level of gene expression. These alterations, in turn, might induce a higher tendency to relapse, and possibly a poorer response to medication. Third, delayed identification of bipolar disorder and misdiagnosis with unipolar depression can lead to the prescription of antidepressant therapy, which can induce rapid cycling, mania, mixed states and treatment resistance (Ghaemi, Ko & Goodwin, 2002). Fourth, misdiagnosis may also lead to inadequate psychoeducation, inappropriate medication regimens (which, in turn, may have a negative effect on outcome) and rejection from clinicians when symptoms are mislabelled as behavioural issues. Finally, untreated illness may interfere with the attainment of age-specific social, psychological and educational developmental goals (Macneil, 2004).

Optimal treatment of the first episode: are there specific treatment guidelines for the early phase of bipolar disorders?

As Malla and Norman (2001) pointed out, early intervention is not only about intervening early; it should also involve the development of specific treatment strategies. Recent developments in early intervention strategies have revealed the need for specific pharmacological guidelines. For example, it has been shown that lower doses of antipsychotic medication have similar efficacy but a much lower risk of side effects in early psychosis than doses usually prescribed to patients with more chronic disorders (Malla & Norman, 2001; Remington, Kapur & Zipursky, 1998). Additionally, in order to improve outcome, first-episode patients need specific psychological treatment programmes geared towards not only the phase of illness but also the stage of psychosocial development and its associated needs and difficulties (Macneil, 2004).

Current guidelines

Current treatment strategies for bipolar disorders have been developed mainly on the basis of studies conducted in populations of patients with chronic disorder (APA, 2002). Unlike in other medical disciplines such as oncology, psychiatry generally does not use staging

models to delineate phase-specific treatment needs. To our knowledge, none of the official guidelines for treatment of bipolar disorders makes mention of specific strategies for the early phase of the illness, neither concerning medication nor regarding psychological approaches (Conus, Berk & McGorry, 2006b). The only guideline elements that can be derived from the most recent version of the *Practice Guidelines for the Treatment of Patients with Bipolar Disorder*, published by the American Psychiatric Association (APA, 2002) and that can apply to the early phase of bipolar disorders can be summarized as follows.

1. Mood stabilizers (lithium or valproate) should be used during the acute manic phase and continued for at least 6 months after a single manic episode, or 18 months in children and adolescents.

2. Antipsychotic medication should be used in association with mood stabilizers according to the severity of the episode and/or the presence of psychotic symptoms.

3. When entering the maintenance phase of the treatment, need for ongoing antipsychotic medication should be reassessed. Although atypical antipsychotic drugs are sometimes considered for maintenance therapy, definitive evidence that their efficacy as maintenance treatment is comparable to that of lithium or valproate is still missing.

It is worth noting that this last recommendation is likely to change given the recent publication of evidence that atypicals indeed do have maintenance efficacy. For example, olanzapine has been shown to have comparable efficacy to lithium (Tohen *et al.*, 2005), and has been reported to be superior to placebo in prevention of mania, depression and overall relapse in randomised designs (Tohen *et al.*, 2003a,b, 2004).

In addition, a few recent publications have proposed guidelines for the treatment of first-episode psychosis but some of the proposed strategies still need to be studied in the frame of randomized controlled trials (Lambert *et al.*, 2003; National Early Psychosis Project, 1998; Royal Australian and New Zealand College of Psychiatrists, 2005; International Early Psychosis Association Writing Group, 2005). The guidelines published by the Canadian Network for Mood and Anxiety Treatments (Yatham *et al.*, 2005) provide more up-to-date information regarding issues such as the role of atypical antipsychotic medication in the acute and maintenance phases. Nevertheless, they also fail to address the issues specifically related to the early phase of the disorder.

Current practice

These limited guidelines do not seem to reflect current practice for the treatment of first-episode mania, principally regarding the use of antipsychotic medication. Despite the availability of benzodiazepines to help to control agitation in the acute phase, and regardless of the above-mentioned recommendation that antipsychotic drugs should be used only during acute manic phases with psychotic features, or in particularly severe manic or mixed episodes, antipsychotic drugs remain the most commonly prescribed adjunctive treatment for mania (Conus & McGorry, 2002). Zarate *et al.* (2000) found that patients with first-episode mania were as likely as those with first-episode non-affective psychosis to receive antipsychotic drugs, although usually at lower dosage. Moreover, they found that 77% of these patients with first-episode mania received antipsychotic medication at discharge and 25% were still receiving it at the 6-month follow-up. In populations with chronic disorder and 6 months after hospitalization for a manic episode, 68% to 95% of patients who have been prescribed antipsychotic drugs are still taking them, and usage in up to 67% has been observed during the maintenance phase (Sernyak *et al.*, 1994; Verdoux *et al.*, 1996). This is a matter of concern for various reasons. First, bipolar patients have a high susceptibility to tardive dyskinesia if they take typical antipsychotic drugs (Keck, McElroy & Strakowski, 2000). Second, if these drugs rather than benzodiazepines are used for acute control of behaviour, they tend to be prescribed at high dosages and this can induce extrapyramidal syndromes and lead to prolonged alienation of patients from treatment. Additionally, Craig *et al.* (2004) found that patients who were prescribed typical antipsychotic medication ended up with poorer scores on the Global Assessment of Functioning (APA, 1994) at outcome and spent less time in remission. Zarate *et al.* (2000) also found that prolonged prescription of typical neuroleptic drugs after remission of mania had a detrimental effect (increased risk of side effects, dysphoria, depressive symptoms, shorter time to depressive relapse). Atypical antipsychotic agents constitute a promising alternative to typical neuroleptics for use in acute bipolar mania (Mensink & Sloof, 2004). Their mood-stabilizing capacities still need to be studied (Mahli *et al.*, 2005). Unfortunately, atypical antipsychotic drugs also induce side effects, such as somnolence, hyperprolactinaemia, osteoporosis, dyslipidaemia, weight gain and diabetes, and even extrapyramidal symptoms (Mahli *et al.*, 2005).

Guidelines for prescription of mood stabilizers

Because of the high risk of relapse after a first manic episode and the deleterious effect of multiple episodes on outcome, current guidelines suggest maintenance therapy should be proposed after a first manic episode (Yatham *et al.*, 2005). Additionally, the notion that mood stabilizers have a primary neuroprotective function is gaining currency (Hennion *et al.*, 2002). There is ample neuroimaging data regarding structural changes in bipolar disorder (Monkul, Mahli & Soares, 2005), and recent data suggest that atypical agents prevent structural changes in first-episode psychosis (Lieberman *et al.*, 2005). Similarly, there are data suggesting that lithium and valproate can prevent tissue loss in the amygdala in paediatric bipolar disorders (Chang *et al.*, 2005). If further research confirms these findings, it could strongly support the idea of early initiation of maintenance therapy. However, considering the difficulties most young patients have accepting a diagnosis of bipolar disorder after a first manic episode, the poor adherence rates to lithium in first-episode cohorts and the risk of a rebound episode on abrupt discontinuation, this guideline is often hard to follow in clinical practice.

Treatment adherence

Finally, another dimension of pharmacological treatment, namely adherence to prescribed medication, deserves specific attention. Non-adherence to treatment is known to be an important problem in any medical or psychiatric condition and has been identified as one of the major risk factors for relapse in bipolar disorders.

Basco and Rush (1995) showed that the rate of non-adherence with mood stabilizers was close to 50%. In a cohort of 101 patients hospitalized for acute mania, Keck *et al.* (1996) demonstrated that 64 (64%) were non-adherent to their medication in the month prior to admission. They also found that treatment adherence was associated with higher rates of recovery and more rapid recovery (Keck *et al.*, 1998). In first-episode patients, the rate of non-adherence seems to be even higher and is reported by some authors to be as high as 57% (Cochran, 1984). Among the 83 bipolar patients in a cohort of 109 patients with a first episode of an affective disorder, Strakowski *et al.* (1998) reported that 41% were fully adherent, 26% partially and 33% totally non-adherent. Craig *et al.* (2004) found that 43% of patients were non-adherent to mood stabilizers at 6 months. These numbers might be explained by various factors. First, denial is an associated feature of the illness. It is common for individuals to have a number of episodes before accepting the implications of the recurrent nature of the illness. Furthermore, lifestyle change involved in taking prophylactic medication represents a major challenge, especially for young people. This underlines the need to develop psychosocial interventions aimed at the specific needs of this group of individuals (Macneil, 2004). The impact of non-adherence on outcome of first-episode mania has not been well studied. Strakowski *et al.* (1998) found that syndromal recovery was more likely to occur for patients with full adherence than for those with partial adherence. The impact of total non-adherence is more difficult to assess because non-adherent patients tend to drop out of research studies altogether. Moreover, non-adherence rarely occurs in isolation and is often combined with other poor prognostic factors such as substance abuse, and might then have an indirect as well as a direct effect on outcome. It is, however, possible that adherence may be a marker of other behaviours or illness characteristics modulating outcome.

Case vignette

Amanda was admitted for the first time when she was 19 years old. She had become progressively agitated and restless over the last month, and hardly slept more than 3 hours a night during the few days preceding admission. She was spending most evenings going out partying without experiencing any feelings of tiredness. On the day of admission, she got into an argument in a shop after she had tried on clothes for more than 2 hours and pretended to leave with various items without paying. On the ward she was over-familiar with the nursing staff, disinhibited and irritable, and her thoughts were accelerated. After long negotiations, she finally accepted medication and was given benzodiazepine first and then sodium valproate. While manic symptoms decreased, she agreed she had gotten carried away at some point but rejected the idea of having had a manic episode. She said she was feeling better than ever and that she had finally overcome her shyness. After discharge, she rapidly discontinued medication, and told her case manager that it made her feel depressed and tired. She also said she missed the time when she was feeling high, and she minimized her disturbed behaviour before admission.

Defining targets for early intervention in bipolar disorders

Based on the previous two sections, it seems clear that early intervention strategies are justified in the treatment of bipolar disorders. However, as mentioned, one of the main challenges in the development of such strategies is to formulate a better definition of the various stages of the disorder, which leads from a vulnerability status to the initial onset-phase and then to the full-blown disorder. The task is made difficult by the nature of the disorder and its cyclical aspects. First, the initial manifestation of bipolar disorders can take many shapes, ranging most commonly from depressive episodes of varying intensity to mania of abrupt onset, both of which can be very hard to diagnose (Berk *et al.*, 2006). In many other cases, onset may be much less clear-cut and manifest as ill-defined mood disturbances. Even though the sensitivity of such symptoms may be significant, their specificity is very low, and they may be very hard to distinguish from manifestations of early adolescence, normal reactions to life events, or early signs of other disorders.

Therefore, one of the main challenges is to diagnose these initial manifestations properly in order to determine which one will eventually lead towards bipolar disorder and, thus, to initiate proper treatment as soon as possible. In this context it may prove useful to apply a combined strategy: (1) to develop a better characterization of the signature of bipolar depression, allowing prospective identification of bipolarity in individuals presenting with depression; (2) to gather more extensive knowledge about initial manic manifestations of the disorder; and (3) to explore and define the more progressive forms of onset, which by analogy with early psychosis could be defined as the 'initial prodrome' to bipolar disorder.

Bipolar depression

As discussed above, depression is the most common type of onset in bipolar I patients (Perugi *et al.*, 2000). Additionally, in bipolar disorder, the bulk of morbidity is in the depressive phase of the disorder. Finally, the ratio of depressive to manic episodes in bipolar I disorder is 3:1, whereas in bipolar II disorder the ratio of depression to hypomania is 47:1 (Judd *et al.*, 2002). This creates a scenario where young people with developing bipolar disorder present with depression and are inevitably at risk of being misdiagnosed as unipolar. This is a concern, considering that antidepressants can induce mania, mixed states and rapid cycling in susceptible individuals; that antidepressant-induced manias are more likely to be dysphoric than euphoric (Berk & Dodd, 2005); that mania in young people is indeed more likely to be dysphoric (Wozniak, Biederman & Richards., 2001); and finally, that suicidal risk is disproportionately high in mixed states (Berk & Dodd, 2005). For these reasons, the development of strategies allowing an accurate and early diagnosis of bipolarity in depressed young individuals is critical and is an important target for early intervention.

First-episode mania

A major reason for latency between onset and treatment in bipolar disorders is the failure to identify mania in young patients, which can be explained by various factors. First, the clinical presentation of mania is frequently atypical in adolescents and young adults, with high rates of mixed episodes, as evidenced by irritability and increase in energy and flight of ideas rather than euphoria and grandiosity (Akiskal *et al.*, 2003; Wozniak *et al.*, 2001). Second, mild mania is uncommonly a source of distress and, therefore, seldom a focus of clinical attention. Third, disruptive behaviour in mania can overlap phenomenologically with personality disorders: symptoms and diagnosis can easily be mistaken for cluster B personality traits and disorders in patients with recurrent and long-standing behavioural disturbances, unstable personal relationships and periodic affective symptoms (Tryer & Brittlebank, 1993). Akiskal (1981) showed that secondary personality dysfunction can develop in the context of prolonged affective disturbances and can be confused with personality disorder. Fourth, there is also a high rate of comorbidity and overlap with manifestations of other disorders, such as attention deficit hyperactivity disorder, anxiety, substance-use disorder and antisocial behaviour (Wozniak *et al.*, 2001). Finally, younger patients present with a higher rate of psychotic symptoms (Joyce, 1984), more often of a mood-incongruent nature (McGlashan, 1988). For example, in a sample of 108 patients with first-episode psychotic mania treated at EPPIC between 1987 and 1995, Conus *et al.* (2004) found high rates of mood-incongruent psychotic symptoms, persecutory delusions and Schneiderian symptoms, not only in those with a diagnosis of schizoaffective disorder (100%, 86%, and 81%, respectively) but also in those with a diagnosis of bipolar disorder (74%, 69%, and 59%, respectively). Such a presentation leads to a high rate of misdiagnosis, most often with schizophrenia, but also with conduct disorders, attention deficit hyperactivity disorder and antisocial or borderline personality disorders. Clinicians need to be more aware of these elements in order to be able to consider a diagnosis of mania, even if the clinical presentation is not dominated by euphoria and grandiosity; this, in turn, may allow an earlier and more accurate identification of bipolar disorders.

Initial prodrome to bipolar disorder

As mentioned above, in many cases it appears that bipolar disorders develop in a progressive manner. As a first step, it might prove useful to apply the concepts of 'prodrome' and 'onset' to bipolar disorders as they have been used for psychosis in general and schizophrenia in particular. The 'prodrome' can be defined as the period of disturbance that represents a deviation from a person's previous experience and behaviour, prior to the development of the threshold features of a disorder. By comparison, the 'onset' can be more difficult to define in bipolar spectrum disorders. For example, it might become clear only much later and retrospectively that an initial depressive episode was actually the first manifestation of a bipolar I disorder.

As a first approach, it might prove useful to draw an analogy between first-episode mania and first-episode psychosis. The first psychotic episode must occur for the clinician to make the diagnosis of a psychotic disorder (and is absolutely necessary, for example, for schizophrenia to be diagnosed) and gives coherence to earlier manifestations of the illness once they can be put in the context of the prodromal phase. Similarly, the first manic episode marks the diagnosis of a bipolar I disorder. What happens during the pre-manic phase – episodes of subthreshold or threshold depression, hypomania or anxiety syndromes, for example – could be considered as the initial prodrome to bipolar I disorders and become a key target for early intervention. However, a key challenge is that, as in prodromal schizophrenia, potential early symptoms of bipolar disorder such as depression and anxiety are both widespread and of low specificity. Additionally, they are more likely to follow an intermittent, rather than a continuous, pattern. Mild mania, while specific, is ego-syntonic, rarely distressing and consequently seldom reported. Moreover, such definitions have limitations and are difficult to apply to other disorders of the bipolar spectrum, such as bipolar II disorders. Nevertheless, they might allow the exploration of the initial phase of the illness and be further refined and adapted at a second stage.

Where do we go from here?

In summary, treatment of the early phase of bipolar disorders currently lacks specificity, and most published guidelines fail to differentiate treatment strategies early in the course from those recommended for later stages. The important issues of inaccurate and delayed identification of the disorder, delayed prescription of mood stabilizers, unclear ideal duration of mood-stabilizer treatment, high use of antipsychotic medication and, finally, poor adherence to treatment have been described above. Additionally, there are specific psychological and social issues associated with the onset phase of the disorder that are not specifically addressed by currently available psychological interventions. All these elements suggest there is an urgent need for research and development in early intervention in bipolar disorders. Various strategies that could be applied to face this challenge within the broader framework of early intervention strategies in psychiatry are discussed below.

Earlier identification of bipolar disorders

Earlier identification of the disorder would allow psychological and pharmacological treatment to be commenced sooner, with the potential to reduce the neurobiological and psychosocial collateral damage caused by prolonged duration of untreated illness. Additionally, medication could be introduced in a phase where it may be more efficacious. Two strategies might have an impact on delayed identification of bipolar disorders: improved identification of first-episode mania and of bipolar depression.

Improved identification of first-episode mania

Mania often has an atypical mixed or dysphoric presentation during adolescence and early adulthood. Clinicians should be more aware of this problem, and replication and extension of studies focusing on the particular clinical presentation of first-episode mania are useful in this regard. However, such studies aiming at identifying and refining the characterization of discrete syndromes have their limitations. As mentioned by McGorry (1995a), current categorical classifications for mental disorders do not fit well with the clinical presentation of initial psychotic disorders; this certainly also applies to affective psychoses and bipolar disorders. It may, therefore, prove useful to develop diagnostic approaches based on a dimensional concept. In this frame, the 'affective dimension' of a clinical presentation may constitute a valid and useful additional target for early intervention.

Identification of bipolar depression

There is currently limited knowledge regarding the characteristics of depressive episodes that might presage the future development of bipolar illness. Strober and Carlson (1982) examined a cohort of 60 adolescents with major depression and found that the presence of mood-congruent psychotic features, psychomotor retardation, rapid onset and pharmacologically induced hypomania was associated with a higher risk of developing bipolar illness. More recently, Berk *et al.* (2004) reviewed the literature relevant to this issue and pointed out the following features of bipolar depression: early age of onset, abrupt onset/offset, psychomotor retardation (altered emotional reactivity, delay in verbal response, slowed movements), melancholic symptoms (worthlessness, unvarying mood, marked anhedonia), atypical depressive symptoms (hypersomnia, hyperphagia, leaden paralysis) and other features such as irritability, mixed states, lability and high level of recurrence. A new Bipolar Depression Rating Scale has been developed that should contribute to resolving this issue (Berk *et al.*, 2007). Screening instruments for hypomania such as the Mood Disorder Questionnaire (Hirschfeld *et al.*, 2003a) would also be a valuable additional component to routine care to detect potential bipolarity in young individuals presenting with depressive symptoms.

Identification of the initial prodrome to bipolar disorders

While an important body of literature has been published on the warning signs of manic relapses, the 'initial prodrome' to bipolar disorders has received little attention. Various approaches can be proposed to explore this phase of the illness. Akiskal *et al.* (1985) prospectively followed 68 juvenile offspring or siblings of bipolar patients with mood symptoms. They observed an often insidious onset of bipolar disorder in

late childhood, adolescence or early adulthood, with relatively minor oscillations in mood that were mainly depressive in nature. It could be argued, however, that the restriction of the study to offspring of bipolar patients might limit the relevance of the findings to be only applicable for patients with a family history of bipolar disorder, which is not true for all bipolar patients. The most systematic and detailed study of the initial prodrome to bipolar disorder to date comes from Egeland *et al.* (2000), who as part of a broader Amish study examined medical histories of 58 bipolar I patients. They were able to identify a range of symptoms and behaviours predating the onset of illness: episodic changes in mood (depressed mood 53%, anger dyscontrol 38%, irritable mood 33%) and energy (increased energy 47%, decreased energy 38%) were the most consistently reported. These were followed by bold/intrusive behaviours (29%), excessive behaviours (28%), conduct problems (28%), decreased sleep (26%), crying (26%) and oversensitivity (24%). The strengths of this study are its inclusion only of patients formally diagnosed with bipolar disorder, and its use of data spontaneously provided during the early phase of illness. However, it is limited by its reliance on file data rather than on a standardized interview, and by the fact that social history was provided by informants rather than by the patients themselves. This may have led to an overemphasis on observable behavioural changes and neglect of depression or more subjective aspects of prodrome and onset. Additionally, the study was conducted within an Amish population; young people who develop bipolar disorders and live in more standard conditions are highly likely to have an added smoke-screen of substance abuse added into the clinical picture, making early diagnosis even more difficult. A study is currently underway at EPPIC that aims to assess retrospectively the 12 months preceding a first manic episode in a cohort with a first episode of bipolar mania, in order to identify possible clinical markers of an at-risk mental state (Conus *et al.*, 2006c).

In contrast to these retrospective studies, Thompson *et al.* (2003) have provided prospectively collected data about the development of manic episodes in three patients who developed bipolar I or II disorder during their treatment in a clinic specializing in patients at ultra high risk of developing psychosis (Yung *et al.*, 2003). A review of the case descriptions reveals that all three patients presented with an initial depressive episode and reported some degree of anxiety and paranoia prior to their inclusion in the clinic. Other symptoms that either emerged or were evident during the three patients' 12 months of treatment included mood swings (in two), racing thoughts (in two), increased activity/energy (in two), decreased energy/tiredness (in two), disturbed sleep (in two), distractibility/difficulty concentrating (in two), and perceptual changes (in two). A range of comorbid diagnoses were also present. These symptoms are generally in keeping with those of the retrospective reports (Egeland *et al.*, 2000) but it is important to note that there were no specific prodromal features that clearly distinguished patients who developed bipolar disorder from those who developed other psychoses such as schizophrenia. Other limitations of this study include its very small sample size and its focus on early psychosis rather than exclusively on bipolar disorders, which implies the use of assessment tools that may not have been specific enough to capture various aspects of the pre-manic mood prodrome.

It is important to note that this approach, as well as the methods used in studies mentioned above, have important limitations; for example, none of them used a matched control group of participants who do not go on to develop bipolar disorder, and there are problems with retrospective recall as it introduces subjective bias and also relies upon the patient's memory. Additionally, Bellivier *et al.* (2003) demonstrated in a consecutive series of 368 patients that it is possible to differentiate, based on the age of onset, three subgroups of bipolar disorders: (1) an early age of onset group (mean age 17.4 years), (2) those with a medium age of onset (mean age 25.1 years), and (3) those with late age of onset (mean age 40.4 years). This may further complicate the exploration of the prodromal phase, since it is likely that each of these subgroups go through distinct and specific prodromal phases. For example, it has been shown that the 'early presentation' category tends to be associated with early comorbid forms of presentation, higher levels of functional impairments and more frequent psychotic symptoms

(Carlson, Bromet & Sievers, 2000). However, despite these difficulties and limitations, these works open a new field of research and pave the way for more sophisticated research protocols. Once potential high-risk profile(s) for bipolar disorders can be defined, the next step would be to explore their validity and specificity in the context of larger prospective high-risk studies.

Development of specific guidelines for the treatment of the early phase of bipolar disorders

Pharmacological treatment

Pharmacological treatment of the early phase of bipolar disorders needs to be more extensively studied in order to develop phase-specific guidelines. Each phase defined above may then constitute a specific stage of the disorder where distinct treatment strategies would apply.

The identification of patients going through a *prodromal phase* would allow the study of biological events occurring during this critical phase (e.g. modifications of brain structure or gene expression) or the identification of psychosocial factors that might be linked to the emergence and development of the disorder. This, in turn, could lead to the development of potential preventive strategies such as neuroprotective agents, psychosocial interventions or primary prevention of secondary substance-use disorder (Thompson *et al.*, 2003). If identification of *bipolar depression* can be improved, the issue of initiation of mood stabilizers in young people with a suspected bipolar basis to their depression could be explored. This would contribute to avoidance of the risk of development of mixed or dysphoric mania and consequent suicidal tendencies under antidepressant treatment. No such trials have been conducted though they are strongly needed (Baldessarini *et al.*, 2003; Geller *et al.*, 2004). In *first-episode mania*, it would be useful to compare the efficacy and effectiveness of mood stabilizers as well as to define the ideal duration of prophylaxis after a first manic episode. Studies are needed on antipsychotic treatment (1) to define the need for, and the optimal duration of, antipsychotic treatment both in psychotic and non-psychotic mania; (2) to compare typical and atypical antipsychotic drugs in terms of safety as well as efficacy; and (3) to compare the efficacy and effectiveness of various atypical antipsychotic drugs in both the acute and the maintenance phases. Regarding this last issue, a file audit study recently conducted at EPPIC explored response to treatment in a non-randomized non-controlled naturalistic setting and showed that olanzapine had a higher efficacy than risperidone in first-episode affective (mainly manic) psychoses, leading to lower scores on the Clinical Global Impression scale (Guy, 1976) at the end of the trial, a higher rate of global improvement on this scale and a higher rate of remission of positive symptoms (Lambert *et al.*, 2005). Similarly, the comparative efficacy and effectiveness of mood stabilizers in this population has not been documented. Finally, it is necessary to examine whether atypical agents or traditional mood stabilizers have neuroprotective properties in first-episode patients. The confirmation of the capacity of such agents to prevent the neurostructural, neurocognitive and functional consequences of illness would indeed constitute a critical element in helping to define when, and for how long, they should be prescribed.

Psychological approaches

It must be emphasized that the treatment of the early phase of bipolar disorders should involve considerably more than providing medication. Indeed, there has been recognition of this by a number of organizations including the British Association of Psychopharmacology, the World Federation of Biological Psychiatry and the American Psychiatric Association (Jones, Sellwood & McGovern, 2005). The 1990 US National Institute of Mental Heath (NIMH) report (Prien & Potter, 1990, p. 149) succinctly acknowledged '... it is clear that pharmacotherapy alone does not meet the needs of many bipolar patients'.

In recent years, there has been a growth in research on psychological interventions for bipolar disorder. Specifically, recent reviews have found that individual cognitive–behavioural therapy can have an impact on the symptoms of bipolar disorder, medication

adherence, social functioning and likelihood of relapse (Gonzalez-Pinto *et al.*, 2004; Huxley, Parikh & Baldessarini, 2000; Jones, 2004; Scott & Gutierrez, 2004). Although none of these studies was designed specifically for a first-episode population, an emphasis on the importance of early intervention is supported by the finding by Scott *et al.* (2006) in the largest randomized controlled trial of cognitive–behavioural therapy for bipolar disorder to date, which indicated that this approach was more effective for people who had fewer episodes.

However, the population with first-episode bipolar disorder can provide a clinician with a number of challenges as patients often present with poor insight and high rates of comorbidity with alcohol (Conus & McGorry, 2002) and substance use (Ernst & Goldberg, 2004). Therefore, the clinician may face potential engagement difficulties with a first-episode population, which should be addressed before commencing a psychological intervention. It may be that a focus on the person's explanatory model of their situation, assistance with practical issues (including addressing accommodation, financial and legal issues), and joint goal setting may be required and may assist with enhancing engagement.

Awareness of developmental issues is also essential when providing psychological interventions for people with first-episode bipolar disorder, given that most people develop the disorder in their late teens and early twenties (Burke *et al.* 1990; Hirschfeld, Lewis & Vornik, 2003b; Lish *et al.*, 1994). Specifically, the clinician should attend to the impact of the disorder on the person's developmental trajectory, including their ability to develop independence, and should 'pitch' information or therapeutic interventions appropriately to the person's cognitive and emotional level, and involve family members, who may play a considerable role in the person's life in the treatment process.

It is now commonly accepted that psychoeducation should be regarded as a key element of good practice in the treatment of bipolar disorders. As Colom *et al.* (2003) showed, psychoeducation prevents relapses and hospital admission in euthymic bipolar patients. Psychoeducation as it is conducted today in bipolar disorder integrates the following elements: early detection of the illness (Perry *et al.*, 1999), promotion of regular and adequate lifestyles (Frank *et al.*, 1999), the improvement of therapeutic adherence (Scott & Tacchi, 2002) and treatment of symptoms and the resolution of problems (Lam *et al.*, 2003). All of these elements should be integrated in psychoeducation programmes for bipolar disorders.

However, standardized psychoeducation may require modification for working with a first-episode population. Many individuals with first-episode bipolar disorder may be unwilling to accept their diagnosis, and simply distributing pre-packaged handout material without an understanding of the person's level of insight or an explanatory model may at best be ineffective and at worst damage engagement and the therapeutic relationship, increase likelihood of dropout or lead to catastrophization and over-identification with the disorder. Therefore, it appears that psychoeducation should occur with a strong awareness of what McGorry (1995b, p. 320) referred to as the 'psychoeducational needs' of the person, and should involve '... the provision of the right kind of information, provided flexibly and sensitively to each individual ...'.

In a cohort of 87 patients with first-episode bipolar mania, 35 (41%) failed to reach symptomatic remission after 12 months despite a generally good syndromic recovery, and only 34 (39%) returned to their premorbid level of functioning (Conus *et al.*, 2006a). Patients who remained symptomatic suffered mainly from anxiety, particularly social phobia and restriction of social interactions. Additionally, a significant proportion of patients abused illicit substances and failed to adhere to medication.

Emphasis on functional recovery needs to address these comorbid difficulties and may also involve practical assistance around social and vocational functioning, including liaison with employment, educational and voluntary services to assist people in returning to their level of premorbid functioning. Planning for returning to work or study, including managing anxiety, discussion around how the person will explain their absence and identifying potential stressors, can be valuable. In addition, encouraging return to regular sleep and activity schedules can be important prior to recommencing work or study, as these are often disrupted by the disorder.

Relapse-prevention work with people in the first episode can be challenging, as lack of insight, denial and minimization may be more likely in this population, than in a population who have experienced multiple episodes. Rather than simple symptom monitoring, which can create unnecessary hypervigilance and 'false positives' following a first episode in individuals and their families, attending to the *meaning* associated with risk of relapse can be a valuable intervention. Specifically, identifying the person's beliefs about likelihood of relapse, their perceived control over this and the anticipated outcome should a relapse occur can be an extremely useful focus for psychological intervention.

In summary, psychological interventions with first-episode bipolar disorder can include:

- a strong emphasis on engagement and the importance of developing a positive therapeutic relationship, which can be challenging in the first episode
- awareness of the impact of developmental issues on the presentation of the disorder and its treatment
- involving family members where appropriate, given the likely importance of family members for a first-episode population
- psychoeducation, provided with awareness of its potential impact on the person's sense of self and understanding of the potentially protective nature of denial, and managing this sensitively
- relapse prevention, including discussion of associated affect and the person's beliefs around the likelihood and potential impact of relapse
- emphasis on functional recovery, given that this has been largely neglected to date.

Conclusions

While confirming the dearth of early-intervention strategies and the absence of guidelines for the treatment of the first stages of bipolar disorders, the arguments developed in this chapter show that the principles guiding the approach of early psychosis may also be relevant to bipolar disorders. Specific targets can be identified that need to be defined more clearly in order to provide a framework for future research trials.

Once initiated, this domain of research would open the door to numerous other areas of investigation (brain structure, cognition, functional neurochemistry and neuroprotection) that could both improve our understanding of the nature of bipolar disorders and lead to the development of new treatment approaches of higher efficacy.

REFERENCES

Akiskal, H. S. (1981). Subaffective disorders: dysthymic, cyclothymic and bipolar II disorders in the 'borderline' realm. *Psychiatric Clinics of North America*, **4**, 25–46.

Akiskal, H. S. (1999). Bipolarity: beyond classic mania. *Psychiatric Clinics of North America*, **22**, 512–703.

Akiskal, H. S., Downs, J., Jordan, P. *et al.* (1985). Affective disorders in referred children and younger siblings of manic depressives. Mode of onset and prospective course. *Archives of General Psychiatry*, **42**, 996–1003.

Akiskal, H. S., Hantouche, E. G., Azorin, J. M. *et al.* (2003). Clinical characterization acute mania: data in 1090 patients – 'EPIMAN-II'. *Bipolar Disorders*, **5**(Suppl 1), 27.

APA (1994). *Diagnostic and Statistical Manual of Mental Disorders*, 4th edn. Washington, DC: American Psychiatric Press.

APA (2002). Practice guideline for the treatment of patients with bipolar disorder (revision). *American Journal of Psychiatry*, **159**, 4–50.

Angst, J. (1985). Switch from depression to mania: a record study over decades between 1920 and 1982. *Psychopathology*, **18**, 140–54.

Angst, J., Felder, W. & Lohmeyer, B. (1980). Course of schizoaffective psychoses: results of a followup study. *Schizophrenia Bulletin*, **6**, 579–85.

Baethege, C., Smolka, M. N., Grushka, P. *et al.* (2003). Does prophylaxis-delay in bipolar disorder influence outcome? Results from a long-term study of 147 patients. *Acta Psychiatrica Scandinavica*, **107**, 260–7.

Baldessarini, R. J., Tondo, L. & Hennen, J. (2003). Treatment latency and previous episodes: relationship to pretreatment morbidity and response to maintenance treatment in bipolar I and II disorders. *Bipolar Disorders*, **5**, 169–79.

Basco, M. R. & Rush, A. J. (1995). Compliance with pharmacology in mood disorders. *Psychiatric Annals*, **25**, 269–79.

Bellivier, F., Golmard, J. L., Rietschel, M. *et al.* (2003). Age at onset in bipolar I affective disorder: further evidence for three subgroups. *American Journal of Psychiatry*, **160**, 999–1001.

Berk, M. & Dodd, S. (2005). Are treatment emergent suicidality and decreased response to antidepressants in younger patients due to bipolar disorder being misdiagnosed as unipolar depression? *Medical Hypotheses*, **65**, 39–43.

Berk, M., Malhi, G. S., Mitchell, P. B. *et al.* (2004). Scale matters: the need for a Bipolar Depression Rating Scale (BDRS). *Acta Psychiatrica Scandinavica*, **422**(Suppl), 39–45.

Berk, M., Berk, L., Moss, K., Dodd, S. & Malhi, G. S. (2006). Diagnosing bipolar disorder: how can we do it better? *Medical Journal of Australia*, **184**, 459–62.

Berk, M., Malhi, G. S., Cahill, C. *et al.* (2007). The Bipolar Depression Rating Scale (BDRS): its development, validation and utility. *Bipolar Disorder*, **9**, 571–9.

Burke, K. C., Burke, J. D., Regier, D. A., Rae, D. S. (1990). Age at onset of selected mental disorders in five community populations. *Archives of General Psychiatry*, **47**, 511–18.

Carlson, G. A., Bromet, E. J. & Sievers, S. (2000). Phenomenology and outcome of subjects with early- and adult-onset psychotic mania. *American Journal of Psychiatry*, **157**, 213–19.

Chang, K., Karchemskiy, A., Barnea-Goraly, N. *et al.* (2005). Reduced amygdala gray matter volume in familial pediatric bipolar disorder. *Journal of the American Academy of Child and Adolescent Psychiatry*, **44**, 565–73.

Cochran, S. D. (1984). Preventing medical noncompliance in the outpatient treatment of bipolar affective disorders. *Journal of Consulting and Clinical Psychology*, **52**, 873–8.

Colom, F., Vieta, E., Martinez-Aran, A. *et al.* (2003). A randomized trial on the efficacy of group psychoeducation in the prophylaxis of recurrence in bipolar patients whose disease is in remission. *Archives of General Psychiatry*, **60**, 402–7.

Conus, P. & McGorry, P. D. (2002). First episode mania: a neglected priority for early intervention. *Australian and New Zealand Journal of Psychiatry*, **36**, 158–72.

Conus, P., Abdel-Baki, A., Harrigan, S., Lambert, M. & McGorry, P. D. (2004). Schneiderian first rank symptoms predict poor outcome within first episode manic psychosis. *Journal of Affective Disorders*, **81**, 259–68.

Conus, P., Cotton, S., Abdel-Baki, A. & McGorry, P. D. (2006a). Symptomatic and functional outcome 12 months after a first episode of psychotic mania: barriers to recovery in a catchment area sample. *Bipolar Disorders*, **8**, 221–31.

Conus, P., Berk, M. & McGorry, P. D. (2006b). Pharmacological treatment in the early phase of bipolar disorders: what stage are we at? *Australian and New Zealand Journal of Psychiatry*, **40**, 199–207.

Conus, P., Berk, M., Hallam, K., Lucas, N. & Ward, J. (2006c). The prodrome to first episode psychotic mania: results of a retrospective study. *Schizophrenia Research*, **86**(Suppl), 37.

Coryell, W., Scheftner, W., Keller, M. *et al.* (1993). The enduring psychosocial consequences of mania and depression. *American Journal of Psychiatry*, **150**, 720–7.

Craig, T. J., Grossman, S., Mojtabai, R. *et al.* (2004). Medication use patterns and 2-year outcome in first-admission bipolar disorders with psychotic features. *Bipolar Disorders*, **6**, 406–15.

Dion, G. L., Tohen, M., Anthony, W. A. & Waternaux, C. S. (1988). Symptoms and functioning of patients with bipolar disorder six months after hospitalisation. *Hospital and Community Psychiatry*, **39**, 652–7.

Egeland, J. A., Blumenthal, R. L., Nee, J., Sharpe, L. & Eddincott, J. (1987). Reliability and relationship of various ages of onset criteria for major affective disorders. *Journal of Affective Disorders*, **12**, 159–65.

Egeland, J. A., Hostetter, A. M., Pauls, D. L. & Sussex, J. N. (2000). Prodromal symptoms before onset of manic-depressive disorder suggested by first hospital admission histories. *Journal of the American Academy of Child and Adolescent Psychiatry*, **39**, 1245–52.

Ernst, C. L. & Goldberg, J. F. (2004). Clinical features related to age at onset in bipolar disorder. *Journal of Affective Disorders*, **82**, 21–7.

Frank, E., Swartz, H. A., Mallinger, A. G. *et al.* (1999). Adjunctive psychotherapy for bipolar disorder: effects of changing treatment modality. *Journal of Abnormal Psychology*, **108**, 579–87.

Geller, B., Tillman, R., Craney, J. L. & Bolhofner, K. (2004). Four-year prospective outcome and natural history of mania in children with a prepubertal and early adolescent bipolar disorder phenotype. *Archives of General Psychiatry*, **61**, 459–67.

Ghaemi, S. N., Ko, J. Y. & Goodwin, F. K. (2002). 'Cade's disease' and beyond: misdiagnosis, antidepressant use, and a proposed definition for bipolar spectrum disorder. *Canadian Journal of Psychiatry*, **47**, 125–34.

Goldberg, J. F. & Ernst, C. L. (2002). Features associated with the delayed initiation of mood stabilizers at illness onset in bipolar disorder. *Journal of Clinical Psychiatry*, **63**, 985–91.

Gonzalez-Pinto, A., Gonzalez, C., Enjuto, S. *et al.* (2004). Psychoeducation and cognitive-behavioral therapy in bipolar disorder: an update. *Acta Psychiatrica Scandinavica*, **109**, 83–90.

Goodwin, F. K. & Jamison, K. R. (1990). *Manic–Depressive Illness*. New York: Oxford University Press.

Guy, W. (1976). *ECDEU Assessment Manual for Psychopharmacology*, revised. [*DHEW Publication* No. (ADM) 76–338.] Rockville MD: National Institute of Mental Health.

Harrow, M., Goldberg, J. F., Grossman, L. S. & Meltzer, H. Y. (1990). Outcome in manic disorders. *Archives of General Psychiatry*, **47**, 665–71.

Hennion, J. P., el-Masri, M. A., Huff, M. O. & el-Mailakh, R. S. (2002). Evaluation of neuroprotection by lithium and valproic acid against ouabain-induced cell damage. *Bipolar Disorders*, **4**, 201–6.

Hirschfeld, R. M., Calabrese, J. R., Weissman, M. M. *et al.* (2003a). Screening for bipolar disorder in the community. *Journal of Clinical Psychiatry*, **64**, 53–9.

Hirschfeld, R. M., Lewis, L. & Vornik, L. A. (2003b). Perceptions and impact of bipolar disorder: how far have we really come? Results of the National Depressive and Manic Depressive Association 2000 Survey of Individuals with Bipolar Disorder. *Journal of Clinical Psychiatry*, **64**, 161–74.

Huxley, N. A., Parikh, S. V. & Baldessarini, R. J. (2000). Effectiveness of psychosocial treatments in bipolar disorder: state of the evidence. *Harvard Review of Psychiatry*, **8**, 126–40.

International Early Psychosis Association Writing Group (2005). International clinical practice guidelines for early psychosis. *British Journal of Psychiatry*, **187**(Suppl. 48), 120–4.

Jones, S. (2004). Psychotherapy of bipolar disorder: a review. *Journal of Affective Disorders*, **80**, 101–14.

Jones, S. H., Sellwood, W. & McGovern, J. (2005). Psychological therapies for bipolar disorder: the role of model-driven approaches to therapy integration. *Bipolar Disorders*, **7**, 22–32.

Joyce, P. R. (1984). Age of onset in bipolar affective disorder and misdiagnosis as schizophrenia. *Psychological Medicine*, **14**, 145–9.

Judd, L. L., Akiskal, H. S., Schettler, P. J. *et al.* (2002). The long-term natural history of the weekly symptomatic status of bipolar I disorder. *Archives of General Psychiatry*, **59**, 530–7.

Keck, P. E., McElroy, S. L., Strakowski, S. M. *et al.* (1996). Factors associated with pharmacological noncompliance in patients with mania. *Journal of Clinical Psychiatry*, **57**, 292–7.

Keck, P. E., McElroy, S. L., Strakowski, S. M. *et al.* (1998). 12-month outcome of patients with bipolar disorder following hospitalisation for a manic or mixed episode. *American Journal of Psychiatry*, **155**, 646–52.

Keck, P. E., McElroy, S. L. & Strakowski, S. M. (2000). Antipsychotics in the treatment of mood disorders and risk of tardive dyskinesia. *Journal of Clinical Psychiatry*, **61** (Suppl 4), 33–8.

Kraepelin, E. (1919). *Dementia Praecox*. New York: Churchill Livingstone.

Kukopulos, A., Reginaldi, D., Laddomada, P. *et al.* (1980). Course of the manic–depressive cycle and changes caused by treatments. *Pharmacopsychiatric Neuropsychopharmakologie* **13**, 156–67.

Lam, D. H., Watkins, R., Hayward, P. *et al.* (2003). A randomised controlled study of cognitive therapy for relapse prevention for bipolar affective disorder: outcome of the first year. *Archives of General Psychiatry*, **60**, 145–52.

Lambert, M., Conus, P., Lambert, T. & McGorry, P. D. (2003). Pharmacotherapy of first-episode psychosis. *Expert Opinion on Pharmacotherapy*, **4**, 717–50.

Lambert, M., Conus, P., Eide, P. *et al.* (2005). Treatment of early psychosis with olanzapine or risperidone (TEPOR study): a medical record review study in 367 non-affective and affective first-episode psychosis patients admitted to the Early Psychosis Prevention and Intervention Centre (EPPIC) in Melbourne Australia between 1998–2000. *Pharmacopsychiatry*, **38**, 1–8.

Lieberman, J. A., Tollefson, G. D., Charles, C. *et al.* for the HGDH Study Group (2005). Antipsychotic drug effects on brain morphology in first-episode psychosis. *Archives of General Psychiatry*, **62**, 361–70.

Lish, J. D., Dime-Meenan, S., Whybrow, P. C., Price, R. A. & Hirschfeld, R. M. (1994). The National Depressive and Manic–depressive Association (DMDA) survey of bipolar members. *Journal of Affective Disorders*, **31**, 281–94.

Macneil, C. (2004). Cognitive behavioural therapy with bipolar disorder: theory and reality with a first episode population. *Schizophrenia Research*, **70**(Suppl 1), 92.

Mahli, G. S., Berk, M., Bourin, M. *et al.* (2005). Atypical mood stabilizers: a 'typical' role for atypical antipsychotics. *Acta Psychiatrica Scandinavica*, **426**, 29–38.

Malla, A. M. & Norman, R. M. (2001). Treating psychosis: is there more to early intervention than intervening early? *Canadian Journal of Psychiatry*, **46**, 645–8.

McGlashan, T. H. (1988). Adolescent versus adult onset of mania. *American Journal of Psychiatry*, **145**, 221–3.

McGorry, P. D. (1995a). A treatment relevant classification of psychotic disorders. *Australian and New Zealand Journal of Psychiatry*, **29**, 555–8.

McGorry, P. D. (1995b). Psychoeducation in first episode psychosis: a therapeutic process. *Psychiatry*, **58**, 313–28.

McGorry, P. D. & Jackson, H. J. (1999). *The Recognition and Management of Early Psychosis: A Preventive Approach.* Cambridge, UK: Cambridge University Press.

Mensink, G. J. R. & Sloof, C. J. (2004). Novel antipsychotics in bipolar and schizoaffective mania. *Acta Psychiatrica Scandinavica*, **109**, 405–19.

Monkul, E. S., Malhi, G. S. & Soares, J. C. (2005). Anatomical MRI abnormalities in bipolar disorder: do they exist and do they progress? *Australian and New Zealand Journal of Psychiatry*, **39**, 222–6.

National Early Psychosis Project (1998). *Australian Guidelines for Early Psychosis.* Melbourne: University of Melbourne.

Perry, A., Tarrier, N., Morriss, R., McCarthy, E. & Limb, K. (1999). Randomised controlled trial of efficacy of teaching patients with bipolar disorder to identify early symptoms of relapse and obtain treatment. *British Medical Journal*, **318**, 149–53.

Perugi, G., Micheli, C., Akiskal, H. S. *et al.* (2000). Polarity of the first episode, clinical characteristics, and course of manic depressive illness: a systematic retrospective investigation of 320 bipolar I patients. *Comprehensive Psychiatry*, **41**, 13–18.

Post, R. M. (1992). Transduction of psychosocial stress into the neurobiology of recurrent affective disorder. *American Journal of Psychiatry*, **149**, 999–1010.

Post, R. M., Leverich, G. S., Altshuler, L. *et al.* (2003). An overview of recent findings of the Stanley Foundation Bipolar Network (Part I). *Bipolar Disorders*, **5**, 310–19.

Prien, R. F. & Potter, W. Z. (1990). NIMH workshop report on treatment of bipolar disorder. *Psychopharmacology Bulletin*, **26**, 409–27.

Remington, G., Kapur, S. & Zipursky, R. B. (1998). Pharmacotherapy of first-episode schizophrenia. *British Journal of Psychiatry*, **172**, 66–70.

Royal Australian and New Zealand College of Psychiatrists (2005). Royal Australian and New Zealand College of Psychiatrists clinical practice guidelines for the treatment of schizophrenia and related disorders. *Australian and New Zealand Journal of Psychiatry*, **39**, 1–30.

Roy-Byrne, P., Post, R. M., Uhde, T. W., Porcu, T. & Davis, D. (1985). The longitudinal course of recurrent affective illness: life chart data from research patients at the NIMH. *Acta Psychiatrica Scandinavica*, **317**(Suppl), 1–34.

Scott, J. & Gutierrez, M. J. (2004). The current status of psychological treatments in bipolar disorders: a systematic review of relapse prevention. *Bipolar Disorders*, **6**, 498–503.

Scott, J. & Tacchi, M. J. (2002). A pilot study of concordance therapy for individuals with bipolar disorders who are non-adherent with lithium prophylaxis. *Bipolar Disorders*, **4**, 386–92.

Scott, J., Paykel, E., Morriss, R. *et al.* (2006). Cognitive-behavioural therapy for severe and recurrent bipolar disorders: randomised controlled trial. *British Journal of Psychiatry*, **188**, 313–20.

Sernyak, M. J., Griffin, R. A., Johnson, R. M. *et al.* (1994). Neuroleptic exposure following inpatient treatment of acute mania with lithium and neuroleptics. *American Journal of Psychiatry*, **151**, 133–5.

Strakowski, S. M., Keck, P. E., McElroy, S. L. *et al.* (1998). Twelve-month outcome after first hospitalisation for affective psychosis. *Archives of General Psychiatry*, **55**, 49–55.

Strober, M. & Carlson, G. (1982). Bipolar illness in adolescents with major depression: clinical, genetic, and psychopharmacologic predictors in a three- to four-year prospective follow-up investigation. *Archives of General Psychiatry*, **39**, 549–55.

ten Have, M., Vollebergh, W., Bijl, R. & Nolen, W. A. (2002). Bipolar disorder in the general population in the Netherlands (prevalence, consequences and care utilisation): results from the Netherlands Mental Health Survey and Incidence Study (NEMESIS). *Journal of Affective Disorder*, **68**, 203–13.

Thompson, K. N., Conus, P., Ward, J. L. *et al.* (2003). The initial prodrome to bipolar affective disorder: prospective case studies. *Journal of Affective Disorder*, **77**, 79–85.

Tohen, M., Waternaux, C. M. & Tsuang, M. T. (1990a). Outcome in mania. *Archives of General Psychiatry*, **47**, 1106–11.

Tohen, M., Waternaux, C. M., Tsuang, M. T. & Hunt, A. T. (1990b). Four-year follow-up of twenty-four first-episode manic patients. *Journal of Affective Disorders*, **19**, 79–86.

Tohen, M., Stoll, A. L., Strakowski, S. M. *et al.* (1992). The McLean First-Episode Psychosis Project: six-month recovery and recurrence outcome. *Schizophrenia Bulletin*, **18**, 273–82.

Tohen, M., Strakowski, S. M., Zarate, C. *et al.* (2000a). The McLean–Harvard First-Episode Project: 6-month symptomatic and functional outcome in affective and nonaffective psychosis. *Biological Psychiatry*, **48**, 467–76.

Tohen, M., Hennen, J., Zarate, C. *et al.* (2000b). Two-year syndromal and functional recovery in 219 cases of first-episode major affective disorder with psychotic features. *American Journal of Psychiatry*, **157**, 220–8.

Tohen, M., Marneros, A., Bowden, C. L. *et al.* (2003a). Olanzapine vs. lithium in relapse prevention in bipolar disorder: a randomized double-blind controlled 12-month clinical trial. *Bipolar Disorders*, **5**(Suppl 1), 89.

Tohen, M., Bowden, C. L., Calabrese, J. R. *et al.* (2003b). Olanzapine's efficacy for relapse prevention in bipolar disorder: a randomized double-blind, placebo-controlled 12-month clinical trial. *Bipolar Disorders*, **5**(Suppl 1), 89.

Tohen, M., Chengappa, K., Suppes, T. *et al.* (2004). Relapse prevention in bipolar I disorder: 18-month comparison of olanzapine plus mood stabiliser v. mood stabiliser alone. *British Journal of Psychiatry*, **184**, 337–45.

Tohen, M., Greil, W., Calabrese, J. R. *et al.* (2005). Olanzapine versus lithium in the maintenance treatment of bipolar disorder: a 12-month, randomized, double-blind, controlled clinical trial. *American Journal of Psychiatry*, **162**, 1281–90.

Tryer, S. P. & Brittlebank, A. D. (1993). Misdiagnosis of bipolar affective disorder as personality disorder. *Canadian Journal of Psychiatry*, **38**, 587–9.

Tsuang, M. T., Woolson, R. F. & Fleming, J. A. (1979). Long term outcome of major psychoses: I schizophrenia and affective disorders compared with psychiatrically symptom-free surgical controls. *Archives of General Psychiatry*, **36**, 1295–301.

Verdoux, H., Gonzales, B., Takei, N. & Bourgeois, M. (1996). Survey of prescribing practice of antipsychotic maintenance treatment for manic–depressive outpatients. *Journal of Affective Disorders*, **38**, 81–7.

Wozniak, J., Biederman, J. & Richards, J. A. (2001). Diagnostic and therapeutic dilemmas in the management of pediatric-onset bipolar disorder. *Journal of Clinical Psychiatry*, **62**(Suppl 14), 10–15.

Yatham, L. N., Kennedy, S. H., O'Donovan, C. *et al.* for the Canadian Network for Mood and Anxiety Treatments. (2005) Canadian Network for Mood and Anxiety Treatments (CANMAT) guidelines for the management of patients with bipolar disorder: consensus and controversies. *Bipolar Disorders*, **7**(Suppl 3), 5–69.

Yung, A. R., Phillips, L. J., Yuen, H. P. *et al.* (2003). Psychosis prediction: 12-month follow up of a high-risk ('prodromal') group. *Schizophrenia Research*, **60**, 21–32.

Zarate, C. A., Tohen, M., Land, M. & Cavanagh, S. (2000). Functional impairment and cognition in bipolar disorder. *Psychiatric Quarterly*, **71**, 309–29.

Zis, A. P., Grof, P., Webster, M. & Goodwin, F. K. (1980). Prediction of relapse in recurrent affective disorder. *Psychopharmacological Bulletin*, **16**, 47–9.

The critical period: other psychopathology and comorbidity

Substance misuse in first-episode psychosis

Darryl Wade, Leanne Hides, Amanda Baker and Dan Lubman

Introduction

Substance misuse is one of the most challenging issues for clinicians in the management and treatment of first-episode psychosis (FEP). The aims of this chapter are to (1) review current knowledge about substance misuse and regular tobacco use in FEP, (2) describe hypotheses that have been proposed to explain the high rate of substance misuse among individuals with psychosis, (3) review the evidence for the efficacy of psychological interventions for substance misuse and regular tobacco use in psychosis, and (4) provide guidance to clinicians in implementing psychological interventions for substance misuse in FEP. In the current chapter, substance misuse refers to substance abuse or dependence, although low levels of substance use may be associated with problems in people with severe mental disorders (Kavanagh, Mueser & Baker, 2003a).

Substance misuse and regular tobacco use in first-episode psychosis

Rate and patterns

Individuals with psychotic disorders are at increased risk for substance misuse compared with individuals with other common psychiatric disorders (Regier *et al.*, 1990) and the general population (Degenhardt & Hall, 2001; Regier *et al.*, 1990). Consistent with these findings, individuals with FEP have a significantly higher rate of substance misuse than their non-psychotic peers (DeLisi *et al.*, 1991; Hambrecht & Häfner, 1996).

Estimates of the rate of lifetime substance misuse in individuals treated for FEP have varied widely, ranging from 10% (Verma *et al.*, 2002) to 74% (Lambert *et al.*, 2005), with most studies in Australia and the USA reporting a rate of at least 40% (DeLisi *et al.*, 1991; Lambert *et al.*, 2005; Rabinowitz *et al.*, 1998; Strakowski *et al.*, 1998; Wade *et al.*, 2005). The observed rate of substance misuse is likely to be influenced by the prevalence of substance misuse in the general community as well as other factors such as diagnostic and sampling methods and the demographic characteristics of the sample (Blanchard *et al.*, 2000). For example, the high rate of substance misuse reported in two recent studies from Australia (Lambert *et al.*, 2005; Wade *et al.*, 2005) probably reflects the predominance of participants with known risk factors for substance misuse including male gender, younger age and social disadvantage.

Cannabis and alcohol are the most frequently misused substances, and misuse of two or more substances is relatively common (Hambrecht & Häfner, 1996; Lambert *et al.*, 2005; Rabinowitz *et al.*, 1998; Sorbara *et al.*, 2003; Wade *et al.*, 2005). For example, Wade *et al.* (2005) reported the following rates of lifetime substance misuse in a group of 126 young persons with FEP: cannabis 63.5%, alcohol 27.8%, amphetamines 18.3%, hallucinogens 12.7%, opioids 12.7%, benzodiazepines 2.4% and inhalants 1.6%. More than half (58.9%) of a group of 90 patients with a history of substance misuse engaged in polysubstance misuse that was defined as the presence of two or more of cannabis, alcohol or other substance misuse. Cigarette smoking is also common among individuals with FEP, and substance misusers are particularly prone to

The Recognition and Management of Early Psychosis: A Preventive Approach, ed. Henry J. Jackson and Patrick D. McGorry.
Published by Cambridge University Press. © Cambridge University Press 2009.

regular tobacco use (Rabinowitz *et al.*, 1998; Wade *et al.*, 2005). For example, Wade *et al.* (2005) reported that 77.0% of all individuals with FEP and 93.3% of individuals with comorbid substance misuse had a history of daily tobacco use.

Temporal order and course of substance misuse and regular tobacco use

The onset of substance misuse precedes the onset of positive symptoms of psychosis in most individuals with comorbid substance misuse and FEP (Hambrecht & Häfner, 1996; Rabinowitz *et al.*, 1998; Sevy *et al.*, 2001; Wade *et al.*, 2005). However, this common temporal sequence may simply represent the typical order of onset of both disorders and is not necessarily an indication that substance misuse is aetiologically significant (Blanchard *et al.*, 2000). Regular tobacco use often predates the onset of substance misuse in FEP (Wade *et al.*, 2005).

Many individuals with FEP achieve remission and/ or a reduction in the severity of substance misuse following entry to treatment (Addington & Addington, 2001; Lambert *et al.*, 2005; Wade *et al.*, 2006a) and a significant reduction in substance use is likely to be associated with improved clinical outcome (Lambert *et al.*, 2005). Relatively few individuals commence substance misuse following entry to treatment (Lambert *et al.*, 2005; Wade *et al.*, 2006a). Of most concern is that a significant proportion of individuals persist with substance misuse despite involvement with treatment services (Addington & Addington, 2001; Hides *et al.*, 2006; Lambert *et al.*, 2005; Sorbara *et al.*, 2003; Strakowski *et al.*, 1998; Wade *et al.*, 2006a). Strakowski *et al.* (1998) reported that at least half of the individuals with affective FEP and a history of substance misuse persisted with substance misuse during the 12-month period following treatment entry. In contrast with substance misuse, the rate of regular tobacco use appears to remain relatively stable following entry into treatment for FEP. Wade *et al.* (2006a) reported that three-quarters of 103 individuals in a group reported daily tobacco use prior to and during the first 15 months of treatment for FEP (76.7% and 75.7%, respectively).

Correlates and consequences of substance misuse

Male gender and younger age have been frequently linked with substance misuse in FEP (Cantwell *et al.*, 1999; Hambrecht & Häfner, 1998; Linszen, Dingemans & Lenior, 1994; Wade *et al.*, 2005). Generally, there is a lack of consistent associations between substance misuse and a range of other sociodemographic variables, although drug misuse has been associated with unemployment (Wade *et al.*, 2005) and a lower level of education (Strakowski *et al.*, 1998).

Limited evidence suggests that substance misuse is associated with better premorbid social functioning in individuals with chronic psychosis (Arndt *et al.*, 1992; Dixon *et al.*, 1991). However, this has not been confirmed in studies of substance misuse in FEP (Linszen *et al.*, 1994; Rabinowitz *et al.*, 1998; Sevy *et al.*, 2001; Van Mastrigt, Addington & Addington, 2004; Wade *et al.*, 2005). The inconsistent findings between studies of FEP and more chronic psychosis may reflect methodological factors such as selection bias. It is also feasible that the greater availability of illicit substances in more recent times has negated poor social adjustment as an impediment to substance use in younger clients. Similar to individuals with chronic psychosis (e.g. Mueser *et al.*, 1999), substance misuse in FEP has been associated with antisocial traits and behaviours (Hambrecht & Häfner, 1996; Rabinowitz *et al.*, 1998).

At initial presentation for FEP, substance misuse does not appear to be associated with the severity of positive, negative or depressive symptoms (Linszen *et al.*, 1994; Sevy *et al.*, 2001; Wade *et al.*, 2005) or the duration of untreated psychosis (Norman & Malla, 2002; Wade *et al.*, 2005). However, persistent substance misuse following entry to treatment is associated with a range of adverse outcomes, including more-severe positive psychotic symptoms (Hides *et al.*, 2006; Lambert *et al.*, 2005; Linszen *et al.*, 1994; Sorbara *et al.*, 2003; Wade *et al.*, 2006b) and an increased rate of inpatient admission (Sorbara *et al.*, 2003; Wade *et al.*, 2006b). For example, Hides *et al.* (2006) found that increased frequency of cannabis use was associated with a shorter time to relapse of positive symptoms among 69 individuals with recent-onset psychosis during a 6-month follow-up period. Wade *et al.* (2006b) found that substance misuse (primarily cannabis), particularly heavy misuse, was associated with increased risk of inpatient admission, relapse of positive symptoms and a shorter time to relapse of positive symptoms among 103 individuals with FEP during a 15-month follow-up period. The link between substance misuse and positive symptoms may reflect the neurobiological effects of substances on dopaminergic pathways (Voruganti *et al.*, 2001), although other explanations are possible such as stressful life events influencing both substance misuse and positive symptoms. Non-adherence to prescribed antipsychotic and other medications is a frequent corollary of substance misuse in FEP (Coldham, Addington & Addington, 2002; Lambert *et al.*, 2005; Strakowski *et al.*, 1998) and represents an additional risk factor for relapse of positive symptoms (Robinson *et al.*, 1999).

Suicidal ideation and behaviours are common in FEP (Nordentoft *et al.*, 2002) and individuals with co-occurring substance misuse are particularly vulnerable (Verdoux *et al.*, 2001). The increased rate of suicidality among substance misusers may represent direct (e.g. overdose) or indirect (e.g. hopelessness secondary to positive symptoms) effects of substance misuse, or a common factor such as certain personality traits may predispose some individuals to both suicidality and substance misuse (Gut-Fayand *et al.*, 2001).

Male gender, younger age, incomplete secondary school and unemployment have all been associated with regular tobacco use in FEP (Wade *et al.*, 2005). Regular tobacco use is known to be associated with an increased risk of smoking-related diseases and premature death among individuals with psychosis compared with the general population (Brown, Barraclough & Inskip, 2000).

Hypotheses to explain the high rate of substance misuse in individuals with psychosis

A number of hypotheses have been proposed to explain the high rate of co-occurring psychosis and substance misuse (see reviews by Blanchard *et al.*, 2000; Mueser, Drake & Wallach, 1998). These hypotheses include that

(1) psychosis increases the risk of substance misuse, (2) substance misuse increases the risk of psychosis, and (3) common factors increase the risk of both disorders. Of course, more than one hypothesis may help to explain the relationship between substance misuse and psychosis in any given individual.

Psychosis causes substance misuse

The self-medication hypothesis (Khantzian, 1985) proposes that individuals with psychosis are more prone to substance misuse because they selectively misuse particular substances in order to 'treat' specific symptoms of the psychotic illness. However, several lines of evidence tend not to support the self-medication hypothesis. As highlighted above, substance use typically begins before the onset of positive symptoms, relatively few individuals commence substance misuse after treatment entry and misuse of more than one substance is relatively common. Other evidence indicates that individuals with psychotic disorders have similar patterns of substance misuse to the rest of the community, albeit at higher rates (Degenhardt & Hall, 2001; Regier *et al.*, 1990). Individuals with psychosis most commonly report using substances to relieve feelings of dysphoria, anxiety and boredom, rather than specific psychotic symptoms or medication side effects (Dixon *et al.*, 1991; Green, Kavanagh & Young, 2004; Spencer, Castle & Michie, 2002), and the type of substance used does not appear to be associated with the experience of psychotic symptoms (Hamera, Schneider & Deviney, 1995). Despite a lack of evidence for the self-medication hypothesis, the possibility remains that individuals may use substances at times to help them to cope with the dysphoria associated with a range of psychosocial problems, including poverty, trauma, family conflict, cognitive impairments, limited coping skills, poor academic performance and lack of vocational opportunities.

Substance use causes psychosis

The hypothesis that substance use is a risk factor for psychosis has received support from a number of recent longitudinal cohort and population-based studies of cannabis use and later development of psychosis.

The largest individual study undertaken (Andreasson *et al.*, 1987) examined the link between cannabis use and later schizophrenia in a cohort of 45 570 Swedish conscripts, who were followed up through a national psychiatric case register. A dose–response relationship was found between self-reported cannabis use at 18 years of age and later inpatient admission for schizophrenia during the 15-year follow-up period. Heavy cannabis users (50 occasions or more) were six times more likely to be hospitalized for schizophrenia than non-users, although the risk of developing schizophrenia was substantially reduced after adjustment for potential confounds. A 27-year follow-up (Zammit *et al.*, 2002) of the same cohort ($n = 50\,087$) reported that the association between cannabis use and schizophrenia could not be explained by a range of potential confounders, including sociability personality traits and amphetamine use. In a 20-year follow-up study of 1265 children from Christchurch, Fergusson, Horwood & Swain-Campbell (2003) reported that individuals who met criteria for cannabis dependence at 21 years of age were over twice more likely to report psychotic symptoms, even after controlling for previous psychotic symptoms (at age 18) and a range of other confounds including other drug use. Similarly, within the Dunedin birth cohort, cannabis users (three times or more) by age 15 and 18 years had higher rates of psychotic symptoms at 26 years of age compared with non-users and were more likely to meet criteria for schizophreniform disorder (Arseneault *et al.*, 2002). Recent meta-analyses of relevant studies suggest that cannabis use is associated with an approximate twofold increase in the relative risk of developing schizophrenia or other psychosis outcome (see Arseneault *et al.*, 2004; Henquet *et al.*, 2005; Semple, McIntosh & Lawrie, 2005).

Catechol-*O*-methyltransferase is an enzyme involved in the metabolism of dopamine, a neurotransmitter heavily implicated in the pathogenesis of schizophrenia. However, its ability to metabolize dopamine is substantially affected by a functional polymorphism that codes for a substitution of methionine (Met) for valine (Val) (Lachman *et al.*, 1996). Using data from the Dunedin cohort, Caspi *et al.* (2005) have recently shown that carriers of the allele encoding Val were more likely to experience psychotic symptoms and develop schizophreniform disorder if they began to use cannabis during adolescence, whereas there was no increase in risk among individuals carrying two copies of the allele encoding Met, nor among adult-onset cannabis users. This suggests that for at-risk individuals (e.g. those with specific genetic polymorphisms or a strong family history of psychosis), adolescence represents a critical period of vulnerability to the effects of psychoactive substance use.

The evidence suggests that cannabis use, particularly adolescent onset and heavy use in vulnerable individuals, is a risk factor for later psychosis including schizophrenia. However, the lack of a significant increase in the incidence of schizophrenia despite an increase in the rate of cannabis use in the general community suggests that cannabis is a contributing factor rather than the sole and sufficient cause of schizophrenia (Degenhardt, Hall & Lynskey, 2003). Indeed, Arseneault *et al.* (2004) have suggested that eliminating cannabis use entirely would only reduce the incidence of schizophrenia by around 8%.

Common risk factors for psychosis and substance misuse

It is plausible that the high rate of substance misuse among individuals with psychosis reflects common biological, personality or environmental factors. Some researchers have suggested that substance misuse and psychosis are both independent manifestations of a common neurobiological factor, and that the increased rate of substance misuse among individuals with psychosis reflects the impact of neuropathological changes of the psychotic illness on areas of the brain that mediate drug reward and reinforcement (Chambers, Krystal & Self, 2001). However, research evidence linking brain pathology with co-occurring substance misuse and psychosis has not been forthcoming.

Certain personality traits have been implicated in the aetiology of co-occurring substance misuse and psychosis (reviewed by Hides, Lubman & Dawe, 2004). As noted above, substance misuse in individuals with psychosis has been linked with antisocial personality disorder (Mueser *et al.*, 1999) as well as related personality traits of sensation seeking, impulsivity and negative affectivity

(Blanchard *et al.*, 1999; Dervaux *et al.*, 2001; Gut-Fayand *et al.*, 2001; Liraud & Verdoux, 2000). However, it is not clear whether these personality features are a common risk factor for both substance misuse and psychosis, or an additional risk factor for substance misuse in individuals with psychotic disorders in a manner similar to the general population.

Studies of psychological interventions for substance misuse in psychosis

Psychological interventions that target risk factors for poor outcome are an important component of optimal treatment during the critical years following diagnosis of psychosis (Lewis, Tarrier & Drake, 2005). The high rate of co-occurring substance misuse and FEP and its links with poor clinical outcome indicate that psychological interventions for substance misuse should be a high priority for affected individuals. Psychological interventions developed for substance misuse in FEP or recent-onset psychosis (Edwards *et al.*, 2003; Kavanagh *et al.*, 2003b) have much in common with interventions developed for individuals with more established psychotic illnesses (e.g. Baker, Bucci & Kay-Lambkin, 2004). Common elements of these interventions include using therapeutic strategies that match the motivational state of the individual, adopting a harm-minimization rather than abstinence-based approach, and using communication and therapeutic strategies that take account of the information-processing problems often experienced by individuals with psychosis. In addition, most interventions are based on principles of motivational interviewing and/or cognitive-behavioural therapy (CBT) (see below).

Relatively few randomized controlled trials of psychological interventions for substance misuse in individuals with psychosis have been conducted (reviewed by Drake *et al.*, 2004). Several trials have evaluated single-session interventions to improve engagement with treatment. Two of these trials have shown that a single session of motivational interviewing is more effective than standard care in assisting individuals with psychosis to attend subsequent therapy (Martino *et al.*, 2000, Swanson, Pantalon & Cohen, 1999),

although a more recent trial (Baker *et al.*, 2002) failed to replicate these findings when subsequent treatment involved a specialist 'dual diagnosis' service.

Only two randomized controlled trials have evaluated psychological interventions designed to reduce substance use and/or improve clinical outcome during the early course of psychosis. Edwards *et al.* (2006) evaluated a 10-session cannabis-focused intervention consisting of psychoeducation, motivational interviewing and CBT that was delivered over 3 months in individuals with stabilized FEP who continued to use cannabis. No significant differences were found between the 24 individuals who received the cannabis-focused intervention and the 23 receiving psychoeducation in cannabis use, symptom severity or general functioning at the end of treatment or at 6-months after the intervention. Both groups showed a similar reduction in cannabis use during the follow-up period. Despite the lack of a standard-care control condition in the study, the findings suggest that relatively simple interventions such as psychoeducation may be useful to reduce cannabis use in FEP. Kavanagh *et al.* (2004) evaluated a motivational interviewing intervention (six to nine sessions within 10 days) for substance misuse in 25 individuals admitted to hospital for FEP or recent-onset psychosis. Follow-up assessments were undertaken at 6 weeks and at 3, 6 and 12 months following initial assessment. The primary outcome was a rating of abstinence or substantial improvement on all substances. Based on analyses for 'treated' individuals, significantly more individuals who received at least some of the motivational interview intervention showed improvement in substance use at 6 and 12 months following initial assessment compared with individuals who received standard care. However, differences in outcome between the two groups were no longer significant when intention-to-treat analyses were performed. Despite lack of control of therapist time, the findings suggest that a relatively brief motivational interviewing intervention may be an effective means to improve engagement as well as motivation to address problematic substance use in some individuals with recent-onset psychosis.

Several randomized controlled trials of interventions for substance misuse among samples with established psychotic disorders have been undertaken. Baker *et al.*

(2006a) found that 65 outpatients with regular substance use who were offered 10 weekly sessions of motivational interviewing–CBT reported greater improvement in depressive symptoms at 6 months and better general functioning at 12 months after the initial assessment compared with the 65 individuals who received standard care. Both groups showed a similar reduction in frequency of substance use during the 12-month follow-up period. James *et al.* (2004) reported that the 29 individuals who were willing to discuss their problematic substance use at weekly motivation-based group sessions over 6 weeks showed significant reductions in global psychopathology, drug use problems and antipsychotic medication dose at 3 months after intervention compared with the 29 individuals who received a single educational session. Barrowclough *et al.* (2001) reported that 18 substance misusers allocated to a programme of motivational interviewing, CBT and a family intervention for up to 9 months showed an improvement in general functioning, a reduction in the severity of positive symptoms and a lower rate of psychotic relapse at 12 months (following initial assessment) compared with the group of 18 individuals who received standard care. The intervention group had a greater percentage of days abstinent from all substances relative to baseline at all time points, although the differences were not statistically significant. At 18 months following initial assessment, the intervention group maintained improvements in general functioning and had less-severe negative symptoms compared with controls, but there were no significant differences between groups on substance use measures (Haddock *et al.*, 2003).

It is difficult to draw firm conclusions about the efficacy of psychological interventions for substance misuse in individuals with psychosis based on findings from these trials. The few trials undertaken have significant methodological limitations, including small sample size, high attrition, lack of adequate control conditions and failure to specify primary outcomes. In addition, the psychological intervention in several trials was associated with only modest benefits in reducing substance use and/or improving other outcomes compared with the control condition. Further large and well-designed trials are needed to assess the efficacy of psychological interventions for comorbid substance

misuse and psychosis and to determine the adequate 'dosage' and relative benefit of different components of these interventions. Despite the methodological limitations of the studies undertaken to date, the results seem to indicate that relatively brief interventions (including assessment of substance use and ongoing monitoring as delivered in 'control' conditions) can lead to clinical and functional improvements for some individuals with co-occurring substance misuse and psychosis.

Few randomized controlled trials have evaluated cigarette smoking cessation interventions among individuals with psychosis and none of these has been undertaken solely among individuals with FEP. A pilot study by Evins *et al.* (2001) found that nine individuals allocated to 12 weeks of bupropion plus a CBT group intervention had a higher rate of significant smoking reduction at the end of treatment compared with individuals who received placebo plus CBT. George *et al.* (2002) found that 16 individuals randomized to 10 weeks of bupropion plus a group intervention had a higher rate of smoking abstinence at the end of treatment compared with 16 individuals who received placebo plus a group intervention. However, there was no difference between groups at 6 months after the intervention. Another study by George *et al.* (2000) randomized individuals to a specialized group therapy programme for smokers with schizophrenia ($n = 28$) or a generic group therapy programme designed for smokers in the general community ($n = 17$). All participants were offered 10 weekly sessions of group therapy and 10 weeks of nicotine replacement therapy using a transdermal patch. The findings showed little difference between groups in smoking abstinence at the end of treatment or at 6 months after the intervention.

Baker *et al.* (2006b) reported the results of a larger trial among 298 regular smokers with a psychotic disorder residing in the community. Individuals were randomized to an eight session, individually administered smoking cessation intervention consisting of nicotine replacement, motivational interviewing and CBT ($n = 147$) or a routine care control condition ($n = 151$). Intention-to-treat analyses revealed no significant differences between the treatment and control groups in abstinence rates during the 12 months following initial assessment. However, a significantly higher proportion of smokers who completed all treatment sessions had quit smoking at 3, 6 and 12 months. There was a strong dose–response relationship between treatment session attendance and smoking reduction status, with half of those who completed the intervention programme achieving a 50% or greater reduction in daily cigarette consumption across the follow-ups, compared with less than one-fifth of the controls. These findings demonstrate the utility of an intervention combining nicotine replacement with motivational interviewing–CBT among people with a psychotic disorder. Cigarette smoking cessation interventions among individuals with FEP are worthy of evaluation.

Providing psychological interventions for substance misuse in first-episode psychosis

Psychological interventions for substance misuse need to be provided within an integrated and comprehensive approach to treatment of FEP. Integrated treatment provided by a single service, as opposed to a 'split' treatment provided by separate mental health and drug and alcohol services, enables a more consistent approach to clinical management and can reduce the burden on individuals and carers. Moreover, there is emerging evidence that integrated treatment programmes can improve outcomes for affected individuals (Drake *et al.*, 2004), although there is a lack of well-designed randomized controlled trials (Jeffery *et al.*, 2000). Many individuals with co-occurring substance misuse and FEP require a comprehensive treatment service that provides continuity of care and takes responsibility for addressing multiple needs including stable accommodation, financial and legal assistance, medical and dental treatment, educational and vocational support, and opportunities for social and community-based activities. A comprehensive approach to treatment also includes family interventions to improve relatives' knowledge and capacity to cope with common problems associated with co-occurring substance misuse and FEP (Gleeson *et al.*, 1999).

Stepped care, that is, the provision of simpler interventions with more intensive interventions offered later depending on a client's response to earlier interventions (Kay-Lambkin, Baker & Lewin, 2004), provides a useful framework for considering the initial provision of psychological interventions for co-occurring substance misuse and FEP. Some individuals will require only relatively brief interventions, such as assessment and basic information to assist them to reduce or cease substance misuse, while others will require more intensive interventions such as psychoeducation, motivational interviewing and CBT to achieve these goals. Ongoing assessment is required during the initial treatment period to track substance use and associated problems in order to guide the most appropriate intensity of psychological interventions. However, some individuals with persistent and more severe substance misuse will require a longer-term treatment approach that includes interventions such as assertive case management, medical treatment, accommodation support and family interventions.

The following information is intended to provide an overview of assessment and treatment issues relevant to provision of psychological interventions for substance misuse in FEP. Interested readers are encouraged to seek more detailed information from published treatment manuals (e.g. Baker *et al.*, 2004; Graham *et al.*, 2004; Hinton *et al.*, 2002).

Engagement

A primary goal of initial assessment and treatment is engagement. Efforts to engage an individual can be a difficult task during the initial acute phase of FEP when the person is often distressed and suspicious of others. Engagement can be enhanced by a calm, warm and professional manner; a genuine interest in the young person and curiosity about their interests and opinions including their explanatory model of psychosis; and a willingness to listen to the individual's concerns and to provide prompt assistance with urgent practical issues such as financial, accommodation or legal problems.

Initial assessment

All individuals presenting with FEP require a comprehensive biopsychosocial assessment to develop a formulation of the individual's presenting problems and to determine appropriate treatment interventions. It is essential that all individuals with FEP are assessed for co-occurring substance misuse, owing to the high rate of substance misuse found in this population and the associated negative outcomes. Initial assessment of substance misuse is usually undertaken as part of a comprehensive psychiatric assessment in FEP, including routine biomedical investigations. From the outset, an empathic and professional approach can assist with efforts to engage the young person with the assessment process. Many individuals are willing to provide details about substance use because they perceive it as a 'normal' activity that is widespread among their peers. An explanation of the purpose of the assessment and the confidentiality of personal information can reassure individuals with concerns about legal sanctions if they disclose details of illicit substance use. Carers and others in close contact with the individual can often provide accurate information about substance use and any adverse effects. Box 14.1 provides an overview of important information to collect in an initial assessment of substance use in FEP.

A number of screening instruments for substance use have been found to be useful in the assessment of substance misuse in psychosis. These include the Alcohol Use Disorders Identification Test (Saunders *et al.*, 1993), the Dartmouth Assessment of Lifestyle Instrument (Rosenberg *et al.*, 1998), and the Alcohol, Smoking and Substance Involvement Screening Test (WHO ASSIST Working Group, 2002).

Diagnostic instability during the early course of psychosis necessitates some caution in making diagnostic judgements during the initial assessment period. In those with psychotic symptoms complicated by substance use, premature diagnosis of substance-induced psychosis may result in inadequate or delayed treatment for individuals later diagnosed with schizophrenia or another primary psychotic disorder (Arendt *et al.*, 2005). Hence, the priority of initial assessment should be to identify treatment-relevant syndromes (such as psychosis, substance misuse and depression) rather than to make definitive diagnoses (McGorry *et al.*, 2003). The accuracy of diagnosis can be improved with longitudinal assessment of treatment response as

---

Box 14.1. Initial assessment of substance use in first-episode psychosis

- Types of substance used, including alcohol, cannabis, amphetamines, sedatives, hallucinogens, inhalants, opioids, cocaine and tobacco
- Frequency, pattern, mode (e.g. intravenous), social context (e.g. self or with others) and duration of substance use
- Negative consequences of substance use, including problems with mental health, physical health, family or friends, finances, educational or vocational pursuits, housing, legal issues
- The presence and severity of a dependence syndrome, including tolerance and withdrawal symptoms
- The temporal onset of psychosis and substance use
- Interactions between psychosis and substance use
- The presence of risks to the individual (e.g. accidental or deliberate overdose, unsafe injecting practice) or others (e.g. aggressive behaviour while intoxicated or withdrawing; neglect of children)
- Reasons for using substances
- Motivation to change substance use
- Urine drug screen, routine bloods (including liver function tests) and screening for blood-borne viruses (with counselling where appropriate).

---

well as the interaction between psychotic symptoms and substance misuse.

Motivation to address substance misuse

An important factor to assess is the individual's level of motivation to address substance use (Miller & Rollnick, 2002, Mueser & Drake, 2003). Osher and Kofoed (1989) have described four stages of treatment characterized by different motivational states: engagement, persuasion, active treatment and relapse prevention. In the engagement stage, the individual is not engaged with treatment and is unwilling to discuss substance use. In the persuasion stage, the individual is engaged with treatment but is not committed to making changes to substance use. In the active treatment stage, the individual is making an attempt to reduce substance use and to address problems associated with substance use. In relapse prevention, the individual has not experienced any recent problems related to substance use. Assessment of preparedness for treatment is important because the types of intervention to consider are linked to the individual's level of motivation, and attempts by a clinician to provide interventions that are inappropriate for the current stage of treatment are likely to be met with resistance. Measures that may be useful to assess a client's motivation to address substance use include the Readiness to Change (Rollnick *et al.*, 1992) questionnaire and the Stages of Treatment Scale (McHugo *et al.*, 1995).

Assessment feedback

Providing the individual with personalized feedback about the assessment is an opportunity to develop a shared understanding of the individual's current problems, including the role of substance use in the development and maintenance of those problems. Young people with FEP should be provided with feedback on the frequency, quantity and impact of their substance use. It is important to check the accuracy of the information (e.g. 'Does that sound right?') and to promote further dialogue with the individual regarding their substance use (e.g. 'Can you tell me a bit more about your substance use?'). Feedback about the assessment is also an opportunity to provide information about psychosis and the treatment of psychosis, the interaction between psychosis and substance use, and the risks to mental and physical health associated with substance use and tobacco use. Abstinence or low levels of substance use should be reinforced by providing psychoeducational material on the mental health consequences of substance use as well as information on the advantages of continued abstinence, such as fewer symptom exacerbations. Useful links to internet sites that provide relevant information sheets about these topics are provided in Box 14.2.

Psychoeducation

The individual's explanatory model of psychosis is often the starting point for a dynamic exchange of ideas between a client and a clinician during the process of psychoeducation in FEP (McGorry, 1995). Topics

---

> **Box 14.2.** Useful internet sites for information sheets and other resources related to substance and tobacco use
>
> - Early Psychosis Prevention and Intervention Centre: information about psychosis and other mental health issues: http://www.eppic.org.au
> - SANE: information about psychosis and other mental health issues including the association between psychosis and cannabis: http://www.sane.org
> - Australian Drug Foundation: information about a wide range of topics related to substance and tobacco use: http://druginfo.adf.org.au
> - Quit Victoria: information about health effects of tobacco use and ceasing tobacco use: http://www.quit.org.au

---

to be covered in psychoeducation include an explanation of psychotic and other symptoms, risk factors for psychosis, the course of illness, the rationale for ongoing treatment and support, and stigma associated with mental illness.

The issue of substance use is a significant issue in psychoeducation for individuals with FEP. The clinicians should elicit the individual's knowledge about the adverse consequences of substance use (e.g. 'What do you know about the effects of [substance] on mental health?'). Later, the clinician can provide advice and suggestions while providing an opportunity for the individual to disagree (e.g. 'Would it be OK if I gave you some information about [substance] and its relationship to mental health?'). Key 'messages' for the clinician to convey about substance use in FEP include: substance use is relatively common among individuals with FEP; substance use is a component risk factor for psychosis in vulnerable individuals and is unlikely to cause psychosis by itself; regular substance use is a risk factor for poor clinical outcomes, including relapse and rehospitalization as well as other psychosocial problems; and a significant number of individuals reduce or cease substance use following the onset of FEP.

Clinicians should provide relevant information about antipsychotic and other medications, including anti-craving (e.g. acamprosate) or drug substitution (e.g. nicotine replacement) medications, to assist the individual to make an informed decision about treatment options. Common concerns that individuals have about medications include doubts about the efficacy or safety of the medication, not wanting to take 'unnatural' substances, the risk of becoming addicted to the medication and being reminded of problems. Clinicians should anticipate these concerns and address them by listening to the individual, providing information to correct misconceptions about medication and planning regular reviews of treatment response and side effects. The recommended practice of using low-dose antipsychotic medications for FEP can reduce the likelihood of extrapyramidal side effects that make individuals less likely to adhere to antipsychotic medication. Motivation-based interventions may also assist with improving adherence to medication (Kemp *et al.*, 1998).

Harm minimization

Harm minimization strategies are particularly useful for individuals not motivated to make a change in their substance use or with a goal for controlled use (see Box 14.3). The provision of information about harm minimization strategies can assist the individual to reduce the harmful effects associated with substance use and can help to build motivation to change in individuals who plan to continue using substances. For individuals who inject substances, information regarding safe injecting practices and associated risky behaviours is a priority given the high risk of bloodborne viral infections among young people with serious mental illness (Hercus, Lubman & Hellard, 2005).

Motivational interviewing

Motivational interviewing has been defined as 'a client centred, directive method for enhancing intrinsic motivation to change by exploring and resolving ambivalence' (Miller & Rollnick, 2002, p. 25). Using an empathic and non-judgemental approach, the clinician employs specific strategies to assist the individual to improve their recognition of substance-related problematic behaviours and to begin the process of change. First, the clinician seeks to develop a discrepancy between an individual's current behaviours and

---

Box 14.3. General harm minimization strategies

- Being informed of the effects of particular substances
- Not using substances when distressed or alone
- Not using multiple substances at the same time
- Using safer modes of administration of drugs
- Using an initial 'test' of a drug to avoid overdose or other complications
- Not using substances when driving a car or in other potentially hazardous situations
- Being aware of safer sex practices
- Not sharing needles
- Being informed about healthy nutrition
- Having a plan to access personal or emergency support if required.

---

achieving important personal goals (e.g. heavy cannabis use may make it less likely that an individual will stay out of hospital and maintain employment). Avoiding language that could be perceived by the client as judgemental (such as 'problems' and 'bad aspects of use'), the clinician asks the individual to list the 'good things' and 'not so good things' about substance use and to describe what their life would be like if they were to reduce their substance use. Second, the clinician 'rolls with resistance' and avoids arguments about the individual's views or behaviours to maintain a collaborative working relationship. Resistance from an individual is often expressed as irritation or anger and is a signal for the clinician to use reflective listening and other techniques to reduce the defensiveness of the individual. Third, supporting self-efficacy is achieved by reinforcing efforts that individuals have previously made to change behaviour or improve their well-being. Typically, individuals make a decision about whether or not they wish to commit to reducing substance use after several sessions of motivational interviewing, which may occur intermittently over the course of treatment.

Cognitive–behavioural therapy

If an individual expresses a commitment to change their substance use, the clinician can assist the individual to develop specific goals (e.g. complete abstinence or limits on the frequency, quantity or money spent on substance use) and to work toward achieving their goals using CBT and other therapeutic strategies.

Common strategies to assist individuals with their efforts to address substance use include:

- set realistic, achievable and short-term goals that are clearly defined in behavioural terms
- provide regular monitoring of attempts to achieve goals
- engage supportive others to assist the individual with their plan to reduce substance use
- encourage the individual to keep a list of reasons for wanting to change substance use to help to maintain motivation
- provide a personalized handout of the plan to reduce substance use
- identify high-risk situations for substance use
- provide education about cravings and withdrawal symptoms and practice coping strategies to manage these difficulties
- teach the individual to challenge cognitions associated with substance use (e.g. positive drug use expectancies) and/or negative affective states and to use problem solving to address high-risk situations
- practise refusal skills for use in high-risk situations
- develop a plan to deal with a lapse of problematic substance use.

Maintenance of successful reduction of substance use requires regular monitoring and reinforcement of successful strategies to avoid problematic substance use.

Conclusions

Substance misuse and regular tobacco use among young people with FEP are associated with a range of negative effects on both mental and physical health, as well as social functioning. The initial treatment period following diagnosis of a psychotic disorder provides an opportunity to alleviate client and carer burden associated with problematic substance use in FEP. The most urgent task is to develop effective psychosocial interventions that can be implemented within well-resourced treatment and support services in order to provide maximum

opportunity to affected individuals for recovery and participation in the wider community.

REFERENCES

Addington, J. & Addington, D. (2001). Impact of an early psychosis programme on substance use. *Psychiatric Rehabilitation Journal*, **25**, 60–7.

Andreasson, S., Allebeck, P., Engstrom, A. & Rydberg, U. (1987). Cannabis and schizophrenia. A longitudinal study of Swedish conscripts. *Lancet*, **ii**, 1483–6.

Arndt, S., Tyrrell, G., Flaum, M. & Andreasen, N. C. (1992). Comorbidity of substance abuse and schizophrenia: the role of premorbid adjustment. *Psychological Medicine*, **22**, 379–88.

Arendt, M., Rosenberg, R., Foldager, L., Perto, G. & Munk-Jorgensen, P. (2005). Cannabis-induced psychosis and subsequent schizophrenia-spectrum disorders: follow-up study of 535 incident cases. *British Journal of Psychiatry*, **187**, 510–15.

Arseneault, L., Cannon, M., Poulton, R. *et al.* (2002). Cannabis use in adolescence and risk for adult psychosis: longitudinal prospective study. *British Medical Journal*, **325**, 1212–13.

Arseneault, L., Cannon, M., Witton, J. & Murray, R. M. (2004). Causal association between cannabis and psychosis: examination of the evidence. *British Journal of Psychiatry*, **184**, 110–17.

Baker, A., Lewin, T., Reichler, H. *et al.* (2002). Motivational interviewing among psychiatric in-patients with substance use disorders. *Acta Psychiatrica Scandinavica*, **106**, 233–40.

Baker, A., Bucci, S. & Kay-Lambkin, F. (2004). *Intervention for Alcohol, Cannabis and Amphetamine Use among People with a Psychotic Illness*. [NDARC Technical Report No. 193.] Sydney: National Drug and Alcohol Research Centre.

Baker, A., Bucci, S., Lewin, T. J. *et al.* (2006a). Cognitive-behavioural therapy for substance use disorders in people with psychotic disorders: randomised controlled trial. *British Journal of Psychiatry*, **188**, 439–48.

Baker, A., Richmond, R., Haile, M. *et al.* (2006b). Randomised controlled trial of a smoking cessation intervention among people with a psychotic disorder. *American Journal of Psychiatry*, **163**, 1934–42.

Barrowclough, C., Haddock, G., Tarrier, N. *et al.* (2001) Randomized controlled trial of motivational interviewing, cognitive behaviour therapy, and family intervention for patients with comorbid schizophrenia and substance use disorders. *American Journal of Psychiatry*, **158**, 1706–13.

Blanchard, J. J., Squires, D., Henry, T. *et al.* (1999). Examining an affect regulation model of substance abuse in schizophrenia: the role of traits and coping. *Journal of Nervous and Mental Disease*, **187**, 72–9.

Blanchard, J. J., Brown, S. A., Horan, W. P. & Sherwood, A. R. (2000). Substance use disorders in schizophrenia: review, integration, and a proposed model. *Clinical Psychology Review*, **20**, 207–34.

Brown, S., Barraclough, B. & Inskip, H. (2000). Causes of the excess mortality of schizophrenia. *British Journal of Psychiatry*, **177**, 212–17.

Cantwell, R., Brewin, J., Glazebrook, C. *et al.* (1999). Prevalence of substance misuse in first-episode psychosis. *British Journal of Psychiatry*, **174**, 150–3.

Caspi, A., Moffitt, T. E., Cannon, M. *et al.* (2005). Moderation of the effect of adolescent-onset cannabis use on adult psychosis by a functional polymorphism in the catechol-*O*-methyltransferase gene: longitudinal evidence of a gene x environment interaction. *Biological Psychiatry*, **57**, 1117–27.

Chambers, R. A., Krystal, J. H. & Self, D. W. (2001). A neurobiological basis for substance abuse comorbidity in schizophrenia. *Biological Psychiatry*, **50**, 71–83.

Coldham, E. L., Addington, J. & Addington, D. (2002). Medication adherence of individuals with a first episode of psychosis. *Acta Psychiatrica Scandinavica*, **106**, 286–90.

Degenhardt, L. & Hall, W. (2001). The association between psychosis and problematical drug use among Australian adults: findings from the National Survey of Mental Health and Well-being. *Psychological Medicine*, **31**, 659–68.

Degenhardt, L., Hall, W. & Lynskey, M. (2003). Testing hypotheses about the relationship between cannabis use and psychosis. *Drug and Alcohol Dependence*, **71**, 37–48.

DeLisi, L. E., Boccio, A. M., Riordan, H. *et al.* (1991). Familial thyroid disease and delayed language development in first admission patients with schizophrenia. *Psychiatry Research*, **38**, 39–50.

Dervaux, A., Bayle, F. J., Laqueille, X. *et al.* (2001). Is substance abuse in schizophrenia related to impulsivity, sensation seeking, or anhedonia? *American Journal of Psychiatry*, **158**, 492–4.

Dixon, L., Haas, G., Weiden, P. J., Sweeney, J. & Frances, A. J. (1991). Drug abuse in schizophrenic patients: clinical correlates and reasons for use. *American Journal of Psychiatry*, **148**, 224–30.

Drake, R. E., Mueser, K. T., Brunette, M. F. & McHugo, G. J. (2004). A review of treatments for people with severe mental illnesses and co-occurring substance use disorders. *Psychiatric Rehabilitation Journal*, **27**, 360–74.

Edwards, J., Hinton, M., Elkins, K. & Athanasopoulos, O. (2003). Cannabis and first-episode psychosis: the CAP project. In

H. L. Graham, A. Copello, M. J. Birchwood & K. T. Mueser (eds.), *Substance Misuse in Psychosis: Approaches to Treatment and Service Delivery*. Chichester, UK: John Wiley, pp. 283–304.

Edwards, J., Elkins, K., Hinton, M. *et al.* (2006). Randomized controlled trial of a cannabis-focused intervention for young people with first-episode psychosis. *Acta Psychiatrica Scandinavica*, **114**, 109–17.

Evins, A. E., Mays, V. K., Rigotti, N. A. *et al.* (2001). A pilot trial of bupropion added to cognitive behavioral therapy for smoking cessation in schizophrenia. *Nicotine and Tobacco Research*, **3**, 397–403.

Fergusson, D. M., Horwood, L. J. & Swain-Campbell, N. R. (2003). Cannabis dependence and psychotic symptoms in young people. *Psychological Medicine*, **33**, 15–21.

George, T. P., Ziedonis, D. M., Feingold, A. *et al.* (2000). Nicotine transdermal patch and atypical antipsychotic medications for smoking cessation in schizophrenia. *American Journal of Psychiatry*, **157**, 1835–42.

George, T. P., Vessicchio, J. C., Termine, A. *et al.* (2002). A placebo controlled trial of bupropion for smoking cessation in schizophrenia. *Biological Psychiatry*, **52**, 53–61.

Gleeson, J, Jackson, H. J., Stavely, H. & Burnett, P. (1999). Family intervention in early psychosis. In P. D. McGorry & H. J. Jackson (eds.), *The Recognition and Management of Early Psychosis*. Cambridge, UK: Cambridge University Press, pp. 376–406.

Graham, H. L., Copello, A., Birchwood, M. J. *et al.* (2004). *Cognitive-behavioural Integrated Treatment (C-BIT): A Treatment Manual for Substance Misuse in People with Severe Mental Health Problems*. Chichester, UK: John Wiley.

Green, B., Kavanagh, D. & Young, R. M. (2004). Reasons for cannabis use in men with and without psychosis. *Drug and Alcohol Review*, **23**, 445–53.

Gut-Fayand, A., Dervaux, A., Olie, J. *et al.* (2001). Substance abuse and suicidality in schizophrenia: a common risk factor linked to impulsivity. *Psychiatry Research*, **102**, 65–72.

Haddock, G., Barrowclough, C., Tarrier, N. *et al.* (2003). Cognitive-behavioural therapy and motivational intervention for schizophrenia and substance misuse: 18-month outcomes of a randomised controlled trial. *British Journal of Psychiatry*, **183**, 418–26.

Hambrecht, M. & Häfner, H. (1996). Substance abuse and the onset of schizophrenia. *Biological Psychiatry*, **40**, 1155–63.

Hambrecht, M. & Häfner, H. (1998). Are symptoms observed differently in male and female first-episode patients? *Schizophrenia Research*, **29**, 186.

Hamera, E., Schneider, J. K. & Deviney, S. (1995). Alcohol, cannabis, nicotine, and caffeine use and symptom distress in schizophrenia. *Journal of Nervous and Mental Disease*, **183**, 559–65.

Henquet, C., Murray, R., Linszen, D. & van Os, J. (2005). The environment and schizophrenia: the role of cannabis use. *Schizophrenia Bulletin*, **31**, 608–12.

Hercus, M., Lubman, D. I. & Hellard, M. (2005). Blood borne viral and sexually transmissible infections among psychiatric populations: what are we doing about them? *Australian and New Zealand Journal of Psychiatry*, **39**, 849–55.

Hides, L., Lubman, D. & Dawe, S. (2004). Models of co-occurring substance misuse and psychosis: are personality traits the missing link? *Drug and Alcohol Review*, **23**, 425–32.

Hides, L., Dawe, S., Kavanagh, D. J. & Young, R. M. (2006). Psychotic symptom and cannabis relapse in recent-onset psychosis: a prospective study. *British Journal of Psychiatry*, **189**, 137–43.

Hinton, M., Elkins, K., Edwards, J. & Donovan, K. (2002). *Cannabis and Psychosis: An Early Psychosis Treatment Manual*. Melbourne: Early Psychosis Prevention and Intervention Centre.

James, W., Preston, N. J., Koh, G. *et al.* (2004). A group intervention which assists patients with dual diagnosis reduce their drug use: a randomized controlled trial. *Psychological Medicine*, **34**, 983–90.

Jeffery, D. P., Ley, A., McLaren, S. & Siegfried N. (2000). Psychosocial treatment programmes for people with both severe mental illness and substance misuse. *Cochrane Database of Systematic Reviews*, **2**, CD001088. [DOI: 10.1002/14651858.CD001088].

Kavanagh, D. J., Mueser, K. T. & Baker, A. (2003a). Management of comorbidity. In M. Teesson & H. Proudfoot (eds.), *Comorbid Mental Disorders and Substance Use Disorders: Epidemiology, Prevention and Treatment*. Canberra: Commonwealth of Australia, pp. 78–120.

Kavanagh, D. J., Young, R., White, A. *et al.* (2003b). Start over and survive: a brief intervention for substance misuse in early psychosis. In H. L. Graham, A. Copello, M. J. Birchwood & K. T. Mueser (eds.), *Substance Misuse in Psychosis: Approaches to Treatment and Service Delivery*. Chichester, UK: John Wiley, pp. 244–58.

Kavanagh, D. J., Young, R., White, A. *et al.* (2004). A brief motivational intervention for substance misuse in recent-onset psychosis. *Drug and Alcohol Review*, **23**, 151–5.

Kay-Lambkin, F. J., Baker, A. L. & Lewin, T. J. (2004). The 'co-morbidity roundabout': a framework to guide assessment and intervention strategies and engineer change among people with comorbid problems. *Drug and Alcohol Review*, **23**, 407–23.

Kemp, R., Kirov, G., Everitt, B., Hayward, P. & David, A. (1998). Randomised controlled trial of compliance therapy: 18-month follow-up. *British Journal of Psychiatry*, **172**, 413–19.

Khantzian, E. (1985). The self-medication hypothesis of addictive disorders: focus on heroin and cocaine dependence. *American Journal of Psychiatry*, **142**, 1259–64.

Lachman, H. M., Papolos, D. F., Saito, T. *et al.* (1996). Human catechol-*O*-methyltransferase pharmacogenetics: description of a functional polymorphism and its potential application to neuropsychiatric disorders. *Pharmacogenetics*, **6**, 243–50.

Lambert, M., Conus, P., Lubman, D. I. *et al.* (2005). The impact of substance use disorders on clinical outcome in 643 patients with first-episode psychosis. *Acta Psychiatrica Scandinavica*, **112**, 141–8.

Lewis, S. W., Tarrier, N. & Drake, R. J. (2005). Integrating non-drug treatments in early schizophrenia. *British Journal of Psychiatry*, **187**, 65–71.

Linszen, D. H., Dingemans, P. M. & Lenior, M. E. (1994). Cannabis abuse and the course of recent-onset schizophrenic disorders. *Archives of General Psychiatry*, **51**, 273–9.

Liraud, F. & Verdoux, H. (2000). Which temperamental characteristics are associated with substance use in subjects with psychotic and mood disorders? *Psychiatry Research*, **93**, 63–72.

Martino, S., Carroll, K. M., O'Malley, S. S. & Rounsaville, B. J. (2000). Motivational interviewing with psychiatrically ill substance abusing patients. *American Journal on Addictions*, **9**, 88–91.

McGorry, P. D. (1995). Psychoeducation in first-episode psychosis: a therapeutic process. *Psychiatry*, **58**, 313–28.

McGorry, P., Killackey, E., Elkins, K., Lambert, M. & Lambert, T. (2003). Summary: Australian and New Zealand clinical practice guideline for the treatment of schizophrenia. *Australasian Psychiatry*, **11**, 136–47.

McHugo, G. J., Drake, R. E., Burton, H. L. & Ackerson, T. H. (1995). A scale for assessing the stage of substance abuse treatment in persons with severe mental illness. *Journal of Nervous and Mental Disease*, **182**, 164–7.

Miller, W. & Rollnick, S. (2002). *Motivational Interviewing: Preparing People for Change*. New York: Guilford Press.

Mueser, K. T. & Drake, R. E. (2003). Integrated dual disorder treatment in New Hampshire (USA). In H. L. Graham, A. Copello, M. J. Birchwood & K. T. Mueser (eds.), *Substance Misuse in Psychosis: Approaches to Treatment and Service Delivery*. Chichester, UK: John Wiley, pp. 93–105.

Mueser, K. T., Drake, R. E. & Wallach, M. A. (1998). Dual diagnosis: a review of aetiological theories. *Addictive Behaviours*, **23**, 717–34.

Mueser, K. T., Rosenberg, S. D., Drake, R. E. *et al.* (1999). Conduct disorder, antisocial personality disorder and substance use disorders in schizophrenia and major affective disorders. *Journal of Studies on Alcohol*, **60**, 278–84.

Nordentoft, M., Jeppesen, P., Abel, M. *et al.* (2002). OPUS study: suicidal behaviour, suicidal ideation and hopelessness among patients with first-episode psychosis – one-year follow-up of a randomised controlled trial. *British Journal of Psychiatry*, **181**, 98–106.

Norman, R. M. G. & Malla, A. K. (2002). Examining adherence to medication and substance use as possible confounds of duration of untreated psychosis. *Journal of Nervous and Mental Disease*, **190**, 331–4.

Osher, F. C. & Kofoed, L. L. (1989). Treatment of patients with psychiatric and psychoactive substance use disorders. *Hospital and Community Psychiatry*, **40**, 1025–30.

Rabinowitz, J., Bromet, E. J., Carlson, L. G., Kovasznay, B. & Schwartz, J. E. (1998). Prevalence and severity of substance use disorders and onset of psychosis in first-admission psychotic patients. *Psychological Medicine*, **28**, 1411–19.

Regier, D. A., Farmer, M. E., Rae, D. S. *et al.* (1990). Comorbidity of mental disorders with alcohol and other drug abuse. Results from the Epidemiologic Catchment Area (ECA) study. *Journal of the American Medical Association*, **264**, 2511–18.

Robinson, D., Woerner, M. G., Alvir, J. M. J. *et al.* (1999). Predictors of relapse following response from a first episode of schizophrenia or schizoaffective disorder. *Archives of General Psychiatry*, **56**, 241–7.

Rollnick, S., Heather, N., Gold, R. & Hall, W. (1992). Development of a short 'readiness to change' questionnaire for use in brief, opportunistic interventions among excessive drinkers. *British Journal of Addiction*, **87**, 743–54.

Rosenberg, S. D., Drake, R., Wolford, G. L. *et al.* (1998). Dartmouth Assessment of Lifestyle Instrument (DALI): a substance use disorder screen for people with severe mental illness. *American Journal of Psychiatry*, **155**, 232–8.

Saunders, J. B., Aasland, O. G., Babor, T. F., de le Fuente, J. R. & Grant, M. (1993). Development of the alcohol use disorders identification test (AUDIT). WHO collaborative project on early detection of persons with harmful alcohol consumption. *Addiction*, **88**, 791–804.

Semple, D. M., McIntosh, A. M. & Lawrie, S. M. (2005). Cannabis as a risk factor for psychosis: systematic review. *Journal of Psychopharmacology*, **19**, 187–94.

Sevy, S., Robinson, D. G., Holloway, S. *et al.* (2001). Correlates of substance misuse in patients with first-episode schizophrenia and schizoaffective disorder. *Acta Psychiatrica Scandinavica*, **104**, 367–74.

Sorbara, F., Liraud, F., Assens, F., Abalan, F. & Verdoux, H. (2003). Substance use and the course of early psychosis: a 2-year follow-up of first-admitted subjects. *European Psychiatry*, **18**, 133–6.

Spencer, C., Castle, D. & Michie, P. T. (2002). Motivations that maintain substance use among individuals with psychotic disorders. *Schizophrenia Bulletin*, **28**, 233–47.

Strakowski, S. M., Keck, P. E., McElroy, S. L. *et al.* (1998). Twelve-month outcome after a first hospitalization for affective psychosis. *Archives of General Psychiatry*, **55**, 49–55.

Swanson, A. J., Pantalon, M. V. & Cohen, K. R. (1999). Motivational interviewing and treatment adherence among psychiatric and dually diagnosed patients. *Journal of Nervous and Mental Disease*, **187**, 630–5.

Van Mastrigt, S., Addington, J. & Addington, D. (2004). Substance misuse at presentation to an early psychosis program. *Social Psychiatry and Psychiatric Epidemiology*, **39**, 69–72.

Verdoux, H., Liraud, F., Gonzales, B. *et al.* (2001). Predictors and outcome characteristics associated with suicidal behaviour in early psychosis: a two-year follow-up of first-admitted subjects. *Acta Psychiatrica Scandinavica*, **103**, 347–54.

Verma, S. K., Subramaniam, M., Chong, S. A. & Kua, E. H. (2002). Substance abuse in schizophrenia: a Singapore perspective. *Social Psychiatry and Psychiatric Epidemiology*, **37**, 326–8.

Voruganti, L. N. P., Slomka, P., Zabel, P., Mattar, A. & Awad, A. G. (2001). Cannabis induced dopamine release: an in-vivo SPECT study. *Psychiatry Research Neuroimaging*, **107**, 173–7.

Wade, D., Harrigan, S., Edwards, J. *et al.* (2005). Patterns and predictors of substance use disorders and daily tobacco use in first-episode psychosis. *Australian and New Zealand Journal of Psychiatry*, **39**, 892–8.

Wade, D., Harrigan, S., Edwards, J. *et al.* (2006a). Course of substance misuse and daily tobacco use in first-episode psychosis. *Schizophrenia Research*, **81**, 145–50.

Wade, D., Harrigan, S., Edwards, J. *et al.* (2006b). Substance misuse in first-episode psychosis: 15-month prospective follow-up study. *British Journal of Psychiatry*, **189**, 229–34.

WHO ASSIST Working Group (2002). The alcohol, smoking, and substance involvement screening test (ASSIST): development, reliability and feasibility. *Addiction*, **97**, 1183–94.

Zammit, S., Allebeck, P., Andreasson, S., Lundberg, I. & Lewis, G. (2002). Self reported cannabis use as a risk factor for schizophrenia in Swedish conscripts of 1969: historical cohort study. *British Medical Journal*, **325**, 1199–204.

15

Suicide prevention in first-episode psychosis

Paddy Power and Jo Robinson

Of all the forms of human suffering, few compare with the pain that leads some to think of suicide as a means of relief ... Such a person needs support and inspiration but this is not enough. The deeply depressed person also needs a set of methods to use in order to rebuild his or her sense of purpose, meaning and skills in dealing with what life has to offer ... means by which to move from the darkness of self destruction to a better life.

Aaron Beck (1996).

Introduction

Suicide is one of the most tragic and often unspoken consequences of psychotic disorders. Conservative calculations of suicide rates in psychosis yield depressing statistics. Between 4% and 10% of people with schizophrenia and 6% and 15% of people with affective psychosis will eventually commit suicide (Brown, 1997; Inskip, Harris & Barraclough, 1998; Palmer, Pankratz & Bostwick, 2005; Siris, 2001). It is the commonest cause of unnatural death for people with these illnesses during their first 10 years of follow-up (Craig, Ye & Bromet, 2006) and accounts for a sizeable proportion (20–37%) of all suicides (Burgess *et al.*, 2000; Hiroeh *et al.*, 2001; Hunt *et al.*, 2006) associated with mental illness. Among adolescents, schizophrenia alone accounts for almost one-third of all youth suicides (Hunt *et al.*, 2006).

The numbers dying from suicide is of pandemic proportions. The World Health Organization (WHO) estimates that one million people commit suicide annually worldwide, with on average one death occurring every 40 seconds and one suicide attempt every 2 seconds (WHO, 2007). With psychotic disorders such as schizophrenia (7–12% suicides) and bipolar disorder (24% suicides) responsible for over a third of suicides associated with mental illness (Heilä, 1999; Hiroeh *et al.*, 2001) and as much as a fifth of all suicides (Gupta & Guest, 2002; Heilä & Lönnqvist, 2003; Milne, Matthews & Ashcroft, 1994), conservative estimates indicate that 200 000 people with psychosis die each year by suicide (that is one person every 3 minutes).

For a country with a population of 50 million, half a million of its population will suffer from schizophrenia (1% prevalence) and 25 000 will eventually kill themselves if current rates (5%; Palmer *et al.*, 2005) continue. If one includes people with bipolar disorder (0.5–1.5% prevalence; 6–15% suicide rate, contributing to 11% of all suicides; Gupta & Guest, 2002), this figure is likely to reach at least 40 000 suicides. Broadening the scope further to encompass all psychotic disorders (prevalence 3% population; Perälä *et al.*, 2007), the numbers dying by suicide could well be double this figure.

Similarly, in a country (population of 50 million) with annual suicide rates of 15/100 000, psychotic disorders will account for approximately 1500 of the 7500 people who commit suicide each year. At local catchment area population sizes of 250 000, one would expect seven or eight suicides each year amongst those with psychosis, with one of the largest groups being young males in the first 5 years of illness. Estimating the number of suicides among patients with first-episode psychosis (in their first 3 years in treatment), one would expect, on average, nearly two suicides annually in this catchment area and over 375 first-episode suicides nationally – based

The Recognition and Management of Early Psychosis: A Preventive Approach, ed. Henry J. Jackson and Patrick D. McGorry.
Published by Cambridge University Press. © Cambridge University Press 2009.

on incidence of psychosis of at least 25/100 000 (Kirkbride *et al.*, 2006; Power *et al.*, 1998; Proctor, Mitford & Paxton, 2004) and an average suicide rate of 5.5% observed in the first 5 years of follow-up in 18 first-episode studies (Heilä & Lönnqvist, 2003). Suicides among patients with first-episode psychosis would, therefore, represent 5% of the national deaths from suicide.

The ripple effect of each of these individual suicides has the potential to permeate through generations within a family, a service and the wider community, representing a graphic symbol of anger, regret, hopelessness and despair. Such tragic deaths may become a focus of identification for those who become similarly afflicted, for example, offspring. This is a cycle that can be broken with the hope of new treatments, earlier intervention, better outcomes, less stigma and alienation, and proper support during the recovery for patients and carers.

The factors that contribute to these tragic deaths are complex. Prediction is especially fraught and it would be unwise to overgeneralize the importance of any one risk factor, particularly as most patients will experience some degree of suicidal ideation during the course of their psychotic illness (Power *et al.*, 2003). Acute psychotic symptoms, although important, may only contribute directly to approximately 10% of suicides (Nordentoft *et al.*, 2002). The majority of suicides may have far more to do with the social, psychological and emotional impact of patients' illnesses. Hopelessness and depression during the recovery phases are key mediators. These factors might even be considered normative responses given the often profound adjustments and challenges patients face during recovery.

For many, suicide is only a fleeting consideration. However, for a sizeable minority, suicide becomes a serious and persistent preoccupation over days and weeks. These patients need particularly close monitoring during these phases, together with targeted interventions to address their depression and hopelessness. The fact that the majority of these patients do not go on to complete suicide is perhaps a testament to the help, support and treatment that they receive. Sadly, for a small number, even the best of interventions will fail to prevent the inevitable. Clinicians and carers have to

accept that, despite their best efforts, they cannot always protect every patient from the impact of their illness. An open dialogue with carers about the risks may well limit the impact and distress experienced by those left behind after such distressing incidents.

There is encouraging evidence that the general process of early intervention can reduce this risk of suicide in psychosis (McGorry, Henry & Power, 1998). Particular treatments – both medical and psychological – have also been shown to reduce levels of suicidality in psychosis. Finally, risk-management strategies may provide additional safeguards by identifying and monitoring those at highest risk.

This chapter covers the literature on suicide and early psychosis, highlighting approaches to risk assessment and management. It focuses on interventions that have been shown to provide promising results in suicide prevention in early psychosis. These strategies should all be seen as an integral part of wider national strategies in suicide prevention. Suicide owing to psychosis represents a sizeable component of the overall morbidity of suicide in the general population and there is considerable scope with better interventions to reduce its risk.

What is the process of suicidality in psychosis?

Not all self-inflicted deaths in psychosis are suicides in the true sense. For a legal determination of death by suicide several criteria need to be fulfilled. The death must be (1) unnatural, (2) self-inflicted, and (3) with intent (O'Carrol *et al.*, 1996). The level of 'intent' is measured by evidence indicating that the person intended (1) to take the action, (2) to harm himself/herself by that action, (3) to die as a result of that action, and (4) at the time of the action was capable of understanding the likely consequences of the action.

During the non-psychotic state

Even in non-psychotic states, it may be difficult to determine whether a death was intentional, as people attempting suicide frequently experience considerable

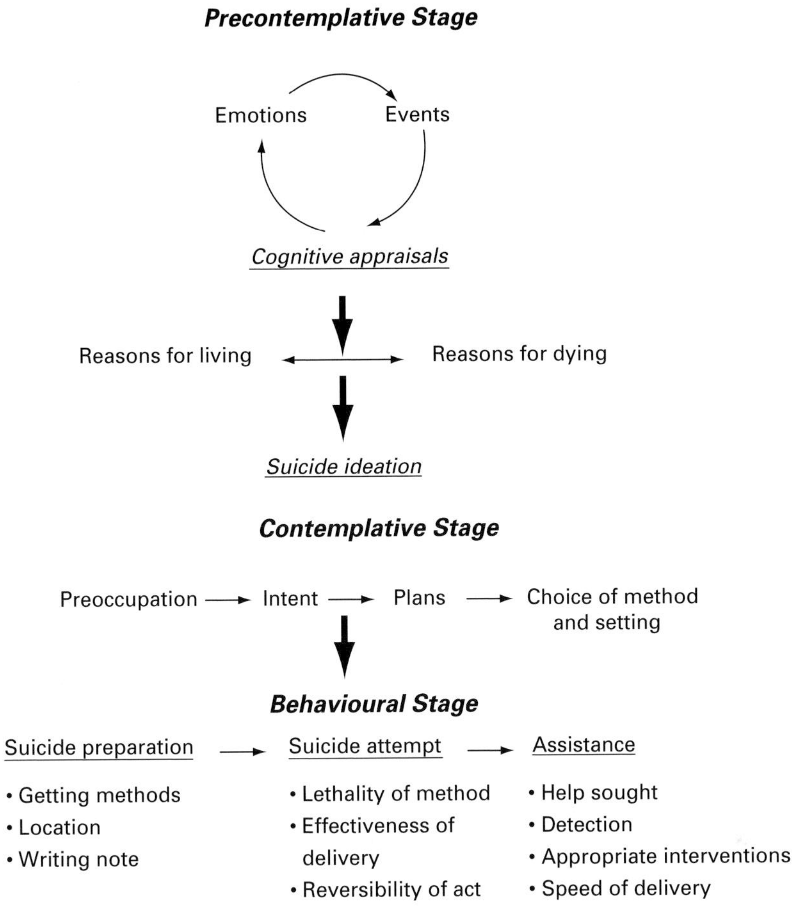

Precontemplative Stage

Emotions   Events

Cognitive appraisals

Reasons for living   ←→   Reasons for dying

Suicide ideation

Contemplative Stage

Preoccupation → Intent → Plans → Choice of method and setting

Behavioural Stage

Suicide preparation → Suicide attempt → Assistance

- Getting methods
- Location
- Writing note

- Lethality of method
- Effectiveness of delivery
- Reversibility of act

- Help sought
- Detection
- Appropriate interventions
- Speed of delivery

Fig. 15.1. Cognitive model of suicidality.

ambivalence about death (Andriessen, 2006). As with any form of violence, the intentions may be more complex than self-destruction alone. Hopelessness is often cited as a fundamental factor, but in clinical practice it is only one of the many emotions described by suicidal patients. Anger, self-loathing, shame, revenge, anxiety, fear, panic, emptiness, resignation, reckless abandon and a wish to escape an impossible situation all can complicate the suicidal state. These emotions may arise as a response to assumptions prompted by external events, thereby shifting the balance between wanting to live to wanting to die, potentially creating a state of increasing suicidality. This state drives the momentum

from ambivalence to preoccupation with death, to actual intent/motive, to formal plans and choice of method, to preparatory behaviours and, finally, to the suicide act. The lethality of the act is heavily dependent on chance, the reversibility of the method chosen and whether help is sought and available in time. Figure 15.1 represents a model of suicide behaviour.

During the psychotic state

However, during acute psychotic states, the process of intentional self-destruction is potentially more complex, disturbed, ego-dystonic, dichotomous and disorganized. The psychotic experience and process may drive self-destructive urges. The confusion, embarrassment and emotional distress of psychosis may precipitate feelings of hopelessness and despair. Delusional and paranoid interpretations may motivate thoughts of escape by suicide. Command hallucinations may prompt intent and plans. Yet despite these experiences, a person may maintain a relatively intact sense of self-preservation and help-seeking, thereby minimizing the risk of acting upon these experiences. However, the psychotic process may also inhibit self-preservation. Disorganized thinking may impair insight, judgement, problem solving and help-seeking. A disregard for personal safety may result in unintentionally lethal actions, for example jumping off buildings or into water, wandering in front of traffic, reckless driving, fire-setting, exposure to exploitation/assault and threatening armed police. Profound neglect in catatonic states may result from refusal to eat or drink, prolonged exposure to the elements and fatal blood clots from immobilization. In such situations, relatively mild or even unintentional self-destructive urges might easily result in lethal consequences.

Methods chosen

Methods of suicide (and suicide attempt) in people with psychosis are typically violent and include methods such as hanging, jumping in front of a moving vehicle or from a high place and cutting one's wrists (Harkavy-Friedman *et al.*, 1999; Hunt *et al.*, 2006). During acute psychosis, the methods chosen may be more bizarre and opportunistic, for example, self-immolation with inflammable hairsprays. Fire safety, cigarette lighters, hanging points, sharps, glass and electrical appliances should all be routinely part of any risk-management policy in residential units accommodating acutely psychotic patients.

When does suicide tend to occur in first-episode psychosis?

The early stages of illness are critical. Suicide is much more likely to occur during the first years of illness (Inskip *et al.*, 1998; Westermeyer, Harrow & Marengo,

1991), particularly during the early years after diagnosis (Brown, 1997; Mortensen & Juel, 1993). Two percent of young patients with first-episode psychosis will commit suicide during these first 2 years (Krausz, Muller-Thomsen & Maasen, 1995). Those with a younger age of onset are especially at risk (particularly males) (Krauzs *et al.*, 1995; Westermeyer *et al.*, 1991). Even the first prodrome of psychosis carries a high risk. However, up to three-quarters of suicides in psychosis actually happen during the early recovery phases, usually within several months of discharge from hospital (Craig *et al.*, 2006; Drake *et al.*, 1984; Hunt *et al.*, 2006). Table 15.1 lists some of the factors involved in each phase of illness. 'Depression' and 'loss of a significant other' are the two commonest reasons given by patients attempting suicide during these phases (Harkavy-Friedman *et al.*, 1999).

Prodrome phase

Suicide in the prodromal phase of the first episode is under-recognized and poorly studied. Young people with prodromal symptoms or 'at-risk mental states' suffer relatively moderate levels of psychopathology and distress during the turmoil of emerging psychosis. Only a fraction of these individuals seek professional help at the time, and even if they do the risks are commonly overlooked. In one of the few specialized clinics for these patients (the Personal Assessment and Crisis Evaluation Clinic in Melbourne), 22 (91.5%) of a small sample of 25 clients were experiencing suicidal ideation at presentation and six (24%) had actually made a suicide attempt (Adlard, 1997). Two of the clinic's patients, who later dropped out of follow-up, went on to commit suicide within 6 months.

First-episode acute phase

By the time the first episode emerges, 50% will have experienced recent thoughts of suicide (Nordentoft *et al.*, 2002) and 25% will have attempted suicide before they first presented to mental health services (Addington *et al.*, 2004; Nordentoft *et al.*, 2002). In a study of self-harm among 495 first-episode patients in the UK, suicide attempt was one of the main factors for

Table 15.1. Suicide responses to phase of psychosis

Illness phase	Types of suicidal reactions
Pre-illness	Reactions to deprivations, traumas, adjustment difficulties, comorbid conditions, personality
Prodrome	Reaction to precipitating stresses, mood changes and deterioration during prodrome
Acute psychotic phase	Command hallucinations
	Acting on delusional ideas
	Disorganized thinking/risk taking leading to unintentional self-harm
	Escape from fear/distress caused by psychotic experiences
	Escape from mental anguish of depression
	Impact of consequences, deprivations, losses caused by illness
Early recovery phase	Impact of insight, stigma and significant losses
	Persistent distressing psychotic symptoms
	Part of post-psychotic depressive phase
	Debilitating negative features
	Treatment or service effects (side effects, poor continuity, etc.)
Late recovery phase	Repeated failures to re-engage in previous role functioning
	Impact of isolation, rejection, losses and enduring social disabilities
	Disengagement or lack of adequate support services
Relapse phase	Reaction to precipitating triggers of relapse
	Insight into consequences of relapse
	Direct response to psychotic experiences and distress

presentation to mental health services (Harvey et al, 2006). A third of patients presented with an immediate risk of self-harm, with over a quarter of these patients deliberately harming themselves at the time. Self-harm at first presentation was more likely among those with depressive psychosis, psychomotor retardation, and longer duration of untreated psychosis.

In a study of suicidal ideation among first-episode patients attending the Early Psychosis Prevention and Intervention Centre (EPPIC) in Melbourne, 65% reported experiencing active suicidal ideation within the first month of presentation. For most, this is fleeting and mild. However, 15% reported feeling seriously suicidal with intent. The average severity of suicidality among the first-episode population appears to resolve rapidly within the first 3 months of treatment but then rises again back to the high levels from the fourth month onwards, before finally falling again at about 18 months follow-up (Power, 2004).

In patients with non-affective psychosis, this fluctuating course of suicidality may represent the coalescing of two distinct phases. The initial peak of suicidality at first presentation (Fig. 15.2) may represent the more acute influence of psychotic features on self-harm behaviours, which responds quickly to treatment in most patients (e.g. command hallucinations, escape behaviours, delusionally motivated self-harm, or accidental self-harm owing to confused disorganized thought processes). The second more prolonged peak of suicidality (Fig. 15.2) may be a reaction to the slow uphill struggle most patients experience in the first 1–2 years. In addition, it may represent the effect of a gradually accumulating smaller group of relapsing psychotic patients.

Suicidality in patients with depressive psychosis may follow a somewhat different course to those with non-affective psychosis. Suicidal ideation will tend to mirror depressive swings in mood. However, patients may be at greatest risk of acting upon these ideas when their depression begins to lift in response to initial treatment and as they regain sufficient energy, concentration and motivation. Once past this critical high-risk phase, one generally sees a gradual resolution of suicidality as the depressive features subside – for most people within 2 or 3 months of starting treatment. The occasional

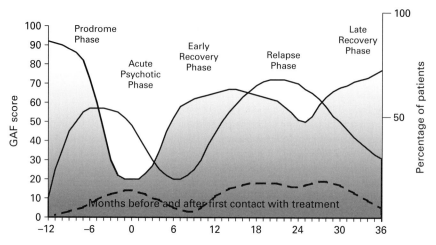

Fig. 15.2. Representative time line of the course of suicidality in non-affective psychosis: percentage per month with suicidal ideation (—) and suicide attempts (- -). GAF, Global Assessment of Functioning.

chronic/treatment-resistant depressed psychotic patient is a particular concern and should merit serious and prompt consideration for electroconvulsive therapy (ECT) as they pose an exceptionally high risk of suicide. Patients with manic psychosis may initially represent a significant risk of unintentional self-harm during the acute manic phase, but then a more serious risk of suicide as they grapple to repair the damage wrought by their episode, or if they slip into a prolonged post-manic–depressive phase.

Recovery phase

It is not surprising that patients become suicidal during the recovery phase, as this is the period when patients emerge from their acute psychosis to face some of the most difficult adjustments to the illness as they struggle to recover normal cognitive and emotional/social functioning. Males appear to take longer than females to regain premorbid level of functioning after their first episode of psychosis (Power *et al.*, 1998). Recovery may be a slow, frustrating and disheartening process for individuals, particularly if they are acutely aware of their own loss of potential. The emergence of insight, hopelessness and depression are features that are particularly evident in the early months after the first

episode of psychosis (Birchwood *et al.*, 2000) and are associated with suicidal ideation and attempts (Addington, Addington & Patten, 1998; Amador *et al.*, 1996; Aquilar *et al.*, 1997).

An additional feature of this recovery phase is that it is commonly the time when acute clinical and social support/attention/supervision is gradually withdrawn in the belief that the high-risk acute phase has abated. The patient is expected to return to coping with everyday stresses, despite the fragility of their functioning and the magnitude of changes they have to accommodate. The risk is that the patient is prematurely exposed to the very stresses and triggers that precipitated the psychosis in the first place. The responses of family and social support systems may be crucial during this period. Rejection, alienation and stigma may add to a patient's sense of distress, loss, hopelessness and despair.

Certain additional factors may increase the risk of suicide during the recovery phase: higher premorbid intelligence quotient, higher socioeconomic background, higher expectations, relatively greater degree of deterioration, loss, stigma, poorer social support and social exclusion/rejection have all been shown to increase the risk of suicide for those with schizophrenia (Siris, 2001).

Relapse phase

Given that psychotic illnesses tend to be relapsing in the majority of patients (Robinson *et al.*, 1999) (most relapses occur between the end of the first year and the third year of follow-up), the realization and psychological impact of relapse may induce profound despair and hopelessness. Preparing patients for the possibility of relapse and empowering them with a range of strategies to deal effectively with relapses may well ameliorate the depressing impact of these episodes as well as hopefully reducing the risk of relapse overall. As yet, however, there is no study of the effect of relapse-prevention counselling on suicide during follow-up.

Suicide risk assessments and formulation in early psychosis

So which patients are at highest risk of suicide in early psychosis (Table 15.2) and what are the most important risk factors to consider? As with non-psychotic conditions, the greater the number of risk factors an individual has, the higher the risk of suicide. Levels of psychopathology, hopelessness, suicidal ideation and a history of suicide attempts appear to be most predictive of later suicide (Nordentoft *et al.*, 2002). Nevertheless, for first-episode patients there may be little illness history to rely upon. The assessing clinician will need to consider the effect of a wide range of more subtle risk factors and extrapolate into the future to identify other potential risk factors downstream, for example, the risk of a patient losing his or her partner or custody of a child and how the patient might react.

The initial suicide risk assessment

Suicide risk assessment and formulation is central to patients' initial clinical assessment, and all mental health clinicians should be trained to a level of basic competence before they undertake any unsupervised assessments of newly presenting first-episode patients. Such assessments require a considerable degree of skill, sensitivity and experience. Ideally, initial assessments should be conducted in pairs so each clinician can cross-reference

Table 15.2. Risk factors for suicide in schizophrenia and bipolar affective disorder

Risk factor	Schizophrenia	Bipolar affective disorder
Age		
Male:female	1.6:1	
Single/separated	↔	
Childless	Trend ↑	
Ethnicity (white)	↑	
Unemployed	↔	
Higher education	Trend ↑	
Higher intelligence quotient	↑	
Living alone	↑	
Recent loss	↑↑	
Family history of depression	↑	↑
Family history of suicide	↑	↑
Childhood loss and deprivations	↔	
Long-term physical illness	↔	
Young age of illness onset	↑	↑
Early stage of illness (< 5 years)	↑	↑
Substance use	↑	↑
Poor treatment adherence	↑	
Compulsory admissions	↑	
Past depressive episodes	↑	↑
Suicide attempts in past	↑↑	↑↑
Recent suicidal ideation	↑↑↑	↑↑↑
Fear of mental disintegration	↑↑	
Agitation	↑	
Worthlessness	↑	
Hopelessness	↑	
Command hallucinations	↑	
Hallucinations	Protective	
Delusions	Protective	
Insight	↔	
Negative symptoms (Flat affect)	Protective	

↑, increased; ↓, decreased, ↔, equivocal.
Based on Hawton *et al.* (2005a,b).

and collaborate in building the initial formulation and plan. Any clinical record should routinely incorporate suicide risk assessment and formulation as part of the initial assessment documentation.

Box 15.1. Questions to ask during the initial risk assessment

General enquiries about suicide

How does what is happening make you feel?

Does it get you down?

How frightening is it?

Does it make you feel so upset that you think you might lose control?

What do you feel like doing when that happens?

Have you felt as if life is not worth living?

Have you had thoughts of ending it all?

What has happened to make you to want do this yourself?

What things have you thought of doing?

Have you actually make any plans?

What steps have you taken already?

When are you planning to do it?

What things are stopping you from doing it?

Do you think you have any alternative options?

What do you think will help?

Do you think it will get better?

Have you ever felt this bad before?

Have you ever tried to commit suicide before?

What happened?

What helped you recover?

Did you ask anyone for help at the time?

Does anyone else know about this?

Psychotic-related experiences

Voices or passivity phenomena

Does anyone ever tell you to harm yourself or do something risky?

What do they tell you to do?

Does it make you feel like doing it?

Do you have any control over it?

How difficult is it to resist?

Have you ever done what they say?

What would happen if you don't?

Paranoid delusions

Do you think others want to kill/seriously harm you?

What do you think they will do to you?

Do you believe that you have no escape?

Manic delusions

Do you think you are invincible?

What are some of the most superhuman things you can do?

Depressive delusions

Do you feel very guilty?

Does it make you want to end your live?

What have you done that makes you feel so bad?

Will anything help?

What are the critical questions clinicians should ask about suicide in the initial interviews? Such enquiries (Box 15.1) are best left until well into an interview when the clinician has hopefully had time to develop rapport and an understanding of some of the issues. Ideally, the clinician should determine where the person is situated along the spectrum of suicidality from *ideation, intent, plans, actions* and *accessing means* (Fig. 15.1; Schwartz, 2000). The interviewer should identify the triggering event and explore the patient's underlying rationale for considering suicide and try to ascertain the level of distress, anger, panic, loss of control, emptiness, hopelessness and despair. Studies suggest that clinicians significantly underestimate suicidal patients' feelings of loss of control, panic and emptiness prior to suicide attempts and, instead, tend to focus on emotions of hopelessness and despair (Schnyder *et al.*, 1999).

Plenty of time should be allowed in the later part of the interview to explore the risk assessment further if the patient reveals more immediate serious levels of suicidality as the clinician may have to re-evaluate the management plan and devote time to liaising with all those involved (e.g. if it prompts admission to hospital). Time should also be set aside for debriefing patients after any discussion about suicide, as not infrequently such enquiries will prompt patients to re-evaluate their reasons for living.

If the patient has been suicidal in the past, a detailed account should be recorded of each episode and suicide attempt. This should form the template for future risk assessments, so a chronological record can be maintained throughout a patient's contact with services. The details should be checked with family, carers and other agencies involved so a comprehensive picture is developed.

Some patients will be very guarded at the initial assessment, fearful that if they mention being suicidal then they will be immediately hospitalized. To avoid this, it is helpful to explain that fleeting thoughts of suicide are a common reaction to the mental 'pain' or anguish that accompanies an acute episode. It is important to reassure patients that these feelings will tend to subside once they get help and treatment, that most people do not act upon such thoughts, and that they can be managed at home as long as certain safeguards

Box 15.2. Initial suicide risk assessment and formulation

Historical risk factors		Current suicidal factors		Future/potential risks	
Previous suicide ideation	□	Depressed/agitated	□	Discharge from hospital	□
Previous suicide attempts	□	Hopelessness/guilt	□	Disengage from treatment	□
Family history of suicide	□	Bizarre risk-taking delusions	□	Poor treatment response	□
Family history of psychosis	□	Command hallucinations	□	Relapse of psychosis/depression	□
Personality disorder	□	Suicidal/morbid thoughts	□	Persistent substance use	□
Substance-use disorder	□	Suicidal plans	□	Threatened serious loss	□
Single/separated/live alone	□	Access to lethal means	□	High expressed emotion/critical atmosphere	□
Unemployment/inactive	□	Refusing help or treatment	□	Social isolation/rejection	□
Serious traumas or abuse	□	Impulsive/unpredictable	□	Unstable accommodation	□
Summary: absent/mild/moderate/severe		Summary: absent/mild/moderate/severe		Summary: absent/mild/moderate/severe	

Suicide risk formulation (reason for high risk: nature, severity, immediacy and reversibility of the risk)

Initial risk management plan (supervision, reviews, removal of means, engagement, treatment and stress resolution)

Client and carers' view of initial management plan (acknowledgement of risk, willingness to collaborate)

---

are in place. It is essential to negotiate an agreement that they will inform carers or staff as soon as it becomes unbearable so more help can be provided.

Mute, partly catatonic or extremely guarded patients should be managed with great caution, particularly if they manifest high levels of stress, agitation, perplexity and unpredictability. Their confused behaviour may result in self-injurious actions, such as, wandering in front of traffic or fire setting. Hospitalization is generally the safest option unless 24-hour supervised care can be provided at home.

Suicide risk-assessment schedules

There are a large number of assessment schedules now available to rate indicators of suicidality – for a review of these see Goldston (2000). Although very useful as an aid to a comprehensive clinical suicide risk assessment, they cannot be relied upon on their own and no schedules exist that are specifically designed to assess suicide risk in psychosis. Some schedules include direct measures of suicide intent (Scale for Suicide Ideation: Beck, Kovacs & Weissman, 1979; Suicide Intent Scale: Beck, Schuyler & Herman, 1974a; Adolescent Suicide Questionnaire: Pearce & Martin, 1994), while others assess indirect measures that can be broadly divided into either state (Hopelessness Scale: Beck *et al.*, 1974b;

the Reasons for Living Inventory: Linehan *et al.*, 1983), or trait measures of suicide risk. Other scales include the Youth Assessment Checklist (Martin, 1995); Kienhorst's Assessment Checklist (Kienhorst *et al.*, 1990); Lethality of Suicide Attempts Rating Scale (Smith, Conroy & Ehler, 1984); the suicidality subscale of the K-SADS (Orvaschel *et al.*, 1982); and, finally, the suicidality subscale of Health of the Nation Outcome Scales (Wing, 1994). Their particular value is in providing an objective measure of suicidality that can be monitored and reviewed during follow up.

The initial risk formulation and provisional risk management plan

Ideally, the initial formulation and provisional risk management plan should be developed collaboratively at the first meeting with the patient, carers and other agencies involved. At the end of the assessment, the clinician should check with the client that they have understood correctly why they have been feeling suicidal and together work out sensible ways of managing the risks over the subsequent few days. Risk assessment forms (Box 15.2) can provide a helpful summary and clearly identifiable record of the assessment formulation and plan. Contingencies should also be discussed and 24-hour emergency contact details provided in case the patient becomes an immediate risk. Potential means (e.g. ropes, tablets) should be made inaccessible and carers should always be involved in the risk management plan.

Occasionally, patients will object to carers being informed, but our recommendation is that carers must always be informed from the outset if there is serious immediate risk (no one will respect one's 'ethical' principles after the event, particularly if the information could have saved the patient's life). If the patient is hospitalized, then all staff on each shift should be made clearly aware of an individual patient's risk and the level of supervision/observation required, for example, one-to-one nursing at arm's length.

Additional factors to consider during the risk assessment

As a more comprehensive formulation of suicide risk is built up during the initial interviews, it is helpful to explore the wider influence of the patient's biological, psychological and social circumstances.

Biological markers of suicide risk

The influence of genetics, neurochemical alterations, certain chronic illnesses, medications and substances of abuse should all be considered in the assessment of suicide risk. Genotyping opens up possibilities but as yet provides only very limited value as markers of risk or treatment response (e.g. to clozapine).

Genes and neurochemistry

A family history of suicide attempts is an important independent risk factor for suicide (Brent & Mann, 2005). This familial risk for suicide may be partly associated with low cerebrospinal fluid levels of concentrations of 5-hydroxyindoleacetic acid (5-HIAA; the primary metabolite of serotonin), which may be a familial marker of anxiety and impulsivity/aggression (Korn *et al.*, 1995; Spirito & Esposito, 2006). Relatively low 5-HIAA concentrations in cerebrospinal fluid were first reported by Asberg, Traskman & Thoren (1976) in unipolar depressed patients who were suicidal.

However, the picture in schizophrenia and bipolar disorders is more inconsistent (Van Praag, 1986). Gene–environment interactions are complex and, as yet, such genetic markers alone yield low predictive values, in the order of 10% (Mann *et al.*, 2006).

Other biological measures have yet to demonstrate proven efficacy. These include tritiated imipramine binding, urinary 17-hydroxycorticosteroids, urinary norepinephrine-to-epinephrine (noradrenaline-to-adrenaline) ratio, dexamethasone suppression test, thyroid-stimulating hormone response to thyrotrophin-releasing hormone, corticotrophin-releasing factor and low serum cholesterol levels. Even combining two of the most promising tests (the dexamethasone suppression test, which measures adrenal gland response to adrencorticotrophic hormone, and the 5-HIAA assessment) still yields low predictive values of 25% at most (Mann *et al.*, 2006).

Alcohol and other drugs

Alcohol abuse is associated with an increased risk of suicide attempts in first-episode psychosis (Verdoux *et al.*, 1999) and may mediate this risk through its depressogenic effects, impairment of problem-solving skills, complication of adverse life events as well as aggravation of impulsive personality traits, possibly through effects on serotonergic neurotransmission (Brady, 2006). Substance abuse greatly increases this risk and polysubstance users are at highest risk, with more than a six-fold higher risk of suicide attempts compared with non-users (Verdoux *et al.*, 1999). Any clinical assessment of suicide risk should include a detailed account of the association between suicidal thoughts and attempts and the use of alcohol or drugs, so that this can be factored into the patient's suicide risk treatment and risk management plan.

Chronic illnesses

Chronic debilitating illnesses carry an independent risk of suicide and their effects on patients' suicidality and self-esteem should not be underestimated even in younger patients. Chronic illness is a contributing factor in approximately 10% of suicides (Whitlock, 1986). Psychosis is more likely to occur in certain illnesses, such as diabetes mellitus, autoimmune disorders and multiple sclerosis. Diabetes, in particular, poses a concern given the challenge managing it in adolescence, the significant risk of overdose with self-administered insulin and the increased risk of developing diabetes with atypical antipsychotic medications.

Medication

A number of medications have been implicated as suicidogenic. Whether these associations are causal or merely coincidental remains unclear, but certain antidepressants should be used cautiously in suicidal patients, particularly adolescents. Side effects of akathisia and dysphoria with antipsychotic drugs and antidepressants may have a role in suicide in schizophrenia (Hansen & Kingdom, 2006). However, one of the main risks with these medications is toxicity in an overdose. The newer antipsychotic and antidepressant medications would, therefore, be preferable. Clinicians should, nonetheless, enquire about stockpiles of medication at patients' homes, ensure that these are removed and that only short prescriptions are dispensed and stored, preferably kept by carers.

Stressful life events, coping style, personality and psychological risk factors

Patients with schizophrenia report higher levels of adverse life events (such as childhood abuse) than the general population (Fennig *et al.*, 2005). There is a heightened risk of suicide during the immediate aftermath of events such as major losses, separations, bereavements, unemployment, debts, homelessness, recent arrest and imprisonment (Kerkhof & Diekstra, 1995). Certain individuals are more prone to react in a suicidal manner because of personality factors such as increased predisposition to aggression and impulsivity, while others may react to such external stresses by internalizing blame and avoiding help through an acute sense of shame and stigma. Fennig *et al.* (2005) reported that a subgroup of adolescent patients with psychosis and who attempted suicide did not actually experience more life events overall but were more prone to perceive the events they experienced as

negative or to have a greater impact. Identifying the recent losses, their impact on the patient, their coping style and their experience with previous traumas will help with an assessment of how an individual is likely to react to future complications of the illness. New stresses may re-ignite unresolved traumas from the past or provoke intolerable fears for their future. It is important that these issues are identified early before such ruminations fester and eventually become a rationale for ending their lives.

Wider family, social and cultural risk factors

Patients' attitudes towards suicide are likely to be strongly determined by their family and cultural background. The prevalence of suicide and self-harm behaviour varies considerably between countries (Fig. 15.3) and between ethnic or social groups within the same country (Raleigh, 1996). In Western countries, youth suicidality has reached epidemic proportions, with 30% of teenagers reporting having considered suicide and 10% having attempted suicide (Evans *et al.*, 2005). Youth suicide rates (age 15–24 years) are highest in eastern and western Europe, Scotland, Ireland and New World countries, including Australia, New Zealand, Canada and the USA (Australian Institute for Suicide Research and Prevention, 2003) and lower in southern Europe and Asia (except for Japan and Singapore, where rates are exceptionally high (Fig. 15.3).

In many cases, these at-risk individuals represent an underclass of the 'have nots' and most vulnerable, whose lives are characterized by a sense of failure, stigma, shame, rejection, abandonment and social exclusion. Suicide and self-harm behaviours may, in some respect, represent a coping style or learnt response to adversity. Psychosis is just one more example of social adversity and suicide its potential solution. In some, suicide may even symbolize their own final victory over adversity, by not surrendering to ignominy, and for some, it may even represent a glorified martyrdom or ultimate sacrifice.

A family history of suicide is not just a genetic marker of risk but is likely to represent within a family the relative's final battle with their illness. In our

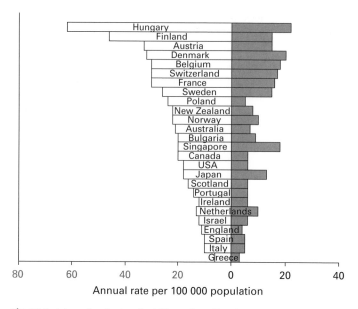

Fig. 15.3. International rates of suicide: males □ Females ▪.

own experience, a group that is especially worrying involves patients whose parent committed suicide during their childhood and who also struggled with a similar illness.

Within a mental health service population, social groups may form around common identities, and occasionally a preoccupation with death may come to symbolize a group's raison d'être. Such networks might prove highly risky to the most vulnerable members of the group, who act out group fantasies. With the Internet, there is additional potential for such networks to form through chat rooms and instant messaging. For young people, text messages or webcam may be a far more natural choice of communicating their suicide intent than any traditional suicide note.

Unfortunately, close family members and primary carers are often unaware of their relatives' suicide preoccupations or attempts. In one large study, relatives knew of suicide attempts in only a third of cases (Rascón *et al.*, 2004). They had limited knowledge of the risk of suicide in schizophrenia and failed to recognize any tendency towards suicide in their relatives.

Service and treatment risk factors

There is evidence that systemic changes and dislocations within and between services contribute to suicide – the process of deinstitutionalization has not been without its many victims (Munk, 1999). Poorly coordinated case management, disorganized services, delayed responses, poor communication, abrupt patient transfers, lack of risk management monitoring, inadequate resources and poorly trained and demoralized staff have all been implicated in critical inquiries regarding suicides. Contributing factors to suicide cited in association with inpatient units include harsh, punitive and degrading practices (e.g. the use of seclusion, straight jackets, physical restraint, unnecessary intramuscular medication); poor collaboration about dose regimens; excessive side effects; and badly designed inpatient units with poor observation, inappropriate fixtures, stigmatizing and demoralizing environments and an inappropriate mix of patient populations. For newly presenting first-episode patients, exposure to such practices and settings can have a traumatizing impact, contributing to a sense of hopelessness and demoralization. Regardless of the setting, just the experience of psychosis is enough to induce symptoms of post-traumatic stress disorder in over a third of patients (McGorry *et al.*, 1991). More recent enquiries suggest that the picture is improving (Appleby et al, 2006). Nonetheless, in this national review, mental health teams estimated that almost a quarter of suicides among their clients were preventable.

Even good treatments and therapies themselves are not without their risks. The dysphoric effects of medications have been implicated together with side effects such as akathisia. Unsupervised stores of medications also pose a risk of overdose. But risks are not confined to pharmacotherapies alone. Psychological interventions contain inherent 'side effects'. Insight-oriented therapies may, in some patients, only compound depressive reactions to the experience of psychosis and undermine their natural tendency towards sealing-over and denial. Fragile dependencies on therapists may be shattered by unexpected changes in staff or by leave arrangements.

Protective factors

Protective factors in suicide rarely get a mention in the literature and tend to be overlooked in risk assessments. However, it is important to remember that some of these protective factors may only be state rather than trait dependent. State-protective factors may include core symptoms of the illness that, if treated, may then actually expose the person to greater risk of suicide during the resolution phase of illness, such as acute manic symptoms (Shaffer *et al.*, 1988), the presence of thought disorder (Apter *et al.*, 1988) and negative symptoms in schizophrenia (Fenton & McGlashan, 1991). A patient who is suicidal during the acute phase of illness may pose an even greater risk of acting upon these thoughts during the recovery phase when these protective symptoms are removed. Complicating personality traits such as obsessional traits may be associated with a reduced risk of suicide compared with other traits such as borderline and antisocial features.

Suicide risk management

Suicide risk management strategies within a service can be broadly divided into those that are universal (preventive), selective strategies (screening and monitoring) and indicated interventions or therapies for those at highest risk (Table 15.3). Universal strategies target the whole clinic population with risk prevention: service model, accessibility, policies and facility design. Even though these universal approaches are likely to have limited effect at an individual level, they may significantly shift the general risk of suicide within a service and have as much impact as indicated interventions and treatments. To have maximum impact on reducing suicide risk, services need to strike a balance between these universal, selective and indicated interventions. The following section deals with these three approaches in more detail starting with selective interventions (universal preventive strategies are described last).

Selective interventions

Routine risk monitoring

Routine risk assessment and management systems should be an integral part of any mental health service. An alert should be triggered within the service for any patient assessed to be a suicide risk and the service should remain on high alert until a formal review has determined that the risk has subsided. These patients should then be considered for one or more specific interventions to reduce the risk (see section below on specific interventions).

This basic monitoring of risk should be regularly reviewed and, given the transient nature of suicidality, it should happen particularly during (1) the transition from prodrome to psychosis, (2) the early phase of recovery, (3) early relapse if it occurs, and (4) during phases when there are rapid fluctuations in mental state. Comprehensive reassessments of suicide risk should be made after any behaviour suggestive of a suicide attempt. This should trigger a reappraisal of the care plan and a formal review with the patient, carer, treating team and any other agencies involved. The increased risk should also trigger more frequent contact with the

Table 15.3. Risk prevention, management and interventions

Risk management strategies	Components
Universal prevention	
Service models	Early detection and intervention, assertive outreach
Design and safety modifications to service facilities	Hanging points; electrical supply safety circuits; fire safety systems; storage systems for glass and knives; clear lines of observation
Policies and supervision regarding medication	Fortnightly dispensing for high-risk patients; supervision and storage of medication by carers
Policies and supervision of transfers between teams	Close monitoring of transfers from one service to another; assertive follow-up of clients lost to follow-up
Staff training and supervision	Mandatory risk assessment training
Rehabilitative options	Appropriately paced support with reintegration into vocational and educational activities; social support and peer groups; attention to physical healthcare
Social care options	Supervised accommodation: support options; access to living support grants; liaison with criminal justice and prison services
Indicated risk management	
Regular risk assessments or at key transitions	
Brief risk review	*Routine*: monthly by case manager/doctor
	Additional: before planned drop in contact/supervision; before planned increase in responsibilities; at setback in recovery plans/significant adversity
Full risk assessment	*Routine*: entry and discharge from service
	Additional: on admission and discharge from hospital; on transfer from one team to another; on transfer from one case manager to another; after suicide attempt or worsening suicidality; on relapse of psychosis; if significant depression
Service-wide risk monitoring systems	Zoning; TREAT (see text for fuller description of both)
Selective interventions for those at highest risk	
Crisis intervention for suicidal patients	Staffing with sufficient capacity for emergency outreach assessments; emergency access to senior clinicians for assessment and decisions about risk management; prompt access to safe and secure settings with close supervision, e.g. hospital/triage unit; use of 1: 1 nursing observation in hospital; debriefing patient and carers
Pharmacotherapy for suicidal patients	Temporary addition of benzodiazepines to alleviate distress; addition of antidepressants; atypical antipsychotic drugs; electroconvulsive therapy in severe intractable psychosis at high risk
Psychological options	Cognitive–behavioural therapy for depression, suicidality, persistent symptoms, traumas and post-traumatic stress disorder, after suicide attempts or other stresses; substance dependence/abuse counselling; family work for high expressed emotion or dysfunctional families
Audit and suicide reviews	Routine debriefing and internal reviews

service until the risk has subsided, mediated ideally via one of the risk management systems described below. The full risk assessment should be reviewed again whenever a transfer occurs from one team to another, for example at discharge from hospital.

Examples of systems of risk monitoring

The *zoning system* (Ryrie *et al.*, 1997; Table 15.4) is one of a number of risk management systems available in mental health services, but it is recommended because

Table 15.4. Zoning (traffic light) system for risk management in community teams

Zone	Category	Minimum monitoring
Red	Acutely psychotic or depressed patients who are at significant risk to self or others	Minimum weekly face-to-face reviews by case manager and fortnightly reviews by doctor
	Patients who have dropped out of contact or are at immediate risk of disengagement	Prompt home visits if fail to attend
	New patients being assessed or recently discharged from hospital	Daily case review at team handover and weekly team meetings
Amber	Recovering patients with either residual symptoms or significant disability but who do not pose an immediate risk to self or others; need assertive follow-up and monitoring of treatment adherence	Minimum fortnightly face-to-face reviews by case manager and monthly reviews by doctor; prompt reminders and contact if fail to attend
		Regular case reviews at weekly team meetings
Green	Recovered patients who are either back to normal functioning or are engaged in daytime activities; motivated to attend for follow-up and treatment	Minimum monthly face to face reviews by case manager and 2-monthly reviews by doctor; prompt reminders and contact if fail to attend; 3-monthly case reviews at weekly team meetings.
Hospital	Patients temporarily in hospital while acutely psychotic or depressed; co-working with inpatient team	Weekly reviews by case manager in hospital; attendance at ward rounds and discharge planning meetings

of its ease of administration and usefulness in clinical practice. It has been successfully introduced in early intervention services such as the Lambeth Early Onset service in London (Power *et al.*, 2007) and includes both inpatient and community risk management protocols.

Patients are categorized at daily team handovers into three levels of risk (low, green; moderate, amber; high, red) (Ryrie *et al.*, 1997). This assessment is supplemented by a risk assessment questionnaire undertaken when the team makes initial contact with the patient. All new patients to one of the teams are placed in the red zone until the multidisciplinary team decides otherwise. A highly visible board/chart is kept in each team base with a list of the team's patients in each of the three zones. Any clinician may move a patient up into a higher risk zone at any time if they are concerned about the patient but a patient zone may not be downgraded until the team has made a decision to do so at its regular multidisciplinary clinical review meeting. The zoning system is linked to a patient management protocol that determines the intensity of supervision and frequency

of observations/contact; for example, an inpatient in the red zone must have a nurse accompany them while on leave (if on red zone and high-profile observations then no leave is permitted and whereabouts must be confirmed every 15 minutes). The system also determines the frequency of risk assessment reviews and means that red zone patients are frequently evaluated and discussed at each team meeting and shift handovers. It is also a useful audit and management tool for evaluating service demand, incidents, caseloads and staffing levels.

A further example of a risk identification and management system is the Treatment Resistance and Early Intervention Team (TREAT) employed by EPPIC in Melbourne. The team's role includes identification of those patients at high risk of suicide. This is done using a simple screening measure – the suicidality subscale of the Brief Psychiatric Rating Scale, which has previously been found to be effective in its ability to identify young people with first-episode psychosis at risk of suicide (Power *et al.*, 2003). Patients are screened on a monthly basis by their case manager, in addition to any risk assessments that are conducted as part of routine clinical practice. Those who score 4 or above on the scale are identified as high risk and are then presented to a multidisciplinary meeting by their case manager, during which recommendations are made for their continued treatment.

Indicated interventions: specific treatments for those identified at highest risk

The suicide risk assessment and formulation should guide the clinician in recommending a range of specific treatment options to address the suicide risk issues faced by a particular patient. This is not a 'one-size-fits-all' remedy and certain therapies (e.g. clozapine, CBT or family therapies) may be wholly inappropriate for a given individual even if research evidence generally supports their use in suicidal patients. The formulation should determine whether the patient's suicidality is driven by (1) the acute symptoms of psychosis; (2) complicating mood disturbance; (3) preexisting comorbid conditions, such as personality disorder; (4) the individual's internal psychological reaction to the impact of their illness; (5) external factors such as reactions of significant others and losses; (6) post-traumatic stress features related to a previous suicide attempt or death of a significant other; and, finally, (7) suicide pacts between patients. Tailoring individual packages of interventions to address these various risk factors will avoid a 'one-size-fits-all' approach and will better identify the specific goals of suicide risk reduction.

The additional suicide preventive effect of these additional specific therapies is small (Bronisch, 1996; van der Sande *et al.*, 1997b) and it is essential to ensure that optimal standard treatment interventions for psychosis are already in place – simply engaging patients better in standard treatment will reduce the risk of suicide (Dahlsgaard, Beck & Brown, 1998). De Hert *et al.* (2001) reported in their study of 63 suicides of patients with schizophrenia that those who committed suicide were seven times less likely to comply with treatment than matched control patients. Heilä (1999) examined suicides among patients with schizophrenia

($n = 92$) and noted that over half of the patients were either not prescribed adequate antipsychotic treatment or were not using it at the time of their death. The National Confidential Inquiry into Suicide in the UK noted that of the 960 people with schizophrenia who died by suicide between 1996 and 2000, nearly a third (30%) were non-compliant with their medication (Hunt *et al.*, 2006). Side effects of medication were common and the report recommended that all patients who were non-compliant with 'typical' antipsychotic medication owing to side effects should be offered atypical medication as an alternative (Appleby *et al.*, 2001).

Acute suicide risk containment

Staff and carers should have clear guidelines outlining how they should respond to someone identified at imminent risk. Services should ensure that contact details of all senior staff are readily available to all staff, and all carers should have clear written advice about who to contact in an emergency. The immediate priority is to ensure the patient's safety, adequate supervision and the removal of potential methods of self-harm. Staff should apply the principle of the least-restrictive intervention needed to achieve a safe and effective outcome (Schwartz, 2000). In less-acute situations, this might just involve increasing the frequency of contact and support.

In very-high-risk situations, the patient may need to be promptly accompanied and moved to a place of safety, such as hospital. Senior staff should be readily available to provide further assessment and consultation regarding the most appropriate options. Extra staff may need to be called upon for assistance. Patients' belongings should be searched to remove potentially harmful contents. All staff on a shift should be made aware of the imminent risk, the level of supervision required and any restrictions imposed to prevent access to means of self-harm (e.g. cigarette lighters, cords, sharps). Places of containment (e.g. hospital bedrooms) should be designed to minimize risk of self-harm by removal of obstacles to lines of vision, hanging points, curtain/blind cords, breakable fittings and glass, and by the installation in rooms of individual trip switches, smoke detectors, observation panels, night lighting and reverse barrier doors. Teams may need to enlist extra staff at short notice to cover 1:1 observations and these staff should have personal alarms for emergencies. Routine systems should be in place to allow team leaders to approve funds for these extra staff immediately. The treating team should review the risk management and treatment plan as soon as possible (e.g. within the next working day) to determine what specific treatments (Table 15.3) should be recommended.

Pharmacological and physical treatments

Antitypical antipsychotic drugs. Preliminary trials of the newer antipsychotic drugs, in particular those with dopamine D_2 and serotonin 5-HT_2 receptor antagonist activity (e.g. risperidone, quetiapine, olanzapine, sertindole), indicate that they may have a suicide preventive effect compared with conventional antipsychotic drugs (Kerwin & Bolonna, 2004), possibly through their favourable impact on side effects, negative symptoms, anxiety and depression. In a large case–control study of 756 patients with schizophrenia-spectrum disorders, Barak *et al.* (2004) reported that atypical antipsychotic drugs were 3.5 times less likely to be associated with suicide attempts than conventional antipsychotic drugs.

Clozapine. Approximately one quarter of schizophrenia patients who commit suicide are treatment resistant (Heilä, 1999). Meltzer and Okayli (1995) recommend that clozapine should be prescribed early in patients with 'treatment resistant' psychosis to reduce the risk of suicide. They reported that 35 (40%) of 88 patients treated with clozapine became less suicidal according to indicators such as the number of suicide attempts and the severity of suicidal ideation. A subsequent much larger study (InterSePT Study) also suggested that clozapine may have a specific effect on reducing suicidal ideation (Meltzer, 2005).

Antidepressants. Though antidepressants are frequently (11–43%) prescribed with antipsychotic medication in schizophrenia, there are few studies of their effects and none in the first episode (Micallef, Fakra & Blin, 2006), even though the prevalence of depressive symptoms is high (Birchwood *et al.*, 2000). In schizophrenia and schizoaffective disorders, the combined use of antidepressants and antipsychotic medication during the acute psychotic phase has been shown to delay the resolution of, or even exacerbate, psychotic symptoms (Kramer, Vogel & Dijohnson, 1989; Prusoff, Williams & Weissman, 1979). However, treatment in post-psychotic depression does appear to be beneficial (Siris, 2001), in reducing both depressive symptoms and rates of psychotic relapse, particularly for those who respond early to these treatments. Of the selective serotonin-reuptake inhibitors (SSRIs), only sertraline has been studied, showing limited benefits or equivocal findings (Micallef *et al.*, 2006). However, in depressive psychosis, there is clear evidence in favour of the combined use of antidepressant and antipsychotic drugs (Parker *et al.*, 1992; Spiker *et al.*, 1985). The SSRIs (in combination with an antipsychotic drug) produce lower side effects than the older tricyclic antidepressants (Rothschild *et al.*, 1993).

Lithium. Lithium has been shown to be associated with lower rates of suicide in affective disorders (Coppen, 1994), but reports of its efficacy in first-episode psychosis are lacking.

Electroconvulsive therapy. This is the most effective treatment available for affective psychosis (Mukherjee, Sacheim & Schur, 1994; Parker *et al.*, 1992), the disorder that carries the highest risk of suicide (Blumenthal, 1990). In five of six studies reviewed by Tanney (1986), ECT appeared to have a preventive effect on suicide behaviours, although none focused specifically on early psychosis. However, ECT should be reserved as a second-line treatment, except in emergency situations when the patient is at very high risk. In first-episode psychosis, ECT is undertaken in less than 5% of patients (Power *et al.*, 1998).

Psychological interventions

Individual and group-based CBT interventions that focus on enhancing adaptation and recovery from psychosis (e.g. Drury *et al.*, 1996; Jackson *et al.*, 2001; Kemp *et al.*, 1996) would be expected to minimize the risk of suicide. However, so far only one of these interventions (LifeSPAN, see below) has been designed with suicide in mind, and the impact of the other interventions on suicidality has yet to be studied. A few other cognitive interventions have been developed for non-psychotic suicidal patients (Freeman & Reinecke, 1993; Perris, 1994; Salkovkis, Atha & Storer, 1990; Shearin & Linehan, 1994; van der Sande *et al.*, 1997a), but their actual impact on suicidality is very limited (van der Sande *et al.*, 1997b).

LifeSPAN therapy was designed specifically for acutely suicidal young patients with psychosis (Power *et al.*, 2003). It is a 10-session individual CBT intervention provided by clinical psychologists in addition to standard clinical care. The initial sessions are devoted to an analysis of the patient's suicidality in order to identify the main contributing psychological factors. Then a plan is collaboratively negotiated to address the short-term issues (e.g. recent losses, hopelessness, guilt and shame) and long-term issues (e.g. premorbid traumas, abuse, bereavement, self-esteem, gender identity issues). As far as possible, the short-term issues are the focus of the remaining sessions. Counsellors should proceed particularly slowly with addressing these issues, adopting a stress-diathesis model of suicidality, and being especially sensitive to patients' vulnerabilities at this stage of recovery (Schwartz, 2000). Patients' executive functions and coping strategies may be significantly impaired by their illnesses. Furthermore, they may have reached their limit in accommodating additional stresses, particularly as belief in recovery may yet to be realized. Long-term issues are best left until the patient is sufficiently recovered and stable. The final couple of sessions are devoted to a reanalysis, developing a long-term suicide risk management plan with contingencies, and then a handover in a joint interview with the patient's case manager and carer.

The LifeSPAN therapy was evaluated in a small randomized controlled trial of 42 patients offered either Life SPAN or standard therapy in the EPPIC programme (Power *et al.*, 2003). LifeSPAN was associated with significant reductions in levels of hopelessness, suicidal ideation and improved quality of life scores.

These improvements were maintained at follow-up 6 months later. However, there was no reduction in suicide attempts and one patient in each arm of the trial committed suicide within 6 months of follow-up. It highlighted the challenges of working with this very-high-risk group and the importance of not relying on one aspect of treatment in suicide prevention.

Psychosocial interventions

Potential psychosocial interventions may include psychosocial interventions that reduce 'hopelessness', particularly during the early recovery phase; the provision of intensive support post-discharge from hospital; minimizing the potentially disruptive impact of an episode of mental illness on the person's social milieu; protecting the person's developmental trajectory and sense of 'self' via interventions that support peer relationships, work and vocational involvements; and introducing successful role models (Lipschitz, 1995).

Given that the social network of those with psychosis often constricts to a small group of concerned relatives, interventions such as psychoeducation and therapies that reduce critical 'expressed emotion' have been suggested by Lipschitz (1995) in order to reduce the risk of suicide.

Self-help

A number of books have been written for both suicidal patients and survivors of suicide. The most comprehensive self-help book is *Choosing to Live* (Ellis & Newman, 1996), which is a step-by-step survival guide for acutely suicidal patients, using CBT approaches. It is a rather ambitious book that might be more suited to clinicians and carers as the average suicidal patient is unlikely to have the sustained motivation to read all of its 171 pages. Other books include *Stronger than Death: When Suicide Touches Your Life* (Chance, 1997), and *Questions and Answers about Suicide* (Lester, 1989).

There are also a number of organizations with helpful internet sites, including the American Association of Suicidology (http://www.cyberpsych.org/aas.htm), the Suicide Education and Information Centre (www.suicideinfo.ca), SAVE (the Suicide Awareness Voices of

Education; http://www.save.org) and Friends for Survival (http://www.friendsforsurvival.org/suggested_books.htm).

Universal strategies: service-wide suicide prevention

Raising staff awareness, protocols and providing training in suicide prevention

Raising confidence and skills among staff and carers in detecting, assessing and managing suicide risk is integral to any risk management strategy. Training programmes to address this have been shown to provide a significant reduction in suicide rates (Rihmer, Rutz & Pihlgren, 1995). They involve staff at all levels within a service – even reception, switchboard and administrative staff who come into regular contact with patients. They should also include carers, family (Rascón *et al.*, 2004) and patients themselves. At the very least, they should form part of the basic 'first aid' training and induction to new members.

Clear procedures should be in place in the event of emergencies so concerns can be directed easily and quickly to the staff member who is clinically responsible so that the risk can be contained until extra help arrives, for example, by having duty systems for emergencies, well-rehearsed protocols, good channels for communication and supervision, clear lines of clinical accountability and crisis assessment procedures. Even providing simple protocols for staff and crisis cards for carers/patients with emergency numbers may go a long way in reducing the potential for patients, carers and staff to becoming lost in the system as they try to find help during a crisis; it may even reduce readmissions to hospital (Sutherby *et al.*, 1999).

There are a wide variety of more formal training programmes and modules for suicide prevention – some of which have been evaluated with good effect. They range from simple brief introductory workshops for non-health professionals (Davidson & Range, 1999), through training modules for primary care physicians (Green & Gask, 2005) and training workshops for front-line clinical staff (Fenwick *et al.*, 2004) to web-based public health training packages (Stone, Barber & Potter, 2005).

Debriefing and service reviews

Debriefing and support after a serious suicide attempt or completed suicide are a basic part of any mental health service. Suicides are an inevitable occurrence despite everyone's best efforts, and it is essential that support is provided promptly, not just for the bereaved family and friends but also for other patients in the service and for any staff directly involved. Copy cat suicides are not uncommon (McKenzie *et al.*, 2005) and being bereaved by suicide is a known risk factor for future suicidal behaviour among friends and family of the deceased. Hence, adequate debriefing may go a long way to reducing the risk of subsequent morbidity for all involved (Schwartz, 2000). The support needs to continue well after the funeral and involve formal debriefing sessions. It should be provided again when issues are re-ignited by anniversaries and around the time of the subsequent coroner's inquest.

Service-wide annual internal reviews of serious untoward incidents are very helpful in bringing to light trends or areas of concern that might prompt changes in policy or resources, for example, policies on the presence of cigarette lighters in inpatient units. However, such case reviews/audits need to be handled sensitively and the identities of individual patients and staff protected to avoid undue blame or criticism.

Models of mental health service provision

Early intervention services may by their very nature reduce the risk of suicide (Harkavy-Friedman, 2006; McGorry *et al.*, 1998) by detecting patients earlier, maintaining assertive engagement, providing more psychosocial recovery and relapse-prevention programmes, and streaming their patients into youth-appropriate settings.

To what extent can strategies for early detection make a difference to suicides occurring even before first contact with services? Given the high prevalence of suicidality at first presentation, there is no doubt that a small proportion of people in the prodrome or with undetected psychosis commit suicide even before they are known to services. There is also evidence that the longer the duration of untreated psychosis the greater the risk of suicide attempts (Clarke *et al.*, 2006; Verdoux *et al.*, 2001). There are encouraging findings that early detection may reduce this risk. Melle *et al.* (2006) demonstrated that the early detection programme employed by the Early Treatment and Intervention in Psychosis study in Norway appeared to pick up patients significantly earlier in their period of untreated psychosis and was associated with a reduction in the measures of suicidality (plans or attempts) before first contact. The rate of attempted suicides in the month preceding first contact was 1% in patients in the area with the early detection programme versus 10% in patients from the areas without the programme.

What effect might the engagement and psychosocial strategies of services for early intervention have on suicidality during the 'critical' follow-up period (typically 3 years)? Again, there is encouraging evidence that suicide rates within such services are lower than the average 5.5% rates seen in the first 5 years of follow-up of previous cohorts of patients with first-episode psychosis (Heilä & Lönnqvist, 2003). In the first year of follow-up of recent early intervention services, the reported suicide rate was 0.3% in the OPUS trial (Bertelsen *et al.*, 2007), 0.4% in the Calgary Early Psychosis Programme (Addington *et al.*, 2004), 0.2% for each year of follow-up in EPPIC (Power, 2004), and 0.18–0.21% for each year of follow-up in the Lambeth Early Onset (LEO) service. After 3 years of follow-up in the OPUS trial (3 years is the limit for most early intervention services), suicide rates were significantly lower in those randomized to the early intervention service (0.36%) than in those randomized to standard services (1.45%) and by 5 years, the suicide rates were 1.15% and 1.5%, respectively (Bertelsen *et al.*, 2007). A more marked differential was seen for deaths from all causes in this study (including suspected suicides): 0.36% in the early intervention group and 3% in the standard group by 3 years and 2.2% and 3.8%, respectively, by 5 years of follow-up. Whether this differential can be maintained after leaving the early intervention service is yet to be confirmed. It is possible that suicide rates slip back to the normal rate when patients are discharged or transferred from such services (Bertelsen *et al.*, 2007).

Other service models have varying impacts. Services with poor continuity of care have relatively higher rates of suicide (Desai, Dausey & Rosenhack, 2005). Service models such as 'assertive outreach' or 'home treatment', and the use of community treatment order legislation, may have an impact on reducing suicide through facilitating better engagement in treatment and closer supervision with aftercare for those most at risk (Power, 1999). More general factors within health services are policies and resources that improve risk assessment, management and interagency communication. For example, the Care Programme Approach in the UK has a mandated system of risk assessment, care plans and regular multiagency review. Improving communication across health agencies via electronic record systems may also reduce the risks.

Adequate social services and social policies

Social policies and services have an important role in negating the marginalization of young people with psychotic disorders, by providing safety net services, such as youth housing and vocational support services; introducing antidiscrimination legislation; funding services to support carers and advocacy organizations; promoting health education; and controlling media coverage of suicides. Limiting access to lethal methods of suicide is also critical, and there is good evidence to suggest that this does lead to a reduction in suicide rates at a population level (Mann *et al.*, 2005). This includes car exhaust modifications, domestic gas modifications, restrictions and fencing around potential jumping points, limiting access to household poisons, gun control legislation and regulations to reduce the availability of 'lethal' prescriptions of medications.

The future of suicide prevention in psychosis

As the focus of suicide prevention moves towards earlier intervention and prevention, it will shift attention to patients at a younger age and earlier stage in the development of their psychosis. This will inevitably challenge clinicians' skills of identifying those most at risk and it will alter the way services and treatments are provided. The evidence base for identifying which patients are at most risk of suicide, and when, is still very rudimentary and far more research is needed to highlight the relevant importance of, and the complex interplay between, risk factors. Markers of gene–environment risk offer the promise of better predictive power, and there is considerable potential to develop better actuarial models of prognosis. However, in their rudimentary form these have the risk of entrapping a large proportion of first-episode patients into overly restrictive practices as well as leading to potential stigmatization, for example, raising insurance premiums, restricting access to accommodation or limiting job opportunities.

Despite the major impact that psychosis contributes to the national rates of suicide, there is still little study of the suicide-preventive effects of specific pharmacological or psychological interventions in psychosis. This is in dire need of attention, even if it is a particularly challenging area to study.

Conclusions

There is a greater awareness that the early years of psychosis represent a period of highest risk for suicide and that early intervention strategies may reduce this risk. However, early intervention services will only have a limited impact on suicide rates in the absence of comprehensive risk management strategies to identify and monitor patients at highest risk. A simple zoning system of risk that determines the intensity of care provision may be one such model. Once identified, patients need ready access to specific interventions that are likely to minimize their risk. Interventions such as certain medication treatments, cognitive therapies and psychosocial/family interventions may have an important role, but further evidence is needed to prove their effectiveness in suicide prevention. Finally, the mainstay of suicide prevention in psychosis is making sure good quality care and treatment is available as early as possible, all delivered by well-trained staff in non-stigmatizing settings and working closely with carers and agencies – promoting not just a sense of recovery and hope but also sensible management of the psychosis and the risks involved. If early intervention services can indeed deliver on these goals, then

there is considerable potential for significant reduction in patients' risk of suicide and more generally will dispel the spectre of tragedy that has traditionally pervaded these conditions.

REFERENCES

Addington, D., Addington, J. & Patten, S. (1998). Depression in people with first-episode schizophrenia. *British Journal of Psychiatry*, **172**(Suppl 33), s90–2.

Addington, J., Williams, J., Young, J. & Addington, D. (2004). Suicide behaviour in early psychosis. *Acta Psychiatrica Scandinavica*, **109**, 116–20.

Adlard, S. (1997). An Analysis of Health Damaging Behaviours in Young People at High Risk of Psychosis. Fellowship dissertation, Royal College and New Zealand College of Psychiatrists, Melbourne.

Amador, X. F., Freidman, J. H., Kasapis, C. *et al.* (1996). Suicidal behaviour in schizophrenia and its relationship to awareness of illness. *American Journal of Psychiatry*, **153**, 1185–8.

Andriessen, K. (2006). On 'intention' in the definition of suicide. *Suicide and Life-Threatening Behaviour*, **36**, 533–8.

Appleby, L., Shaw, J., Sherratt, J. *et al.* (2001). *Safety First: Five-year Report of the National Confidential Inquiry into Suicide and Homicide by People with Mental Illness.* London: The Stationary Office.

Appleby, L., Shaw, J., Kapur, N. *et al.* (2006). *Avoidable Deaths: Five Year Report into the National Confidential Inquiry into Suicide and Homicide by People with Mental Illness.* London: The Stationary Office.

Apter, A., Bleich, A., Plutchik, R., Mendelsohn, S. & Tyano, S. (1988). Suicidal behaviour, depression and conduct disorder in hospitalised adolescents. *Journal of the American Academy of Child and Adolescent Psychiatry*, **27**, 696–9.

Aquilar, E. J., Haas, G., Manzanera, F. G. *et al.* (1997). Hopelessness and first-episode psychosis: a longitudinal study. *Acta Psychiatrica Scandinavica*, **96**, 25–30.

Asberg, M., Traskman, L. & Thoren, P. (1976). 5-HIAA in the cerebrospinal fluid: a biochemical suicide predictor? *Archives of General Psychiatry*, **33**, 1193–7.

Australian Institute for Suicide Research and Prevention (2003). *International Suicide Rates: Recent Trends and Implications for Australia.* Canberra: Australian Government Department of Health and Ageing.

Barak, Y., Mirecki, I., Knobler, H. Y., Natan, Z. & Aizenberg, D. (2004). Suicidality and second generation antipsychotics in schizophrenia patients: a case-controlled retrospective study during a 5-year period. *Psychopharmacology*, **175**, 215–19.

Beck, A., Schuyler, D. & Herman, I. (1974a). Development of suicidal intent scales. In A. T. Beck, H. C. P. Resnik & D. Lettieri (eds.), *The Prediction of Suicide*. Bowie, MD: Charles Press, pp. 5445–56.

Beck, A., Weissman, A., Lester, D. & Trexler, L. (1974b). The measurement of pessimism: the Hopelessness Scale. *Journal of Consulting and Clinical Psychology*, **44**, 861–5.

Beck, A. T. (1996). Foreword. In T. E. Ellis & C. F. Newman (eds.), *Chosing to Live*. Oakland, CA: New Harbinger, pp. ix–xi.

Beck, A. T., Kovacs, M. & Weissman, A. (1979). Assessment of suicidal ideation: the Scale for Suicide Ideation. *Journal of Consulting and Clinical Psychology*, **47**, 343–52.

Bertelsen, M., Jeppesen, P., Petersen, L. *et al.* (2007). Suicidal behaviour and mortality in 547 first-episode psychotic patients: the OPUS trial. *British Journal of Psychiatry*, **51** (Suppl), s140–6.

Birchwood, M., Iqbal, Z., Chadwick, P. & Trower, P. (2000). Cognitive approach to depression and suicidal thinking in psychosis: ontogeny of post-psychotic depression. *British Journal of Psychiatry*, **177**, 516–21.

Blumenthal, S. (1990). Youth suicide: risk factors, assessment, and treatment of adolescent and young adult suicidal patients. *Psychiatric Clinics of North America*, **13**, 511–56.

Brady, J. (2006). The association between alcohol misuse and suicidal behaviour. *Alcohol and Alcoholism*, **41**, 473–8.

Brent, D. A. & Mann, J. J. (2005). Family genetic studies, suicide, and suicidal behaviour. *American Journal of Medical Genetics: Seminars in Medical Genetics*, **133**, 13–24.

Bronisch, T. (1996). The relationship between suicidality and depression. *Archives of Suicide Research*, **2**, 235–54.

Brown, S. (1997). Excess mortality of schizophrenia: a meta-analysis. *British Journal of Psychiatry*, **171**, 502–8.

Burgess, P., Pirkis, J., Morton, J. & Croke, E. (2000). Lessons from a comprehensive clinical audit of users of psychiatric services who committed suicide. *Psychiatric Services*, **51**, 1555–60.

Chance, S. (1997). *Stronger than Death: When Suicide Touches Your Life*. New York: W. W. Norton.

Clarke, M., Whitty, P., Browne, S. *et al.* (2006). Suicidality in first episode psychosis. *Schizophrenia Research*, **86**, 221–5.

Coppen, A. (1994). Depression as a lethal disease: prevention strategies. *Journal of Clinical Psychiatry*, **55**(Suppl), 37–45.

Craig, T. J., Ye, Q. & Bromet, E. J. (2006). Mortality among first-admission patients with psychosis. *Comprehensive Psychiatry*, **47**, 246–51.

Dahlsgaard, K. K., Beck, A. T. & Brown, G. K. (1998). Inadequate response to therapy as a predictor of suicide. *Suicide and Life-Threatening Behaviour*, **28**, 197–204.

Davidson, M. W. & Range, L. M. (1999). Are teachers of children and young adolescents responsive to suicide prevention training modules? Yes. *Death Studies*, **23**, 61–71.

De Hert, M., McKenzie, K. & Peuskens, J. (2001). Risk factors for suicide in young people suffering from schizophrenia: a long-term follow-up study. *Schizophrenia Research*, **47**, 127–34.

Desai, R. A., Dausey, D. J., Rosenhack, R. A. (2005). Mental health service delivery and suicide risk: the role of individual patient and facility factors. *American Journal of Psychiatry*, **162**, 311–18.

Drake, R. E., Gates, C., Cotton, P. G. & Whitaker, A. (1984). Suicide among schizophrenics: who is at risk? *Journal of Nervous and Mental Disease*, **172**, 613–17.

Drury, V., Birchwood, M., Cochrane, R. & MacMillan, F. (1996). Cognitive therapy and recovery from acute psychosis: a controlled trial: I. Impact on psychotic symptoms. *British Journal of Psychiatry*, **169**, 593–601.

Ellis, T. E. & Newman, C. F. (1996). *Choosing to Live*. Oakland, CA: New Harbinger.

Evans, E., Hawton, K., Rodham, K. & Deeks, J. (2005). The prevalence of suicidal phenomena in adolescents: a systematic review of population-based studies. *Suicide and Life-Threatening Behaviour*, **35**, 239–50.

Fennig, S., Horesh, N., Aloni, D., Apter, A., Weizman, A. & Fennig, S. (2005). Life events and suicidality in adolescents with schizophrenia. *European Child and Adolescent Psychiatry*, **14**, 454–460.

Fenton, W. & McGlashan, T. (1991). Natural history of schizophrenia subtypes. *Archives of General Psychiatry*, **48**, 969–77.

Fenwick, C. D., Vassilas, C. A., Carter, H. & Haque, M. S. (2004). Training health professionals in the recognition, assessment and management of suicide risk. *International Journal of Psychiatry in Clinical Practice*, **8**, 117–21.

Freeman, A. & Reinecke, M. A. (1993). *Cognitive Therapy of Suicide Behaviour: A Manual for Treatment*. New York: Springer.

Goldston, D. (2000). *Assessment of Suicidal Behaviours and Risk Among Children and Adolescents*. [Technical Report submitted to NIMH under Contract No 263-MD-909995. Bethesda, MB: National Institutes of Mental Health.

Green, G. & Gask, L. (2005). The development, research and implementation of STORM (Skills-based Training on Risk Management). *Primary Care Mental Health*, **3**, 207–13.

Gupta, R. D. & Guest, J. F. (2002). Annual cost of bipolar disorder to UK society. *British Journal of Psychiatry*, **180**, 227–33.

Hansen, L. & Kingdom, D. (2006). Akathisia as a risk factor for suicide. *British Journal of Psychiatry*, **188**, 192.

Harkavy-Friedman, J. M. (2006). Can early detection of psychosis prevent suicidal behaviour? *American Journal of Psychiatry*, **163**, 768–70.

Harkavy-Friedman, J. M., Restifo, K., Malaspina, D. *et al.* (1999). Suicidal behaviour in schizophrenia: characteristics of individuals who had and had not attempted suicide. *American Journal of Psychiatry*, **156**, 1276–8.

Harvey, S. B., Dean, K., Morgan, C. *et al.* (2006). How often does deliberate self-harm precipitate first presentation to services with psychosis? Findings from the AESOP Study, *Schizophrenia Research*, **86**, S56–7.

Hawton, K., Sutton, L., Haw, C., Sinclair, J. & Deeks, J. (2005a). Schizophrenia and suicide: systematic review of risk factors. *British Journal of Psychiatry*, **187**, 9–20.

Hawton, K., Sutton, L., Haw, C., Sinclair, J. & Harris, L. (2005b). Suicide and attempted suicide in bipolar disorder: a systematic review of risk factors. *Journal of Clinical Psychiatry*, **66**, 693–704.

Heilä, H. (1999). Suicide in schizophrenia: a review. *Psychiatria Fennica*, **30**, 47–57.

Heilä, H. & Lönnqvist, J. (2003). The clinical epidemiology of suicide in schizophrenia. In R. M. Murray, P. B. Jones, E. Susser, J. Van Os & M. Cannon (eds.), *The Epidemiology of Schizophrenia*. Cambridge, UK: Cambridge University Press, pp. 288–316.

Hiroeh, U., Appleby, L., Mortensen, P. & Dunn, G. (2001). Death by homicide, suicide, and other unnatural causes in people with mental illness: a population-based study. *Lancet*, **358**, 2110–12.

Hunt, I. M., Kapur, N., Windfuhr, K. *et al.* (2006). Suicide in schizophrenia: findings from a national clinical survey. *Journal of Psychiatric Practice*, **12**, 139–47.

Inskip, H., Harris, E. C. & Barraclough, B. (1998). Lifetime risk of suicide for affective disorder, alcoholism and schizophrenia. *British Journal of Psychiatry*, **172**, 35–7.

Jackson, H., McGorry, P., Henry, L. *et al.* (2001). Cognitively-oriented psychotherapy for early psychosis. *British Journal of Clinical Psychology*, **40**, 57–70.

Kemp, R., Hayward, P., Applewhaite, G., Everitt, B. & David, A. (1996). Compliance therapy in psychotic patients: randomised controlled trial. *British Medical Journal*, **312**, 345–9.

Kerkhof, A. J. & Diekstra, R. F. (1995). How to evaluate and deal with acute suicide risk. In R. F. Diekstra, W. Gulbinat, I. Kienhorst & D. de Leo (eds.), *Preventive Strategies on Suicide*. Leiden: E. J. Brill, pp. 97–119.

Kerwin, R. W. & Bolonna, A. A. (2004). Is clozapine antisuicidal? *Expert Review of Neurotherapeutics*, **4**, 187–90.

Kienhorst, C. W. M., deWilde, E. J., van den Bout, J. *et al.* (1990). Self-report suicidal behaviour in Dutch secondary education students. *Suicide and Life Threatening Behaviour*, **20**, 101–12.

Kirkbride, J. B., Fearon, P., Morgan, C. *et al.* (2006). Heterogeneity in incidence rates of schizophrenia and other psychotic syndromes: findings from the 3-center AESOP study. *Archives of General Psychiatry*, **63**, 250–8.

Korn, M. L., Brown, S. L., Kotler, M., Gordon, M. & Van Praag, H. M. (1995). Biological aspects of suicide. In R. F. Diekstra, W. Gulbinat, I. Kienhorst & D. de Leo (eds.), *Preventive Strategies on Suicide*. Leiden: E. J. Brill, pp. 311–37.

Kramer, M., Vogel, W. & Dijohnson, C. (1989). Antidepressants in 'depressed' schizophrenic inpatients. A controlled trial. *Archives of General Psychiatry*, **46**, 922–8.

Krausz, M., Muller-Thomsen, T. & Maasen, C. (1995). Suicide among schizophrenic adolescents in the long-term course of illness. *Psychopathology*, **28**, 95–103.

Lester, D. (1989). *Questions and Answers about Suicide*. Philadelphia, PA: Charles Press.

Linehan, M., Goodstein, J., Nielsen, S. & Chiles, J. (1983). Reasons for staying alive when you are thinking of killing yourself: the Reasons for Living Inventory. *Journal of Consulting and Clinical Psychology*, **51**, 276–86.

Lipschitz, A. (1995). Suicide prevention in young adults (age 18–30). *Suicide Prevention: Toward the Year 2000*, **25**, 155–70.

Mann, J. J., Apter, A., Bertolote, J. *et al.* (2005). Suicide prevention strategies: a systematic review. *Journal of the American Medical Association*, **294**, 2064–74.

Mann, J. J., Currier, D., Stanley, B. *et al.* (2006). Can biological tests assist prediction of suicide in mood disorders? *International Journal of Neuropsychopharmacology*, **9**, 465–74.

Martin, G. (1995). *Youth Assessment Checklist*. Bedford, South Australia: Flinders Medical Centre, Child and Adolescent Mental Health Service.

McGorry, P. D., Chanen, A., McCarthy, E. *et al.* (1991). Post-traumatic stress disorder following recent-onset psychosis: an unrecognized post-psychotic syndrome. *Journal of Nervous and Mental Disease*, **179**, 253–8.

McGorry, P. J., Henry, L. & Power, P. (1998). Suicide in early psychosis: could early intervention work? In R. Kosky & H. Eshkevari (eds.), *Suicide Prevention: The Global Context*. New York: Plenum Press, pp. 103–10.

McKenzie, N., Landau, S., Kapur, N. *et al.* (2005). Clustering of suicides among the mentally ill: suicide may be contagious. *British Journal of Psychiatry*. **187**, 476–80.

Melle, I., Johannesen, J. O., Friis, S. *et al.* (2006). Early detection of the first episode of schizophrenia and suicidal behaviour. *American Journal of Psychiatry*, **163**, 800–4.

Meltzer, H. Y. (2005). Suicidality in schizophrenia: pharmacologic treatment. *Clinical Neuropsychiatry: Journal of Treatment Evaluation*, **2**, 76–83.

Meltzer, H. & Okayli, G. (1995). The reduction of suicidality during clozapine treatment in neuroleptic resistant schizophrenics. *American Journal of Psychiatry*, **152**, 183–90.

Micallef, J., Fakra, E. & Blin, O. (2006). Intérêt des antidépresseurs chez le patient schizophrène présentant un syndrome dépressif. [Use of antidepressant drugs in schizophrenic patients with depression; Abstract in English.] *L'Encéphale*, **32**, 263–9.

Milne, S., Matthews, K. & Ashcroft, G. W. (1994). Suicide in Scotland 1988–1989. Psychiatric and physical morbidity according to primary care case notes. *British Journal of Psychiatry*, **165**, 541–4.

Mortensen, P. & Juel, K. (1993). Mortality and causes of death in first admitted schizophrenic patients. *British Journal of Psychiatry*, **163**, 183–9.

Mukherjee, S., Sackeim, H. & Schur, D. (1994). Electroconvulsive therapy of acute manic episodes: a review of 50 years experience. *American Journal of Psychiatry*, **151**, 169–76.

Munk, J. P. (1999). Has deinstitutionalization gone too far? *European Archives of Psychiatry and Clinical Neuroscience*, **249**, 136–43.

Nordentoft, M., Jeppesen, P., Abel, M. *et al.* (2002). OPUS study: suicidal behaviour, suicidal ideation and hopelessness among patients with first-episode psychosis. One-year follow-up of a randomised controlled trial. *British Journal of Psychiatry*, **181**(Suppl 43), s98–106.

O'Carrol, P., Berman, A., Maris, M. *et al.* (1996). Beyond the tower of Babel: a nomenclature for suicidology. *Suicide and Life-Threatening Behaviour*, **26**, 237–52.

Orvaschel, H., Puig-Antich, J., Chambers, W. J., Tabrizi, M. A. & Johnson, R. (1982). Retrospective assessment of pre-pubertal major depression with the Kiddie-SADS-E. *Journal of the American Academy of Child and Adolescent Psychiatry*, **21**, 392–7.

Palmer, B. A., Pankratz, V. S. & Bostwick, J. M. (2005). The lifetime risk of suicide in schizophrenia: a reexamination. *Archives of General Psychiatry*, **62**, 247–53.

Parker, G., Roy, K., Hadzi-Pavlovic, D. & Pedic, F. (1992). Psychotic depression: a meta-analysis of physical treatments. *Journal of Affective Disorders*, **24**, 17–24.

Pearce, C. & Martin, G., (1994). Predicting suicide attempts among adolescents. *Acta Psychiatrica Scandinavica*, **90**, 324–8.

Perälä, J., Suvisaari, J., Saarni, S. I. *et al.* (2007). Lifetime prevalence of psychotic and bipolar I disorders in a general population. *Archives of General Psychiatry*, **64**, 19–28.

Perris, C. (1994). Cognitive therapy in the treatment of patients with borderline personality disorders. *Acta Psychiatrica Scandinavica*, **89** (Suppl), 69–72.

Power, P. (1999). *Outpatient Commitment: Is it Effective*. MD Thesis, University of Melbourne.

Power, P. (2004). Suicide prevention in first episode psychosis. In P. McGorry & J. Gleeson (eds.), *Psychological Interventions in Early Psychosis*. Chichester: John Wiley, pp. 175–89.

Power, P., Elkins, E., Adlard, S. *et al.* (1998). An analysis of the initial treatment phase of first episode psychosis. *British Journal of Psychiatry*, **172** (Suppl 33), s71–7.

Power, P., Bell, R., Mills, R. *et al.* (2003). Suicide prevention in first episode psychosis: the development of a randomised controlled trial of cognitive therapy for acutely suicidal patients with early psychosis. *Australian and New Zealand Journal of Psychiatry*, **37**, 414–20.

Power, P., McGuire, P., Iacoponi, E. *et al.* (2007). Early intervention in the real world: Lambeth Early Onset (LEO) and Outreach and Support in South London (OASIS) service. *Early Intervention in Psychiatry*, **1**, 97–103.

Proctor, S. E., Mitford, E. & Paxton R. (2004). First episode psychosis: a novel methodology reveals higher than expected incidence: a reality based population profile in Northumberland, UK. *Journal of Evaluation in Clinical Practice*, **10**, 539–47.

Prusoff, B., Williams, D. & Weissman, M. (1979). Treatment of secondary depression in schizophrenia: a double blind, placebo controlled trial of amitriptyline added to perphenazine. *Archives of General Psychiatry*, **36**, 569–75.

Raleigh, V. S. (1996). Suicide patterns and trends in people of Indian subcontinent and Caribbean origin in England and Wales. *Ethnicity and Health*, **1**, 55–63.

Rascón, G. L., Gutiérrez, L. M. D. L., Valencia, C. M. *et al.* (2004) Family perception of the suicide attempt and suicidal ideation of relatives with schizophrenia. *Salud Mental*, **27**, 44–52.

Rihmer, Z., Rutz, W. & Pihlgren, H. (1995). Depression and suicide on Gotland: an intensive study of all suicides before and after a depression-training programme for general practitioners. *Journal of Affective Disorders*, **35**, 147–52.

Robinson, D., Woerner, M. G., Alvir, J. M. J. *et al.* (1999). Predictors of relapse following response from a first episode of schizophrenia or schizoaffective disorder. *Archives of General Psychiatry*, **56**, 241–7.

Rothschild, A. J., Samson, J. A., Bessette, M. P. & Carter-Campbell, J. T. (1993). Efficacy of the combination of fluoxetine and perphenazine in the treatment of psychotic depression. *Journal of Clinical Psychiatry*, **54**, 338–42.

Ryrie, I., Hellard, L., Kearns, C. *et al.* (1997). Zoning: a system for managing case work and targeting resources in community mental health teams. *Journal of Mental Health UK*, **6**, 515–23.

Salkovkis, P., Atha, C. & Storer, D. (1990). Cognitive behavioural problem solving in the treatment of patients who repeatedly attempt suicide: a controlled trial. *British Journal of Psychiatry*, **157**, 871–6.

Schnyder, U., Valach, L., Bichsel, K. & Michel, K. (1999). Attempted suicide: do we understand the patients' reasons. *General Hospital Psychiatry*, **21**, 62–9.

Schwartz, R. C. (2000). Suicidality in schizophrenia: implications for the counselling profession. *Journal of Counselling and Development*, **78**, 496–9.

Shaffer, D., Garland, A., Gould, M., Fisher, P. & Trautman, P. (1988). Preventing teenage suicide: a critical review. *Journal of the American Academy of Child and Adolescent Psychiatry*, **27**, 675–87.

Shearin, E. N. & Linehan, M. M. (1994). Dialectical behaviour therapy for borderline personality disorder: theoretical and empirical foundations. *Acta Psychiatrica Scandinavica*, **89** (Suppl), S61–8.

Siris, S. (2001). Suicide and schizophrenia. *Journal of Psychopharmacology*, **15**, 127–35.

Smith, K., Conroy, R. W. & Ehler, B. D. (1984). Lethality of Suicide Attempt Rating Scale. *Suicide and Life-Threatening Behaviour*, **14**, 215–42.

Spiker, D. G., Weiss, J. C., Dealy, R. S. *et al.* (1985). The pharmacological treatment of delusional depression. *American Journal of Psychiatry*, **142**, 430–5.

Spirito, A. & Esposito, S. C. (2006). Attempted and completed suicide in adolescence. *Annual Review of Clinical Psychology*, **2**, 237–66.

Stone, D. M., Barber, C. W. & Potter, L. (2005). Public health training online: the National Center for Suicide Prevention training. *American Journal of Preventive Medicine*, **29**(Suppl 2), 247–51.

Sutherby, K., Szmukler, G. I., Halpern, A. *et al.* (1999). A study of 'crisis cards' in a community psychiatric service. *Acta Psychiatrica Scandinavica*, **100**, 56–61.

Tanney, B. L. (1986). Electroconvulsive therapy and suicide. In R. Maris (eds.), *Biology of Suicide*. New York: Guilford Press, pp. 116–40.

van der Sande, R., van Roojijen, L., Buskens, E. *et al.* (1997a). Intensive inpatient and community intervention versus routine care after attempted suicide. A randomised controlled intervention study. *British Journal of Psychiatry*, **171**, 35–41.

van der Sande, R., Buskens, E., Allart, E., van der Graaf, Y. & van Engeland, H. (1997b). Psychosocial intervention following suicide attempt: a systematic review of treatment interventions. *Acta Psychiatrica Scandinavica*, **96**, 43–50.

van Praag, H. (1986). Biological suicide research: outcome and limitations. *Biological Psychiatry*, **21**, 1305–23.

Verdoux, H., Liraud, F., Gonzales, B. *et al.* (1999). Suicidality and substance misuse in first-admitted subjects with psychotic disorder. *Acta Psychiatrica Scandinavica*, **100**, 389–95.

Verdoux, H., Liraud, F., Gonzales, B. *et al.* (2001). Predictors and outcome characteristics associated with suicidal behaviour in early psychosis: a two-year follow-up of first-admitted subjects. *Acta Psychiatrica Scandinavica*, **103**, 347–54.

Westermeyer, J., Harrow, M. & Marengo, J. (1991). Risk for suicide in schizophrenia and other psychotic and non-psychotic disorders. *Journal of Nervous and Mental Disease*, **179**, 259–66.

Whitlock, F. A. (1986). Suicide and physical illness. In A. Roy (eds.), *Suicide*. Baltimore, MD: Williams & Wilkins, pp. 151–70.

Wing, J. K. (1994). *Health of the Nation Outcome Scale: HoNOS Field Trials*. London: Royal College of Psychiatrists, Research Unit.

World Health Organization (2007). *Suicide Prevention*. Geneva: World Health Organizaion (http://www.who.int/mental_health/prevention/suicide/suicideprevent/en/index.html).

16

Emotional and personality dysfunctions in early psychosis

Max Birchwood, John Gleeson, Andrew Chanen, Louise K. McCutcheon, Shona M. Francey and Maria Michail

Emotion and psychosis

During the 1800s, when the concept of psychosis was first introduced, it was used to refer to severe mental illness – illness of the mind – and was regarded as a subcategory of neuroses, which at that time were characterized by an organic aetiology. However, this soon changed, especially after the introduction of the term 'psychoneurosis' by Damerow, which signified the unity of psychosis and neurosis under the assumption that they both share an organic aetiology (Beer, 1996). The concept of psychoneurosis also underwent changes in meaning, especially after the influence of psychoanalytical theory. According to Freud, neuroses were characterized by an underlying, unconscious etiology and in that respect were related to psychoses which signified '... a disturbance between the ego and the outside world' (cited in Beer, 1996, pp. 241–2). Subsequently, the concept of psychoneurosis was reversed from having an organic to having a psychological meaning.

During the twentieth century, the relationship between psychosis and neurosis was neglected. Instead, theories about the dichotomy between the two concepts, primarily based on their distinct etiological origins, were receiving considerable attention. Kraepelin (1919) was among the most influential in classifying neuroses, which were initially regarded as conditions of physical cause. Later on, however, he postulated that neuroses were partly characterized by a psychogenic (e.g. nervous exhaustion) and partly by a constitutional (e.g. hysteria) nature (Beer, 1996). This distinction between psychosis and neurosis was further developed by Karl Jaspers in his book *General Psychopathology* (1963); he argued for a clear and sharp distinction between neurosis, psychosis and psychopathy on the basis of the pervasiveness of the illness. Specifically, he suggested that neuroses are psychic deviations that, unlike the psychoses, which are more pervasive, do not affect the individual as a whole. He, therefore, justified the differentiation between affective disorder and mental illness on the assumption that the former is meaningful and allows empathy whereas the latter is understandable, that is 'madness'. In terms of diagnosis and treatment of schizophrenia, therefore, Jaspers adopted a hierarchical approach wherein affective symptoms are 'trumped' by the presence of positive symptoms, giving way to the now familiar distinction between affective and non-affective psychosis. Following Jaspers, Schneider (1959) also advocated the separation of neurosis from psychopathology of psychosis, which he referred to as mental abnormalities. The primary experiences – the first-rank symptoms – included thought disorder, auditory hallucinations, replacement of will and delusional perceptions. These symptoms, in the absence of 'organic' problems, were the ones used to determine the diagnosis of schizophrenia. It is evident, therefore, how the role of emotion in psychosis has been neglected, as emotional problems have been considered either as part and parcel of the schizophrenic symptomatology or merely as an 'accessory' to the primary symptoms – hallucinations and delusions.

Recently, there have been signs of a renewed marriage or at least courtship between psychosis and neurosis, based on substantial evidence from research and clinical practice showing that emotional dysfunction is pervasive in psychosis, even before symptom formation

The Recognition and Management of Early Psychosis: A Preventive Approach, ed. Henry J. Jackson and Patrick D. McGorry.
Published by Cambridge University Press. © Cambridge University Press 2009.

(Birchwood, 2003; Freeman & Garety, 2003). We will argue in this chapter that emotional dysfunction in early psychosis is inappropriately understood as a comorbidity and that, on the contrary, it is an endemic feature of this supposedly 'non-affective' disorder.

Emotional dysfunction prior to the onset of psychosis

Important sources of evidence regarding the prominent role of emotion in psychosis are studies examining the developmental precursors and risk factors that lead to the development of psychosis. Largely adopting retrospective methods, these studies aimed to identify those premorbid factors whose presence might enhance the probability of transition to psychosis in individuals at high risk. Driven by evidence regarding the presence of premorbid developmental and social impairment in adults with schizophrenia, Hollis (2003) set out to investigate the nature of this impairment in children and adolescents with first-episode psychosis (FEP) and the possibility of continuity with psychotic symptoms. Higher rates of premorbid dysfunction were reported in those individuals who went on to develop schizophrenia particularly affecting the area of social development. Among those developmental precursors measured by the General Developmental Scale, the Premorbid Adjustment Scale and the Childhood Behaviour Scale, evidence of emotional dysfunction and associated disabilities were most prominent. Social anxiety as well as social withdrawal and isolation were documented more commonly in individuals with schizophrenia than in those with other psychoses. These findings supported the epidemiological study of Tien and Eaton (1992). In their prospective study of psychopathological precursors for schizophrenia, they documented the association of anxiety, specifically social phobia and social withdrawal, panic attacks and obsessive–compulsive disorder, with increased risk for the development of schizophrenia as classified in the *Diagnostic and Statistical Manual of Mental Disorders*, 3rd edition (DSM-III; APA, 1980). One of the most important attempts, though, to identify those factors predicting the onset of schizophrenia and to compare the premorbid characteristics of those

high-risk individuals who went on to develop psychosis and those who did not, is the Edinburgh High-Risk Study (Johnstone *et al.*, 2005; Miller *et al.*, 2002). Young individuals aged 16–24 years were identified as being at increased risk for developing schizophrenia through having two or more affected first-degree relatives. Johnstone *et al.* (2005) reported the most significant predictive factors to be the presence of schizotypal cognitions and social withdrawal, social anxiety and introversion. It, therefore, seems that poor social adjustment combined with emotional problems, particularly social anxiety and signs of introversion, have been consistently detected in the developmental trajectory of those individuals who later develop psychosis. Yung *et al.* (2004) also implicated the role of depression among the factors predicting psychosis within an ultra-high-risk group of 104 young people. After reporting a transition rate of 34.6%, the authors were interested in identifying and delineating the clinical features that distinguished those individuals at enhanced risk who eventually developed full-blown psychotic symptoms from those who did not. Among the significant predictors, including poor functioning, long duration of symptoms and reduced attention, elevated levels of depression were highly prevalent and predictive, confirming previous findings of the presence of emotional problems among those subthreshold clinical features proceeding to the onset of psychosis.

Research supports a consistent pattern of emotional dysfunction in the developmental trajectory of those individuals who go on later to develop psychosis. Among those factors manifest in the premorbid developmental and social period, elevated levels of depression as well as social anxiety and the associated social withdrawal and isolation have been very prevalent, thereby indicating that emotional disturbance is a highly significant part and can precede the development of psychosis.

Emotional dysfunction in the prodromal phase

The term 'prodrome' refers to a period of non-specific symptoms and increasing impairment in functioning experienced before the emergence of a frank psycho-sis (Yung *et al.*, 2004). Among those signs that charac-terize this period (e.g. attenuated psychotic symptoms and sleep disturbances), research has consistently shown that emotional problems, and particularly depressed mood, anxiety and irritability, affect the majority of individuals (Häfner *et al.*, 1999; Yung & McGorry, 1996). Yung and McGorry (1996) in their review of the nature of prodromal signs and symp-toms of schizophrenia and affective psychosis have reported that mood-related problems, anxiety as well as restlessness, have been extensively documented in studies examining the clinical and psychopathological features of the initial phase of psychosis. In their study investigating the prodromal characteristics of people with FEP using a retrospective method, Yung and McGorry (1996) confirmed that, aside from atte-nuated psychotic symptoms and behavioural changes, these individuals reported elevated levels of depres-sive and neurotic problems. Häfner *et al.* (1999), in the ABC study of the early course of schizophrenia, reported two symptom categories that characterized this initial phase: negative and affective dimensions. The most frequently occurring prodromal sign repor-ted in their sample was depression, followed by symptoms of anxiety and worry. Indeed, depression was evident in 82% of individuals and was reported to emerge as early as 52 months prior to first admission and to follow a continuous course. Häfner *et al.* (1999) found that those individuals with depression scored higher on specific and non-specific neurotic syn-dromes as well as the psychosis-specific syndrome assessed by the Present State Examination (Wing *et al.*, 1974); however, no prognostic implications were found over a 5-year course. These early findings by Häfner *et al.* (1999) were confirmed by a more recent study which found that 81% of people with FEP, were troubled by depressed mood associated with lack of self-confidence and feelings of guilt for at least 2 weeks prior to first admission. Further-more, those individuals tended to show higher levels of positive, negative and depressive symptoms during their first episode compared with those who did not suffer from depression in the early stages (Häfner *et al.*, 2005).

Emotional dysfunction during the acute phase of psychosis

Depression

Recent attempts to validate the phenomenological domains of psychotic disorder have employed a dimen-sional approach derived from factor analytic studies of psychosis symptoms. Early three-factor models (posi-tive, negative and disorganization: Liddle *et al.*, 1993) have given way to more complex models. McGorry *et al.* (1998) using a large sample with FEP found a robust and clinically valid four-factor solution, com-prising depression and mania in addition to 'positive' and 'negative' symptoms. The dimension of depressive symptoms included feelings of hopelessness, worth-lessness, depressed mood and guilt, which were very prominent among individuals with FEP. Further, such studies continue to confirm that depression, in partic-ular, is a distinct dimension of schizophrenia (Murray *et al.*, 2005).

Although prevalence rates of depression may range greatly from study to study, all reported esti-mates, some varying from 22% to 75% depending on the criteria used (Koreen *et al.*, 1993), are very high. Indeed, symptoms such as loss of interest or plea-sure, concentration difficulties, hypersomnia/insom-nia and psychomotor agitation or retardation were consistently present in the majority of psychotic patients (Wassink *et al.*, 1999). These symptoms were reported to occur at the height of psychosis, namely the acute phase, and to resolve as the psy-chosis remitted. Therefore, they seem to follow the same course as the psychotic symptoms, particularly the positive symptoms (i.e. hallucinations and delu-sions), suggesting that they are a common psychopa-thological feature of schizophrenia (Birchwood *et al.*, 2000a; House, Bostock & Cooper, 1987; Johnson, 1981; Koreen *et al.*, 1993). Furthermore, depressive symptoms have been reliably distinguished both from negative symptoms and akinesia, which are regarded as the result of neuroleptic medication (Birchwood *et al.*, 2000a; House *et al.*, 1987; Koreen *et al.*, 1993), thus challenging the concept of 'phar-macogenic depression'.

Post-psychotic depression

Depressive symptoms can also occur after the onset of psychosis, once the psychotic symptoms have waned, giving rise to the concept of post-psychotic depression (PPD). This is a relatively common clinical state emerging in the aftermath of acute psychotic symptoms, with prevalence rates reaching up to 50% of those examined (McGlashan & Carpenter, 1976). What is even more surprising is the high frequency of PPD in patients with FEP (50%) compared with those with multiple relapses (32%), which underlines the complexity and pervasiveness of the disorder (Birchwood *et al.*, 2000a). Attempts to describe the course pattern of PPD suggest that its onset occurs concurrently with psychosis but it becomes clinically prominent only after the psychotic symptoms subside (Green *et al.*, 1990; McGlashan & Carpenter, 1976). Thus, it seems to develop independently of positive and negative symptoms challenging further the notion that depression in psychosis is merely a by-product of medication (Birchwood *et al.*, 2000a).

Overall, two course patterns of depression in psychosis have been reported: depression that occurs during acute psychosis and relapse, following the same course as positive symptoms, and depression that appears in the aftermath of acute psychotic symptoms (i.e. PDD). The emergence of post-psychotic symptoms remains unaffected by the course and outcome of depressive symptoms during the acute phase (Birchwood *et al.*, 2000a), suggesting that different processes underlie the development of these types of symptom in schizophrenia.

Social anxiety

Anxiety disorders, and particularly symptoms of social anxiety, are among the most prevalent disturbances manifest in people with psychosis, exerting a significant impact upon the course and outcome of the disorder (Cossof & Häfner, 1998; Tibbo *et al.*, 2003). Despite the fact that prevalence rates differ from study to study, as a result of the use of different diagnostic criteria (Cossof & Häfner, 1998 (citing Fenton & McGlashan, 1986); Emsley *et al.*, 1999), the occurrence of social anxiety in the course of psychosis is elevated, affecting predominantly

women and FEP patients (Emsley *et al.*, 1999). Recent estimates of its prevalence in individuals with mental illness range between 8.2% and 36.3% (Cassano *et al.*, 1999; Cossof & Häfner, 1998; Davidson *et al.*, 1993; Goodwin *et al.*, 2003; Pallanti, Quercioloi & Hollander, 2004; Penn *et al.*, 1994), depending on the sample used (inpatients versus outpatients) and the clinical criteria. Taking into consideration the highly impairing nature of social phobia, as well as the serious psychopathological implications entailed, it is possible that its manifestation during the course of psychosis inevitably leads to a poorer outcome of the disorder and impacts upon the ability to form relationships. The pervasiveness of social phobia in schizophrenia led Roth (1991; cited in Davidson *et al.*, 1993) to identify the need for a careful distinction between psychosis presenting with social sensitivity and a 'psychotic' social phobia, which could be regarded as a severe form of this illness. The importance of this distinction is best seen in terms of administering accurate therapeutic treatments, which in the case of comorbidity may call for separate management of the two disorders.

The nature of the link between emotion and psychosis

Interaction of symptoms

Freeman and Garety (2003), examining the connection between neurosis and psychosis, have provided a thorough review of evidence regarding the direct influence of emotion in the development/maintenance of delusions and hallucinations, which may occur through two routes: (1) the content of delusions and hallucinations reflect the content of emotional concerns, and (2) delusions and hallucinations share common maintaining processes with emotional disorders (Freeman & Garety, 2003).

Content of delusions/hallucinations as a reflection of the content of emotional disorders

Evidence for the association between emotion and psychosis come from studies examining the direct role of emotion in the formation of positive symptoms and, particularly, delusions and hallucinations (Freeman & Garety, 2003). Freeman, Garety & Kuipers (2001), aiming to formulate a cognitive model of persecutory delusions examined the central role of anxiety in the development of persecutory delusions. Their cognitive framework was based on the stress–vulnerability model and suggested that the development of delusions follows a life event or stressor that triggers increased arousal. This arousal subsequently causes anomalous experiences (e.g. hearing voices), especially in individuals with a vulnerability to psychosis. Anomalous experiences can be triggered through three routes: (1) the life event or stressor directly causes these anomalies, (2) emotional disturbances may mediate the relationship between stressors and anomalies, or (3) cognitive distortions manifest in psychosis may be triggered and subsequently cause these anomalous experiences. Attempts to provide a meaning for these experiences are then triggered, in which preexisting beliefs about the self, the world and others play a prominent role. It is suggested, that persecutory delusions are formed when individuals hold maladaptive beliefs about themselves and the world around them; examples include when they believe that they deserve to be harmed and punished, or that they are vulnerable and, therefore, an easy target, or when they perceive others around them as hostile and threatening. These dysfunctional beliefs are expected to be closely linked to premorbid anxiety and depression, and in this background, context can influence the formation of persecutory delusions. Anxiety involves the anticipation of threat and danger, which can be physical, social or psychological, and also involves intense worry about the consequences such a threat will entail. Similar themes underlie persecutory delusions that refer to perceived danger or harm intended to be inflicted upon the individual by the persecutor. In that respect, Freeman *et al.* (2001) have suggested that anxiety is likely to play an important role in the formation of persecutory delusions since their content reflects the thematic content of anxiety disorders. In an analogous attempt to provide a cognitive formulation of voices, Birchwood and Chadwick (1997) showed how the relationship between the patient and his/her voices generated the affective and behavioural responses of the individual. More specifically, beliefs about the voice's power and authority were found to determine the coping strategies in which the patient engaged and were also associated with levels of depression. Similarly, earlier findings reported that beliefs about the voices' omnipotence were closely related to emotional distress (Chadwick & Birchwood, 1994). For example, if the voice was regarded as malevolent, it would cause significant distress to the individual and most probably be resisted (Chadwick & Birchwood, 1994), thereby triggering the activation of a defensive mechanism in the form of involuntary subordination or passive aggression.

Similar maintenance processes in delusions, hallucinations and emotion

Studies investigating the role and implications of emotional disorders in psychosis have also provided evidence regarding the impact of emotional processes and mechanisms on the formation and maintenance of delusions and hallucinations. Freeman and his colleagues (2001; Freeman, Garety & Phillips, 2000) have focused particularly on the role of anxiety in persecutory delusions, mainly because of the common themes that underlie the two (e.g. anticipation of danger or threat) and have demonstrated how cognitive distortions evident in individuals with anxiety disorders are also manifested in people with persecutory delusions. It is known that anxiety disorders are characterized by selective bias towards threat-related information (Mansell & Clark, 1999). In their study examining the presence of similar cognitive distortions in people with persecutory delusions, Freeman *et al.* (2001) found that, as with individuals with anxiety disorders, people with persecutory delusions exhibited high levels of internal processing bias towards threat stimuli during the scanning of a number of pictures depicting neutral, happy or threat information. This confirms previous findings by Bentall and Kaney (1989), who, using an Emotional Stroop task, reported signs of selective bias towards threat-related information in persecutory-deluded individuals. Further evidence regarding the presence of similar processes in emotional disorders and delusions refers to the use of safety behaviours and their role in the maintenance of paranoid delusions (Freeman *et al.*, 2001). The authors argued that a situation perceived by paranoid individuals as entailing threat or danger could lead them to act in such a way as to avoid the threat and seek safety. However, the use of safety behaviours does not only trigger the maintenance of cognitive distortions evident in paranoid thinking but was also found to be associated with elevated levels of anxiety.

Aside from delusions, the role of emotion in *triggering* hallucinations via similar cognitive dysfunctions has also received attention; yet, research evidence seems to be rather scarce. Morrison and Haddock (1997), in a study examining the nature and presence of self-focus attention in schizophrenia, found that patients with auditory hallucinations scored higher than schizophrenic patients without hallucinations on the Private Self-Consciousness Subscale of the Self-Consciousness Scale (Fenigstein, Scheier & Buss, 1975). This indicates that the self-focus attention evident in individuals with anxiety disorders is also implicated in schizophrenia and might be crucial, as Frith (1979) suggested, in the understanding of positive symptoms. Moreover, the fact that the loudness of auditory hallucinations, as measured by a self-report hallucinations questionnaire, was associated with higher levels of self-focus attention implies that the degree of this cognitive distortion might be a predictor of hallucinator status. Further evidence demonstrating the presence of cognitive biases in schizophrenia analogous to those observed in anxiety disorders comes from a study by Baker and Morrison (1998). They investigated the presence of attributional biases and metacognitive beliefs in patients with auditory hallucinations during a source monitoring task and after administering questionnaires about metacognition. Evidence of misattributional bias in which internal events were attributed to an external source was evident in voice hearers, who also scored higher on beliefs about the uncontrollability of their thoughts and the corresponding danger than a non-clinical sample and schizophrenic patients without auditory hallucinations. The fact that such metacognitive beliefs were found to be associated with external attributions may render patients vulnerable to interpret their voices in a threatening way, thereby raising the

possibility of the role of metacognitive beliefs in the maintenance of auditory hallucinations. However, it is not known whether these metacognitive beliefs are merely a by-product of hallucinations.

The research seems to demonstrate similarities in the themes that characterize, and the mechanisms that underlie, emotional disorders, delusions and hallucinations. Research showing that cognitive distortions evident in anxiety disorders are also shared by patients with persecutory delusions and/or auditory hallucinations indicates that factors triggering the development and maintenance of anxiety might also be implicated in the formation and persistence of positive psychotic symptoms. A plausible relationship between emotional and psychotic disorders, however, raises the need to identify and delineate the exact psychological processes and pathways involved in the manifestation of emotional dysfunction.

Shared developmental pathways

A further indication of covariation of emotion and psychosis comes from the finding that the social risk factors for psychosis (e.g. deprivation, urbanicity, ethnic density, trauma) are the same as those for emotional dysfunction in the (non-psychotic) population. Birth cohort (e.g. Isohanni *et al.*, 1998) and retrospective (e.g. Jones *et al.*, 1993) studies reveal that FEP is often preceded by social difficulty and emotional disorder as well as a low level of 'psychotic' experiences stretching back into early adolescence (Poulton *et al.*, 2000). These childhood antecedents of a developing psychosis will unfold in a social environment, and there is now considerable evidence that social context influences morbidity and outcome, for example urban living, including deprivation (Pederson & Mortensen, 2001; van Os *et al.*, 2003); membership of marginalized social groups (Bhugra, Bhamra & Taylor, 1997; Fearon *et al.*, 2006); the impact of migration (Bhugra, 2000); and the (favourable) correlates of 'developing nation' status (Harrison *et al.*, 2001). Childhood trauma and problems of parental attachment are vulnerability factors for the development of emotional dysfunction in adulthood (Brown *et al.*, 1990). Elevated levels of sexual, physical and emotional abuse have been consistently reported in the developmental trajectory of individuals suffering from depression and social anxiety (Fombonne *et al.*, 2001; Harrington *et al.*, 1990; Pine *et al.*, 1998). Evidence of a high rate of traumatic history, including sexual abuse (Read & Argyle, 1999), unwanted pregnancy (Myhrman *et al.*, 1996) and dysfunctional parental attachment (Parker *et al.*, 1998; Tiernari, 1994), has also been documented in people with psychosis. Such traumatic experiences may render patients prone to PPD and other emotional disorders.

Developmental psychopathology (Rutter & Sroufe, 2000) shows continuity exists between early emotional functioning and later adaptation. Psychopathological disturbances emerging in adulthood (e.g. anxiety, depression, risk of suicide) are usually preceded by emotional and behavioural problems rooted in childhood and early adolescence (Fombonne *et al.*, 2001; Hofstra, Ende & Verhulst, 2001; Rao *et al.*, 1995). These problems develop in a dimensional and not a categorical way, and they are influenced by the social and familial context (Rutter & Sroufe, 2000). There is also considerable *dis*continuity between adolescent and adult emotional functioning; for example, Andrews and Brown (1995) showed that positive life events in late adolescence can serve to restore a disturbed developmental trajectory back to within normal limits. The domains of emotional functioning also interact; for example, social anxiety increases the developmental risk of adolescent depression (Stein *et al.*, 2001). A strong case can, therefore, be made that the variance in 'comorbid' emotional disorder in FEP is a product, in part, of these unfolding, disturbed developmental pathways, triggered by the psychosis diathesis and the social risk factors for psychosis (Fig. 16.1b). Figure 16.1a represents the more 'classical' model of emotional dysfunction in psychosis.

Emotion as a psychological reaction to psychosis and its symptoms

Here the emphasis is on psychosis and psychotic symptoms as a challenging or traumatic life event that requires adaptation by individuals and their families. Post-psychiatric depression is known to occur some months after recovery from the acute episode. It can be predicted by how patients appraise the personal threat of this shattering life event: where the individual appraises psychosis as leading to *loss* of social goals, roles and status; as a source of *shame*; and from which escape is thwarted (i.e. *entrapment* by a supposed malignant disorder). This predicts the later emergence of PPD with hopelessness (Birchwood *et al.*, 2000a). In the study reported by Birchwood *et al.* (2000a), the first episode of psychosis had a high rate of PPD (over 50%), which was linked to heightened awareness of the diagnosis and its implications. Where symptoms persist, depression has been traced to the *perceived* power of voices (Birchwood *et al.*, 2000b) and of persecutory delusions (Freeman *et al.*, 2001), and to the *subjective* experience of negative symptoms. In general, the distress occasioned by persisting symptoms has been shown to operate through a 'psychological filter'; those patients with more positive self-schema seem able to withstand the threat of voices or other persecutors (Birchwood *et al.*, 2000b; Freeman *et al.*, 2001).

With regard to traumatic reactions, evidence suggests that there is no link with the 'objective' trauma of psychosis (e.g. compulsory admission), as would be required for a DSM-IV diagnosis (APA, 1994; McGorry *et al.*, 1991). In non-psychotic post-traumatic stress disorder, attention now focuses on the *perceived* threat of traumatic events and how people cope; in psychosis, patients may perceive themselves at risk of injury or death from supposed persecutors (Freeman *et al.*, 2001), voices (Birchwood *et al.*, 2000b) or from others in a disturbed psychiatric ward, but its impact on trauma is as yet unknown.

Social anxiety and the shame and stigma of mental illness

Social anxiety could be triggered as a psychological response to a stigmatized illness and particularly as a result of shame-related appraisals arising from mental illness. It is known that social evaluative concerns are the core feature of (non-psychotic) social anxiety. People with social anxiety appear particularly vulnerable to threats to their social status, usually triggered by the possibility of being scrutinized and negatively evaluated because of perceived failed social performance.

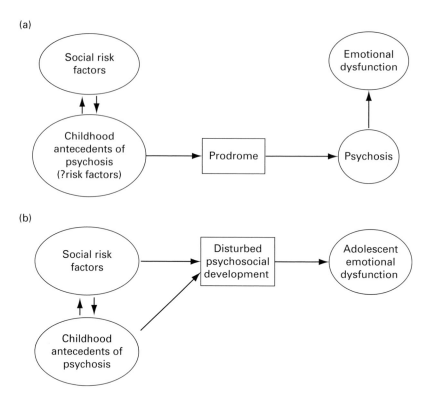

Fig. 16.1. Psychosis (a) and developmental (b) pathways to emotional dysfunction. (a) Emotional dysfunction as a consequence of psychosis. (b) Emotional dysfunction as an endemic feature of the developmental trajectory of psychosis.

However, social anxiety can be triggered by many qualities perceived as socially unattractive (e.g. having an eating disorder). Psychosis is considered to be a highly stigmatized condition (Haghighat, 2001) and patients perceive themselves to be shamed and socially subordinated by others because of their illness and patient status (Birchwood *et al.*, 1993, 2000b), leading to feelings of humiliation, loss of social status and entrapment (Rooke & Birchwood, 1998). Fear of other people discovering the mental illness and the consequences this will entail – social shame and exclusion – triggers attempts to conceal the stigmatized identity in the form of submissiveness, avoidance and withdrawal from social interactions. It is argued, therefore, that shame about mental illness and fear of being devalued and rejected by others once the diagnosis is revealed underlie the development and maintenance of social anxiety and avoidance.

A cognitive model of social anxiety in psychosis

The model presented in Fig. 16.2 provides an account of the development and maintenance of social anxiety in psychosis (Birchwood *et al.*, 2007). It is based on the cognitive model of Clark and Wells (1995) but incorporates the shame appraisals suggested to play a critical role in the emergence of social anxiety in psychosis.

On entering a social situation, and even before that, psychotic individuals have endorsed and accepted the cultural stereotypes attached to their illness. Based on that information, they draw attention to themselves (self-focus attention) and how they think they appear during a social interaction in order to create a mental image of how they believe others see them. Soon, this distorted mental self-representation turns into catastrophic thinking about the way their behaviour is perceived and interpreted by others. So, for example,

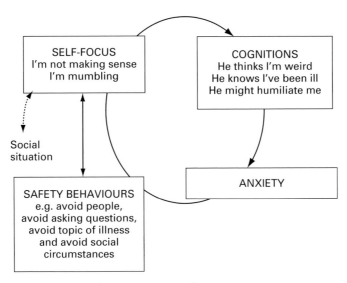

Fig. 16.2. A cognitive model of social anxiety (Birchwood *et al.*, 2007).

if they think that 'I'm mumbling, I'm not making any sense', this leads to catastrophic cognitions like, 'People must think I am weird, they probably know I have a mental illness', which subsequently triggers anxiety symptoms (e.g. sweating, trembling). Fear of their illness being revealed and the consequences of being stigmatized and shamed by the mental illness (e.g. social exclusion, marginalization) leads people with psychosis to engage in safety behaviours. For example, they may avoid talking about their mental illness, avoid asking questions during social interactions, stay on the edge of groups to avoid attracting attention, or even completely withdraw from social situations. These safety behaviours are aimed at reducing the perceived danger; however, most of the time they prevent individuals from disconfirming their unfounded beliefs and, moreover, contaminate social interactions by promoting patterns of avoidance and withdrawal.

In a similar vein, the problems of fear and social avoidance in the context of active psychotic symptoms may be traced to the supposed threat posed by others; patients with persecutory delusions often deal with the perceived threat to their well-being through avoidance of high-risk social encounters. In cognitive therapy, this is one of a class of 'safety behaviours' that function to reduce threat (Freeman *et al.*, 2001). Social

disengagement can also be traced to the content of command hallucinations that can directly undermine trust in others. The therapeutic emphasis in this pathway focuses on patients' appraisals (beliefs, cognitions) of the threat posed by the diagnosis, by voices and by perceived social shame.

Implications for cognitive–behaviour therapy of early psychosis

How times have changed! It was not long ago that talking to people about their psychotic beliefs was deemed impossible or harmful. Cognitive–behaviour therapy (CBT) for psychosis (CBTp) is now recommended by the UK National Institute for Clinical Excellence (NICE, 2002, p. 16) to 'reduce psychotic symptoms, increase insight and promote medication adherence'. This mainly British innovation has been built on some 20 randomized controlled trials (Tarrier & Wykes, 2004) using predominantly standard psychosis outcomes (e.g. Positive and Negative Symptom Scale, relapse). Development of CBTp has mirrored the evaluation methodology for neuroleptic drugs and has reestablished psychotherapy for psychosis as a credible treatment. It has succeeded. But was this the right approach and are we moving in the right direction? The development and evaluation of CBTp has tended to follow the drug metaphor in the way it has pragmatically applied an intervention that has been successful in one disorder (in this case depression) to another (psychosis), and applied the same criteria for success (e.g. reduction in psychosis symptoms and relapses). We have been part of this development, but we believe that this has led to many unintended consequences that cannot be rectified without a decisive change of course.

Contemporary CBTp began in the 1980s with the work of Tarrier and colleagues, helping patients to cope with their symptoms (Tarrier *et al.*, 1993). At the same time, Chadwick and Lowe (1990) showed that it was possible to 'reality test' delusional beliefs. Then the full armamentarium of CBT followed, emphasizing individual formulation and bringing in the assumptions and techniques used in depression, including an emphasis on dysfunctional thinking styles, early trauma and so on. As in so many areas of psychiatry, practice has run ahead of theory. One of the main consequences is well highlighted by Turkington, Kingdon & Turner (2003), who express concern that CBTp now refers to a wide range of CBT treatments varying in length and emphasis, and they have called for greater precision in identifying their active elements, arguing for further trials with better control groups and process measures to assist in this process.

What is cognitive behaviour therapy?

The CBT approach for emotional disorders has its own well-validated assumptions about their origins (maladaptive cognitions) as arising from certain adverse life circumstances. At the heart of this is the link between thinking and emotion/behaviour: that emotional and behavioural responses are largely influenced by the cognitive appraisals made. Recent evidence suggests that cognition and emotion can mutually influence one another. In retrospect, it is curious, and seems to have gone unnoticed, that a therapy for (and theory of) affective disorder was considered appropriate for a 'non-affective' illness. It is even more curious that only a minority of CBTp trials measure distress and emotional dysfunction as a secondary outcome, and only one

has measured it as a primary outcome (Birchwood & Trower, 2006). Is this still CBT? Or has CBTp strayed from its conceptual roots and become something else?

Cognitive–behaviour therapy for (emotional dysfunction in) psychosis

We believe that further large-scale pragmatic CBTp trials as currently designed (beyond those in progress) will not shed further light on the active agents of CBTp nor initiate a process that will improve the effectiveness or specificity of CBTp; in fact, it risks doing the opposite. The next generation of CBTp needs to focus on theory-driven studies of reducing emotional dysfunction and/or behavioural anomaly in psychosis, including studies of treatments, which may be effective in ameliorating distress but may also impact secondarily on the psychotic phenomena themselves.

These studies might include a number of foci for CBT.

The reduction of distress, depression and problem behaviour associated with persecutory delusions and voices. Trower *et al.* (2004), for example, reduced compliance with command hallucinations and distress without a reduction in voice activity.

Anxiety, depression and interpersonal difficulty in those at high risk of developing psychosis. Morrison *et al.* (2004) in their randomized controlled trial of CBT to prevent transition to psychosis in a high-risk group focused principally on these problems, not the attenuated psychosis symptoms that defined the high-risk group.

The relapse prodrome to prevent relapse. Gumley *et al.* (2004) demonstrated a reduction in relapse by working with the earliest (affective) signs of relapse and how patients catastrophized them.

'Comorbid' depression and social anxiety. This would include a focus on individuals' appraisals of the diagnosis and its stigmatizing consequences (Birchwood *et al.*, 2007; Iqbal *et al.*, 2000).

For reduction of stress reactivity. This should increase resilience to life stress and prevent relapse (Myin-Germeys, Delespaul & van Os, 2005).

The increase of self-esteem and social confidence (Hall & Tarrier, 2003).

We believe that the future development and improvement of CBT requires us to move decisively away from the neuroleptic metaphor. Neuroleptics do what neuroleptics do. We believe that the future of CBT lies in understanding the (cognitive) interface between emotion and psychosis and in developing interventions to resolve emotional/behavioural dysfunction alone or as a means of preventing or mitigating psychosis and its positive symptoms. In this way, CBT can sit alongside the neuroleptic drugs but with a distinctive and complementary emphasis, not simply wheeled out when neuroleptics fail, as a substitute in extra time.

Borderline personality disorder: a neglected issue in first-episode psychosis

It is well established that 'poor premorbid adjustment' is associated with a range of adverse outcomes in both FEP and chronic psychosis (van Mastrigt & Addington, 2002). Descriptions of this construct include factors such as sociability and withdrawal, peer relationships, ability to function outside of the nuclear family and capacity to form age-appropriate intimate sociosexual ties (Cannon-Spoor, Potkin & Wyatt, 1982). Yet, discussion has tended to underemphasize the relationship of these factors to personality, especially personality disorder. Nevertheless, one might infer that poor premorbid adjustment involves personality pathology and that it is common in individuals with FEP. Yet, clinical guidelines spend little time addressing this (National Early Psychosis Project Clinical Guidelines Working Party, 1998; Work Group on Borderline Personality Disorder, 2001).

Of all the personality disorders, borderline personality disorder (BPD) is a particularly salient yet neglected problem in FEP. First, it is the most common and serious of the personality disorders in clinical practice (Work Group on Borderline Personality Disorder, 2001) and, second, historical descriptions of BPD arose as an attempt to describe a group of 'in between' patients on the 'border' of psychosis and neurosis (Stone, 2005).

There is little research available regarding the co-occurrence and combined trajectory of BPD and psychosis, and commentary from a clinical perspective is sparse. This is surprising, because in our experience, clinical teams commonly face significant and sometimes overwhelming diagnostic and treatment conundrums when young people present with both features of BPD and psychotic symptoms. The growing trend towards the streaming of patients into specialist FEP programmes, based upon initial diagnosis, adds impetus to the need to resolve these potential impasses. The problem extends, of course, beyond diagnosis because, unfortunately, there is almost no discussion within either FEP treatment guidelines (National Early Psychosis Project Clinical Guidelines Working Party, 1998) or BPD guidelines (McGlashan, 2002) to assist clinicians in considerations regarding treatment for this group of patients.

In our view, the case for an improved understanding of the overlap and combined trajectories of these disorders is clear-cut. First, both disorders in their own right are associated with high levels of functional impairment, morbidity and mortality (Paris, 2004; Siris, 2001; Skodol et al., 2002; Yen et al., 2004). For example, the suicide rate in psychosis has been estimated at 10%, with the risk skewed towards the early years after diagnosis (Siris, 2001), compared with a rate of approximately 8% in BPD (Pompili et al., 2005). High rates of co-occurring mood, anxiety and substance-use disorders are commonly found in BPD (McGlashan et al., 2000; Zanarini et al., 2005). It stands to reason that the combination of BPD and psychosis might lead to significantly worse outcomes. Second, treatments and service provision models might differ for this subgroup, as the FEP model is predicated upon a return to a previous level of, usually, good premorbid functioning (Edwards et al., 1994). For the majority of FEP patients, this is entirely appropriate. However, the interpersonal difficulties, affect dysregulation and impulsivity associated with BPD are likely to have a negative effect upon the therapeutic alliance during the recovery phase of FEP, making conventional treatments more difficult to apply.

In this situation, the risk of treatments being ineffective or even leading to iatrogenic harm remains significant. For example, standard FEP treatment guidelines, with a strong emphasis upon illness-based psychoeducation (National Early Psychosis Project Clinical

Guidelines Working Party, 1998), might consolidate the patient's unhealthy externalization of interpersonal problems or unwittingly elicit rebellious anger and rejection of treatment. A further example relates to the prescribing of antipsychotic medications. In our clinical experience, this can be somewhat arbitrarily based upon spurious judgements regarding the saliency of symptoms, particularly perceptual disturbances (van der Zwaard & Polak, 2001). The prevailing views of clinicians regarding the validity of psychotic symptoms in BPD might result, on the one hand, in undertreatment of psychotic symptoms or, on the other hand, in inadequate consideration of interventions for problematic interpersonal features. Surveys of treatment received by these patients across different treatment settings would be illuminating.

The conceptualization of co-occurring psychosis and borderline personality disorder

The co-occurrence of BPD and FEP has not been discussed from a theoretical perspective in the literature. Instead, discussions have tended to be framed either from a BPD perspective, in which psychosis is often conceptualized as an epiphenomenon, or from a predominantly psychosis illness model, in which personality is usually viewed as a potential vulnerability or complicating factor.

Psychotic symptoms in borderline personality disorder

Within DSM-IV, the diagnosis of BPD includes the presence of transient, stress-related paranoid ideation or severe dissociative symptoms – an acknowledgement that borderline traits and psychotic features coexist (APA, 1994). The rare empirical studies that have examined the prevalence of this co-occurrence support this assumption (Links, Steiner & Mitton, 1989; Pope *et al.*, 1985) and suggest that psychotic features combined with BPD share a specific link through affective disturbances. However, the relationship between the two syndromes remains far from clear. Historically,

the conceptualization of the association and overlap between the disorders has been complex, and it has been confused by varying a-priori assumptions and divergent uses of the term 'borderline' in relation to both personality and psychosis (Bech, 1994). The relationship has tended to be conceptualized from the perspectives of varying psychoanalytic schools (Sidhar, 1979). For example, psychotic symptoms in the context of BPD have been characterized as 'pseudo neurotic schizophrenia' (Axel, 1955; Hoch & Polatin, 1949), and debate has continued as to whether these phenomena can best be conceptualized as 'dissociative', 'psychosis-like' or 'true' psychotic symptoms (Silk *et al.*, 1989).

Personality in first-episode psychosis

We have discussed earlier in this chapter how, from a psychosis perspective, premorbid adjustment might relate to personality, especially personality disorder. The influence of stable personality traits upon the course of FEP (discussed in Ch. 19) has been a small field of enquiry. From a categorical perspective, this has included antisocial personality disorder (Dingemans, Lenior & Linszen, 1998), and from a dimensional perspective, lower agreeableness and neuroticism have been implicated in a poorer course of symptoms in FEP (Gleeson *et al.*, 2005; Horan *et al.*, 2005). However, to our knowledge, there are no published studies of the potential pathoplastic relationship between BPD and FEP.

The prevalence of comorbidity

The study of 'comorbidity' in FEP affords the specific advantage of minimizing the confounding effects of treatment and selection biases (Keshavan & Schooler, 1992). However, studies of comorbidity in FEP have unfortunately rarely reported on the prevalence and stability of axis II diagnoses or features (Sim *et al.*, 2004; Strakowski *et al.*, 1993), although, from a BPD perspective, recent research has highlighted the relative stability over a 2-year period of BPD traits in non-psychotic older adolescent outpatients (Chanen *et al.*, 2004) and studies of FEP have indicated that personality can be measured reliably (Horan *et al.*, 2005).

A small number of empirical studies of FEP have examined the overlap and relationships between BPD and a diagnosis of psychosis. The Chestnut Lodge follow-up studies, for example, reported that BPD did not emerge as a specific risk factor for subsequent schizophrenia despite its high rate in schizophrenia (Fenton & McGlashan, 1989; McGlashan, 1983), but its co-occurrence in schizophrenia may be associated with lower rates of recovery (Torgalsboen, 1999).

Hogg and colleagues (1990) reported on the prevalence of personality disorders and personality disorder traits, as defined by DSM-III (APA, 1980), in 40 patients with recent-onset schizophrenia who were assessed during their recovery phase (Hogg *et al.*, 1990). Using the Structured Interview for DSM-III Personality Disorders (Pfohl, Stangl & Zimmerman, 1983), 13% of the sample was diagnosed with BPD, with 58% having at least one personality disorder diagnosis. Unfortunately, inter-rater reliability for specific diagnoses could not be obtained, but overall agreement on the instrument was poor. A recent prospective study of new admissions to the Early Psychosis Prevention and Intervention Centre (EPPIC) indicated that 20% met criteria for a comorbid diagnosis of BPD (Francey *et al.*, 2006). A description of a patient with such 'comorbidity' is given in the case vignette.

Case vignette

Shelley is a 16-year-old girl who lives with her mother and younger sister. She was referred to EPPIC by her school counsellor after she complained over a 2-month period of hearing abusive voices inside her head and seeing images of her dead grandfather. Shelley described a long history of an unhappy family life, beginning with the death of her biological father when she was 4 years old and violent physical abuse allegedly perpetrated by her stepfather when she was aged 8 to 12. Through Shelley's early childhood years, her mother struggled with alcohol abuse, resulting in Shelley receiving inconsistent basic care and developing a precocious and rebellious pattern of relating to all major adult figures in her life. Shelley has a long-standing problem with anger outbursts at home, resulting in damage to furniture and physical altercations with her sister. She has been experimenting with cannabis since the age of 13 and more recently has been taking ecstasy. She describes an unstable and rapidly shifting group of friendships and interests since primary school. She also complains of a long-standing pattern of intermittent and brief periods of intense sadness, self-loathing and overwhelming anxiety, which have been associated with two attempts to hang herself over the previous year. She has commenced secretly cutting her upper legs with a razor blade over the last 2 years. Shelley is angry and dismissive towards EPPIC staff, saying that no one could possibly understand her. There is no persistent depressed mood.

The therapeutic implications of the borderline personality disorder–psychosis controversy

The lack of conceptual clarity regarding the BPD–psychosis relationship, coupled with the paucity of empirical treatment trials of their co-occurrence, has resulted in diagnostic confusion. Furthermore, clinical guidelines for BPD (McGlashan, 2002; Paris, 2002) and for psychosis (National Early Psychosis Project Clinical Guidelines Working Party, 1998) provide little by way of consensus-based treatment recommendations for their co-occurrence. In order to resolve this uncertainty, there is an urgent need to develop and pilot potential psychotherapeutic interventions for co-occurring psychotic symptoms and BPD. In our view, an appropriate therapeutic model would be flexible enough to be incorporated into existing case management-based service structures for FEP. It should provide a framework for clinicians to share an understanding of the patient's interpersonal problems and should facilitate greater awareness of the risk of inadvertent collusion with patients' problematic patterns; this, in our experience, often results in interprofessional disputes among teams along an 'illness' versus 'non-illness' divide. One candidate intervention for this purpose is cognitive analytic therapy (CAT: Ryle & Kerr, 2002).

Cognitive analytic therapy

Over a 25-year period, CAT has evolved into a brief psychotherapy with particular relevancy for the treatment of BPD (Ryle, 2004; Ryle & Golynkina, 2000). In the course of its development, CAT has integrated a range of psychotherapeutic orientations, including a reformulation of object relations theory, Kellyian personal construct theory, and cognitive and developmental psychology frameworks (Ryle & Kerr, 2002).

The evolution of CAT commenced with Ryle's interest in addressing the paucity of rigorous outcome research into psychodynamic therapy, which motivated him to operationalize and measure stable problematic patterns of inter-relating (Ryle, 2004). The CAT approach reconceptualized the object relations account of the development of the self and the process of internalization of early interpersonal experiences. According to CAT, the self develops in the process of relating (or *proceeding* in relation) to others, particularly caregivers (Ryle & Kerr, 2002). However, CAT diverges from attachment and object relations theory in its conceptualization of the process and outcome of development. The 'phenotypic self' develops by interacting to acquire, over the early years of life, a repertoire of 'more or less adaptive reciprocal role procedures in which knowledge memory, feeling, meaning and action are linked' (Ryle & Kerr, 2002, p. 34). Reciprocal roles in CAT are defined as relatively discrete sequences of behaviour, which incorporate emotions, memories and cognitions, and which are enacted inter- and intrapersonally. These role procedures both anticipate and elicit their reciprocal, for example *critically controlling* in response to *passively complying*, and serve as a 'template' through which events are understood.

Vygotsky's 'activity theory' significantly shaped the evolution of CAT (Ryle & Bennink-Bolt, 2002). From his perspective, the self is constituted by early, socially meaningful, sign-mediated interpersonal experiences, which commence with pre-verbal interactions between infant and caregiver, before progressing to verbal dialogues. These dialogues are constituted by a range of voices, internalized and transmuted to the child predominantly, but not exclusively, by caregivers (Ryle & Kerr, 2002).

Cognitive analytic therapy in borderline personality disorder

According to Ryle and Kerr (2002), the *linking* of the 'more or less adaptive' repertoire of roles underpins a unified subjective sense of self and a concomitant continuity in experience. The failure to achieve this integration, which is associated with highly restricted and inflexible reciprocal roles, results in dissociated and rapidly switching 'self-states' and impoverished continuity of experience, associated with a deficit in self-reflection that is typical in BPD (Ryle, 1997).

Therapy, which is highly collaborative, structured and time limited, aims to assist the patient to achieve greater integration by recognizing and revising their dysfunctional procedures, reciprocal roles and switches in self states. This process is aided by the introduction of therapy tools, including a narrative reformulation letter and a reformulation diagram. Transference and countertransference are reconceptualized as specific examples of reciprocal role enactments and reciprocations, and as opportunities to encourage recognition and revision of problematic reciprocal roles.

Cognitive analytic therapy in psychosis

Recently, Kerr and colleagues have argued that CAT theory may explain the contribution of interpersonal stress and psychological variables to specific psychotic phenomenology (Kerr, Birkett & Chanen, 2003). They outlined the parallels between psychotic phenomenology and CAT's conceptualization of problematic reciprocal roles. They argued, for example, that subtle information-processing deficits in infancy and childhood might elicit rejecting, critical or depriving patterns of caregiving, which would lead to internalization of problematic and restricted reciprocal roles, thereby creating 'internal expressed emotion'. The neurodevelopmental impact of stress (whether externally or internally generated), mediated through endocrinological functioning in response to persistent problematic interpersonal enactments and reciprocations, theoretically results in further exacerbation to information-processing capacity in the vulnerable older adolescent. Eventually, this contributes to the development of acute psychotic states. In more severe psychotic states, CAT would understand psychotic symptoms and phenomena to represent the jumbled, amplified or distorted enactments of the individual's repertoire of reciprocal roles.

An integrated theoretical account of both BPD and psychosis has been developed with CAT, making it wellplaced to offer a useful model for intervention in co-occurring BPD and FEP. Moreover, CAT has recently proven successful in a randomized controlled trial of early intervention in BPD at the Helping Young People Early (HYPE) Clinic, ORYGEN Youth Health (A. Chanen, unpublished data). A pre-pilot of CAT for co-occurring BPD and psychosis has also recently been safely conducted at EPPIC under the leadership of HYPE and supported by the Association of Cognitive Analytic Therapy (UK), including the completion of a skills training programme in CAT for a number of EPPIC clinicians.

Given the claims that CAT can provide an overarching theoretical account of vulnerability to and phenomenology of both conditions and the claim that it can provide a practical therapeutic intervention for both disorders, a pilot trial of CAT for co-occurring BPD and psychosis is underway at ORYGEN. A similar project is under development by colleagues in Sheffield, UK. The ORYGEN project seeks to build upon work carried out at EPPIC in the mid to late 1990s, developing a psychological model of and intervention for recovery from FEP (Henry, 2004). This model has much in common with the CAT approach, including an emphasis upon the real experience of the patient and the development of a collaborative therapeutic relationship. Some limitations of this model include the lack of a fully integrated theory of the self, along with the absence of both a theory and techniques for managing severe disturbances in the therapeutic and other interpersonal relationships.

The research questions include:

- is CAT a safe treatment option for patients with co-occurring BPD (or subthreshold BDP) and psychotic symptoms, in terms of exacerbations in psychopathology?
- is CAT a feasible treatment option for patients with co-occurring BPD (or subthreshold BPD) and psychotic symptoms, in terms of proportion of therapy sessions attended?

The primary aims of the study are (1) to refine an appropriate form of CAT for patients diagnosed with FEP and comorbid BPD or subthreshold BPD, (2) to produce a treatment manual, and (3) to evaluate the safety and feasibility of CAT for this group. Secondary aims are (1) to check the validity of outcome measures and (2) to explore the effects of CAT in relation to psychopathology, psychosocial functioning and quality of life over a 6-month follow-up period. Results may provide an important contribution to this difficult and complex area of clinical need.

The pilot study, which is currently underway, is being conducted as a randomized controlled trial of CAT combined with treatment as usual compared with the latter alone for 16 young outpatients, aged 15 to 24 years inclusive, who have been diagnosed with comorbid BPD and early psychosis (in full or partial remission). The rater, who will be independent of treatment, will not be blind to treatment allocation owing to practical constraints and limited resources for conducting the pilot study. Baseline, end of treatment and 6-month outcome data will be collected.

Conclusions

Emotional dysfunction and personality disorder represent significant problems that co-occur in young people who develop a psychosis. The key theme of this chapter is that these difficulties are misleadingly referred to as 'comorbidities', as this tends to render them subordinate status in the hierarchy of symptoms. It is now clear not only that these 'comorbidities' are pervasive in FEP but also that they can represent either a manifestation of the psychosis diathesis itself or the consequence of shared social risk factors. There are also emerging ideas about how emotional dysfunction and the emerging psychosis experience, for example, interact in the development of formal, distressing psychosis and need for care. In treatment terms, therefore, the use of cognitive and related therapies might be more profitably focused on these 'comorbidities' rather than on the psychosis symptoms themselves (Birchwood & Trower, 2006). This, we believe, is the challenge that lies ahead.

REFERENCES

APA (1980). *Diagnostic and Statistical Manual of Mental Disorders*, 3rd edn. Washington, DC: American Psychiatric Press.

APA (1994). *Diagnostic and Statistical Manual of Mental Disorders*, 4th edn. Washington, DC: American Psychiatric Press.

Andrews, B. & Brown, G. W. (1995). Stability and change in low self-esteem: the role of psychosocial factors. *Psychological Medicine*, **25**, 23–31.

Axel, M. (1955). 10 borderline cases: a report on the question of pseudoneurotic schizophrenia. *Psychiatric Quarterly*, **29**, 555–87.

Baker, A. C. & Morrison, P. A. (1998). Cognitive processes in auditory hallucinations: attributional biases and metacognition. *Psychological Medicine*, **28**, 1199–208.

Bech, P. (1994). The borderline syndromes of depression, mania and schizophrenia: the coaxial or temperamental approach. *Acta Psychiatrica Scandinavica*, **89**(Suppl), 45–9.

Beer, M. D. (1996). The dichotomies: psychosis/neurosis and functional/organic: an historic perspective. *History of Psychiatry*, **vii**, 231–55.

Bentall, R. & Kaney, S. (1989). Content specific information processing and persecutory delusions: an investigation using the emotional Stroop test. *British Journal of Medical Psychology*, **62**, 355–64.

Bhugra, D. (2000). Migration and schizophrenia. *Acta Psychiatrica Scandinavica Supplementum*, **102**, 68–73.

Bhugra, D., Bhamra, J. & Taylor, P. (1997). Users views of a drop-in project for the homeless. *International Journal of Social Psychiatry*, **43**, 95–103.

Birchwood, M. (2003). Editorial: pathways to emotional dysfunction in psychosis. *British Journal of Psychiatry*, **182**, 373–5.

Birchwood, M. & Chadwick, P. (1997). The omnipotence of voices: testing the validity of a cognitive model. *Psychological Medicine*, **27**, 1345–53.

Birchwood, M. & Trower, P. (2006). The future of cognitive-behavioural therapy for psychosis: not a quasi-neuroleptic. *British Journal of Psychiatry*, **188**, 107–8.

Birchwood, M., Mason, R., MacMillan, F. & Healy, J. (1993). Depression, demoralization and control over psychotic illness: a comparison of depressed and non-depressed patients with a chronic psychosis. *Psychological Medicine*, **23**, 387–95.

Birchwood, M., Iqbal, Z., Chadwick, P. & Trower, P. (2000a). Cognitive approach to depression and sucidal thinking in psychosis. 1. Ontogeny of post-psychotic depression. *British Journal of Psychiatry*, **177**, 516–21.

Birchwood, M., Meaden, A., Trower, P. Gilbert, P. & Plaistow, J. (2000b). The power and omnipotence of voices, subordination and entrapment by voices and significant others. *Psychological Medicine*, **30**, 337–44.

Birchwood, M., Trower, P., Brunet, K. *et al.* (2007). Social anxiety and the shame of psychosis. *Behaviour Research and Therapy*, **45**, 1025–37.

Brown, G. W., Andrews, B., Bifulco, A. & Veiel, H. (1990). Self-esteem and depression. 1: Measurement issues and prediction of onset. *Social Psychiatry and Psychiatric Epidemiology*, **25**, 200–9.

Cannon-Spoor, H. E., Potkin, S. G. & Wyatt, R. J. (1982). Measurement of premorbid adjustment in chronic schizophrenia. *Schizophrenia Bulletin*, **8**, 470–84.

Cassano, G. B., Pini, S., Saettoni, M. & Dell'Osso, L. (1999). Multiple anxiety disorder comorbidity in patients with mood spectrum disorders with psychotic features. *American Journal of Psychiatry*, **156**, 474–6.

Chadwick, P. & Birchwood, M. (1994). The omnipotence of voices. A cognitive approach to auditory hallucinations. *British Journal of Psychiatry*, **164**, 190–201.

Chadwick, P. D. & Lowe, C. F. (1990). Measurement and modification of delusional beliefs. *Journal of Consulting and Clinical Psychology*, **58**, 225–32.

Chanen, A. M., Jackson, H. J., McGorry, P. D. *et al.* (2004). Two-year stability of personality disorder in older adolescent outpatients. *Journal of Personality Disorders*, **18**, 526–41.

Clark, D. M. & Wells, A. (1995). A cognitive model of social phobia. In R. G. Heimberg, M. R. Liebowitz & D. A. Hope (eds.), *Social Phobia: Diagnosis, Assessment, and Treatment*, New York: Guilford Press, pp. 69–93.

Cossof, S. J. & Häfner, R. J., (1998). The prevalence of comorbid anxiety in schizophrenia, schizoaffective disorder and bipolar disorder. *Australian and New Zealand Journal of Psychiatry*, **32**, 67–72.

Davidson, J., Hughes, D., George, L. & Blazer, D. (1993). The epidemiology of social phobia: findings from the Duke Epidemiological Catchment Area Study. *Psychological Medicine*, **23**, 709–18.

Dingemans, P. M. A. J., Lenior, M. E. & Linszen, D. H. (1998). Personality and schizophrenia relapse. *International Clinical Psychopharmacology*, **13**(Suppl 1), 89–95.

Edwards, J., Francey, S. M., McGorry, P. D. & Jackson, H. J. (1994). Early psychosis prevention and intervention: evolution of a comprehensive community-based specialised service. *Behaviour Change. Special Issue: Behaviour Therapy and Schizophrenia I*, **11**, 223–33.

Emsley, R., Oostihuizen, P., Joubert, A., Roberts, M. & Stein, D. J. (1999). Depressive and anxiety symptoms in patients with schizophrenia and schizophreniform disorder. *Journal of Clinical Psychiatry*, **60**, 747–51.

Fearon, P., Kirkbride, J., Morgan, C. *et al.* (2006). Incidence of schizophrenia and other psychoses in ethnic minority groups: results from MRC AESOP study. *Psychological Medicine*, **36**, 1541–50.

Fenigstein, A., Scheier, M. F. & Buss, A. H. (1975). Public and private self-consciousness. Assessment and theory. *Journal of Consulting and Clinical Psychology*, **43**, 522–7.

Fenton, W. S. & McGlashan, T. H. (1989). Risk of schizophrenia in character disordered patients. *American Journal of Psychiatry*, **146**, 1280–4.

Fombonne, E., Wostear, G., Cooper, V., Harrington, R. & Rutter, M. (2001). The Maudsley long-term follow-up of child and adolescent depression. 1. Psychiatric outcomes in adulthood. *British Journal of Psychiatry*, **179**, 210–17.

Francey, S. M., Jovev, M., Phassouliotis, C. *et al.* (2006). Co-morbid borderline personality disorder and first episode psychosis: how many and what happens? *Schizophrenia Research*, **86**(Suppl), 113.

Freeman, D. & Garety, P. (2003). Connecting neurosis and psychosis: the direct influence of emotion on delusions and hallucinations. *Behaviour Research and Therapy*, **41**, 923–47.

Freeman, D., Garety, P. & Phillips, M. L. (2000). An examination of hypervigilance for external threat in individuals with generalized anxiety disorder and individuals with persecutory delusions using visual scan paths. *Quarterly Journal of Experimental Psychology*, **53A**, 549–67.

Freeman, D., Garety, P. A. & Kuipers (2001). Persecutory delusions: developing and understanding of belief and maintenance of emotional distress. *Psychological Medicine*, **31**, 1293–306.

Frith, C. D. (1979). Consciousness, information processing and schizophrenia. *British Journal of Psychiatry*, **34**, 225–35.

Gleeson, J. F., Rawlings, D., Jackson, H. J. & McGorry, P. D. (2005). Agreeableness and neuroticism as predictors of relapse after first-episode psychosis: a prospective follow-up study. *Journal of Nervous and Mental Disease*, **193**, 160–9.

Goodwin, D. R., Amador, F. X., Malaspina, D. *et al.* (2003). Anxiety and substance use comorbidity among inpatients with schizophrenia. *Schizophrenia Research*, **61**, 89–95.

Green, M., Nuechterlein, K., Ventura, J. & Mintz, J. (1990). The temporal relationship between depressive and psychotic symptoms in recent-onset schizophrenia. *American Journal of Psychiatry*, **147**, 179–82.

Gumley, A., O'Grady, M., Power, K. & Schwannauer, M. (2004). Negative beliefs about self and illness: a comparison of individuals with psychosis with and without comorbid social anxiety disorder. *Australian and New Zealand Journal of Psychiatry*, **38**, 960–4.

Häfner, H., Loffler, W., Mauer, K., Hambrecht, M. & an der Heiden, W. (1999). Depression, negative symptoms, social stagnation and social decline in the early course of schizophrenia. *Acta Psychiatrica Scandinavica*, **100**, 105–18.

Häfner, H., Mauer, K., Trendler, G. *et al.* (2005). Schizophrenia and depression: challenging the paradigm of two separate diseases – a controlled study of schizophrenia, depression and healthy controls. *Schizophrenia Research*, **77**, 11–24.

Haghighat, R. (2001). A unitary theory of stigmatization: pursuit of self-interest and routes to destigmatization. *British Journal of Psychiatry*, **178**, 207–15.

Hall, P. L. & Tarrier, N. (2003). The cognitive–behavioural treatment of low self-esteem in psychotic patients: a pilot study. *Behaviour Research and Therapy*, **41**, 317–32.

Harrington, R., Fudge, H., Rutter, M., Pickles, A. & Hill, J. (1990) Adult outcomes of childhood and adolescent depression: I. Psychiatric status. *Archives of General Psychiatry*, **47**, 465–73.

Harrison, G., Hopper, K., Craig, T. *et al.* (2001). Recovery from psychotic illness: a 15 and 25 year international follow-up study. *British Journal of Psychiatry*, **178**, 506–17.

Henry, L. (2004). Psychological intervention in recovery from early psychosis: cognitively oriented psychotherapy. In J. Gleeson & P. D. McGorry, (eds.), *Psychological Interventions in Early Psychosis: A Treatment Handbook*. Chichester, UK: John Wiley, pp. 63–80.

Hoch, P. & Polatin, P. (1949). Pseudoneurotic forms of schizophrenia. *Psychiatric Quarterly*, **23**, 248–76.

Hofstra, M., Ende, J. & Verhulst, F. (2001). Adolescents' self-reported problems as predictors of psychopathology in adulthood: 10-year follow-up study. *British Journal of Psychiatry*, **179**, 203–9.

Hogg, B., Jackson, H. J., Rudd, R. P. & Edwards, J. (1990). Diagnosing personality disorders in recent-onset schizophrenia. *Journal of Nervous and Mental Disease*, **178**, 194–9.

Hollis, C. (2003). Developmental precursors of child and adolescent-onset schizophrenia and affective psychoses: diagnostic specificity and continuity with symptom dimensions. *British Journal of Psychiatry*, **182**, 37–44.

Horan, W. P., Subotnik, K. L., Reise, S. P., Ventura, J. & Nuechterlein, K. H. (2005). Stability and clinical correlates of personality characteristics in recent-onset schizophrenia. *Psychological Medicine*, **35**, 995–1005.

House, A., Bostock, J. & Cooper, J. (1987). Depressive symptoms in the year following onset of a first schizophrenic illness. *British Journal of Psychiatry*, **151**, 773–9.

Iqbal, Z., Birchwood, M., Chadwick, P. & Trower, P. (2000). Cognitive approach to depression and suicidal thinking II. Testing the validity of a social ranking model. *British Journal of Psychiatry*, **177**, 522–8.

Isohanni, I., Jarvelin, M-R., Nieminen, P. *et al.* (1998). School performance as a predictor of psychiatric hospitalization in adult life. A 28 year follow-up in the Northern Finland 1966 birth cohort. *Psychological Medicine*, **28**, 967–74.

Jaspers, K. (1963). *General Psychopathology*. J. Hoenig & M. W. Hamilton (trans.). Chicago, IL: University of Chicago Press.

Johnson, W. (1981). Studies of depressive symptoms in schizophrenia. I. The prevalence of depression and its possible causes. *British Journal of Psychiatry*, **139**, 89–101.

Johnstone, C. E., Ebmeier, P. K., Miller, P., Owens, G. C. D. & Lawrie, M. S. (2005). Predicting schizophrenia: findings from the Edinburgh High-Risk Study. *British Journal of Psychiatry*, **186**, 18–25.

Jones, P. B., Bebbington, P. E., Foerster, A. *et al.* (1993). Premorbid social underachievement in schizophrenia: results from the Camberwell Collaborative Psychosis Study. *British Journal of Psychiatry*, **162**, 65–71.

Kerr, I. B., Birkett, P. B. C. & Chanen, A. (2003). Clinical and service implications of a cognitive analytic model of psychosis. *Australian and New Zealand Journal of Psychiatry*, **37**, 515–23.

Keshavan, M. S. & Schooler, N. R. (1992). First-episode studies in schizophrenia: criteria and characterization. *Schizophrenia Bulletin*, **18**, 491–513.

Koreen, A., Siris, S., Chakos, M. *et al.* (1993). Depression in first-episode schizophrenia. *American Journal of Psychiatry*, **150**, 1643–8.

Kraepelin, E. (1919). *Dementia Praecox*. New York: Churchill Livingstone.

Liddle, P. F., Barnes, T. R. E., Curson, D. A. & Patel, M. (1993). Depression and the experience of psychological deficits in schizophrenia. *Acta Psychiatrica Scandinavica*, **88**, 243–7.

Links, P. S., Steiner, M. & Mitton, J. (1989). Characteristics of psychosis in borderline personality disorder. *Psychopathology*, **22**, 188–93.

Mansell, W. & Clark, D. (1999). How do I look to others? Social anxiety and processing of the observable self. *Behavioural Research and Therapy*, **37**, 419–34.

McGlashan, T. H. (1983). The borderline syndrome. 2. Is it a variant of schizophrenia or affective-disorder? *Archives of General Psychiatry*, **40**, 1319–23.

McGlashan, T. H. (2002). The borderline personality disorder practice guidelines: the good, the bad, and the realistic. *Journal of Personality Disorders*, **16**, 119–21.

McGlashan, T. H. & Carpenter, W. (1976). An investigation of the postpsychotic depressive symptom. *American Journal of Psychiatry*, **133**, 14–19.

McGlashan, T. H., Grilo, C. M., Skodol, A. E. *et al.* (2000). The Collaborative Longitudinal Personality Disorders study:

baseline axis I/II and II/II diagnostic co-occurrence. *Acta Psychiatrica Scandinavica*, **102**, 256–64.

McGorry, P., Chanen, A., McGarthy, E. *et al.* (1991). Posttraumatic stress disorder following recent-onset psychosis. *Journal of Nervous and Mental Disease*, **179**, 253–8.

McGorry, P. D., Bell, R. C., Dudgeon, P. C. & Jackson, H. J. (1998). The dimensional structure of first episode psychosis: an exploratory factor analysis. *Psychological Medicine*, **28**, 935–47.

Miller, P., Byrne, M., Hodges, A. *et al.* (2002). Schizotypal components in people at high risk of developing schizophrenia: early findings from the Edinburgh High-Risk Study. *British Journal of Psychiatry*, **180**, 179–84.

Morrison, A. & Haddock, G. (1997). Self-focused attention in schizophrenic patients. *Personality and Individual Differences*, **23**, 937–41.

Morrison, A. P., French, P., Walford, L. *et al.* (2004). Cognitive therapy for the prevention of psychosis in people at ultra-high risk. *British Journal of Psychiatry*, **185**, 291–7.

Murray, V., McKee, I., Miller, P. M. *et al.* (2005). Dimensions and classes of psychosis in a population cohort: a four-class, four-dimension model of schizophrenia and affective psychoses. *Psychological Medicine*, **35**, 499–510.

Myhrman, A., Rantakallio, P., Isohanni, M., Jones, P. & Partanen, U. (1996). Unwantedness of a pregnancy and schizophrenia in the child. *British Journal of Psychiatry*, **169**, 637–40.

Myin-Germeys, I., Delespaul, P. & van Os, J. (2005). Behavioural sensitization to daily life stress in psychosis. *Psychological Medicine*, **35**, 733–41.

National Early Psychosis Project Clinical Guidelines Working Party (1998). *Australian Clinical Guidelines for Early Psychosis*. Melbourne: National Early Psychosis Project, University of Melbourne.

NICE (2002). *Schizophrenia: Core Intervention in the Treatment and Management of Schizophrenia in Primary and Secondary Care*. London: National Institute for Clinical Excellence.

Pallanti, S., Quercioloi, L. & Hollander. E. (2004). Social anxiety in outpatients with schizophrenia. A relevant cause of disability. *American Journal of Psychiatry*, **161**, 53–8.

Paris, J. (2002). Clinical practice guidelines for borderline personality disorder. *Journal of Personality Disorders*, **16**, 107–8.

Paris, J. (2004). Introduction to the special feature on suicide and borderline personality disorder. *Journal of Personality Disorders*, **18**, 213–14.

Parker, G., Roussos, J., Hadzi-Pavlovic, D. *et al.* (1998). The development of a refined measure of dysfunctional parenting and assessment of its relevance in patients with affective disorders. *Psychological Medicine*, **27**, 1193–203.

Pederson, C. B. & Mortensen, P. B. (2001). Evidence of a dose-response relationship between urbanicity during upbringing and schizophrenia risk. *Archives of General Psychiatry*, **58**, 1039–46.

Penn, L. D., Hope, A. D., Spaulding, W. & Kucera, J. (1994). Social anxiety in schizophrenia. *Schizophrenia Research*, **11**, 277–84.

Pfohl, B., Stangl, D. & Zimmerman, M. (1983). *The Structured Interview for DSM-III Personality Disorders (SIDP)*. Iowa City, IA: University of Iowa Hospitals and Clinics.

Pine, D., Cohen, P., Gurley, D., Brook, J. & Ma, Y. (1998). The risk for early adulthood anxiety and depressive disorders in adolescents with anxiety and depressive disorders. *Archives of General Psychiatry*, **55**, 56–64.

Pompili, M., Girardi, P., Ruberto, A. & Tatarelli, R. (2005). Suicide in borderline personality disorder: a meta-analysis. *Nordic Journal of Psychiatry*, **59**, 319–24.

Pope, H. G., Jonas, J. M., Hudson, J. I., Cohen, B. M. & Tohen, M. (1985). An empirical study of psychosis in borderline personality disorder. *American Journal of Psychiatry*, **142**, 1285–90.

Poulton, R., Caspi, A., Moffitt, T. E. *et al.* (2000). Children's self-reported psychotic symptoms and adult schizophreniform disorder: a 15 year longitudinal study. *Archives of General Psychiatry*, **57**, 1053–8.

Rao, U., Ryan, N., Birmaher, B. *et al.* (1995). Unipolar depression in adolescence: clinical course in adulthood. *Journal of American Academy of Child and Adolescent Psychiatry*, **34**, 566–78.

Read, J. & Argyle, N. (1999). Hallucinations and thought disorder among adult psychiatric inpatients with a history of child abuse. *Psychiatric Services*, **50**, 1467–72.

Rooke, O. & Birchwood, M. (1998). Loss, humiliation and entrapment as appraisals of schizophrenic illness: a prospective study of depressed and non-depressed patients. *British Journal of Clinical Psychology*, **37**, 259–68.

Rutter, M. & Sroufe, L. A. (2000). Developmental psychopathology: concepts and challenges. *Development and Psychopathology*, **12**, 265–96.

Ryle, A. (1997). The structure and development of borderline personality disorder: a proposed model. *British Journal of Psychiatry*, **170**, 82–7.

Ryle, A. (2004). The contribution of cognitive analytic therapy to the treatment of borderline personality disorder. *Journal of Personality Disorders*, **18**, 3–35.

Ryle, A. & Bennink-Bolt, F. (2002). Cognitive analytic therapy: a Vygotskian development of object relations theory. In I. S. Nolan & P. Nolan (eds.), *Object Relations and Integrative Psychotherapy: Tradition and Innovation in Theory and Practice*, London: Whurr, pp. 126–42.

Ryle, A. & Golynkina, K. (2000). Effectiveness of time-limited cognitive analytic therapy of borderline personality disorder: factors associated with outcome. *British Journal of Medical Psychology Special Issue: Cognitive Analytic Therapy*, **73**(Pt 2), 197–210.

Ryle, A. & Kerr, I. B. (2002). *Introducing Cognitive Analytic Therapy: Principles and Practice*. Chichester, UK: John Wiley.

Schneider, K. (1959). *Clinical Psychopathology*, 5th edn. M. W. Hamilton (trans.). New York: Grune & Stratton.

Sidhar, A. P. (1979). A case of borderline psychosis. *Samiksa*, **33**, 89–105.

Silk, K. R., Lohr, N. E., Westen, D. & Goodrich, S. (1989). Psychosis in borderline patients with depression. *Journal of Personality Disorders*, **3**, 92–100.

Sim, K., Swapna, V., Mythily, S. *et al.* (2004). Psychiatric comorbidity in first episode psychosis: the Early Psychosis Intervention Program (EPIP) experience. *Acta Psychiatrica Scandinavica*, **109**, 23–9.

Siris, S. (2001). Suicide and schizophrenia. *Journal of Psychopharmacology*, **15**, 127–35.

Skodol, A. E., Gunderson, J. G., McGlashan, T. H. *et al.* (2002). Functional impairment in patients with schizotypal, borderline, avoidant, or obsessive-compulsive personality disorder. *American Journal of Psychiatry*, **159**, 276–83.

Stein, M., Fuetsch, M., Muller, N. *et al.* (2001). Social anxiety and the risk of depression. *Archives of General Psychiatry*, **58**, 251–6.

Stone, M. H. (2005). Borderline personality disorder: history of the concept. In M. C. Zanarini (ed.), *Borderline Personality Disorder*. New York: Taylor and Francis, pp. 1–18.

Strakowski, S. M., Tohen, M., Stoll, A. L. *et al.* (1993). Comorbidity in psychosis at 1st hospitalization. *American Journal of Psychiatry*, **150**, 752–7.

Tarrier, N. & Wykes, T. (2004). Is there evidence that cognitive behaviour therapy is an effective treatment for schizophrenia? A cautious or cautionary tale. *Behaviour Research and Therapy*, **42**, 1377–401.

Tarrier, N., Beckett, R., Harwood, S. & Baker, A., (1993). A trial of two cognitive–behavioural methods of treating drug-resistant residual psychotic symptoms in schizophrenic patients I: outcome. *British Journal of Psychiatry*, **162**, 524–32.

Tien, Y. A. & Eaton, W. W. (1992). Psychological precursors and sociodemographic risk factors for the schizophrenia syndrome. *Archives of General Psychiatry*, **49**, 37–46.

Tiernari, P. (1994). Interaction between genetic vulnerability and family environment: the Finnish adoptive family study of schizophrenia. *Acta Psychiatrica Scandinavica*, **84**, 460–5.

Tibbo, P., Swainson, J., Chue, P. & LeMelledo, J. M. (2003). Prevalence and relationship to delusions and hallucinations of anxiety disorders in schizophrenia. *Depression and Anxiety*, **17**, 65–72.

Torgalsboen, A. K. (1999). Comorbidity in schizophrenia: a prognostic study of personality disorders in recovered and non-recovered schizophrenia patients. *Scandinavian Journal of Psychology*, **40**, 147–52.

Trower, P., Birchwood, M., Meaden, A. *et al.* (2004). Cognitive therapy for command hallucinations: randomised controlled trial. *British Journal of Psychiatry*, **184**, 312–20.

Turkington, D., Kingdon, D. & Turner, T. (2003). Effectiveness of a brief cognitive–behavioural therapy intervention in the treatment of schizophrenia. *British Journal of Psychiatry*, **180**, 523–7.

van der Zwaard, R. & Polak, M. A. (2001). Pseudohallucinations: a pseudoconcept? A review of the validity of the concept, related to associated symptomatology. *Comprehensive Psychiatry*, **42**, 42–50.

van Mastrigt, S. & Addington, J. (2002). Assessment of premorbid function in first-episode schizophrenia: modifications to the premorbid adjustment scale. *Journal of Psychiatry and Neuroscience*, **27**, 92–101.

van Os, J., Hanssen, M., Bak, M. R. V. & Vollebergh, W. (2003). Do urbanicity and familial liability coparticipate in causing psychosis? *American Journal of Psychiatry*, **160**, 477–82.

Wassink, T., Flaum, M., Nopoulos, P. & Andreasen, N. (1999). Prevalence of depressive symptoms early in the course of schizophrenia. *American Journal of Psychiatry*, **156**, 315–16.

Wing, J. K., Cooper, J. E. & Sartorius, N. (1974). *Present State Examination*. Cambridge, UK: Cambridge University Press.

Work Group on Borderline Personality Disorder (2001). Practice guideline for the treatment of patients with borderline personality disorder. *American Journal of Psychiatry*, **158**(Suppl 10), 1–52.

Yen, S., Shea, M. T., Sanislow, C. A. *et al.* (2004). Borderline personality disorder criteria associated with prospectively observed suicidal behavior. *American Journal of Psychiatry*, **161**, 1296–8.

Yung, A. R. & McGorry, P. D. (1996). The prodromal phase of first episode psychosis: past and current conceptualizations. *Schizophrenia Bulletin*, **22**, 353–70.

Yung, A. R., Phillips, L. J., Yuen, H. P. & McGorry, P. (2004). Risk factors for psychosis in an ultra-high risk group: psychopathology and clinical features. *Schizophrenia Research*, **67**, 131–52.

Zanarini, M. C., Frankenburg, F. R., Hennen, J., Reich, B. & Silk, K. R. (2005). The McLean Study of Adult Development (MSAD): overview and implications of the first six years of prospective follow-up. *Journal of Personality Disorders Special Issue: Longitudinal Studies*, **19**, 505–23.

The critical period: specific interventions

Family intervention in early psychosis

Catharine McNab and Don Linszen

Introduction

Families caring for people with psychotic illness have been the subject of research and clinical interest for many decades. In large part, however, the available literature is limited to an exploration of the experiences of carers of people with chronic schizophrenia. Further, the primary focus in this field has been on the impact of families on patients, most notably, on caregiver factors that are associated with onset and relapse. Exploration of the impact of caregiving on carers themselves has been limited. This chapter summarizes research on family factors in psychosis, with particular reference to research into first-episode psychosis (FEP). It discusses early research on the role of the family in the aetiology of psychotic disorder; examines later research that conceptualized family environments as possible risk factors for relapse, particularly within the expressed emotion (EE) paradigm; and reviews the application of EE research into the FEP and 'ultra-high-risk' (UHR) groups. This chapter also considers the limited literature regarding the experiences of families of those with FEP, focusing on distress and grief. Finally, it provides an overview of family interventions in the first episode, notes difficulties with implementing family interventions and suggests some guidelines for working with relatives and caregivers of young people with FEP, as well as directions for future research.

Families as the cause of psychotic disorder

Early proposals regarding the role of families in the course of psychotic illness were based on anecdotal or methodologically problematic evidence. These theories focused on the family's role in the origin of schizophrenia. Mothers, in particular, were regarded as 'schizophrenogenic' or having a 'perverted maternal instinct' (Rosen, 1947), which could be associated with overprotectiveness or rejection (Fromm-Reichmann, 1950). Alternatively, relatives, and in particular mothers, were proposed to provide conflicting overt verbal and abstract non-verbal information, which the 'target' patient could neither fully comprehend nor withdraw from. This was proposed as placing patients in a 'double-bind' (Bateson et al., 1956), resulting in psychotic symptoms such as thought disorder and disorganized speech. Lidz et al. (1957) identified 'marital schism' (overt conflicts between the parents) and 'marital skew' (in which the disturbed functioning of one parent was compensated by distorted communication of the other) as the underlying causes of psychotic disorder. Based on these theories, many family interventions in chronic schizophrenia were applied to the families of young people with FEP (Haley, 1980; Lidz, 1973; Palazzoli-Selvini et al., 1978), but the efficacy and appropriateness of this application was not systematically evaluated.

Families and the course of psychotic disorder

More recently, the focus has shifted from family factors contributing to onset to those contributing to relapse. These have included difficulties with families in sharing a focus of conversational attention (communication

The Recognition and Management of Early Psychosis: A Preventive Approach, ed. Henry J. Jackson and Patrick D. McGorry. Published by Cambridge University Press. © Cambridge University Press 2009.

deviance: Miklowitz & Stackman, 1992; Singer & Wynne, 1965; Wynne & Singer, 1963) and the emotional climate in the family, particularly criticism, guilt induction and intrusiveness (affective style: e.g. Miklowitz *et al.*, 1989). Although there is a relatively significant literature focusing on these constructs, research into the construct of EE has dominated the field.

What is expressed emotion?

The development of the construct of EE was prompted by the observation of Brown, Carstairs & Topping (1958) that the prognosis for patients with psychosis appeared to be related to their living situation after discharge. They noted that patients returning from admission to live with spouses or parents fared less well than patients returning to live with siblings or in shared accommodation. At the time, these findings were specific to psychotic disorders and did not generalize to their other categories of depression, epilepsy or 'psychoneurosis'. Further analysis of this association revealed that their findings were particularly strong in families in which a key member (e.g. a parent or spouse), within the context of a semi-structured interview, demonstrated one of three tendencies in their observations of the patient and their perceptions of their relationship with the patient. These included commenting on behaviours or characteristics of the patient that were regarded as annoying or that the respondent resented, making comments suggesting generalized criticism or rejecting attitudes towards the patient and report or demonstration of over-intrusive or self-sacrificing behaviour, exaggerated responses or over-identification with the patient (Leff & Vaughn, 1985). These three characteristics were called criticism, hostility and emotional over-involvement (EOI), respectively, and were known collectively as EE.

The impact of expressed emotion: its predictive validity in formal and informal carers

The attractiveness of the concept of EE lies in its predictive validity. Hooley and Hiller (1998) reviewed meta-analyses in the field and concluded that EE is highly predictive of psychotic relapse, with rates in

families with high EE ranging between 50% and 65%, while those for families with low EE ranged from 23% to 35%. From a meta-analysis, Butzlaff and Hooley (1998) reported a weighted mean effect size in samples of clients with psychotic disorders of 0.3, qualifying as a medium effect size (Cohen, 1992; for additional reviews consistent with this, see Bebbington & Kuipers (1994), Kavanagh (1992) and Parker & Hadzi-Pavlovic (1990)).

Although the EE–relapse link was first explored in relation to psychotic relapse, the predictive validity of EE appears even stronger in other disorders, despite the initial reservations of Brown *et al.* (1958) regarding the construct's generalizability to other disorders. Disorders in which EE predicts worsening symptomatology and/or relapse include depression (e.g. Hinrichsen & Pollack, 1997; Hooley, 1986), bipolar disorder (e.g. Miklowitz *et al.*, 1988), eating disorders (e.g. van Furth *et al.*, 1996), substance use (e.g. O'Farrell *et al.*, 1998), comorbid substance use and psychotic disorder (Pourmand, Kavanagh & Vaughan, 2005) and post-traumatic stress disorder (Tarrier, Sommerfield & Pilgrim, 1999). Expressed emotion also appears to play a role in the prognosis of physical health disorders (reviewed by Vaughn, Leff & Sarner, 1999; Wearden *et al.*, 2000). The focus on a dichotomous outcome variable of relapse–no relapse is, however, far less common in EE research outside of the psychotic disorders.

This relationship between EE and relapse emerges not only across disorders but also across patient gender (cf. King & Dixon, 1999) and many cultures (reviewed by Karno & Jenkins, 1993). The major moderating factor in the link between EE and relapse is the amount of time spent with the target carer: EE is more strongly related to relapse when carers have more contact with patients (e.g. Bebbington & Kuipers, 1994). The size of the relationship between EE and relapse is similar in medication and medication-free conditions (reviewed by Kavanagh, 1992). Suggestions have been made that criticism and hostility are more strongly related to patient functioning than EOI, both longitudinally and cross-sectionally (reviewed by Wearden *et al.*, 2000); however, these findings are inconsistent (e.g. schizophrenia: Breitborde *et al.*, 2007; King & Dixon, 1999; anxiety disorders: Chambless & Steketee, 1999; eating disorders: Szmukler *et al.*, 1985; 'affective disturbance': Bentsen *et al.*, 1996).

The occurrence of EE is not confined to informal care-giving by relatives; formal caregivers, such as case managers and residential care staff, also demonstrate behaviour typical of high and low EE (e.g. Oliver & Kuipers, 1996) although rates of EE are generally lower in this group than amongst informal caregivers (e.g. Barrowclough *et al.*, 2001). Barrowclough *et al.* (2001) suggested that staff may under-report EE through reticence in response to researchers; they may also have less emotional investment in patients than informal carers and, consequently, less strong feelings about patients. When EE is present in formal caregivers, it is primarily based on criticism rather than EOI. High EE in this group has also been associated with outcome, despite generally lower amounts of patient contact than occurs between informal caregivers and patients (e.g. Ball, Moore & Kuipers, 1992; Snyder *et al.*, 1994).

Why does expressed emotion have impact: what are the mechanisms of its link with relapse?

The dominant model of EE suggests that it indicates 'real-world' problematic responses to deteriorating mental state in patients, which may reflect either premorbid characteristics of the carer or specific response styles to symptom exacerbation or to stress more broadly (Brown, Carstairs & Topping, 1962). Expressed emotion is seen as a stressor for patients, interacting with organic vulnerability to cause symptom exacerbation and ultimately relapse (Nuechterlein & Dawson, 1984). This stressor is regarded as particularly salient when evident in key support networks such as the family. Having just one carer who is high in EE is regarded in the literature as likely to provoke this stress. As a result, EE levels of any particular environment are dictated by whether or not *any* member is high in EE: if not, the environment is low EE, and if so, the environment is high EE.

In a more elaborate model of the mechanisms of the EE–relapse link, Tarrier *et al.* (1999) suggested that the stressful environment of EE impairs patients' habituation to arousal, proposed to be a key process in symptom improvement in a range of disorders such as psychosis and post-traumatic stress disorder. Kuipers and colleagues (Garety *et al.*, 2001; Kuipers, 2006; Kuipers

et al., 2006) have suggested that two components of EE, criticism and hostility, increase environmental stress, which together with premorbid schema, causes affective change, particularly anxiety and depressed mood. This, in turn, interacts with reasoning processes and secondary appraisal of symptoms to cause exacerbation in positive psychotic symptoms. By comparison, EOI may be stressful because it implies that patients lack the skill or strengths needed to remedy their own difficulties, possibly reinforcing a sense of futility and failure (Coyne, Wortman & Lehman, 1988).

The strength of the predictive relationship between EE and psychotic relapse is such that Butzlaff and Hooley (1998) have argued for a moratorium on further EE–relapse replication studies in schizophrenia. Despite the consistent findings with respect to the EE–outcome link broadly, it is possible that replication studies are still necessary in novel patient populations. This includes FEP and the putative prodrome, where results appear less consistent.

Expressed emotion and first-episode psychosis and ultra-high-risk patients

It is difficult to evaluate whether EE itself is more prevalent in chronic than first-onset psychotic illness because of at least two factors. The first is the wide range in prevalence of EE levels reported within the chronic mental illness literature. The second is that only one study to date has directly examined differences in EE between chronic and first-episode mental illness. In this study, Bachmann *et al.* (2002) did not detect a difference in EE levels between these two samples in either depressive or psychotic disorder. Non-comparative studies of EE in FEP generally report rates of high EE similar to those in chronic samples. Prevalence of high EE in first-episode populations ranges between 20% and 71% (e.g. Bachmann *et al.*, 2002; Barrelet *et al.*, 1990; Hahlweg *et al.*, 1989; Heikkilä *et al.*, 2002; MacMillan *et al.*, 1987; Nugter *et al.*, 1997; Patterson, Birchwood & Cochrane, 2005; Pourmand *et al.*, 2005; Stirling *et al.*, 1993).

Regardless of levels of high EE, some argue that the nature of the EE construct is such that its predictive validity should extend into the first relapse (Kavanagh,

1992). However, the link is less consistently detected in the FEP group. Studies exploring the EE–relapse relationship in the FEP and UHR groups were detected by PsycINFO and Medline searches using keywords of 'expressed emotion', and 'first episode' or 'prodrom*' or 'early onset', and in the references of papers detected in this way, and are summarized in Table 17.1. Barrelet *et al.* (1990), Jarbin, Gråwe & Hansson (2000), King & Dixon (1999), Leff & Brown (1977), Linszen *et al.* (1996) and Nuechterlein, Snyder & Mintz (1992) detected relationships between EE and outcome in FEP. However, other studies have suggested that EE's impact on outcome is delayed in the FEP group (Huguelet *et al.*, 1995; Lenior *et al.*, 2002); is negligible once controlling for other factors, such as duration of untreated symptoms (MacMillan *et al.*, 1986; cf. Mintz, Mintz & Goldstein, 1987), or is not predictive at all (Nugter *et al.*, 1997; Stirling *et al.*, 1991; Stirling *et al.*, 1993). The evidence for the predictive power of EE in FEP, therefore, appears weaker than that in chronic mental illness (see also Butzlaff & Hooley, 1998).

Given the generally neglected field of early intervention in mania (Conus & McGorry, 2002), it is unsurprising that, to date, there are no studies of EE specifically in populations with first-episode mania. However, those patients with first-episode mania with psychotic features may be included within some of the studies listed in Table 17.1.

Kavanagh (1992) proposed that, given the theories about the mechanisms by which EE causes relapse, it stands to reason that EE would be associated with onset of psychosis. However, in contrast to early psychoanalytically oriented literature, Brown (1985, p. 17, emphasis added) suggested that the construct of EE specifically, and of problematic family interactions generally, was one that he felt was relevant to *relapse* rather than the *onset* of psychotic illness: 'I had not ... been impressed by the many formulations in the psychiatric literature about the fundamental role of patients' relationships with parents in the aetiology of schizophrenia. There appeared to be far too many exceptions for it to provide a *general* theory about origins of the disorder'. This statement, however, has not prevented some exploration of the family as a psychosocial candidate of transition to psychosis, with mixed results. Norton

(1982) found that 91% of her sample of 'disturbed' adolescents with two high-EE parents later received diagnoses of schizophrenia or related disorders (e.g. probable schizophrenia, or borderline or schizoid personality disorder); 25% of those with one high-EE parent and 10% of those with two low-EE parents were similarly diagnosed at follow-up. This finding suggests a very strong role of EE in the onset of psychotic illness broadly defined. Using more recent conceptualizations of UHR, however, O'Brien *et al.* (2006) found no relationship between levels of criticism and outcome at a 3-month follow-up, and a positive relationship between negative symptoms and social functioning, and EOI, warmth and positive comments at both intake and 3 months. These findings suggest that, in this age group, EOI may be beneficial rather than problematic, and clearly require further exploration.

Why is the link between expressed emotion and outcome less consistently detected in first-episode psychosis?

Expressed emotion appears to be less problematic in terms of client outcome in FEP. A number of reasons may account for this, although few have been examined empirically. It may be that measures of EE are less ecologically valid in this group, so that carers report certain behaviours and feelings regarding the patient but do not allow these to translate into interpersonal behaviour. This might be consistent with the conceptualization of EE as a response to symptom behaviour – carers may be more able to censor their interpersonal interactions with patients when these symptoms are new, but allow themselves to speak freely with others (Bachmann *et al.*, 2002). This may particularly be the case with EOI in these samples (e.g. McCarty *et al.*, 2004). Other authors have proposed that EE does not predict relapse in patients with early-onset psychosis because attitudes towards the patient become 'contaminated' by parents experiencing repeated relapses (MacMillan *et al.*, 1986). However, the research reviewed above seems to suggest that EE 'attitudes' are present to the same degree in early-onset and chronic schizophrenia; an alternative explanation is

Table 17.1. Expressed emotion and patient outcome in first-episode psychosis and in patients at ultra-high risk

Authors	Participants	Time of assessment	Expressed emotion: assessment measure and levels	Predictive validity of expressed emotion	Caveats
Leff & Brown, 1977	Pooled data of first-admitted patients in 1972 and 1976 in UK studies (sample size and age unclear)	Unknown	CFI	38% of sample with high EE and 13% with low EE relapsed	
Norton, 1982	'Disturbed' adolescents regarded as at risk of developing psychosis (sample size and age unclear)	Unknown	Unclear	91% of sample with two high-EE parents later received diagnoses of schizophrenia or related disorders (e.g. probable schizophrenia, or borderline or schizoid personality disorder); 25% of those with one high-EE parent and 10% of those with two low-EE parents were similarly diagnosed at follow-up (period unclear)	
MacMillan et al., 1986	Relatives of 82 patients with first-episode schizophrenia (age unclear)	Within 6 weeks of index admission	CFI: 56.82% high EE (very limited EOI)	CC predicted relapse/readmission rates but no longer did so when duration of illness preceding admission and neuroleptic treatment following discharged controlled for	Unclear how relapse/readmission operationalized
Barrelet et al., 1990	36 French-speaking relatives in Geneva of patients (median age 24.5 years) with 'first-admission schizophrenia' (diagnosis of schizophrenia or paranoid psychosis)	Date of assessment unclear ('at intake')	CFI: 66.67% high EE	EE significantly associated with 9-month relapse, probably primarily caused by CC; using the standard EE cutoff 33% high EE relapsed over follow-up period and 0% in low EE, but 'highest statistical difference' between low and high EE obtained with cutoff point between 11 and 13 CC, with relapse rates of 4% in low CC group and 64% in high CC group	First admission (cf. first episode); relapse defined by readmission or 'duration of symptoms for 2 weeks'; severity of symptoms unclear
Stirling et al., 1991	33 patients aged between 16 and 50 (mean age 25 years) with 'recent-onset schizophrenia' and their relatives,	Assessed within 1 month of admission; onset of first episode within previous 2 years	CFI: 43.33% high EE	No significant relationship between EE (either overall or the subscales) and relapse, even when thresholds for high EE altered; relapse over 12-month follow-up occurred in 40% with high EE and 43% with low EE	Relapse poorly defined ('significant exacerbation of symptoms, which usually, though not always, necessitated rehospitalization'; could occur for as little as a week)
Nuechterlein et al., 1992	43 consecutive first-admission and recent-onset patients with schizophrenia (mean age 22.7 years)	Within 1 month of admission	CFI	39% relapsed within 12 months from the high EE group; 0% relapsed from the low EE group	
Stirling et al., 1993	30 patients with 'recent-onset schizophrenia' and their 37 relatives (18-month follow-up of the sample in Stirling et al. (1991))	18 months after initial assessment, outside of the admission context	?:	No significant relationship between initial EE and later relapse, although a significant relationship between EE rating at 18-month follow-up and patient outcome at that point	

Table 17.1. (cont.)

Authors	Participants	Time of assessment	Expressed emotion: assessment measure and levels	Predictive validity of expressed emotion	Caveats
Rund et al., 1995	12 patients	Unclear	CFI/FMSS	No relationship between EE and relapse	
Huguelet et al., 1995	44 first-admission patients with a diagnosis of schizophrenia	Unclear	CFI	EE did not correlate with relapse until 3-year follow-up	34% attrition rate
Nugter et al., 1997	64 family members of patients aged between 15 and 26 years, consecutively admitted in inpatient unit with primary diagnosis of schizophrenia, schizophreniform or schizoaffective disorder and need for continuous antipsychotic medication; living with or in close contact with family; mean age 20 years	Mean of 4-months' post-service entry	FMSS: 52.1% high EE	No predictive validity of EE per se, but unstable EE approached significance in the group that did not receive integrated treatment (including family therapy) such that higher relapse rates were associated with a change in EE levels over 12-months' of follow-up	
King & Dixon, 1999	69 people with schizophrenia aged between 17 and 36 years (mean age 27.9 years)	Unclear	CFI	EE environment significantly associated with relapse; used cutoff of 7 on CC, 3 on EOI and/or 1 on hostility. Best predictors were fathers' CC levels and mothers' EOI 9-month relapse rate: 55%, high EE, 17%, low EE 18-month relapse rate: 55%, high EE; 40%, low EE	
Jarbin et al., 2000	15 adolescents with schizophrenia, schizophreniform disorder, schizoaffective disorder or affective psychosis (mean age 16.4 years)	Date of assessment unclear	FMSS: 33% 'high', 13% 'borderline'	'High' and 'borderline' EE, when combined, showed a trend towards prediction of relapse: high specificity for relapse at 1 (0.8) and 2 (1.0) years, moderate sensitivity (0.5)	Small sample size
O'Brien et al., 2006	26 primary caregivers of 26 people aged between 12 and 35 years (mean age 16.2 years) and identified as at 'ultra high' risk of developing psychosis according to the Structured Interview for Prodromal Symptoms	Date of assessment unclear	CFI: 35% high EE	Caregiver EOI associated with improvement in negative symptoms and social functioning at 3-month follow-up; caregiver positive remarks associated with improvement in negative and disorganized symptoms at follow-up; caregiver warmth associated with improved social functioning at follow-up; CC unrelated to outcome at 3 months	Small sample

CC, critical comments subscale of expressed emotion; CFI, Camberwell Family Interview (Leff & Vaughn, 1985); EE, expressed emotion; EOI, emotional over-involvement; FMSS, Five Minute Speech Sample (Magaña et al., 1986).

that EE 'behaviour' becomes more contaminated, reactive and *entrenched* after repeated episodes.

Alternatively, examination of the cross-cultural validity of the EE–relapse link may provide further insight. Previous research in patients with chronic disorder has suggested that EE's predictive validity may be dependent on cultural norms. Even slightly elevated levels may be sufficient to provoke relapse in cultures with generally lower levels of EE (e.g. Asian and Mexican cultures: Nomura *et al.*, 2005; Wig *et al.*, 1987). Threshold levels of EE may, by comparison, need to be higher in countries in which higher levels of EE are typical (e.g. the Middle East: Heresco-Levy, Greenberg & Dasberg, 1990; Mediterranean countries: Francis & Papageorgiou, 2004). Nevertheless, EE generally continues to retain some prognostic validity once thresholds are altered.

Adolescence may have its own 'parenting culture' in which high EE interactions are widespread. Conflict with parents is regarded as a vital part of adolescence, and emotional over-involvement is probably not uncommon and even appropriate at times in parenting adolescents. Expressed emotion may be seen in early-onset illness as an exacerbation of normative interactions between parents and adolescents, one which is probably quite different from the expected relationship between parents and their adult offspring. For this reason, EE interactions may be less stressful for adolescents in their first episode than they are for older people (Heresco-Levy *et al.*, 1990). This may particularly be the case for EOI. Some authors have suggested that EOI is not predictive of outcome at first episode, because it is either rarely present (Dingemans, Linszen & Lenior, 2002; Kershner, Cohen & Coyne, 1996; MacMillan *et al.*, 1986; cf. Stirling *et al.*, 1991) or more normative (Barrelet *et al.*, 1990). It is possible that the subtle communication of the message of over-involvement, that the individual lacks the ability to manage difficulties on his or her own, is less damaging in childhood and adolescence, as the degree to which autonomy and independence has been encouraged may still be minimal. As Peris and Baker (2000, p. 461) noted: 'the line demarcating normal parental concern and overbearing intrusiveness may be blurred in childhood and adolescence, when psychosis generally emerges'. Wamboldt *et al.* (2000, p. 889) also pointed out that 'the boundary is less clear between helpful, yet increased

emotional support and aid, and excessive, harmful emotional over-involvement' in children and adolescents. Provision of overt support and assistance, rather than promoting independence and autonomy, may be less problematic in early-onset illness during adolescence than in chronic illness. Wamboldt *et al.* (2000) also noted, in particular, that the pathology of 'excessive praise' may be less relevant because it is particularly common in parents of young people, especially children; in their study, EOI generally, and excessive praise in particular, was not associated with behaviour problems or psychopathology. However, the respective impact of the subscales of EE on outcome are rarely explored, and as such we are limited in the degree to which we can draw conclusions about the possibly different effects on outcome of EOI, criticism and hostility in early-onset mental illness. Further research exploring this is required.

The issue of the degree to which EE, and particularly EOI, is problematic for patients is somewhat distinct from whether EE is an understandable 'reaction' to parenting a young person with emerging serious mental illness. Expressed emotion, especially EOI, may be a reasonable response to the parenting of adolescents generally, or to the grief and loss that may accompany the experience of learning that a son or daughter has developed symptoms that mean he or she may experience a difficult and chronic illness. It may also be seen within the context of relationship intimacy research. High EE has been linked with low premorbid and current relationship intimacy (Fearon *et al.*, 1998). A key developmental task of adolescence is a distancing from parents, and hence probably a lowering of levels of intimacy between parent and child. Occurrence of EE could, therefore, be seen as a normative response to parental perception of the diminishing quality of the parent–child relationship. However, 'reasonable' or 'understandable' responses may also be problematic for the targeted individual.

It may also be that the social context of EE differs between the first episode and subsequent episodes. It is generally a parent or a partner who is assessed with reference to EE, given that it was these family members who were integral to the development of the construct. In the initial stages of research into expressed emotion, patients were generally living with relatives, had small social networks and few close relationships (Vaughn *et al.*, 1999). In the first episode, although patients are similarly likely to still be living with their families, for age- rather than symptom-related reasons, relationships other than familial ones are likely to be relatively intact and these may 'dilute' the impact of parental or partner EE. Furthermore, high EE within other relationships, such as friendships, nascent intimate relationships, or general peer networks in the form of bullying, may constitute salient high EE environments that work against low EE within the family context to contribute to relapse. Findings suggesting a link between bullying and both psychotic experiences in non-patients (Lataster *et al.*, 2006; Morrison & Petersen, 2003), and hallucinations in psychosis (Hardy *et al.*, 2005) may provide preliminary support for this suggestion.

Methodological factors may also contribute to findings of a less consistent link. Kavanagh (1992) suggested that there is no reason why EE should not be related as much to the timing of first episodes of psychosis as to subsequent ones: findings to the contrary may be a result of retrospective methodologies, or particularly narrow readings of relapse (see also King & Dixon, 1999). It is also possible that the focus in the psychosis literature on a dichotomous outcome of relapse/no relapse has limited the power of analyses, in contrast to much of the literature linking EE and outcome more broadly defined in childhood and adolescent mental illness. A further methodological issue may be the frequency of the predicted outcome in first-episode populations, in contrast to more chronically affected groups. The highest proportion of 'good outcome' patients will be seen at the first episode, as any case sample including relapsers will automatically lower the proportion of those people who have recovered (Bland, Parker & Orn, 1978). It is possible that EE's predictive power in the first episode is minimized by the lower incidence of relapse in the first episode than later in the course of illness.

In summary, the link between EE and outcome is less consistently detected in FEP than in chronic schizophrenia. A range of factors, including the developmental appropriateness of EE (particularly EOI), degree of interactions outside the immediate family context and methodological issues, may be responsible for this.

This suggests that the proposal of Butzlaff and Hooley (1998) for a moratorium on EE–outcome research, given the demonstrated strength of the link, is less applicable in the first-episode literature. It also suggests that further exploration of EE levels in the first episode might be fruitful, particularly the subscales of EE as they may be linked with different correlates cross-sectionally and differentially predict outcome. Finally, it also indicates that a fuller understanding of the experience of relatives of people with FEP beyond assessment of EE would allow interventions to be appropriately tailored to this particular group.

The course of family experience: distress, experience of caregiving and grief

The previous section indicates that most studies of family members or caregivers of people with psychotic disorder have been provoked by interest in the role of the family in aetiology and relapse (Lowyck *et al.*, 2001). A focus on EE to the exclusion of an analysis of the family's experience of caring for a mentally ill member disregards the importance of the well-being of caregivers in its own right (Fadden, 1998). Furthermore, the family's experience may be linked to patient prognosis and service use beyond any role of EE; for example, levels of family burden appear to have a negative influence on patient medication (Perlick *et al.*, 1999), and frequency of contact with patients (Wasow, 1994; cf. Harvey *et al.*, 2001a), which may, in turn, be linked to difficulties seeking timely care (Cole *et al.*, 1995; Judge *et al.*, 2005) and, ultimately, to higher levels of service use (Becker *et al.*, 1997). It is important to examine relatives' experiences independently of EE. Primary family-related constructs examined within this context have included distress and burden and/or negative experience of caregiving. Grief experiences of caregivers have also been explored, although in much less detail.

The caregiving experience: how distressed are caregivers?

Mental illness caregiving research is dominated by caregivers of heterogeneous groups of people with fairly chronic 'psychiatric disability' broadly defined. This generally includes a significant majority of individuals with schizophrenia-spectrum disorders, but also affective, anxiety and other disorders. Caregiver participants in these studies have normally occupied a caregiving role for some years, ranging from 2 months to 41 years, but with few in the early onset or FEP phase (e.g. Provencher *et al.*, 2003). Studies sampling these groups report that caregivers have a risk of experiencing psychological difficulties that is two to three times higher than that of the general population, with prevalence rates of severe psychological distress in caregivers ranging from 25% to 61% (e.g. Cornwall & Scott, 1996; St Onge & Lavoie, 1997). This level of distress emerges in qualitative research (e.g. Saunders & Byrne, 2002) and structured psychiatric interviews (e.g. Wittmund *et al.*, 2002), as well as in questionnaire measures.

Specific issues in the literature on first-episode psychosis and ultra-high-risk groups

It is possible that the high levels of distress reported by caregivers are a consequence of the chronicity of the caregiving role in these studies, so it may not be general to the experiences of carers in FEP. Indeed, such carers may not even see themselves as 'carers', a point often overlooked in the literature. Findings examining links between duration of caregiving/patient illness and distress levels are equivocal. Gibbons *et al.* (1984) and Martens and Addington (2001) found distress to be highest at first episode and then to fall, and Möller-Leimkühler (2006) reported that scores on a range of measures of distress were lower at 1-year follow-up than at intake. In contrast, Harvey *et al.* (2001b) reported that distress rises as psychosis continues. Additionally, Brown and Birtwhistle (1998) found little variation in distress over a 15-year follow-up period in a group of carers of people with schizophrenia, and Östman and Hansson (2004) found few differences in burden between relatives of people at first admission in comparison to subsequent admissions. The Scottish Schizophrenia Research Group (1992) found that distress reduced after 2 years, but developed again at

5-year follow-up in the first episode. The longitudinal course of distress, therefore, remains unclear.

A small amount of research has specifically explored distress levels in the first-episode group. Qualitative research confirms that carers experience the early phase of caregiving as distressing; however, the trajectory of distress remains unclear. Jungbauer and Angermeyer (2002), in their qualitative study of carers of people with schizophrenia, reported that families remember disorder onset as particularly stressful: the patient's symptomatology emerges suddenly and apparently without reason, and the patient appears significantly different from their 'former self', with associated feelings on the part of carers of weakness, anxiety, loss of control, guilt, shame and confusion. Rolland (1994), however, proposed that distress may increase as strain on family caregivers grows through exhaustion and a building up of caregiving tasks over time.

Quantitative studies examining distress levels of caregivers of patients with FEP are also both scarce and inconsistent, and five studies are summarized in Table 17.2. These studies were detected by PsycINFO and Medline searches using keywords of 'first episode' or 'prodrom*' or 'early onset', and 'burden' or 'distress' or 'depression', and 'family' or 'caregiv*', as well as in the references of papers detected in this way. McCreadie (2001) noted that the disparity between some findings may be accounted for by the difference in time period separating first-episode onset and participation in research, which was up to 2 weeks for the Scottish Schizophrenia Group (1992) study, and up to 2 years for the Tennakoon *et al.* (2000) study. Only one study to date has compared caregivers at different stages of caregiving; Bibou-Nakou, Dikaiou and Bairactaris (1997) reported a trend for caregivers of people with an illness duration of less than 2 years to be more distressed than those who have been caring for longer periods. This suggests a process of accommodation to the emotional demands of caregiving, but the study requires replication. Overall, despite some inconsistent results regarding the short- and long-term course of distress in caregivers, it appears that levels of distress in caregivers of people with recent-onset disorder are at least comparable to those in carers of people with more chronic difficulties.

Table 17.2. Quantitative studies examining distress and burden in caregivers of patients with first-episode psychosis

Authors	Participants	Time of assessment	Distress: assessment measure and levels	Burden: assessment measure and levels
Scottish Schizophrenia Group, 1987	31 relatives of patients	During first week of patient's admission for FEP	GHQ: 77% reached psychiatric caseness	Not assessed
Bibou-Nakou et al., 1997	52 relatives of patients with schizophrenia, divided into 'continuing treatment' (ill at least 2 years) and 'acute' (ill less than 2 years)	Unclear	GHQ: no descriptives reported, but trend for those in the 'acute case' group to have higher distress levels than those in the 'continuing treatment case' group	Not assessed
Tennakoon et al., 2000	40 relatives of patients aged between 18 and 45 years experiencing a first psychotic episode of less than 24 months' duration	Unclear	GHQ: 12% reached 'psychiatric caseness'	No descriptives reported
Addington et al., 2003	238 family members of patients admitted to an early-psychosis programme	As soon as possible after acceptance into service	PGWB: 26% 'severely distressed', 21% 'moderately distressed'	Mean scores of negative experiences of caregiving 87.58 (SD = 33.64), comparable to samples of caregivers of people with chronic mental illness (Szmukler et al., 1996)
Patterson et al., 2005	50 relatives as described in Patterson et al. (2000), 36 at 9-month follow-up	As in Patterson et al. (2000)	No descriptives reported; depression on Calgary Depression Scale for Schizophrenia not significantly associated with EE at initial assessment or follow-up	No descriptives reported; no significant differences between high and low EE on negative experiences of caregiving at initial assessment, but high EOI reported higher burden than low EOI 9-month follow-up: high EE associated with higher levels of total negative burden; this effect entirely linked to EOI in relatives, who recorded nearly 50% higher perceived burden than the low-EOI group (no significant difference between high and low CC)

FEP, first-episode psychosis; GHQ, General Health Questionnaire (Goldberg & Blackwell, 1988); PGWB, Psychological General Well-being Scale (Bech, 1993; Dupuy, 1984); EE, expressed emotion; CC, expressed emotion subscale of 'critical comments'; EOI, expressed emotion subscale of 'emotional overinvolvement'.

Individual differences in the caregiving experience

Szmukler et al. (1996) used a stress and coping paradigm (Lazarus & Folkman, 1984) in developing the only model of caregiving in mental illness. *Stressors* in this instance refer to the patient's illness, behaviours and disabilities, as well as the associated perceived disruption of caregiver life. *Mediating factors*, such as social support, carer personality and quality of family relationships, may all serve to mitigate the impact of stressors upon the appraisal of the caregiving experience. *Appraisal* itself, or the salience of threatening and/or positive components of the caregiving experience (also known as 'burden' or 'negative experiences of caregiving'), in turn, interacts with *coping strategies* in the prediction of outcomes such as psychological and physical health. While these predictors have been explored in some detail in the chronic caregiving literature (e.g. Harvey et al., 2001b; Joyce et al., 2003; Provencher et al., 2003; Scazufca & Kuipers, 1999; St Onge & Lavoie, 1997; Szmukler et al., 1996), as far as we are aware there has been no systematic exploration of predictors of distress in the first episode or UHR caregiving groups.

Other components of the caregiving process: loss and grief

Qualitative research focusing on the 'lived experience' of caregivers of people with chronic, serious mental illness has identified grief and loss as other key components of the caregiving context. Studies suggest that these relatives experience significant levels of grief in response to a range of losses: loss of the premorbid 'version' of the patient, loss of their potential, and loss of hopes and aspirations for the patient's future (e.g. Mohr & Regan-Kubinski, 2001; Osborne & Coyle, 2002; Ozgul, 2004; Ryan, 1993; Tuck et al., 1997). This caregiving grief has been termed 'ambiguous loss' (Adams & Sanders, 2004) or 'disenfranchised grief' (Doka, 1989), given the continuing physical presence of the patient (Shabad, 1989). McElroy (1987) has also focused on the idiosyncratic nature of caring for someone with psychiatric illness, in which the cyclical nature of illness and the periodic reappearance of the patient's 'former self' prolong the experience of grieving (see also Terkelsen, 1987). Although grief has received limited empirical attention, it appears to be a key component of the caregiving experience, even for parents of young people with first-episode mental illness (Godress et al., 2004; Solomon & Draine, 1996), including FEP (Patterson, Birchwood & Cochrane, 2000; Patterson et al., 2005). In this first-episode group, EE, and in particular EOI, has been proposed to be an 'attachment behaviour' that emerges from grief and loss (Patterson et al., 2000, 2005), suggesting that working therapeutically with grief may influence EE levels.

Family interventions in first-episode psychosis

Findings linking EE and outcome in chronic schizophrenia have been used to justify the development of intervention programmes primarily aimed at reducing EE rates, which include psychoeducation, family 'therapy', behavioural modification (e.g. coping strategies, communication skills training), relaxation training, cognitive–behavioural interventions and role play. These interventions have little impact on psychiatric morbidity or social functioning but may impact positively on patient employment and independent living, as well as family burden, knowledge and EE. These interventions reduce total costs by about 20%, and the number needed to treat to produce remission in patients using family intervention has ranged between 2 and 6.5 (de Jesus Mari & Streiner, 1994; Pharoah et al., 2003).

The limited and equivocal data available on the EE–relapse link in the first episode, and on the EE–onset link, suggest that interventions focusing on modifying EE levels in the first episode or UHR groups are somewhat premature, as EE cannot be unequivocally regarded as a risk factor for poor outcome in patients. Interventions may, however, be appropriate in this group in order to serve other goals, such as reducing carer distress, negative experiences of caregiving and grief/loss, and to provide psychoeducation in order to maximize carers' caregiving capacity.

Table 17.3 provides a review of interventions that have been evaluated in the first-episode group specifically. These papers were detected by PsycINFO and Medline searches using as key phrases 'intervention*' or 'treatment', and 'first episode' or 'early onset' or 'prodrom*', and 'famil*'; and through references cited in papers detected in this way. These interventions in the first episode appear effective in enhancing knowledge and understanding of mental illness generally and psychotic illness in particular. However, interventions targeting EE in the first episode are less effective than those in more chronic samples in reducing relapse rates, although they may lead to reductions in both the need for inpatient admission and length thereof (e.g. Zhang *et al.*, 1994). This lesser efficacy of interventions in the first episode may be a consequence of the weaker link between EE and relapse in the first-episode group, as reported above. Alternatively, as family interventions are often compared with 'treatment as usual' in first-episode studies (as many services that conduct these trials are specialist first-episode services), it may be difficult to demonstrate any significant additive effect of family therapy over usual treatment in the absence of large sample sizes.

However, neither of these suggestions – that family interventions are less useful because EE does not predict relapse in the first episode, or because they provide no additive effect in preventing relapse – can account for the fact that family interventions in the first episode are generally less effective than those in chronically affected groups in reducing EE at all (e.g. Lenior *et al.*, 2002; Linszen *et al.*, 1996; Nugter *et al.*, 1997). Nugter *et al.* (1997) explained this with reference to the possible lesser motivation in relatives to 'change' as a consequence of interventions; many may have found it difficult to believe that later episodes would or could occur, so they are less enthusiastic about modifying their behaviour in order to prevent this. Linszen *et al.* (1996) also suggested that the form of typical family interventions may be inappropriate in the first episode. Participants in our study reported that a focus on behavioural family interventions prevented an opportunity to deal with feelings of grief and loss surrounding the onset of psychotic illness in a son or daughter.

It is possible that, although EE is hypothesized to be less entrenched in early psychosis (Patterson *et al.*, 2000), traditional ways of targeting EE are not effective in this group. Interventions may, therefore, be useful in the first episode, not by reducing EE but by preventing its entrenchment by targeting loss and psychological morbidity (Patterson *et al.*, 2000). Interventions may also provide families with resources to enable them to stay involved with patients, thus allowing early recognition of signs of relapse. In fact, Addington and Burnett (2004) have described the broad goals of working with families in the first episode, including maximizing the adaptive functioning of the family; minimizing disruption to family life and the risk of long-term grief, stress and burden; and reducing negative outcomes for the patient.

Stage models of family interventions

The most comprehensive model of family intervention to date is the recovery stage model described by Addington *et al.* (2005), employed in the Toronto First Episode Psychosis Program. Empirical data suggest that treatment according to this model improves psychological well-being and reduces negative experiences of caregiving in caregivers (Addington *et al.*, 2005).

The initial phase of this intervention focuses on managing the experience of families of the first psychotic episode, normally experienced as a 'crisis' given the generally unfamiliar nature of the experience. Goals of this period of assessment and treatment include engaging with the family and developing a good working relationship, collecting a detailed collateral history and assessment of family and patient needs and practical assistance with managing the crisis. An initial explanatory model of psychosis is offered at this stage, but this is generally not detailed in order to prevent overwhelming the support structure. These goals are facilitated by frequent contact and high support from workers, which may include practical and emotional support to minimize the impact of trauma, repeated and clear messages about psychosis and its treatment and education about the role of the family in treatment. Families may also need to be educated regarding principles of confidentiality at this stage.

Table 17.3. Empirically examined interventions for family members of people with first-episode psychosis

Study	Sample	Intervention	Patient outcome	Family outcome	Caveats
Goldstein et al., 1978	Family members of 104 'acute, young schizophrenics' (number of family members unclear)	Crisis-oriented six-session family therapy; content unclear but with aims to (1) allow patient and family to accept the fact of psychosis, (2) allow them to identify some of the probable precipitating stressors, (3) allow them to generalize from this to identification of possible future precipitants, and (4) permit planning on how to minimize or avoid this	Best outcome in the group receiving both family therapy and 'high-dose' fluphenazine; dependent in part on premorbid functioning	Not assessed	
Zhang et al., 1994	78 male patients with FEP (mean age 24 years)	Family intervention contrasted with 'standard care'; family intervention included 18 months of family therapy (both family groups and individual family therapy sessions) once every 3 months, with an emphasis on psychoeducation, early warning signs, stress management, attributing maladaptive behaviour to illness, communication skills training, and reduction of high EE levels; outreach model where necessary	Hospital readmission rates: family intervention 15%, standard care 54%; family therapy and medication additive in preventing readmission	Not assessed	Standard care involved minimal treatment and unlikely to be comparable to current levels of standard care in first-episode services; 'readmission' a restrictive definition of relapse
Linszen et al., 1996	76 patients (mean age 20 years) with 'early-onset schizophrenic disorders' recently discharged after a 3-month inpatient admission, randomized to behavioural family therapy plus individually oriented patient treatment (n = 37) or individually oriented patient treatment alone (n = 39)	18 family sessions over 12 months of behavioural family therapy (focusing on two sessions of psychoeducation, six sessions of communication skills training and nine sessions of problem-solving skills training) plus individually oriented patient treatment (relapse prevention, psychoeducation and neuroleptic drugs); biweekly for the first 5 months, and monthly thereafter; contrasted with individually oriented treatment alone	The combined condition was associated with slightly higher relapse rates (non-significant difference) among families with low EE by the CFI; no differences in patient relapse rates in the high-EE group After 1 year, this trend was no longer evident; when examining only the non-family intervention group, EE was associated with relapse Overall relapse rates were low (16%)	Not assessed	
Lenior et al., 2001 (5-year follow-up of Linszen et al., 1996)	Subset of 64 patients from Linszen et al. (1996); patients with early schizophrenia, 55% in the first episode; randomized to family intervention or routine care (n = 57 at 5-year follow-up)		Intervention condition had no impact on psychotic episodes or social functioning.	Not assessed	

Table 17.3. (cont.)

Study	Sample	Intervention	Patient outcome	Family outcome	Caveats
Lenior et al. (2002) (8-year follow-up of Linszen et al., 1996)	A subsample of 52 participants from Linszen et al. (1996)		Relapse rates reduced overall during the 12-month treatment period but did not differ between two groups at 5-year follow-up; similarly, no difference between the two groups on patient social functioning; however, total time spent in inpatient care reduced in family intervention group Association between psychotic episode and criticism only, and only at 34 months after discharge	No differential effect of family therapy on CFI EE over follow-up, apart from EOI; there was a delayed increase in EOI in treatment group in comparison with the control group	
Pavuluri et al., 2004	34 patients with early-onset bipolar disorder (mean age 11.33 years; range, 5–17)	Child and family-focused CBT; patient psychoeducation and CBT; carer problem solving, carer affect regulation (e.g. anger-management skills), monitoring of possible precipitants to relapse	Reduction in symptoms of attention deficit hyperactivity disorder, aggression, mania, psychosis, depression, sleep disturbance; improvement in global functioning		Open trial without control group; combined intervention so no ability to separate intervention effects with patient from those with the family; younger age group than most first-episode services
Leavey et al., 2004	106 carers of people with a first episode of psychotic illness in the past 6 months (patient demographics unavailable); 57 randomized to treatment, remainder to control	Brief interactive intervention, with a focus on education and advice about disorder; intervention provided within 6 months of first contact with services, over seven sessions, each one about an hour; delivered individually, usually in carer's home Information provided included details of available services, treatment and likely prognosis; education around early warning signs and ways to seek treatment; attempts to enhance coping strategies, problem-solving and communication styles	No differences between the two groups on number of days spent by patients in hospital at follow-up	No differences between the two groups on relatives' satisfaction at 9-month follow-up; some reduction in strain during active intervention only (i.e. at 4-month follow-up but not 9-month follow-up); global reduction in perception of severity of illness	Limited uptake of intervention; only 42% (24 carers) completed intervention, partially completed by 10 others
Jeppesen et al., 2005; Thorupa et al., 2005	Patients with FEP aged between 18 and 45 years (mean age, 25 years) and their family members randomized to 'integrated	Integrated treatment included a family intervention; Family members were invited to join psychoeducational multifamily groups (as per the McFarlane model) focusing on problem-solving	Integrated treatment produced a significantly larger improvement in both negative and positive symptoms, particularly hallucinations, and relatives'	Those in the integrated treatment group reported less distress related to patients' deficits in social role performance and	Integrated treatment also included patient-focused interventions, such as social skills training with a focus on psychoeducation

Reference	Participants	Intervention	Outcome measure	Results	Comparison group
	treatment group' (n = 185) or standard treatment group (n = 140)	procedures; these initially took the form of individual family meetings without the patient and workshops with formal education for four to six families; Multifamily groups met for 1.5 hours bimonthly for 18 months	perception of patients' social role performance	distress related to adverse effects of patients' illness; however, no differences between the groups regarding distress from patients' disturbed behaviour, knowledge about schizophrenia or FMSS EE; carers in the integrated treatment group were more satisfied with treatment	(particularly regarding comorbid substance use), so it is unclear which component of the integrated treatment was most powerful with respect to outcome; only 127 (68.6%) of relatives in the integrated treatment group availed themselves of one or more sessions of family therapy in first year; 94 (50.8%) began multifamily group therapy, and 79 (42.7%) engaged in six or more multifamily group sessions
Addington et al., 2005	185 family members of people (mean age 23 years) experiencing a first episode of psychosis	Recovery model based on stage of recovery of individuals who have experienced FEP (see text for description)		Significant improvement in psychological well-being and negative experiences of caregiving over 3-year follow-up; those with moderate levels of distress improved in first year; those with more severe levels of distress improved in second year	No comparison group
Miklowitz, Biuckians & Richards, 2006	20 adolescents with bipolar disorder (age range unclear)	Family-focused treatment adapted for adolescents; active intervention over a 10-month period consisted of nine sessions of psychoeducation and support for parents, six sessions of communication and problem solving and maintenance 3-monthly sessions for the following 14 months	Significant improvement in patient depression, total mood, parent-rated problem behaviour overall and externalizing and internalizing behaviour		No comparison group
Stærk Buksti et al., 2006	35 relatives of 26 patients aged between 19 and 35 with FEP	Eight sessions consisting of psychoeducation and 'clarification of questions and group dialogue', with the aim of promoting relatives' feelings of competence, reflection and problem solving	Not assessed	Satisfaction high, and highest with group leader's attitude towards relatives, and social intercourse with other relatives	No comparison group

EE, expressed emotion; EOI, emotional overinvolvement; FMSS, Five Minute Speech Sample; CFI, Camberwell Family Interview; FEP, first-episode psychosis; CBT, cognitive-behavioural therapy.

The second phase of the 'family recovery model' focuses on building on the assessment and engagement that has already begun. A component of this assessment is to identify families who remain at high risk for morbidity and those with sustained patterns of interaction likely to interfere with patient outcome. A greater emphasis is made at this stage on increasing the family's knowledge of psychosis and enhancing their coping strategies in response to this. Further information is also provided about the recovery process for patients and the early warning signs for relapse. Mechanisms to reach these goals include support and education programmes (which may be individually delivered or delivered in a group format in a 'family coping group'), identifying problem-solving and coping strategies for dealing with psychosis and more intensive work for those families at higher risk.

The third phase 'consolidates the gains' by encouraging the incorporation of previous knowledge into daily practice. Families are also asked to encourage the patient in their own recovery process, as well as to monitor the patient and manage relapse risk. There is also a focus on attributional work, by readjusting family expectations. Carers are also encouraged at this stage to maintain psychological well-being by incorporating their own supports where possible. Intervention mechanisms at this stage include 'booster sessions', identifying early warning signs in patients, treatment adherence issues and specific problem solving. Broader issues are canvassed at this stage, when family resilience may be re-emerging, such as issues around individuation and independence of adolescents from the family system, and how to manage this when families feel most anxious and protective.

The final phase of 'prolonged recovery' focuses on discharge of the patient and family into primary care services, or into programmes of longer-term care. Particularly in the latter, work may need to focus on changing expectations and developing a consensus around reasonable longer-term prognosis and adaptation to a less than full recovery. While issues of grief and loss likely emerge before this period, it is at this stage that they are likely to be most salient.

A similar stage approach is used at the Early Psychosis Prevention and Intervention Centre (EPPIC) in Melbourne. The initial stage of 'before detection: perceptions and explanations' focuses explicitly on the UHR group; for example, it is possible that attributions formed during this stage about illness behaviours are difficult to shift, particularly given their non-specificity. At this stage then, the primary focus is on access to information about early warning signs and accessible assessment services for early detection. The second stage, 'after detection: grief and loss', is similar to that of the Addington *et al.* (2005) phase of managing crisis. Gleeson *et al.* (1999) have described an additional focus on the need for families to be given space and an opportunity to ventilate and express their concerns. The third stage, 'toward recovery: coping, competence and adaptive functioning', concentrates on maximizing the resources that families may already have (such as a disposition of optimism and a wide range of supports, as well as symptom improvement in the patient) and provides practical and intensive emotional support to develop these qualities as far as possible in those without them, to prevent more chronic depressive and stress-related disorders. The final stage, 'first relapse and prolonged recovery', similar to the final stage in the Addington model, focuses on the impact on family's explanatory models in the case of relapse or 'insufficient' recovery, with associated beliefs on the family's part around long-term burden and loss of expectations for the child. This suggests the need for access to ongoing support and education.

Key components and guidelines for family services in first episode

A number of authors have published widely on this issue of family services in the first episode (see Addington & Burnett, 2004; EPPIC and the Victorian Department of Human Services, 1997; Gleeson *et al.*, 1999; Wright *et al.*, 2004). The key recommendations from these resources regarding services that should be available to families of young people with FEP are summarized below. The reader is referred to these references for more detailed information. It is clear, however, that the respective importance of each of these types of intervention will remain unsettled until

Box 17.1. General principles for working with families with a member with early psychosis

Recognize the phase nature of the patient's illness, and that family work needs to be adaptable and flexible in approach

Recognize that families will have a range of different feelings, worries and questions

Recognize that families need time and an opportunity to deal with the crisis and ensuing stressors

Recognize that the explanations that families have for what has happened to them need to be heard and understood

Recognize that families need a framework for understanding

Recognize that families also need a recovery time and may go through particular stages

Recognize that the family work may change over time, ranging from a maintenance role to dealing with longer-term, ongoing issues

Recognize that family work is a preventive intervention aimed at addressing levels of distress, burden, coping, social functioning and general health for all family members.

Taken with permission from Gleeson *et al.* (1999).

Box 17.2. Family-based treatment aims where a young person in the family has psychosis

Provide a supportive and controlled environment to allow issues surrounding the illness to be discussed sensitively

Support the family in the containment of anxiety

Provide the family with appropriate information about the illness

Help to avoid maladaptive attributions and foster adaptive attributions

Promote healthy family coping

Facilitate service/family alliances

Prevent or reduce relapses

Taken with permission from Wright *et al.* (2004).

studies are conducted evaluating the degree to which each impacts on family and/or patient experience. Boxes 17.1 and 17.2 provide two specific summaries of general principles and treatment aims for working with families where a young person has psychosis.

Supportive interventions

Underpinning the provision of any supportive intervention is the importance of regarding the family as an ally in treatment, and of assuming limited pathology and recognizing that interventions are generally designed to promote preexisting skills rather than to address dysfunction. Shared problem definition, shared decision making and shared responsibility in a collaborative approach are clearly important. Supportive interventions may primarily involve allowing families to discuss in an unstructured way their experiences and misgivings in obtaining psychiatric assistance, including issues such as stigma. They may also be more practical, for example by assisting families to access services in a timely manner, or providing patient transport when families are unable to. Further supportive interventions encourage families to access their own existing support networks, with a focus on the imperative for families to address their own needs in addition to those of the patient. Support may also be useful in allowing exploration of issues of grief and loss, which may be particularly problematic for families of people with a long prodrome or duration of untreated psychosis. Such support may be provided by clinicians and/or by peer-to-peer support workers or carer consultants where appropriate (Dixon *et al.*, 2004). Particular families may require more support than others; the experience of caring for someone with comorbid psychosis and substance use, for example, is likely to be particularly difficult and may require greater levels of support (Dixon, McNary & Lehman, 1995). Other interventions may not be useful prior to the provision of support, given that symptoms of grief and acute stress may prevent families from processing new information about the illness and its treatment.

A particular issue endemic to all services, not just those with a focus on the first episode, is that of patient consent to the provision of services to families. At EPPIC, the general approach is that family-support services are offered to all family members who know that the patient is unwell and are linked in with the service, although the type of service offered may differ when patients refuse family involvement in care. In this instance, families may be offered support from carer consultants, while clinicians may in the immediate term focus on engagement with the patient as, *inter alia*, a means to explore possible reasons for ambivalence regarding family involvement.

Psychoeducation

Psychoeducation is a key component of all interventions and is likely to be required over a significant period of time in order to maximize the likelihood for it to be absorbed and retained. This is somewhat complicated in FEP, given diagnostic heterogeneity and uncertainty in this group. However, families are likely to require information with respect to a range of factors generally assumed by clinicians. These include an understanding of presenting problems as representing an 'illness' emerging within a diathesis–stress model (this may, in turn, assist in assuaging family guilt to some degree, which may then reduce high EE (Bentsen *et al.*, 1998)). The episodic nature of the illness will probably need to be emphasized, with a concomitant focus on management and recovery rather than cure. Current evidence regarding effective treatment should also be communicated, including medication and/or psychological therapies where appropriate. The construct of relapse should also be introduced, although this may at times be difficult given the resistance of some families after initial recovery to the notion that patient symptoms may recur – a parallel to the patient 'sealing over' process (Tait, Birchwood & Trower, 2004). Further psychoeducation regarding general as well as individualized early warning signs may be useful once the possibility of relapse is recognized. Finally, psychoeducation regarding the developmental tasks of adolescence – of separation, individuation and striving for autonomy – may be usefully overted, with discussion around how this may conflict with parental concern and supervision. Again, psychoeducation may be provided by clinicians to individual families or within a multiple family group. Clinicians at EPPIC facilitate 'family and friends' sessions, which are a block of four 2-hour sessions that are delivered weekly and focus on the nature of psychosis, medication, recovery (especially the phase model of

psychosis) and the future (especially on maintaining recovery and managing relapse).

Attributions

Psychoeducation work may detect particular attributions that families hold about a range of salient factors, such as the illness and the patient. Those who have limited experience of psychotic disorders, apart from what they learn from the mainstream media and/or a family history of someone with a chronic course of schizophrenia, are likely to have pessimistic attributional styles regarding the prospect of recovery. Provision of information regarding the generally positive prognosis for those with FEP (e.g. only 10% of EPPIC patients going on to experience severe, treatment-resistant psychosis) may be useful at this time. Further, 'blaming' attributions about aetiology – whether family or patient focused – are likely to emerge during psychoeducation and impair patient and family recovery, particularly given links with EE (reviewed by Barrowclough & Hooley, 2003). An illness model of psychosis, particularly negative symptoms (which may be more likely to be seen as under volitional control (Barrowclough & Hooley, 2003)), may need to be repeatedly emphasized.

Coping strategies

Anecdotally, the key unmet need of families of young people with FEP is information and coping strategies for situations in which the patient is symptomatic (M. Leggatt, September 2005, personal communication). In the face of criticism or sensitivity from an unwell relative, families may also be concerned that they need to develop an entirely new interactional style with the patient for fear of exacerbating symptomatology, and thereby 'walk on eggshells'. This, in turn, is likely to inhibit clear and open communication within the family and may result in systemic resentment that at times flares into anger. Families may need to be encouraged to develop less-heated ways to discuss potentially sensitive topics, as well as maintaining healthy everyday family functioning. It is also likely that at least some of the coping strategies that the family is currently using are effective and useful; reassuring families of this is also indicated (Wright *et al.*, 2004).

Issues of implementation of family interventions into routine clinical practice

Despite the demonstrated efficacy of family interventions, at least in chronic mental illness (Pharoah *et al.*, 2003), few families actually receive these services. Lehman *et al.* (1998) reported that less than 10% of families of outpatients with schizophrenia receive services, and Dixon *et al.* (2001) noted that the use of interventions in routine clinical practice is 'alarmingly limited'. Reasons for this are likely to include time pressure on clinicians, limited funding both to train clinicians in conducting family interventions and actually to conduct them, and limited availability of supervision and support from management and colleagues (Fadden, 1997; Smith & Velleman, 2002). The few services in which work with family and carers has been delivered within this context appear to have made significant financial and organizational investments in all of these areas (e.g. Kelly & Newstead, 2004; Sin *et al.*, 2003).

Additionally, appropriate interventions must be flexible, allowing families to have their particular needs met at any one time (Fadden, 1998). No broad-based intervention is likely to meet the needs of all families, and as such, a 'stepped care' model may be appropriate, where 'high-risk' or 'high-need' families are identified once a basic intervention has been provided. These families could then be offered a more comprehensive treatment package through specialist family services.

Conclusions

A review of the literature suggests that the empirical basis for EE-focused family intervention in early psychosis is unsettled, given the inconsistency of EE-outcome findings in this population. Such a focus in the UHR group is more questionable, given that the limited data to date suggest that some components of EE may be associated with better, rather than worse, prognosis. However, distress, negative experiences of caregiving and grief are features of caregiving in early psychosis, perhaps to similar degrees as in more chronic contexts. Components of interventions that may help to ameliorate these experiences include providing both emotional and practical support, psychoeducation and coaching in specific coping strategies for managing and assisting an unwell relative. Stage-based interventions provide assistance that is appropriately tailored to the family's experience. However, the effective delivery of these interventions relies on key support from mental health services broadly.

Future directions

Future research should initially clarify the needs and experiences of families; for example, just what do families find helpful in caring for a young person with FEP or at UHR? Do FEP families experience different 'stages' in the recovery process that parallel the patient's recovery? Are the experiences of families affected by the provision of psychoeducation and support early in the course of illness? What components of family interventions developed to date are related to positive outcomes for families? It is also clear that the impact of family dynamics on patient prognosis is not well understood in the first episode; further clarification of these issues would be timely. Additionally, there is a dearth of research exploring a family's experiences of caregiving and distress; this should be addressed. The experience of siblings of young people with FEP is yet to be explored in any detail empirically. Further exploration should also be undertaken of predictors of protective and risk factors for prolonged psychiatric morbidity in families, in order to develop 'stepped care' models that accurately identify 'high-risk' or 'high-need' families, who could then be offered more comprehensive treatment packages through specialist family services. Novel interventions (e.g. delivered via the Internet, by telephone or by trained non-clinicians) that can be easily absorbed into, and sustained within, mental health services could also be developed (e.g. Vale, Jelinek & Best, 2005).

Regardless of these, however, the comments made in Gleeson *et al.* (1999, p. 401) continue to apply almost a decade later.

There is sufficient information available from clinical practice and research to suggest guidelines for family work in early psychosis. Families need to be provided with clear and accurate information about psychosis. They need reassurance about the excellent prospects for recovery from the first episode, tempered with appropriate realism about the risks of relapse. They need an opportunity to express their own feelings about their relative's illness and opportunities to ask questions. They need support to work through any anxiety, grief or despair. Finally, they need information about the kind of emotional environment which facilitates recovery, and sometimes they need specific help in working towards such an environment.

REFERENCES

Adams, K. B. & Sanders, S. (2004). Alzheimer's caregiver differences in experience of loss, grief reactions and depressive symptoms across stage of disease: a mixed-method analysis. *Dementia: International Journal of Social Research and Practice*, **3**, 195–210.

Addington, J. & Burnett, P. (2004). Working with families in the early stages of psychosis. In J. F. M. Gleeson & P. D. McGorry (eds.), *Psychological Interventions for Early Psychosis*. Chichester, UK: John Wiley, pp. 99–116.

Addington, J., Coldham, E. L., Jones, B., Ko, T. & Addington, D. (2003). The first episode of psychosis: the experience of relatives. *Acta Psychiatrica Scandinavica*, **108**, 285–9.

Addington, J., Collins, A., McCleery, A. & Addington, D. (2005). The role of family work in early psychosis. *Schizophrenia Research*, **79**, 77–83.

Bachmann, S., Bottmer, C., Jacob, S. *et al.* (2002). Expressed emotion in relatives of first-episode and chronic patients with schizophrenia and major depressive disorder: a comparison. *Psychiatry Research*, **112**, 239–50.

Ball, R. A., Moore, E. & Kuipers, L. (1992). Expressed emotion in community care staff: a comparison of patient outcome in a nine month follow-up of two hostels. *Social Psychiatry and Psychiatric Epidemiology*, **27**, 35–9.

Barrelet, L., Ferrero, F., Szigethy, L., Giddey, C. & Pellizzer, G. (1990). Expressed emotion and first-admission schizophrenia: nine-month follow-up in a French cultural environment. *British Journal of Psychiatry*, **156**, 357–62.

Barrowclough, C. & Hooley, J. M. (2003). Attributions and expressed emotion: a review. *Clinical Psychology Review*, **23**, 849–80.

Barrowclough, C., Haddock, G., Lowens, I. *et al.* (2001). Staff expressed emotion and causal attributions for client problems on a low security unit: an exploratory study. *Schizophrenia Bulletin*, **27**, 517–26.

Bateson, G., Jackson, D. D., Haley, J. & Weakland, J. (1956). Toward a theory of schizophrenia. *Behavioral Science*, **1**, 251–64.

Bebbington, P. & Kuipers, L. (1994). The predictive utility of expressed emotion in schizophrenia: an aggregate analysis. *Psychological Medicine*, **24**, 707–18.

Bech, P. (1993). *Rating Scales for Psychopathology, Health Status and Quality of Life*. New York: Springer-Verlag.

Becker, T., Albert, M., Angermeyer, M. C. & Thornicroft, G. (1997). Social networks and service utilisation in patients with severe mental illness. *Epidemiologia e Psichiatria Sociale*, **6**, 113–25.

Bentsen, H., Boye, B., Munkvold, O. G. *et al.* (1996). Emotional overinvolvement in parents of patients with schizophrenia or related psychosis: demographic and clinical predictors. *British Journal of Psychiatry*, **169**, 622–30.

Bentsen, H., Notland, T. H., Munkvold, O.-G. *et al.* (1998). Guilt proneness and expressed emotion in relatives of patients with schizophrenia or related psychoses. *British Journal of Medical Psychology*, **71**, 125–38.

Bibou-Nakou, I., Dikaiou, M. & Bairactaris, C. (1997). Psychosocial dimensions of family burden among two groups of carers looking after psychiatric patients. *Social Psychiatry and Psychiatric Epidemiology*, **32**, 104–8.

Bland, R. C., Parker, J. H. & Orn, H. (1978). Prognosis in schizophrenia. *Archives of General Psychiatry*, **35**, 72–7.

Breitborde, N. J. K., López, S. R., Wickens, T. D., Jenkins, J. H. & Karno, M. (2007). Toward specifying the nature of the relationship between expressed emotion and schizophrenic relapse: the utility of curvilinear models. *International Journal of Methods in Psychiatric Research*, **16**, 1–10.

Brown, G. W. (1985). The discovery of expressed emotion: induction or deduction? In J. Leff & C. Vaughn (eds.), *Expressed Emotion in Families*. New York: Guilford Press, pp. 7–25.

Brown, G. W., Carstairs, G. M. & Topping, G. G. (1958). Post-hospital adjustment of chronic mental patients. *Lancet*, **ii**, 685–9.

Brown, G. W., Carstairs, G. M. & Topping, G. (1962). Influence of family life on the course of schizophrenic illness. *British Journal of Preventive and Social Medicine*, **16**, 55.

Brown, S. & Birtwistle, J. (1998). People with schizophrenia and their families: fifteen-year outcome. *British Journal of Psychiatry*, **173**, 139–44.

Butzlaff, R. L. & Hooley, J. M. (1998). Expressed emotion and psychiatric relapse. *Archives of General Psychiatry*, **55**, 547–52.

Chambless, D. L. & Steketee, G. (1999). Expressed emotion and behavior therapy outcome: a prospective study with obsessive-compulsive and agoraphobic outpatients. *Journal of Consulting and Clinical Psychology*, **67**, 658–65.

Cohen, J. (1992). A power primer. *Psychological Bulletin*, **112**, 155–9.

Cole, E., Leavey, G., King, M., Johnson-Sabine, E. & Hoar, A. (1995). Pathways to care for patients with a first episode of psychosis: a comparison of ethnic groups. *British Journal of Psychiatry*, **167**, 770–6.

Conus, P. & McGorry, P. D. (2002). First-episode mania: a neglected priority for early intervention. *Australian and New Zealand Journal of Psychiatry*, **36**, 158–72.

Cornwall, P. L. & Scott, J. (1996). Burden of care, psychological distress and satisfaction with services in the relatives of acutely mentally disordered adults. *Social Psychiatry and Psychiatric Epidemiology*, **31**, 345–8.

Coyne, J. C., Wortman, C. B. & Lehman, D. R. (1988). The other side of support: emotional overinvolvement and miscarried helping. In B. H. Gottlieb (eds.), *Marshalling Social Support: Formats, Processes, and Effects*. Thousand Oaks, CA: Sage, pp. 305–30.

de Jesus Mari, J. & Streiner, D. L. (1994). An overview of family interventions and relapse on schizophrenia: meta-analysis of research findings. *Psychological Medicine*, **24**, 565–78.

Dingemans, P. M., Linszen, D. H. & Lenior, M. (2002). Patient psychopathology and parental expressed emotion in schizophrenia revisited. In A. Schaub (eds.), *New Family Interventions and Associated Research in Psychiatric Disorders*. New York: Springer-Verlag, pp. 91–8.

Dixon, L., McNary, S. & Lehman, A. (1995). Substance abuse and family relationships of persons with severe mental illness. *American Journal of Psychiatry*, **152**, 456–8.

Dixon, L., Lucksted, A., Stewart, B. *et al.* (2004). Outcomes of the peer-taught 12-week family-to-family education programme for severe mental illness. *Acta Psychiatrica Scandinavica*, **109**, 207–15.

Dixon, L., McFarlane, W. R., Lefley, H. *et al.* (2001). Evidence-based practices for services to families of people with psychiatric disabilities. *Psychiatric Services*, **52**, 903–10.

Doka, K. J. (1989). *Disenfranchised Grief: Recognizing Hidden Sorrow*. Lexington, MA: Lexington Books.

Dupuy, H. J. (1984). The psychological general well-being (PGWB) index. In N. K. Wenger, M. E. Mattson, C. D. Furberg & J. Elinson (eds.), *Assessment of Quality of Life in Clinical Trials of Cardiovascular Therapies*. New York: Le Jacq, pp. 170–83.

EPPIC and the Victorian Department of Human Services (1997). *Working with Families in Early Psychosis*. Melbourne: Early Psychosis Prevention and Intervention Centre Statewide Services.

Fadden, G. I. (1997). Implementation of family interventions in routine clinical practice following staff training programs: a major cause for concern. *Journal of Mental Health*, **6**, 599–612.

Fadden, G. I. (1998). Family intervention in psychosis. *Journal of Mental Health*, **7**, 115–22.

Fearon, M., Donaldson, C., Burns, A. & Tarrier, N. (1998). Intimacy as a determinant of expressed emotion in carers of people with Alzheimer's disease. *Psychological Medicine*, **28**, 1085–90.

Francis, A. & Papageorgiou, P. (2004). Expressed emotion in Greek versus Anglo-Saxon families of individuals with schizophrenia. *Australian Psychologist*, **39**, 172–7.

Fromm-Reichmann, F. (1950). *Principles of Intensive Psychotherapy*. Chicago, IL: University of Chicago Press.

Garety, P. A., Kuipers, E., Fowler, D., Freeman, D. & Bebbington, P. E. (2001). A cognitive model of the positive symptoms of psychosis. *Psychological Medicine*, **31**, 189–95.

Gibbons, J. S., Horn, S. H., Powell, J. M. & Gibbons, J. L. (1984). Schizophrenic patients and their families: a survey in a psychiatric service based on a DGH unit. *British Journal of Psychiatry*, **144**, 70–7.

Gleeson, J., Jackson, H. J., Stavely, H. & Burnett, P. (1999). Family intervention in early psychosis. In P. D. McGorry & H. J. Jackson (eds.), *The Recognition and Management of Early Psychosis: A Preventive Approach*. New York: Cambridge University Press, pp. 376–406.

Godress, J., Ozgul, S., Owen, C. & Foley-Evans, L. (2004). Grief experiences of parents whose children suffer from mental illness. *Australian and New Zealand Journal of Psychiatry*, **39**, 88–94.

Goldberg, D. P. & Blackwell, P. (1988). *A User's Guide to the General Health Questionnaire*. Windsor, UK: NFER-Nelson.

Goldstein, M. J., Rodnick, E. H., Evans, J. R., May, P. R. & Steinberg, M. R. (1978). Drug and family therapy in the aftercare of acute schizophrenics. *Archives of General Psychiatry*, **35**, 1169–77.

Hahlweg, K., Goldstein, M. J., Nuechterlein, K. H. *et al.* (1989). Expressed emotion and patient–relative interaction in families of recent onset schizophrenics. *Journal of Consulting and Clinical Psychology*, **57**, 11–18.

Haley, J. (1980). *Leaving Home: The Therapy of Disturbed Young People*. New York: McGraw-Hill.

Hardy, A., Fowler, D., Freeman, D. *et al.* (2005). Trauma and hallucinatory experience in psychosis. *Journal of Nervous and Mental Disease*, **193**, 501–7.

Harvey, K., Burns, T., Sedgwick, P. *et al.* (2001a). Relatives of patients with severe psychotic disorders: factors that influence contact frequency. *British Journal of Psychiatry*, **178**, 248–54.

Harvey, K., Burns, T., Fahy, T., Manley, C. & Tattan, T. (2001b). Relatives of patients with severe psychotic illness: factors that influence appraisal of caregiving and psychological distress. *Social Psychiatry and Psychiatric Epidemiology*, **36**, 456–61.

Heikkilä, J., Karlsson, H., Taiminen, T. *et al.* (2002). Expressed emotion is not associated with disorder severity in first-episode mental disorder. *Psychiatry Research*, **111**, 155–65.

Heresco-Levy, U., Greenberg, D. & Dasberg, H. (1990). Family expressed emotion: concepts, dilemmas and the Israeli perspective. *Israel Journal of Psychiatry and Related Sciences*, **27**, 205–15.

Hinrichsen, G. A. & Pollack, S. (1997). Expressed emotion and the course of late-life depression. *Journal of Abnormal Psychology*, **106**, 336–40.

Hooley, J. M. (1986). Expressed emotion and depression: interactions between patients and high- versus low-expressed-emotion spouses. *Journal of Abnormal Psychology*, **95**, 237–46.

Hooley, J. M. & Hiller, J. B. (1998). Expressed emotion and the pathogenesis of relapse in schizophrenia. In M. F. Lenzenweger & R. H. Dworkin (eds.), *Origins and Development of Schizophrenia: Advances in Experimental Psychopathology*. Washington, DC: American Psychological Press, pp. 447–68.

Huguelet, P., Favre, S., Binyet, S., Gonzalez, C. & Zabala, I. (1995). The use of the Expressed Emotion Index as a predictor of outcome in first admitted schizophrenic patients in a French speaking area of Switzerland. *Acta Psychiatrica Scandinavica*, **92**, 447–52.

Jarbin, H. K., Gråwe, R. W. & Hansson, K. (2000). Expressed emotion and prediction of relapse in adolescents with psychotic disorders. *Nordic Journal of Psychiatry*, **54**, 201–5.

Jeppesen, P., Petersen, L., Thorup, A. *et al.* (2005). Integrated treatment of first-episode psychosis: effect of treatment on family burden – OPUS trial. *British Journal of Psychiatry Special Issue: Early psychosis: A Bridge to the Future*, **187**, s85–9.

Joyce, J., Leese, M., Kuipers, E., Szmukler, G., Harris, T. & Staples, E. (2003). Evaluating a model of caregiving for people with psychosis. *Social Psychiatry and Psychiatric Epidemiology*, **38**, 189–95.

Judge, A. M., Perkins, D. O., Nieri, J. & Penn, D. L. (2005). Pathways to care in first episode psychosis: a pilot study on help-seeking precipitants and barriers to care. *Journal of Mental Health*, **14**, 465–9.

Jungbauer, J. & Angermeyer, M. C. (2002). Living with a schizophrenic patient: a comparative study of burden as it affects parents and spouses. *Psychiatry: Interpersonal and Biological Processes*, **65**, 110–23.

Karno, M. & Jenkins, J. H. (1993). Cross-cultural issues in the course and treatment of schizophrenia. *Psychiatric Clinics of North America*, **16**, 339–50.

Kavanagh, D. J. (1992). Recent developments in expressed emotion and schizophrenia. *British Journal of Psychiatry*, **160**, 601–20.

Kelly, M. & Newstead, L. (1996). Family intervention in routine practice: It is possible! *Journal of Psychiatric and Mental Health Nursing*, **11**, 64–72.

Kershner, J. G., Cohen, N. J. & Coyne, J. C. (1996). Expressed emotion in families of clinically referred and nonreferred children: toward a further understanding of the expressed emotion index. *Journal of Family Psychology*, **10**, 97–106.

King, S. & Dixon, M. J. (1999). Expressed emotion and relapse in young schizophrenia outpatients. *Schizophrenia Bulletin*, **25**, 377–86.

Kuipers, E. (2006). Family interventions in schizophrenia: evidence for efficacy and proposed mechanisms of change. *Journal of Family Therapy*, **28**, 73–80.

Kuipers, E., Bebbington, P., Dunn, G. *et al.* (2006). Influence of carer expressed emotion and affect on relapse in non-affective psychosis. *British Journal of Psychiatry*, **188**, 173–9.

Lataster, T., van Os, J., Drukker, M. *et al.* (2006). Childhood victimisation and developmental expression of non-clinical delusional ideation and hallucinatory experiences: victimisation and non-clinical psychotic experiences. *Social Psychiatry and Psychiatric Epidemiology*, **41**, 423–8.

Lazarus, R. S. & Folkman, S. (1984). *Stress, Appraisal, and Coping*. New York: Springer.

Leavey, G., Gulamhussein, S., Papadopoulos, C. *et al.* (2004). A randomized controlled trial of a brief intervention for families of patients with a first episode of psychosis. *Psychological Medicine*, **34**, 423–31.

Leff, J. & Vaughn, C. (1985). *Expressed Emotion in Families: Its Significance for Mental Illness*. New York: Guilford Press.

Leff, J. P. & Brown, G. W. (1977). Family and social factors in the course of schizophrenia. [Letter] *British Journal of Psychiatry*, **130**, 417–20.

Lehman, A. F., Steinwachs, D. M., Dixon, L. B. *et al.* (1998). Translating research into practice: the Schizophrenia Patient Outcomes Research Team (PORT) treatment recommendations. *Schizophrenia Bulletin*, **24**, 1–10.

Lenior, M. E., Dingemans, P. M. A. J., Linszen, D. H., de Haan, L. & Schene, A. H. (2001). Social functioning and the course of early-onset schizophrenia: five-year follow-up of a psychosocial intervention. *British Journal of Psychiatry*, **179**, 53–8.

Lenior, M. E., Dingemans, P. M. A. J., Schene, A. H., Hart, A. A. M. & Linszen, D. H. (2002). The course of parental expressed emotion and psychotic episodes after family intervention in recent-onset schizophrenia. A longitudinal study. *Schizophrenia Research*, **57**, 183–90.

Lidz, T. (1973). *The Origin and Treatment of Schizophrenia*. New York: Basic.

Lidz, T., Cornelison, A. R., Fleck, S. & Terry, D. (1957). The intrafamilial environment of schizophrenic patients: II. Marital schism and marital skew. *American Journal of Psychiatry*, **114**, 241–8.

Linszen, D. H., Dingemans, P., van der Does, J. W. *et al.* (1996). Treatment, expressed emotion and relapse in recent onset schizophrenic disorders. *Psychological Medicine*, **26**, 333–42.

Lowyck, B., de Hert, M., Peeters, E., Gilis, P. & Peuskens, J. (2001). Can we identify the factors influencing the burden on family members of patients with schizophrenia? *International Journal of Psychiatry in Clinical Practice*, **5**, 89–96.

MacMillan, J. F., Gold, A., Crow, T. J., Johnson, A. L. & Johnstone, E. C. (1986). The Northwick Park Study of first episodes of schizophrenia: IV. Expressed emotion and relapse. *British Journal of Psychiatry*, **148**, 133–43.

MacMillan, J. F., Crow, T. J., Johnson, A. L. & Johnstone, E. C. (1987). Expressed emotion and relapse in first episodes of schizophrenia. *British Journal of Psychiatry*, **151**, 320–3.

Magaña, A. B., Goldstein, M. J., Karno, M. *et al.* (1986). A brief method for assessing expressed emotion in relatives of psychiatric patients. *Psychiatry Research*, **17**, 203–12.

Martens, L. & Addington, J. (2001). The psychological well-being of family members of individuals with schizophrenia. *Social Psychiatry and Psychiatric Epidemiology*, **36**, 128–33.

McCarty, C. A., Lau, A. S., Valeri, S. M. & Weisz, J. R. (2004). Parent–child interactions in relation to critical and emotionally overinvolved expressed emotion (EE): is EE a proxy for behavior? *Journal of Abnormal Child Psychology*, **32**, 83–93.

McCreadie, R. G. (2001). Effects of schizophrenia on patients' relatives. *British Journal of Psychiatry*, **178**, 575.

McElroy, E. M. (1987). The beat of a different drummer. In A. B. Hatfield & H. P. Lefley (eds.), *Families of the Mentally Ill: Coping and Adaptation*. New York: Guilford Press, pp. 225–43.

Miklowitz, D. J. & Stackman, D. (1992). Communication deviance in families of schizophrenic and other psychiatric patients: current state of the construct. *Progress in Experimental Personality and Psychopathology Research*, **15**, 1–46.

Miklowitz, D. J., Goldstein, M. J., Nuechterlein, K. H., Snyder, K. S. & Mintz, J. (1988). Family factors and the course of bipolar affective disorder. *Archives of General Psychiatry*, **45**, 225–31.

Miklowitz, D. J., Goldstein, M. J., Doane, J. A. *et al.* (1989). Is expressed emotion an index of a transactional process? I. Parents' affective style. *Family Process*, **28**, 153–67.

Miklowitz, D. J., Biuckians, A. & Richards, J. A. (2006). Early-onset bipolar disorder: a family treatment perspective. *Development and Psychopathology Special Issue: Developmental Approaches to Bipolar Disorder*, **18**, 1247–65.

Mintz, J., Mintz, L. & Goldstein, M. (1987). Expressed emotion and relapse in first episodes of schizophrenia: a rejoinder to Macmillan *et al.* (1986). *British Journal of Psychiatry*, **151**, 314–20.

Mohr, W. K. & Regan-Kubinski, M. J. (2001). Living in the fallout: parents' experiences when their child becomes mentally ill. *Archives of Psychiatric Nursing*, **15**, 69–77.

Möller-Leimkühler, A. M. (2006). Multivariate prediction of relatives' stress outcome one year after first hospitalization of schizophrenic and depressed patients. *European Archives of Psychiatry and Clinical Neuroscience*, **256**, 122–30.

Morrison, A. & Petersen, T. (2003). Trauma, metacognition and predisposition to hallucinations in non-patients. *Behavioural and Cognitive Psychotherapy*, **31**, 235–46.

Nomura, H., Inoue, S., Kamimura, N. *et al.* (2005). A cross-cultural study on expressed emotion in carers of people with dementia and schizophrenia: Japan and England. *Social Psychiatry and Psychiatric Epidemiology*, **40**, 564–70.

Norton, J. P. (1982). Expressed emotion, affective style, voice tone and communication deviance as predictors of offspring schizophrenia-spectrum disorders. Ph.D. thesis, University of California at Los Angeles.

Nuechterlein, K. H. & Dawson, M. E. (1984). A heuristic vulnerability/stress model of schizophrenic episodes. *Schizophrenia Bulletin*, **10**, 300–12.

Nuechterlein, K. H., Snyder, K. S. & Mintz, J. (1992). Paths to relapse: possible transactional processes connecting patient illness onset, expressed emotion, and psychotic relapse. *British Journal of Psychiatry*, **161**, 88–96.

Nugter, A., Dingemans, P., van der Does, J. W., Linszen, D. & Gersons, B. (1997). Family treatment, expressed emotion and relapse in recent onset schizophrenia. *Psychiatry Research*, **72**, 23–31.

O'Brien, M. P., Gordon, J. L., Bearden, C. E. *et al.* (2006). Positive family environment predicts improvement in symptoms and social functioning among adolescents at imminent risk for onset of psychosis. *Schizophrenia Research*, **81**, 269–75.

O'Farrell, T. J., Hooley, J., Fals-Stewart, W. & Cutter, H. S. G. (1998). Expressed emotion and relapse in alcoholic patients. *Journal of Consulting and Clinical Psychology*, **66**, 744–52.

Oliver, N. & Kuipers, E. (1996). Stress and its relationship to expressed emotion in community mental health workers. *International Journal of Social Psychiatry*, **42**, 150–9.

Osborne, J. & Coyle, A. (2002). Can parental responses to adult children with schizophrenia be conceptualized in terms of loss and grief? A case study. *Counselling Psychology Quarterly*, **15**, 307–23.

Östman, M. & Hansson, L. (2004). Appraisal of caregiving, burden and psychological distress in relatives of psychiatric inpatients. *European Psychiatry*, **19**, 402–7.

Ozgul, S. (2004). Parental grief and serious mental illness: a narrative. *Australian and New Zealand Journal of Family Therapy*, **25**, 183–7.

Palazzoli-Selvini, M., Boscolo, L., Cecchin, G. F. & Prata, G. (1978). *Paradox and Counterparadox: A New Model in the Therapy of the Family in Schizophrenic Transaction*. New York: Jason Aronson.

Parker, G. & Hadzi-Pavlovic, D. (1990). Expressed emotion as a predictor of schizophrenic relapse: an analysis of aggregated data. *Psychological Medicine*, **20**, 961–5.

Patterson, P., Birchwood, M. & Cochrane, R. (2000). Preventing the entrenchment of high expressed emotion in first episode psychosis: early developmental attachment pathways. *Australian and New Zealand Journal of Psychiatry*, **34** (Suppl), S191–7.

Patterson, P., Birchwood, M. & Cochrane, R. (2005). Expressed emotion as an adaptation to loss. *British Journal of Psychiatry*, **187**, s59–64.

Pavuluri, M. N., Graczyk, P. A., Henry, D. B. *et al*. (2004). Child- and family-focused cognitive-behavioral therapy for pediatric bipolar disorder: development and preliminary results. *Journal of the American Academy of Child and Adolescent Psychiatry*, **43**, 528–37.

Peris, T. S. & Baker, B. L. (2000). Applications of the expressed emotion construct to young children with externalizing behavior: stability and prediction over time. *Journal of Child Psychology and Psychiatry and Allied Disciplines*, **41**, 457–62.

Perlick, D., Clarkin, J. F., Sirey, J. *et al*. (1999). Burden experienced by caregivers of persons with bipolar affective disorder. *British Journal of Psychiatry*, **175**, 56–62.

Pharoah, F. M., Rathbone, J., Mari, J. J. & Streiner, D. L. (2003). Family intervention for schizophrenia. *Cochrane Database of Systematic Reviews*, **3**, CD000088.

Pourmand, D., Kavanagh, D. J. & Vaughan, K. (2005). Expressed emotion as predictor of relapse in patients with comorbid psychoses and substance use disorder. *Australian and New Zealand Journal of Psychiatry*, **39**, 473–8.

Provencher, H. L., Perreault, M., St-Onge, M. & Rousseau, M. (2003). Predictors of psychological distress in family caregivers of persons with psychiatric disabilities. *Journal of Psychiatric and Mental Health Nursing*, **10**, 592–607.

Rolland, J. S. (1994). *Families, Illness, and Disability: An Integrative Treatment Model*. New York: Basic Books.

Rosen, J. N. (1947). The treatment of schizophrenic psychosis by direct analytic therapy. *Psychiatric Quarterly*, **21**, 3–37.

Rund, B. R., Oie, M., Borchegrevink, T. S. & Fjell, A. (1995). Expressed emotion, communication deviance, and schizophrenia: an exploratory study of the relationship between two family variables and the course and outcome of a psychoeducational treatment programme. *Psychopathology*, **28**, 220–8.

Ryan, K. A. (1993). Mothers of adult children with schizophrenia: an ethnographic study. *Schizophrenia Research*, **11**, 21–31.

Saunders, J. C. & Byrne, M. M. (2002). A thematic analysis of families living with schizophrenia. *Archives of Psychiatric Nursing*, **16**, 217–23.

Scazufca, M. & Kuipers, E. (1999). Coping strategies in relatives of people with schizophrenia before and after psychiatric admission. *British Journal of Psychiatry*, **174**, 154–8.

Scottish Schizophrenia Research Group (1987). The Scottish first episode schizophrenia study: IV. Psychiatric and social impact on relatives. *British Journal of Psychiatry*, **150**, 340–4.

Scottish Schizophrenia Research Group (1992). The Scottish first episode schizophrenia study: VIII. Five-year follow-up: clinical and psychosocial findings. *British Journal of Psychiatry*, **161**, 496–500.

Shabad, P. C. (1989). Vicissitudes of psychic loss of a physically present parent. In D. Dietrich & P. C. Shabad (eds.), *The Problem of Loss and Mourning: Psychoanalytic Perspectives*. Madison, CT: International Universities Press, pp. 101–26.

Sin, J., Moone, N. & Wellman, N. (2003). Incorporating psycho-educational family and carers work into routine clinical practice. *Journal of Psychiatric and Mental Health Nursing*, **10**, 730–4.

Singer, M. T. & Wynne, L. C. (1965). Thought disorder and family relations of schizophrenics: IV. Results and implications. *Archives of General Psychiatry*, **12**, 201–12.

Smith, G. & Velleman, R. (2002). Maintaining a Family Work for Psychosis Service by recognizing and addressing the barriers to implementation. *Journal of Mental Health*, **11**, 471–9.

Snyder, K. S., Wallace, C. J., Moe, K. & Liberman, R. P. (1994). Expressed emotion by residential care operators and residents' symptoms and quality of life. *Hospital and Community Psychiatry*, **45**, 1141–3.

Solomon, P. & Draine, J. (1996). Examination of grief among family members of individuals with serious and persistent mental illness. *Psychiatric Quarterly*, **67**, 221–34.

St Onge, M. & Lavoie, F. (1997). The experience of caregiving among mothers of adults suffering from psychotic disorders: factors associated with their psychological distress. *American Journal of Community Psychology*, **25**, 73–94.

Stærk Buksti, A., Munkner, R., Gade, I. *et al.* (2006). Important components of a short-term family group programme. From the Danish National Multicenter Schizophrenia Project. *Nordic Journal of Psychiatry*, **60**, 213–19.

Stirling, J., Tantam, D., Thomas, P. *et al.* (1991). Expressed emotion and early onset schizophrenia: a one year follow-up. *Psychological Medicine*, **21**, 675–85.

Stirling, J., Tantam, D., Thomas, P. *et al.* (1993). Expressed emotion and schizophrenia: the ontogeny of EE during an 18-month follow-up. *Psychological Medicine*, **23**, 771–8.

Szmukler, G., Eisler, I., Russell, G. F. & Dare, C. (1985). Anorexia nervosa, parental 'expressed emotion' and dropping out of treatment. *British Journal of Psychiatry*, **147**, 265–71.

Szmukler, G. I., Burgess, P., Herrman, H. *et al.* (1996). Caring for relatives with serious mental illness: the development of the Experience of Caregiving Inventory. *Social Psychiatry and Psychiatric Epidemiology*, **31**, 137–48.

Tait, L., Birchwood, M. & Trower, P. (2004). Adapting to the challenge of psychosis: personal resilience and the use of sealing-over (avoidant) coping strategies. *British Journal of Psychiatry*, **185**, 410–15.

Tarrier, N., Sommerfield, C. & Pilgrim, H. (1999). Relatives' expressed emotion (EE) and PTSD treatment outcome. *Psychological Medicine*, **29**, 801–11.

Tennakoon, L., Fannon, D., Doku, V. *et al.* (2000). Experience of caregiving: relatives of people experiencing a first episode of psychosis. *British Journal of Psychiatry*, **177**, 529–33.

Terkelsen, K. G. (1987). The evolution of family responses to mental illness through time. In A. B. Hatfield & H. P. Lefley (eds.), *Families of the Mentally Ill: Coping and Adaptation*. New York: Guilford Press, pp. 151–66.

Thorup, A., Petersen, L., Jeppesen, P. *et al.* (2005). Integrated treatment ameliorates negative symptoms in first episode psychosis: results from the Danish OPUS trial. *Schizophrenia Research*, **79**, 95–105.

Tuck, I., du Mont, P., Evans, G. & Shupe, J. (1997). The experience of caring for an adult child with schizophrenia. *Archives of Psychiatric Nursing*, **11**, 118–25.

Vale, M. J., Jelinek, M. V. & Best, J. D. (2005). Impact of coaching patients on coronary risk factors: lessons from the COACH Program. *Disease Management and Health Outcomes*, **13**, 225–44.

van Furth, E. F., van Strien, D. C., Martina, L. M. L. *et al.* (1996). Expressed emotion and the prediction of outcome in adolescent eating disorders. *International Journal of Eating Disorders*, **20**, 19–31.

Vaughn, C., Leff, J. & Sarner, M. (1999). Relatives' expressed emotion and the course of inflammatory bowel disease. *Journal of Psychosomatic Research*, **47**, 461–9.

Wamboldt, F. S., O'Connor, S. L., Wamboldt, M. Z., Gavin, L. A., & Klinnert, M. D. (2000). The Five Minute Speech Sample in children with asthma: deconstructing the construct of expressed emotion. *Journal of Child Psychology and Psychiatry*, **41**, 887–98.

Wasow, M. (1994). A missing group in family research: parents not in contact with their mentally ill children. *Hospital and Community Psychiatry Special Issue: Violent Behaviour and Mental Illness*, **45**, 720–1.

Wearden, A. J., Tarrier, N., Barrowclough, C., Zastowny, T. R. & Rahill, A. A. (2000). A review of expressed emotion research in healthcare. *Clinical Psychology Review*, **20**, 633–66.

Wig, N. N., Menon, D. K., Bedi, H. *et al.* (1987). Expressed emotion and schizophrenia in North India: I. Cross-cultural transfer of ratings of relatives' expressed emotion. *British Journal of Psychiatry*, **151**, 156–60.

Wittmund, B., Wilms, H. U., Mory, C. & Angermeyer, M. C. (2002). Depressive disorders in spouses of mentally ill patients. *Social Psychiatry and Psychiatric Epidemiology*, **37**, 177–82.

Wright, B., Casswell, G., White, D. & Partridge, I. (2004). Family work in adolescent psychosis: the need for more research. *Clinical Child Psychology and Psychiatry*, **9**, 61–74.

Wynne, L. C. & Singer, M. T. (1963). Thought disorder and family relations of schizophrenics: I. A research strategy. *Archives of General Psychiatry*, **9**, 191–8.

Zhang, M., Wang, M., Li, J. & Phillips, M. R. (1994). Randomised-control trial of family intervention for 78 first-episode male schizophrenic patients: an 18-month study in Suzhou, Jiangsu. *British Journal of Psychiatry*, **165**, 96–102.

18

Enhancing work functioning in early psychosis

Eóin Killackey, Henry J. Jackson, David Fowler
and Keith H. Nuechterlein

Introduction

The period since the mid 1980s has seen the development of a new paradigm aimed at early intervention in first-episode psychoses (FEP). Central to this change in approach has been a discarding of the pessimistic neo-Kraepelinian picture of schizophrenia as a biological disease with inevitable decline, which was not borne out by the findings of long-term outcome studies (Rees *et al.*, 1998). Instead, premised on vulnerability-stress models (Nuechterlein *et al.*, 1992; Zubin & Spring, 1977), the importance of early intervention and the delineation of a 'critical period' (Birchwood & Fiorillo, 2000), in which there was potential to limit the extent of disability caused by the psychotic disorder, was emphasized. The change in focus from reactive management of chronic illness to proactive intervention to prevent or limit chronicity and disability led to reforms and changes in approaches of mental health systems to psychosis around the world (Edwards & McGorry, 2002).

The foundation of the early-intervention model led to improvements in the way in which people with psychosis entered care, the earlier administration of medicine and also to an expansion of psychosocial interventions into the area that Bellack (1986) referred to as 'psychology's forgotten child'. Studies of cognitive–behavioural therapy (CBT) targeting positive symptoms showed some efficacy (Birchwood *et al.*, 1994; Jackson *et al.*, 1996, 2005; McPhillips & Sensky, 1998; Wood *et al.*, 2001), as did some forms of family intervention (Falloon *et al.*, 1985), in reducing relapse and hospitalization. However, it may be argued that both psychosocial and pharmacological interventions were preoccupied with reducing symptoms rather than primarily focusing on the rehabilitation of functioning, particularly vocational functioning. Few studies of either psychosocial or pharmacological interventions in FEP have been primarily concerned with non-symptom-based outcomes.

The inclusion of work functioning as part of the rehabilitation of people with mental illness is not new (Häfner, 1996; Iles, 1928; Overall & Porterfield, 1963; Porter, 2002; Shevalev, 1935). One hundred and forty years ago, Thomas Carlyle recognized that 'work is the grand cure for all the maladies and miseries that ever beset mankind' (Carlyle, 1899 (reprint 1969, p. 455)). In developed countries, the proportion of people with serious mental illness who were working has decreased since the middle of the last century (Marwaha & Johnson, 2004), possibly as a result of a decline in the availability of the types of job once dominated by this group. Availability of more jobs at lower skill levels may explain why there are fewer problems with unemployment among people with psychosis in developing economies. It has been noted that people with mental illness were also more employed during periods of high general employment in the past (Warner, 1986). In developed economies, employment rates are currently high. This factor, and increased appreciation of the potential mental health benefits of work, has seen the genesis of a new motivation – both political and clinical – for facilitating the employment of people with mental illness who wish to work (Bell & Lysaker, 1996). In addition, new evidence-based methods of vocational rehabilitation have been developed

The Recognition and Management of Early Psychosis: A Preventive Approach, ed. Henry J. Jackson and Patrick D. McGorry.
Published by Cambridge University Press. © Cambridge University Press 2009.

(Lehman, 1995). While these approaches have been successfully evaluated in chronically unwell populations (Cook *et al.*, 1996), little attention has been paid to those at the outset of their experience with mental illness (Killackey *et al.*, 2006). This early phase of illness would appear to be a largely unexplored window of opportunity to implement vocational interventions.

This chapter considers some of the consequences of unemployment and barriers to employment for those with psychotic illnesses. It then reviews methods that have been used to address unemployment among the mentally ill. It details the window of opportunity potentially provided by combining early intervention in psychosis with vocational rehabilitation. Finally, three different programmes from around the world that are exploring vocational interventions in young people with FEP are outlined.

Barriers to employment

A consideration of employment in FEP also requires an understanding of some of the barriers faced by those seeking employment. A survey by the Australian Bureau of Statistics (2006) of barriers to employment among the general population of Australia found that the single largest barrier reported was a lack of either qualifications or experience. It is known that, controlling statistically for 'course of illness', having more education is associated with a greater likelihood of being employed for people with psychosis and schizophrenia (Waghorn, Chant & Whiteford, 2003). Because of the period of life in which psychosis typically has its onset, secondary and post-secondary education is often disrupted. The vocational disadvantage of not completing or engaging in these educational tasks at a developmentally appropriate stage is likely to compound over time. This is another reason in favour of early vocational intervention in all mental illnesses, but particularly psychosis, as the psychotic illnesses tend to lead to the worst vocational outcomes (Sturm *et al.*, 1999). Further disincentives to work are also reported both in the literature and by those attempting to work. In some states within the USA, people

who have qualified for federal disability programmes face the prospect of losing access to publicly funded healthcare and medication if they take a minimum wage-paying job, because their regular job is considered to be evidence that they are no longer disabled. In Australia, while people do not lose access to healthcare, they do lose entitlements such as concession cards and benefit payments, leading to an increase in costs greater than the gain in income and creating a situation whereby people are essentially penalized for working. It has been noted that a person transitioning from welfare payments to minimum wage work in Australia faces an effective tax rate of 60%. This compares with the highest income tax rate of 42%, which applies to income over AU$125 000 per year.

One of the advantages of intervening very early in the course of a psychotic disorder is that individuals may not yet have begun accessing publicly funded benefits as they are more likely to be still supported by family or working at a regular paid job. Indeed, data from people who attended our service (Early Psychosis Prevention and Intervention Centre (EPPIC)) in 2004 show that 71% of them were not on benefits.

Unemployment and its consequences in psychotic illness

It is difficult to ascertain the level of employment or unemployment in groups of people with psychotic illnesses. There is little description in many of the studies that have examined employment in psychosis as to what kind of work is engaged in, how many hours are worked, how work was attained and how well it is remunerated. As Marwaha and Johnson (2004, p. 338) stated: 'There is no standard method of describing employment in schizophrenia'. Many studies are only interested in reporting employment status as a descriptive demographic variable, and they have frequently made arbitrary categories of employed and unemployed (Skeate *et al.*, 2002; Velakoulis *et al.*, 1999), while some have also added student and other roles such as housewife (Barnes *et al.*, 2000; Bhugra *et al.*, 1997, 2000).

Even allowing for the vagaries of employment statistics, it would appear that rates of employment for people with schizophrenia are low (Baron & Salzer, 2002; Marwaha & Johnson, 2004; McGorry, 2005) compared with the general population (Baron & Salzer, 2002; SANE, 2002). Low employment rates have not improved over the years, as demonstrated in long-term follow-up studies (Kua *et al.*, 2003; Rees *et al.*, 1998) and by looking at cross-sectional data collected over a period of time (Marwaha & Johnson, 2004). In a recent review, studies conducted in the UK prior to the 1990s generally reported rates of employment between 20% and 30% (mean, 28.22%), whereas studies conducted after 1990 reported employment rates of 4–27% (mean, 13.7%) for people with schizophrenia (Marwaha & Johnson, 2004).

Fewer studies have examined the rate of employment among FEP patients, but the range across 11 international studies reported in Marwaha and Johnson's review (2004; in which first episode was defined as either first presentation or having no previous episode) is from 13% to 65%, with an average of 37% employed. This large range may reflect the heterogeneous nature of FEP samples, or it may be related to variations across the nations and cultural and ethnic groups included in the review. Three studies published since Marwaha and Johnson's (2004) review have found unemployment levels of 43% in Canada (Addington, Young & Addington, 2003), 50.2% in Australia (Lambert *et al.*, 2005) and 39% in Singapore (Sim *et al.*, 2004). In all three studies, participants were patients attending specialized early psychosis services. The mean of 37% employment from the earlier studies and the findings from more recent studies accords well with data gathered recently at EPPIC, which shows that 29% of those with FEP were employed, 25% were in school or other training and 39% were unemployed (Killackey *et al.*, 2006). One argument that might be made is that younger people have a higher unemployment rate than the general population anyway. In fact, in Australia, when the current population unemployment level was 5.1% (Australian Bureau of Statistics, 2005), unemployment among 15–19 year olds was 3.8%, with a further 3.9% not in the labour force; among 20–24 year olds, 4.8% were unemployed, with

8.3% not in the labour force (Long, 2005). These figures suggest that for those experiencing FEP, the level of employment is grossly higher than in the comparable general population.

As noted in the review of Marwaha and Johnson (2004), and echoed in a number of other studies (Arduini *et al.*, 2002; Gupta *et al.*, 1997; Ho, Andreasen & Flaum, 1997; Robinson *et al.*, 2004; Scottish Schizophrenia Research Group, 1992), the initial employment rate tends to decline quite quickly over the first year or so after admission. A consequence of the rapid decline of employment of people with FEP is that they then become dependent on other sources of support, which may be public welfare, family or, in many cases, both. Ho and colleagues (1997) followed an Iowa cohort of 48 people with FEP for 5 years. At the outset, only five people were receiving benefit payments. At the end of the study, 30 others had commenced receiving benefits and only two had stopped receiving payments. The median time from admission to beginning to receive payments was 7 months (Ho *et al.*, 1997). The decline in functioning over time in individuals with schizophrenia is evident not only in the level of employment but also in downward social drift. Several studies have demonstrated that the socioeconomic status of individuals with a psychotic illness drifts lower, compared with either their own earlier status or that of their parents (Agerbo *et al.*, 2004; Cuesta *et al.*, 1995; Lay *et al.*, 2000). The majority of people who develop psychosis do so at a time in their lives when they are just beginning to develop vocational interests and directions. Not surprisingly, the experience of psychosis derails this aspect of their development and either leads or contributes significantly to a rapid decrease in their likelihood of employment.

There is no doubt that psychotic illnesses are also economically expensive for the community. Taking schizophrenia as an example, in Australia, with a population of just under 20 million, the total cost of schizophrenia in 2001 was nearly AU$2 billion or 0.3% of gross domestic product (SANE, 2002). For those with schizophrenia, there was a loss of earnings of AU$487.6 million through unemployment and absenteeism, from which there was a loss to the country of AU$165.7 million in forgone income and sales taxes. In

2001, the cost attributed to people caring for their ill family member or friend was AU$88.1 million. This included money paid to carers by the government and revenue lost because these carers were unable to participate in the paid labour force owing to their carer responsibilities. Accommodation assistance cost another AU$16.2 million. Finally, 85% of people with schizophrenia in Australia were receiving a public welfare benefit, which accounted for another AU$274 million. Interestingly, of those on a public welfare benefit, only 11.8% of patients were on a benefit that indicated they were seeking employment. All others were on a disability or illness payment (SANE, 2002). Therefore, the indirect cost to the Australian nation of people with schizophrenia not working was AU $543.7 million in 2001. Successful vocational intervention in the early phase of psychotic illness would not only have very substantial personal benefits for the individual patients but also have the potential to yield large economic gains for society.

Being employed is desirable for individuals with psychotic illness because it leads to gains in several life domains (Gold *et al.*, 2002; O'Flynn, 2001). These include areas directly influenced by being employed, such as receiving payment, making social contact and having an external structure, as well as indirect consequences such as increasing quality of life, reducing hospitalization, increasing the sense of efficacy in management of illness, participating in the community and having a productive and contributing role (Drake *et al.*, 1996). In the case of people with FEP, being either supported in maintaining their current employment or aided in their vocational development has the potential to lead to lasting and important functional gains (Crowther *et al.*, 2001).

Employment interventions

Over the last 100 years, and particularly in the period since the Second World War, different methods of vocational intervention have been developed. The fact that only one of the three methods that belong to the modern era of psychiatry has been developed chiefly by mental health professionals says a lot about the place

of vocational rehabilitation in the priorities of health systems. The interventions that have been developed are industrial therapy, social firms, the clubhouse model (transitional employment (TE), train and place) and supported employment (SE).

Industrial therapy

Industrial or work therapy refers to the wide range of chores and jobs given to residents of the old institutions in the times before de-institutionalization (Baron & Salzer, 2002; Leff, 2001; Ungerleider & Shadowen, 1966). In re-examining these programmes now, it can be seen that these programmes were inadequate in three key ways, although they did provide an occupation and in some cases might have helped teach new skills. First, the skills taught may not have generalized to other employment situations. Second, the tasks may not have been well suited to the occupational interests of the individual. Third, these jobs often did not offer remuneration that would have been equivalent to that earned in a similar job in the community, if indeed any financial remuneration was offered at all.

As part of the de-institutionalization process, it was recognized that formerly institutionalized people living in the community needed to develop working skills in order to reintegrate into the social and economic life of the general community. This led to the development of two different approaches. In Europe, particularly in Italy, the concept of the social firm was developed (O'Flynn, 2001). In the USA, the clubhouse model of vocational rehabilitation expanded (Anonymous, 1999).

Social firms

Social firms are a particular kind of social enterprise (Morrin, Simmonds & Somerville, 2004). They are not-for-profit businesses that are set up to provide a product or service to the public and in doing so create employment for people who may ordinarily be excluded from the labour market owing to illness or disability. The criteria required of social firms include that at least 25% of employees have the illness or disability targeted by that social firm (e.g. mental illness), that at least 50% of the turnover comes from the market activity of the company and that in these positions people are paid at least award or market wages and given real responsibilities and have the potential to progress through the business (O'Flynn, 2001; Social Firms UK, 2005, 2006). While it may also be envisaged that skills learned in a social firm would eventually be used to find competitive employment, this is often not an aim of the people or organization running the business, who are more likely to see themselves as investing in the training of an individual (Baker, 2005) with the target of developing a sustainable business (Social Firms UK, 2005, 2006).

A report on social firms in the UK noted that 83% of social firms operated in the service sector (Baker, 2005). In Italy, with over 5000 social firms, 58% were in the service sector, 29% in the manufacture of handicrafts and the remainder in areas described as building (4%), commercial (6%) and agricultural (3%) (Ducci, Stentella & Vulterini, 2002).

In 2003, it was noted that there had not been any systematic evaluation of social firms (Boardman *et al.*, 2003). To date, this seems not to have been remedied. This is a great pity because the evidence from industry groups suggests that this is a means by which people with mental illness could find work in an environment that is accommodating to the needs of their illness. There also seems to be longevity of employment, with less than 7% of staff leaving in a 1-year period (Baker, 2005).

The downside to social firms is that, as with any business, a social firm requires a substantial amount of time and energy just to establish, let alone run, successfully. Further, any individual social firm may not fit the vocational needs of an individual. Therefore, successful use of social firms involves not the establishment of one or two businesses but the development of an employment sector. Italy has experienced substantial growth in this sector through the Italian government's mandate and support of its development as a means to create employment for those marginalized by their illnesses, disabilities or circumstances (Ducci *et al.*, 2002). However, without research to examine the economic and health benefits of social firms, there is little leverage to encourage other governments, or those who might be described as social venture capitalists, to invest in the development of the social firm sector.

The Clubhouse model

In comparison with both industrial therapy and social firms, there has been more research describing and examining two other interventions, the clubhouse model and supported employment. Clubhouse programmes typically involve prevocational training and transitional employment. Supported employment, by comparison, emphasizes direct job placement and ongoing support and is best defined in the individual placement and support (IPS) model of Becker and Drake (2003).

The Clubhouse model was started by ex-psychiatric patients at Fountain House in New York in 1948 (Macias *et al.*, 1999). At the clubhouse, members contribute to the club by participating in voluntary work necessary to the running of the club (the Work Ordered Day) (Anonymous, 1999). The members are thus contributing to the club and developing skills necessary to succeed in employment, such as punctuality, confidence and responsibility. After this experience, members have access to a set period of employment in a local company. This transitional employment, which is central to the clubhouse model (Bond, 2004), involves an arrangement through which the company offers a number of positions that the job club guarantees to fill. The job club may then use 12 people, working part-time to fill four full-time positions, so that no individual is required to work full-time. In order to be certified by the International Center for Clubhouse Development (ICCD), clubhouses must have access to a wide range of different employment settings. Finally, at the end of this process, obtaining competitive employment is a potential goal for members (Johnsen *et al.*, 2004). While this has been the traditional clubhouse model of employment (and clubhouses are still misrepresented as offering only TE (McKay, Johnsen & Stein, 2005)), more recently clubhouses have viewed the Work Ordered Day and TE as the first two steps of a hierarchy of vocational interventions that continues on to SE and then independent employment (McKay *et al.*,

2005). A worldwide survey of ICCD-certified club-houses in 2000 found that TE provided 36.6% of job placements, SE provided 26.6% and independent employment provided 36.8% (Johnsen *et al.*, 2002; McKay *et al.*, 2005).

Clubhouse studies

Research on the effectiveness of the clubhouse model in achieving desired outcomes is one of the acknowledged neglected areas in its development over most of the last 50 years (Anonymous, 1999; McKay *et al.*, 2005). This led to a number of criticisms of clubhouses (Bilby, 1992; Drake *et al.*, 1999; Macias, 2001; McKay *et al.*, 2005). The lack of randomized controlled trials of TE (Henry *et al.*, 2001) has possibly also affected the way that it has been viewed in widely cited systematic reviews of employment interventions for people with serious mental illness (Crowther & Marshall, 2001, Crowther *et al.*, 2001).

Three studies (Henry *et al.*, 2001; Macias, 2001; McKay *et al.*, 2005) have examined either ICCD club-house outcomes or compared them with other pro-grammes (Table 18.1). One of these studies is now considered in more detail.

Only one study to date has actually compared ICCD-certified clubhouses with another approach (Macias, 2001). This study, conducted in Massachusetts, was one of eight component projects of the Employment Intervention Demonstration Project and was known as MA-EIDP (Cook *et al.*, 2005); it compared the ICCD club-house intervention and the programme of assertive community treatment (PACT). The latter is an intensive mobile treatment team providing clinical and rehabilita-tion services in the community (Macias, 2001; Stein & Test, 1980). In order to maintain fidelity to the PACT and ICCD models, a participant's willingness to work was not an entry criterion. Thus, 30% of the MA-EIDP sample had no declared interest in working at enrolment into the study. The final sample consisted of 175 people (with employment data available for 174); analyses were con-ducted on an intention-to-treat basis. Measurements were carried out at baseline, and at 6, 12, 18 and 24 months. The outcome of competitive employment included TE because, according to criteria determined

by the US Department of Labor, TE meets the definition of 'competitive employment', even though it has not been viewed as competitive employment by all research-ers of vocational interventions (Crowther *et al.*, 2001) owing to the 'set-aside' nature of its jobs.

Macias (2001) found that PACT and ICCD had simi-lar outcomes on a number of measures, including the number of participants who started competitive work, the number of participants interested in work at base-line who started competitive work, job satisfaction and the amount of time from enrolment until commencing work. The ICCD clubhouse performed better than PACT on measures of days worked, money earned, quality of jobs, hourly rate of pay and job tenure. However, PACT performed better than the ICCD club-house on participant retention. One of the limitations of this study is that transitional and other forms of employment cannot be distinguished. While this may reflect a philosophical orientation of those involved with clubhouses, which equates transitional, supported and independent work outcomes, it complicates com-parison of the two interventions. For example, while the two programmes did not differ significantly in competi-tive employment outcome as Macias (2001) defined it, it would be helpful to know if differences were present if TE was omitted from competitive employment, given that other researchers view TE as non-competitive. Inclusion of cost data, which showed that vocational and total direct costs of the ICCD clubhouse model were less than PACT, was very useful, although tests of the significance of the difference were not reported. It seems likely that costs of PACT are higher because of the assertive outreach nature of this model. Given that employment programmes for the mentally ill are often placed precariously between health and employment systems, the collection and analysis of economic data would be a helpful component of all investigations into the efficacy and effectiveness of these interventions.

Although the benefits of clubhouses extend far beyond their role in employment rehabilitation, they, like social firms, are not easy to establish. Clubhouse budgets in America averaged just over US$400 000 in 1996 (Macias *et al.*, 1999). Apart from cost, one of the other factors that mitigate against clubhouses being established by and for young people with FEP is that

Table 18.1. Clubhouse studies

Study	Period	Interventions	No.	Outcomes	Results
Henry *et al.*, 2001	1988–1994	TE	138	Predictors of TE tenure	Days worked per week: $\beta = 34.07$
					Length of clubhouse membership: $\beta = 66.26$
					Age: $\beta = 2.77$
				Competitive employment	Total hours worked in TE jobs: OR = 2.025
Macias, 2001	1995–2001	CH ($n = 89$) VS. PACT ($n = 86$)	175	Retention (at 24 months)	PACT, 81%; CH, 60%; $p < 0.01$
				Competitive employment	PACT, 64%; CH, 59%; $p =$ ns
				Time to employment (days)	PACT, 242; CH, 212; $p =$ ns
				Duration of employment (days)	PACT, 173; CH, 257; $p < 0.01$
				Total earnings ($)	PACT, 3792; CH, 6052; $p =$ ns
				Hourly earnings ($)	PACT, 6.25; CH, 7.31; $p < 0.01$
				Tenure of position (days)	PACT, 80; CH, 148; $p < 0.01$
		CH TE ($n = 21$) VS. CH non-TE ($n = 54$) VS. PACT ($n = 106$)	181	Job Characteristics	
				Wage per hour ($)	CH TE, 6.88; CH non-TE, 7.48; PACT, 6.24
				Weekly job hours	CH TE, 12.3; CH non-TE, 20.8; PACT, 20.8
				Weeks worked	CH TE, 19.1; CH non-TE, 22.3; PACT, 11.8
				Total hours worked	CH TE, 283; CH non-TE, 491; PACT, 264
				Total earnings ($)	CH TE, 2012; CH non-TE, 4037; PACT, 1754
McKay *et al.*, 2005[a]	1998–2001	CH-based TE, SE and IE	1702	Time to job (days)	IE, 204; TE, 198; SE, 163
				Days employed	IE, 361; TE, 146; SE, 301
				Job earnings ($)	IE, 16 169; TE, 2 130; SE, 9 787
				Hourly earnings ($)	IE, 7.59; TE, 6.34; SE, 6.91
				Days per week	IE, 3.88; TE, 3.7; SE, 3.9
				Hours per week	IE, 21.1; TE, 13.9; SE, 18.3

CH, clubhouse; TE, transitional employment; SE, supported employment; IE, independent employment; OR, odds ratio; PACT, Programme of Assertive Community Treatment.

[a] While McKay *et al.* (2005) presented results as being different, they do not distinguish which of the three groups differ from each other.

clubhouses are the result of communities forming around a common issue. Typically, young people with FEP are still coming to terms with their psychotic experiences and have not developed an identity based around their illness, nor have they necessarily developed the networks or skills required to establish an undertaking like a clubhouse. To establish a clubhouse for young people with FEP would likely involve such significant input from non-consumers that those with FEP might feel little ownership of the project, which would contravene the philosophy central to the clubhouse model.

Individual placement and support

Supported employment is an approach to vocational intervention that is differentiated from prevocational training models by its focus on rapid job search and placement and by continued support following the acquisition of a competitive position (Cook *et al.*, 2005). Supported employment is most specifically defined in the IPS model, which has been developed for people with severe mental illness since the mid 1990s.

The IPS model has seven defining features (Becker & Drake, 2003; Bond, 2004):

1. It is focused on competitive employment in integrated work settings rather than sheltered or transitional employment
2. The service is open to any person with mental illness who chooses to look for work, so that acceptance into the programme is not determined by measures of work readiness or illness variables
3. Job searching commences directly on entry into the programme
4. The IPS programme is integrated with the mental health treatment team, rather than constituting a separate vocational rehabilitation service
5. Potential jobs are chosen based on consumer preference
6. The support provided in the programme continues after employment is obtained, rather than terminating at a set point, as needed by the individual
7. The IPS services are provided in the community, rather than at the mental health or rehabilitation facility.

In contrast to both social firms and clubhouses, which developed largely from collectives of people experiencing mental illnesses, the SE model has been adapted by researchers and clinicians from its previous use in populations with intellectual disability. Consequently, it is the most studied of the various vocational interventions, and the one most supported by systematic research.

Studies on individual placement and support initiatives

In a review of SE (Bond, 2004), nine randomized controlled trials were considered, five of which utilized IPS and four have been published (Drake *et al.*, 1996, 1999; Lehman *et al.*, 2002; Mueser *et al.*, 2004; Table 18.2). Searches of the literature since then reveal no new randomized controlled trials of IPS. One of these studies is now considered in greater detail.

Lehman *et al.* (2002) examined IPS in a trial where 219 participants were randomized to either IPS or to a psychosocial rehabilitation programme that provided work readiness skills training, sheltered work, assistance in job seeking or referral to external vocational services. Although the IPS group in this study achieved a lower rate of competitive employment (27%) than in previous IPS studies, this employment rate was still notably and significantly higher than in the comparison group (7%). Furthermore, when all forms of work were included, the IPS group (42%) still significantly outperformed the comparison group (11%). As in the other studies, those in the IPS group worked more hours, earned more money and moved into employment more quickly (Lehman *et al.*, 2002). This was the first randomized controlled trial conducted after the development of a fidelity scale for IPS (Bond *et al.*, 1997) and this study utilized the scale to show that fidelity to the IPS model was maintained at all points. In discussing their results, particularly in comparison with the earlier studies by Drake *et al.* (1996, 1999), Lehman *et al.* (2002) suggested two main reasons for the lower employment levels in both the IPS and the comparison groups in their study. First, because of a different recruiting process, they suspected that their sample may have been less motivated to work. Second, they noted that their sample included nearly double the number of people with substance-use problems than were included in the second study of Drake *et al.* (1999), a factor that they found was associated with poorer employment outcome. It is noteworthy that illness variables and work motivation may be important factors in the success of the IPS model. Lehman *et al.* (2002) also speculated that neurocognitive variables may be important in maintaining employment once it is gained, and that this may be facilitated by cognitive remediation (Lehman *et al.*, 2002).

Table 18.2. Individual placement and support studies

Study	No.	Conditions (*n*)	Outcomes	Significant results[a]
Drake *et al.*, 1996	143	IPS (74) vs. GST (69)	Competitive employment	IPS (78.1%) > GST (40.3%)
			Hours worked (proportion 20+ hours per week)	IPS (46.6%) > GST (22.4%)
			Total hours	IPS (607) > GST (205)
			Total earnings ($)	IPS (3394) > GST (1077)
			Period to employment (employed within first month)	IPS (15%) > GST (2%)
Drake *et al.*, 1999	152	IPS (76) vs. EVR (76)	Competitive employment	IPS (60.8%) > EVR (9.2%)
			Hours worked (total)	IPS (322) > EVR (28)
			Weeks worked	IPS (15.1) > EVR (1.2)
			Earnings ($)	IPS (1875) > EVR (154)
			Period to employment[b]	IPS (126) > EVR (293)
Lehman *et al.*, 2002	219	IPS (113) vs. PSR (106)	Competitive employment	IPS (27%) > PSR (7%)
			All employment	IPS (42%) > PSR (11%)
			Hours worked	IPS > PSR
			Earnings	IPS > PSR
			IPS fidelity (maximum 75)	69–71
Mueser *et al.*, 2004	204	IPS (68) vs. PSR (67) vs. SBV (69)	Days to first job	IPS (197) < PSR (369)
			No. in competitive employment	ISP (51) > SBV(19) or PSR (12)
			No. working 20+ hours per week	ISP (23) > SBV(9) or PSR (3)
			Total hours worked	ISP (373) > SBV(103) or PSR (40)
			Total wages earned ($)	ISP (2078) > SBV(618) or PSR (239)
			Total weeks worked	ISP (30) > SBV(5) or PSR (3)
			Average weeks per job	ISP (20) > SBV(5) or PSR (3)
			Weeks at longest job	ISP (26) > SBV(5) or PSR (3)

IPS, individual placement and support; GST, group skills training; EVR, enhanced vocational training; PSR, psychosocial rehabilitation; SBV, standard brokered vocational services.
[a] Income in US dollars.
[b] Time in days from study entry to employment.

Studies of IPS show that it is, in general, a more successful vocational intervention than comparison treatments. Two areas of interest that are raised but not resolved by these studies concern the tenure of positions and the role of illness variables in obtaining employment.

Vocational interventions in first-episode psychosis

The first vocational study to focus exclusively on an early-psychosis population was conducted by Rinaldi and colleagues (2004), who reported on a study with a repeated-measures within-subject design of SE with 40 first-episode clients. The results of this study demonstrated that the IPS model was effective with FEP patients. Over 12 months, unemployment fell from 55% to 5% and competitive employment rose from 10% to 41%. In addition, those who were in education or training at baseline were either maintained in their education or training across the intervention or completed it within the time frame. Rinaldi *et al.* (2004) specifically mentioned that the employment specialist was not only seeking out job opportunities but also helping clients to maintain job or training situations.

This initial study suggests that the potential of IPS in FEP is at least as good as it would seem to be from the more extensive research in groups with more established mental illness. It is possible that, because of the earlier stage of life characterizing individuals with FEP, adaptations specific to this age group will need to be made. For example, an intervention may need to focus on education and training outcomes as well as employment ones. Because this phase of life is naturally the beginning of career development, it is possible that vocational interventions in this phase could take a long-term developmental view and seek to support career establishment rather than primarily placing people in jobs. Another challenge in this phase of illness is that people are still likely to be in contact with, and thus comparing themselves with, same-aged peers who have performed better at school or work. This comparison process may lead to feelings of failure or shame. Combining vocational interventions with specific psychological interventions may increase the efficacy of vocational rehabilitation in this age group.

At least three groups in different parts of the world are exploring the possibility of vocational interventions in FEP. Descriptions of these three programmes highlight the way in which vocational interventions are being targeted at young people with FEP.

Vocational intervention at the Early Psychosis and Prevention Centre, Melbourne, Australia

The EPPIC is part of a public mental health service (ORYGEN Youth Health) in Melbourne, Australia, providing treatment to all 15–25 year olds presenting with FEP in a defined catchment area of approximately 1 million people, covering the west and northwest regions of metropolitan Melbourne. The centre works with young people through a case-management system with psychiatric review. Case managers are able to refer clients who wish to find work to a number of federally funded job agencies in the region. In addition to a vocationally oriented group programme at EPPIC, one of the employment agencies provides on-site service to clients one afternoon a week. Despite this range of services being available, clients of EPPIC have no better

employment rates than figures reported in other studies of FEP cohorts (Marwaha & Johnson, 2004), with studies showing around 55% (Killackey *et al.*, 2006) and 50% (Lambert *et al.*, 2005) being employed or in education. Further, unpublished data from a medium-term follow-up study of EPPIC clients show that, while they do not reach the same level of unemployment as groups of people with chronic schizophrenia, their employment rate does not improve over time from its baseline level.

Since the mid 1990s, two major trials of cognitive therapy for early psychosis have been conducted at EPPIC (Jackson *et al.*, 2005, 2008). In reviewing the findings of these studies, it became apparent that while cognitive therapies may have some benefit for symptoms, they did not seem to lead to dramatic functional changes for participants in their daily lives. It was decided to tackle this in a more direct fashion.

As discussed, there is very little guidance in the literature for establishing a vocational intervention programme for young people with FEP (Killackey & Waghorn, 2008). Adding to this difficulty is a truth that is often alluded to rather than directly mentioned, that in Australia, as in many other countries, the employment sector is entirely separate from the mental health sector and very rarely do practitioners in one system have an understanding of the priorities and operations of the other. In reviewing the literature, the IPS model of supported employment appeared to have the most support as an effective intervention.

In order to ascertain the effectiveness of this intervention in young people attending EPPIC, a small randomized pilot study has initially been set up to compare treatment as usual with treatment as usual plus IPS, adhering as closely as possible to the IPS model. The pilot study has a sample size of 40, with 20 in each condition. An employment consultant has been hired to work on this project. She has nearly a decade of experience working in the general and disability employment agency sector. In order to ensure that fidelity to the model was maintained, her office is located within the building that houses the clinical team rather than the research staff and this has led to a high degree of integration into the clinical team. Her caseload is capped at 20 people, allowing her to conduct as much outreach work as is necessary. Most of her hours are spent out of the office with clients. Clients are recruited to the study via case managers when the client expresses an interest in seeking work. While the IPS model would not have acuteness of psychopathology as an exclusion factor, we are limited to accepting those individuals who are able to give informed consent and, therefore, have not been able to work with people in a truly acute phase. For pragmatic reasons, participants receive a 6-month intervention, which is shorter than the open-ended follow-up of the IPS model. As in the IPS model, job searching begins immediately. Because there are some participants for whom training is a desirable outcome, some clients have been placed in courses in order to increase their qualifications for career areas in which they are interested. In this EPPIC study, a placement in a suitable course leading to enhanced career prospects is considered as valid an outcome as a job. Further, because job agencies have access to funds for such courses and other necessary expenses, our employment consultant will often enrol clients in these agencies and, using her experience, advocate and expeditiously navigate the client through the agency. Assessments are intended to be conducted at baseline and at the end of the intervention. The assessment battery examines symptoms, functioning and employment variables. The study has resulted in positive outcomes on all variables of interest for those in the vocational intervention group (Killackey, Jackson & McGorry, 2008). The case vignette illustrates the approach and outcome for one particular client receiving treatment as usual plus IPS.

Case vignette

Daniel was 19 years old. He had been a client of EPPIC at ORYGEN Youth Health for 6 months. Daniel had worked in a number of jobs since leaving school at the age of 15. Most of these jobs involved part-time or casual unskilled work. However, just after turning 17, Daniel became an apprentice mechanic. He held this job for a year and performed well in the role. Despite this, at the time of onset of his psychosis, Daniel was unable to hold onto his job as some of his paranoia related to work colleagues. For the 12 months before coming to EPPIC,

he had been unemployed, living at home and supported by his family. While his recovery was progressing Daniel had mentioned to his case manager that he would like to return to work. His case manager referred him to the Vocational Intervention Project at EPPIC and he was randomized to the vocational intervention condition. The employment consultant met with Daniel. In their meetings, they discussed areas in which he might like to seek employment. The employment consultant also gave him some help updating his resume and they spent some time discussing the pros and cons of disclosing his illness to potential employers. Daniel said that he would like to return to an apprenticeship – not necessarily as a mechanic – but that because of his work history he wanted to gain a qualification and become a skilled worker. The employment consultant was aware of an apprenticeship scheme funded by the federal government. She contacted the coordinator of the scheme and an interview was arranged for Daniel. Daniel and she role-played some interview scenarios. In the meantime, she also gave Daniel some information about the scheme. This information helped Daniel to consider in which area he would like to commence an apprenticeship. With this information and the employment consultant's counsel, he decided on plumbing. On the day of the interview, the employment consultant collected Daniel from home and took him to the interview. In the car, they conducted a final rehearsal of the way in which Daniel would disclose his experience with psychosis as he had decided that he wanted to be upfront about his illness. Daniel was successful with the interview and commenced his apprenticeship with a plumber who worked in the area where Daniel lived. The employment consultant continued to meet with Daniel for the rest of their allotted 6 months in order to help him to resolve any problems that he found in his work. Because he had disclosed his illness, the employment consultant was able to meet with Daniel with the consent of his boss. Three months after starting his employment, the employment consultant noticed some changes in the way that Daniel was speaking to her. At this stage, she was seeing him more frequently than his case manager. Through her increased knowledge of mental illness gained by being based in a clinical team, she recognized that there was a paranoid flavour to what Daniel was saying. She reported this to the case manager who arranged a special out-of-hours appointment for Daniel. As a result of this, it was decided to alter Daniel's medication. The employment consultant was able to help to negotiate with the employer for Daniel to have some time off while the medication was changed. She also ensured that as Daniel returned to work her support of him increased.

The University of California at Los Angeles Aftercare Research Programme: combining individual placement and support with Workplace Fundamentals Module training

At the University of California at Los Angeles (UCLA) Aftercare Research Programme, a randomized controlled trial of vocational intervention in early psychosis is being completed that focuses on the impact of a full implementation of IPS (Becker & Drake, 2003) combined with group skills training with the Workplace Fundamentals Module developed by Charles Wallace at UCLA (Wallace & Tauber, 2004). This 18-month clinical trial, Improving and Predicting Work Outcome in Recent-Onset Schizophrenia, is one of a series of studies of the early phase of schizophrenia within the Developmental Processes in Schizophrenic Disorders Project (Nuechterlein *et al.*, 1992). Patients with a recent first schizophrenic episode are drawn from a wide range of psychiatric hospitals and clinics in the Los Angeles metropolitan area. The age range accepted is 18 to 45 years, but the mean age of those at the UCLA Aftercare Research Programme has been in the range 22–24 years.

Earlier studies within this project had indicated that work functioning often remained impaired after FEP even though the most typical symptom course involved substantial periods of remission of all psychotic symptoms (Nuechterlein *et al.*, 2006). Longitudinal analyses have shown that several key cognitive deficits continued even after clinical symptoms have gone into remission (Nuechterlein *et al.*, 1992) and that more severe cognitive deficits at the beginning of the outpatient treatment were strong predictors of lack of return to work or school by the end of 9 to 12 months (Nuechterlein *et al.*, 2003). The current randomized clinical trial examines whether the individualized vocational intervention provided by IPS, combined with group training focused on skills required in most workplaces, can compensate for the continuing cognitive deficits and improves work recovery during this critical early psychosis period.

In this programme, IPS has been implemented using the set of principles described earlier in this chapter, with the direct collaboration of Deborah Becker and Robert Drake from Dartmouth Medical School. An employment specialist has been integrated into the clinical treatment team of psychiatrists and psychologists who provide medication, group therapy, family education and case management for all patients in the UCLA Aftercare Research Programme. The IPS was adapted to include supported education as well as supported employment, following the IPS principle that placement should be guided by consumer preferences. Return to a regular educational programme was found to be the preferred and most appropriate vocational step for about half of the participants, while the remainder preferred the goal of competitive employment. The services provided by the employment specialist have varied depending on the needs of the individual patient, but have included help with a rapid search for an appropriate job or educational programme, direct aid in placement in a job or school when needed, working after placement with the employer or teacher when such direct aid was allowed by the patient and working behind the scenes to conduct problem solving with patients about issues that arise at work or school. The employment specialist provided most of her IPS services in the community. The IPS fidelity scale (Bond *et al.*, 1997) has been used to document the successful application of the IPS model. The IPS services have been provided to participants throughout the 18-month study, with intensity of services adjusted over time in response to individual needs.

The group skills training component of the vocational intervention has involved the Workplace Fundamentals Module (Wallace & Tauber, 2004), following the format of other social skills training modules developed at UCLA for individuals with severe mental illness (Liberman *et al.*, 1993). This module involves training sessions for small groups in nine skill areas: (1) how work changes your life, (2) learning about your workplace, (3) identifying your own stressors, (4) learning to solve problems, (5) managing symptoms and medications, (6) managing health and hygiene, (7) learning interactions to improve your work, (8) learning to socialize appropriately with co-workers, and (9) learning to find support and proper motivation. For each skill area, training involves an introduction, videotaped demonstration, role-played practice, generation and evaluation of solutions to resource-management problems, generation and evaluation of solutions to outcome problems, completion of within-group task assignments and completion of work-related tasks at home or at the workplace. For the first 6 months, two group skills training sessions are completed each week, usually on the same day. During the remaining 12 months, the frequency of these group sessions is tapered until only monthly 'booster' sessions are conducted.

The comparison group is being provided with vocational rehabilitation services using the 'brokered model' that has been typical of vocational interventions for psychiatric patients in the USA. Similar to the comparison group for a study of IPS in patients with chronic severe psychiatric disorders (Drake *et al.*, 1996), patients with recent-onset schizophrenia in the brokered model group have been provided referrals to state agencies that are separate from the mental health system and that specialize in vocational services. In southern California, these agencies are the State Department of Vocational Rehabilitation, the Southern California Regional Occupational Center and offices for disabled students in the state college system. To enhance a fair comparison of the two vocational intervention models, referrals to these specialized state agencies have been followed up by the case managers and therapists of the UCLA Aftercare Research Programme more vigorously than might typically be undertaken at a community psychiatric clinic. In addition, patients in the brokered model group are provided group training in social and coping skills that is equivalent in time and general format to the Workplace Fundamentals Module but does not focus on skill areas specifically applicable to job and school settings. Participants in this comparison sample have received psychiatric treatment that fully parallels that of the participants in the enhanced work intervention group, including the same medication protocol (risperidone as the standardized starting medication), case management, individual counselling/therapy and family psychoeducation.

Although this UCLA randomized controlled trial is ongoing and final data analyses have not been completed, interim results were presented at the *International Congress on Schizophrenia Research* (Nuechterlein *et al.*, 2005). Based on data from the first 51 patients with recent-onset schizophrenia who had been entered into the study for at least 6 months, the benefits of the enhanced work intervention programme were already highly significant and very notable. In the combined IPS and Workplace Fundamentals Module group 93% had returned to competitive work or regular school within the first 6 months of the study, compared with 50% in the comparison group ($p < 0.001$). Furthermore, involvement in competitive work or school in the remaining 12 months of the study, during which treatment was less intensive, continued to be distinctively different. The interim analyses showed that 93% of individuals in the enhanced work intervention group and 55% of participants in the brokered model group were competitively employed or in regular school during at least part of this 12-month period and most for the majority of this period. Therefore, these preliminary results from the UCLA Aftercare Research Programme indicate the very substantial impact on work recovery that is possible through enhanced work interventions during the early phase of schizophrenia.

The Norfolk Early Intervention Service, UK

As has been noted above, social and vocational recovery from psychosis in traditional services is a critical problem. Local studies monitoring the 2-year outcomes in the UK county of Norfolk from 1998 to 2002, before the introduction of the Early Intervention Service, suggested that only 15% of young people returned to either full-time work or college after FEP, with a further 19% engaged in some part-time activity of this type. This left 66% of young people doing very little in the way of structured activity 2 years after their psychotic episode. This represented a picture of many young people living isolated lives in the community and engaged in few activities, on the whole symptomatically recovered from psychosis but frequently socially avoidant, anxious and depressed. These figures are consistent with recent reviews of studies from elsewhere in the UK and Europe (Marwaha & Johnson, 2004). These outcomes occurred despite the provision of modern pharmacological and psychological treatments focusing on symptomatic recovery from psychosis and suggested that targeting social recovery directly may be needed. A priority focus on targeting social recovery has guided the interventions provided in the Norfolk Early Intervention Service, which now takes all new patients with psychosis from a catchment area of 750 000 people in a mixed urban and rural area. In this service, specialist care is delivered for 2 years, by a multidisciplinary team of 15 case managers (with psychiatric and psychological support), providing social recovery interventions with a combined caseload of approximately 220. An important focus of the service is the development of a social recovery intervention that combines principles of supported employment, assertive case management and CBT, and that can be provided by case managers in routine clinical settings.

An important aspect of targeting social recovery in the early stages is the promotion and instillation of hope for social recovery. This can represent something of an attitude shift from the experience of clients of traditional services in the UK, where we have observed a tendency for many clinicians to be satisfied with the achievement and maintenance of symptomatic recovery from psychosis while being quite cautious about promoting social recovery in psychosis because of concerns over potential risk of relapse. As well as instilling hope, we also take careful account of cultural and age-appropriate norms in setting goals for social recovery. The exact definition of social recovery is often unclear and depends to some degree on cultural values and age-appropriate expectations. While full-time work is commonly regarded as the gold standard marker of social recovery, it may not be a realistic or appropriate aim for all young people, for many of whom a mix of part-time work, college courses and structured voluntary or leisure activity may be culturally acceptable. The offers of assistance most acceptable to young people are those that fit their own values and existing goals and aspirations. Key principles of our programme are identifying the person's preexisting aspirations and instilling hope of returning to a pathway of achieving these. Wherever possible, we assist the person to return to existing college or work activity as soon as possible,

often by negotiating part-time return with employers or educational institutions. This can happen within weeks of the episode, taking careful account of any problems associated with symptoms but offering ways to manage such problems 'in vivo' rather than avoiding situations in which they may occur or insisting on a delay until full recovery takes place.

We find it is useful to integrate CBT interventions to address social anxiety, depression and hopelessness and to manage mild symptoms of paranoia and hallucinations. Our formulation of the problems of young peoples' recovery from psychosis from a cognitive perspective suggests that poor social recovery may be maintained not solely as a product of factors directly associated with psychotic illness (e.g. symptoms and cognitive impairment) and its social consequences (e.g. stigma and lack of social opportunity) but also as a consequence of hopelessness, social anxiety and negative beliefs about self and others. The experience of psychosis and associated social adversity, including hospitalization and social losses, can often be seen by people with psychosis as a traumatic experience, leading to hopelessness, stigmatization and disruption to valued goals and expectations and then to depression and withdrawal from social behaviour. This rationale provides a clear case for using CBT in combination with social interventions to address problems in social recovery in patients whose recovery has become blocked. In such patients, attempts to improve social recovery in psychosis needs to be undertaken sensitively (often as graded exposure and behavioural experiments) so as not to overstimulate and lead to psychosis. Amongst the patients with more complex problems, who may present with a range of issues associated with psychotic symptoms, sensitivity to stress and underlying cognitive deficits, a more sophisticated approach may be required. Our case managers are, therefore, closely supervised and work jointly with trained cognitive therapists as well as being encouraged to adopt assertive case-management practices and work in partnership with specialist supported employment workers in the team.

We already have some good preliminary evidence of the efficacy of this approach from a comparison of the effects of the Norfolk Early Intervention Service with the outcomes at 3, 12 and 24 months from the historical controls. Compared with the 15% who were engaged in substantive part-time (> 15 hours) or full-time educational or work activity in the historical controls, now around 53% of patients have a meaningful range of activity at 1 year, and this is being maintained at 2 years. It is interesting that many of these achievements started emerging as early as the 3-month stage, providing support for the strategy of return to previous activity as soon as it is feasible. This resulted in no worsening of symptoms. We are also currently running a randomized trial of this type of intervention funded by the UK Medical Research Council. This trial focuses on providing an intensive form of the intervention to the subgroup of patients with more complex problems who have not achieved a reasonable social recovery at least 1 year after FEP.

Conclusions

The literature dealing with vocational recovery has focused on three major models. These have been discussed in some detail in this chapter. Well-conducted randomized controlled trials have clearly shown that IPS is the superior approach on a number of parameters; these include number of people obtaining work, tenure of employment and job satisfaction. However, to date, only one published report with patients with early psychosis has appeared in the literature and this was not such a trial (Rinaldi *et al.*, 2004). The FEP represents a key opportunity in which vocational development is one of the major natural tasks for this critical developmental stage. This chapter has described three different programmes, from Australia, the USA and the UK, respectively. Importantly, this international range of programmes demonstrates that vocational recovery in the form of IPS can fit different socio-political systems/contexts. When implemented in early psychosis, IPS seems to achieve higher success rates than it does in the chronic psychotic populations. It can be modified to include educational recovery and this is important as educational attainment is a key factor in employment success (Waghorn *et al.*, 2003).

The challenge ahead is to translate these research findings into everyday clinical practice. There are several obstacles to this: in many places, health, educational and vocational services are funded separately and often do not work closely together; these separate systems often have their own sets of bureaucratic rules and jargon, the integration of which can seem overwhelming; and change is always a potentially difficult thing to manage. Despite the existence of these problems, they can be resolved. Part of this will involve a change in the mindset of clinicians to acknowledge that functional disability is not 'secondary' to psychotic illness but is a primary problem for those with it and one which is not alleviated by attention to symptomatic recovery alone. There will also need to be a recognition by the educational and vocational sectors that models designed for the rehabilitation of physical illnesses do not necessarily translate to mental illnesses. In implementing IPS, mental health clinicians may have to confront their own prejudices about working with colleagues who are not trained in mental health disciplines but have employment sector experience.

People with mental illness repeatedly state that their number one goal is to work and to participate in society. So far, focusing only on symptomatic recovery has failed to achieve this. The integration of approaches for symptomatic and functional recovery is a huge step in the right direction; we need to promote as much recovery as is possible.

REFERENCES

Australian Bureau of Statistics (2005). *Labour Force Australia: November Key Figures*. Canberra: Australian Bureau of Statistics.

Australian Bureau of Statistics (2006). *Barriers and Incentives to Labour Force Participation, Australia, August 2004 to June 2005*. Canberra: Australian Bureau of Statistics.

Addington, J., Young, J. & Addington, D. (2003). Social outcome in early psychosis. *Psychological Medicine*, **33**, 1119–24.

Agerbo, E., Byrne, M., Eaton, W. W. & Mortensen, P. B. (2004). Marital and labor market status in the long run in schizophrenia. *Archives of General Psychiatry*, **61**, 28–33.

Anonymous (1999). The wellspring of the clubhouse model for social and vocational adjustment of persons with serious mental illness. *Psychiatric Services*, **50**, 1473–6.

Arduini, L., Kalyvoka, A., Stratta, P. *et al.* (2002). Subjective experiences in schizophrenia and bipolar disorders. *European Archives of Psychiatry and Clinical Neuroscience*, **252**, 24–7.

Baker, K. (2005). *Mapping the Social Firm Sector 2005*. Redhill, UK: Social Firms.

Barnes, T. R. E., Hutton, S. B., Chapman, M. J. *et al.* (2000). West London first-episode study of schizophrenia: clinical correlates of duration of untreated psychosis. *British Journal of Psychiatry*, **177**, 207–11.

Baron, R. C. & Salzer, M. S. (2002). Accounting for unemployment among people with mental illness. *Behavioural Sciences and the Law*, **20**, 585–99.

Becker, D. & Drake, R. (2003). *A Working Life for People with Severe Mental Illness*. New York: Oxford Press.

Bell, M. & Lysaker, P. (1996). Levels of expectation for work activity in schizophrenia: clinical and rehabilitation outcomes. *Psychiatric Rehabilitation Journal*, **19**, 71–6.

Bellack, A. S. (1986). Schizophrenia: behaviour therapy's forgotten child. *Behaviour Therapy*, **17**, 199–214.

Bhugra, D., Leff, J., Mallett, R., Der, G. B. C. & Rudge, S. (1997). Incidence and outcome of schizophrenia in Whites, African-Caribbeans and Asians in London. *Psychological Medicine*, **27**, 791–8.

Bhugra, D., Hilwig, M., Mallett, R. *et al.* (2000). Factors in the onset of schizophrenia: a comparison between London and Trinidad samples. *Acta Psychiatrica Scandinavica*, **101**, 135–41.

Bilby, R. (1992). A response to the criticisms of transitional employment. *Psychosocial Rehabilitation Journal. Special Issue: The Clubhouse Model*, **16**, 69–82.

Birchwood, M. & Fiorillo, A. (2000). The critical period for early intervention. *Psychiatric Rehabilitation Skills. Special Issue: The British Approach to Psychiatric Rehabilitation*, **4**, 182–98.

Birchwood, M., Smith, J., Drury, V. *et al.* (1994). A self-report insight scale for psychosis: reliability, validity and sensitivity to change. *Acta Psychatrica Scandinavica*, **89**, 62–7.

Boardman, J., Grove, B., Perkins, R. & Shepherd, G. (2003). Work and employment for people with psychiatric disabilities. *British Journal of Psychiatry*, **182**, 467–8.

Bond, G. R. (2004). Supported employment: evidence for an evidence-based practice. *Psychiatric Rehabilitation Journal*, **27**, 345–59.

Bond, G. R., Becker, D. R., Drake, R. E. & Vogler, K. (1997). A fidelity scale for the individual placement and support model of supported employment. *Rehabilitation and Counselling Bulletin*, **40**, 265–84.

Carlyle, T. (1899; reprinted 1969). *Critical and Miscellaneous Essays*, vol. VI. [The Works of Thomas Carlyle, vol. 29.] New York: AMS Press.

Cook, J. A., Pickett, S. A., Razzano, L. *et al.* (1996). Rehabilitation services for persons with schizophrenia. *Psychiatric Annals*, **26**, 97–104.

Cook, J. A., Leff, H. S., Blyler, C. R. *et al.* (2005). Results of a multisite randomized trial of supported employment interventions for individuals with severe mental illness. *Archives of General Psychiatry*, **62**, 505–12.

Crowther, R. E. & Marshall, M. (2001). Employment rehabilitation schemes for people with mental health problems in the North West region: service characteristics and utilisation. *Journal of Mental Health*, **10**, 373–81.

Crowther, R. E., Marshall, M., Bond, G. R. & Huxley, P. (2001). Helping people with severe mental illness to obtain work: systematic review. *British Medical Journal*, **322**, 204–8.

Cuesta, M. J., Peralta, V., Caro, F. & Leon, J. (1995). Is poor insight in psychotic disorders associated with poor performance on the Wisconsin Card Sorting Test? *American Journal of Psychiatry*, **152**, 1380–2.

Drake, R. E., McHugo, G. J., Becker, D. R., Anthony, W. A. & Clark, R. E. (1996). The New Hampshire study of supported employment for people with severe mental illness. *Journal of Consulting and Clinical Psychology*, **64**, 391–9.

Drake, R. E., McHugo, G., Bebout, R. R. *et al.* (1999). A randomized clinical trial of supported employment for inner-city patients with severe mental illness. *Archives of General Psychiatry*, **56**, 627–33.

Ducci, G., Stentella, C. & Vulterini, P. (2002). The social enterprise in Europe: the state of the art. *International Journal of Mental Health*, **31**, 76–91.

Edwards, J. & McGorry, P. D. (2002). *Implementing Early Intervention in Psychosis: A Guide to Establishing Early Psychosis Services*. London: Martin Dunitz.

Falloon, I. R. H., Boyd, J. L., McGill, C. W. *et al.* (1985). Family management in the prevention of morbidity of schizophrenia. *Archives of General Psychiatry*, **42**, 887–96.

Gold, J. M., Goldberg, R. W., McNary, S. W., Dixon, L. B. & Lehman, A. F. (2002). Cognitive correlates of job tenure among patients with severe mental illness. *American Journal of Psychiatry*, **159**, 1395–402.

Gupta, S., Andreasen, N. C., Arndt, S. *et al.* (1997). The Iowa Longitudinal Study of Recent Onset Psychosis: one-year follow-up of first episode patients. *Schizophrenia Research*, **23**, 1–13.

Häfner, H. (1996). Psychiatric rehabilitation: general issues. *European Psychiatry*, **11**, 39s–50s.

Henry, A. D., Barreira, S. B., Brown, J-M. & McKay, C. (2001). A retrospective study of clubhouse-based transitional employment. *Psychiatric Rehabilitation Journal*, **24**, 344–54.

Ho, B-C., Andreasen, N. & Flaum, M. (1997). Dependence on public financial support early in the course of schizophrenia. *Psychiatric Services*, **48**, 948–50.

Iles, U. G. (1928). Farm work for mental cases. *US Veterans Bureau Medical Bulletin*, **4**, 282–5.

Jackson, H. J., McGorry, P. D., Edwards, J. & Hulbert, C. (1996). Cognitively oriented psychotherapy for early psychosis (COPE). In P. Cotton & H. Jackson (eds.), *Early Intervention and Prevention in Mental Health*. Carlton, Australia: Australian Psychological Society, pp. 131–54.

Jackson, H. J., McGorry, P., Edwards, J. *et al.* (2005). A controlled trial of cognitively oriented psychotherapy for early psychosis (COPE) with four-year follow-up readmission data. *Psychological Medicine*, **35**, 1295–306.

Jackson, H. J., McGorry, P. D., Killackey, E. *et al.* (2008). Acute-phase and 1-year follow-up results of a randomised controlled trial of CBT versus befriending for first-episode psychosis: the ACE project. *Psychological Medicine*, **38**, 725–35.

Johnsen, M., McKay, C., Corcoran, J. & Lidz, C. (2002). *Characteristics of Clubhouses Across the World: Findings from the International Survey of Clubhouses 2000*. Worcester, MA: Programme for Clubhouse Research, Center for Mental Health Services Research, University of Massachusetts Medical School.

Johnsen, M., McKay, C., Henry, A. D. & Manning, T. D. (2004). What does competitive employment mean? A secondary analysis of employment approaches in the Massachusetts employment intervention demonstration project. In W. H. Fisher (ed.) *Research on Employment for Persons with Severe Mental Illness*. Oxford: Elsevier, pp. 43–62.

Killackey, E. & Waghorn, G. (2008). The challenge of integrating employment services with public mental health services in Australia: progress at the first demonstration site. *Psychiatric Rehabilitation Journal*, **32**, 63–6.

Killackey, E., Jackson, H., Gleeson, J., Hickie, I. & McGorry, P. (2006). Exciting career opportunity beckons! Early intervention and vocational rehabilitation in first episode psychosis: employing cautious optimism. *Australian and New Zealand Journal of Psychiatry*, **40**, 951–62.

Killackey, E., Jackson, H. J. & McGorry, P. D. (2008). Vocational intervention in first-episode psychosis: individual placement and support v. treatment as usual. *British Journal of Psychiatry*, **193**, 114–20.

Kua, J., Wong, K. E., Kua, E. H. & Tsoi, W. F. (2003). A 20-year follow-up study on schizophrenia in Singapore. *Acta Psychiatrica Scandinavica*, **108**, 118–25.

Lambert, M., Conus, P., Lubman, D. I. *et al.* (2005). The impact of substance use disorders on clinical outcome in 643 patients with first-episode psychosis. *Acta Psychiatrica Scandinavica*, **112**, 141–8.

Lay, B., Blanz, B., Hartmann, M. & Schmidt, M. H. (2000). The psychosocial outcome of adolescent-onset schizophrenia: a 12-year followup. *Schizophrenia Bulletin*, **26**, 801–16.

Leff, J. (2001). Can we manage without the mental hospital? *Australian and New Zealand Journal of Psychiatry*, **35**, 421–7.

Lehman, A. F. (1995). Vocational rehabilitation in schizophrenia. *Schizophrenia Bulletin*, **21**, 645–56.

Lehman, A. F., Goldberg, R., Dixon, L. B. *et al.* (2002). Improving employment outcomes for persons with severe mental illnesses. *Archives of General Psychiatry*, **59**, 165–72.

Liberman, R. P., Wallace, C. J., Blackwell, G. *et al.* (1993). Innovations in skills training for the seriously mentally ill: the UCLA Social and Independent Living Skills Modules. *Innovations and Research*, **2**, 43–60.

Long, M. (2005). *How Young People are Faring: Key Indicators 2005*. Glebe, Australia: Dusseldorp Skills Forum.

Macias, C. (2001). *Final Report Massachusetts Employment Intervention Demonstration Project 'An Experimental Comparison of PACT and Clubhouse'*. New York: Fountain House.

Macias, C., Jackson, R., Schroeder, C. & Wang, Q. (1999). What is a clubhouse? Report on the ICCD 1996 Survey of USA Clubhouses. *Community Mental Health Journal*, **35**, 181–90.

Marwaha, S. & Johnson, S. (2004). Schizophrenia and employment: a review. *Social Psychiatry and Psychiatric Epidemiology*, **39**, 337–49.

McGorry, P. (2005). Royal Australian and New Zealand College of Psychiatrists clinical practice guidelines for the treatment of schizophrenia and related disorders. *Australian and New Zealand Journal of Psychiatry*, **39**, 1–30.

McKay, C., Johnsen, M. & Stein, R. (2005). Employment outcomes in Massachusetts clubhouses. *Psychiatric Rehabilitation Journal*, **29**, 25–32.

McPhillips, M. & Sensky, T. (1998). Coercion, adherence or collaboration? Influences on compliance with medication. In T. Wykes, N. Tarrier & S. Lewis (eds.), *Outcome and Innovation in Psychological Treatment of Schizophrenia*. Chichester, UK: John Wiley, pp. 161–77.

Morrin, M., Simmonds, D. & Somerville, W. (2004). Social enterprise: mainstreamed from the margins? *Local Economy*, **19**, 69–84.

Mueser, K. T., Clark, R. E., Haines, M. *et al.* (2004). The Hartford study of supported employment for persons with severe mental illness. *Journal of Consulting and Clinical Psychology*, **72**, 479–90.

Nuechterlein, K. H., Dawson, M. E., Gitlin, M. *et al.* (1992). Developmental processes in schizophrenic disorders: longitudinal studies of vulnerability and stress. *Schizophrenia Bulletin*, **18**, 387–425.

Nuechterlein, K. H., Subotnik, K. L., Green, M. F. *et al.* (2003). Neurocognitive predictors of work outcome in the initial course of schizophrenia. In *Proceedings of the Annual Meeting of the International Neuropsychology Society*, Honolulu, Hawaii 2003.

Nuechterlein, K. H., Subotnik, K. L., Ventura, J. *et al.* (2005). Advances in improving and predicting work outcome in recent-onset schizophrenia. [In *Proceedings of the International Congress on Schizophrenia Research*, Savannah, Georgia, 2005] Schizophrenia Bulletin, **31**, 530.

Nuechterlein, K. H., Miklowitz, D. J., Ventura, J. *et al.* (2006). Classifying episodes in schizophrenia and bipolar disorder: criteria for relapse and remission applied to recent-onset samples. *Psychiatry Research*, **144**, 153–66.

O'Flynn, D. (2001). Approaching employment: mental health, work projects and the Care Programme Approach. *Psychiatric Bulletin*, **25**, 169–71.

Overall, J. E. & Porterfield, J. L. (1963). Powered vector method of factor analysis. *Psychometrika*, **28**, 415–22.

Porter, R. (2002). *Madness: A Brief History*. Oxford: Oxford University Press.

Rees, S., Mallard, C., Breen, S. *et al.* (1998). Fetal brain injury following prolonged hypoxemia and placental insufficiency: a review. *Comprehensive Biochemical Physiology*, **119A**, 653–60.

Rinaldi, M., McNeil, K., Firn, M. *et al.* (2004). What are the benefits of evidence-based supported employment for patients with first-episode psychosis? *Psychiatric Bulletin*, **28**, 281–4.

Robinson, D. G., Woerner, M. G., McMeniman, M., Mendelowitz, A. & Bilder, R. M. (2004). Symptomatic and functional recovery from a first episode of schizophrenia or schizoaffective disorder. *American Journal of Psychiatry*, **161**, 473–9.

SANE (2002). *Schizophrenia: Costs. An Analysis of the Burden of Schizophrenia and Related Suicide in Australia*. Melbourne, Australia: SANE.

Scottish Schizophrenia Research Group (1992). The Scottish first episode schizophrenia study: VIII. Five-year follow-up:

clinical and psychosocial findings. *British Journal of Psychiatry*, **161**, 496–500.

Shevalev, E. A. (1935). The question of work therapy of neuroses and psychoses. *Problemy Psikhiatrii i Psikhopatologii*, **1935**, 44–67.

Sim, K., Swapna, V., Mythily, S. *et al.* (2004). Psychiatric comorbidity in first episode psychosis: the Early Psychosis Intervention Programme (EPIP) experience. *Acta Psychiatrica Scandinavica*, **109**, 23–9.

Skeate, A., Jackson, C., Birchwood, M. & Jones, C. (2002). Duration of untreated psychosis and pathways to care in first-episode psychosis: investigation of help-seeking behaviour in primary care. *British Journal of Psychiatry*, **181**, s73–7.

Social Firms UK. (2005). *The Values Based Checklist for Social Firms*. Redhill, UK: Social Firms.

Social Firms UK (2006). *About Social Firms*. Redhill, UK: Social Firms.

Stein, L. I. & Test, M. A. (1980). Alternatives to mental hospital treatment: I. Conceptual model treatment programme and clinical evaluation. *Archives of General Psychiatry*, **37**, 392–7.

Sturm, R., Gresenz, C. R., Pacula, R. L. & Wells, K. B. (1999). Labor force participation by persons with mental illness. *Psychiatric Services*, **50**, 1407.

Ungerleider, J. T. & Shadowen, P. J. (1966). The diagnostic and therapeutic value of work. *Hospital and Community Psychiatry*, **December**, 39–43.

Velakoulis, D., Pantelis, C., McGorry, P. D. *et al.* (1999). Hippocampal volume in first-episode psychoses and chronic schizophrenia: a high-resolution magnetic resonance imaging study. *Archives of General Psychiatry*, **56**, 133–41.

Waghorn, G., Chant, D. & Whiteford, H. (2003). The strength of self-reported course of illness in predicting vocational recovery for persons with schizophrenia. *Journal of Vocational Rehabilitation*, **18**, 33–41.

Wallace, C. J. & Tauber, R. (2004). Supplementing supported employment with workplace skills training. *Psychiatric Services*, **55**, 513–5.

Warner, R. (1986). Hard times and schizophrenia. *Psychology Today*, **20**, 50–2.

Wood, A. G., Saling, M. M., Abbott, D. F. & Jackson, G. D. (2001). A neurological account of frontal lobe involvement in orthographic lexical retrieval: an fMRI study. *Neuroimage*, **14**, 162–9.

Zubin, J. & Spring, B. (1977). Vulnerability: a new view of schizophrenia. *Journal of Abnormal Psychology*, **86**, 103–26.

19

Relapse prevention in early psychosis

John Gleeson, Don Linszen and Durk Wiersma

Introduction

The international emergence of programmes for first-episode psychosis (FEP) since the early 1990s represents an important structural reform of the mental health system, allowing a sharper focus on the problems of recognition, early detection, access to care and the need for interventions specific for both phase of illness and the developmental stage of the patient (Edwards & McGorry, 2002). Within the phase-specific framework of FEP, the recovery period has been highlighted as an intensive period of treatment involving an integration of biological and psychosocial interventions (McGorry, 2005). One of the stated goals of many first-episode services throughout the 'critical period' has been the prevention of relapse (Birchwood, 1999). This goal is reflected in a range of clinical guidelines, including the draft consensus statement of the International Early Psychosis Association, which highlighted the risks of relapse: 'Relapse is distressing and may increase the risk of treatment resistance and other "collateral damage", including worsening stigma' (Edwards & McGorry, 2002, p. 153).

Various treatment guidelines for schizophrenia have incorporated relapse prevention as a goal of treatment. For example, the UK's National Institute for Health and Clinical Excellence (NICE) treatment guidelines for schizophrenia emphasize the importance of integrating the prophylactic role of antipsychotic drugs with family-based interventions and cognitive–behavioural therapy (CBT) during maintenance phases (NICE, 2002). In the USA, the Department of Health and Human Services' Schizophrenia Patient Outcomes Research Team recently revised their treatment recommendations. These also give considerable attention to the issue of relapse prevention, although less space appears to be given to the specific role of psychosocial interventions in relapse prevention. Recommendation 4, for example, states: 'Persons who experience acute and sustained symptom relief with antipsychotic medication should continue to receive antipsychotic medication in order to reduce the risk of relapse or worsening of positive symptoms' (Lehman et al., 2004, p. 197). Importantly, the authors qualified this recommendation with the view that: 'The value of maintenance therapy beyond the first year has not been studied extensively' (Lehman et al., 2004, p. 198). Similar emphasis can be seen in the Dutch and Australasian guidelines (McGorry, 2005; Trimbos Institute, 2005).

Therefore, as far as treatment guidelines are an indicator of consensus, there appears to be a common view that the prevention of relapse is a critical target in early psychosis and beyond. What then is the status of the evidence underpinning these recommendations? What are the gaps in the knowledge base in relation to relapse and its prevention, especially in FEP? This chapter addresses these questions, beginning with a critical discussion of contemporary definitions of psychotic relapse and associated assessment criteria. This is followed by a review of relapse rates in the early years after onset of psychosis. Then factors associated with relapse are examined and the current knowledge regarding the prevention of relapse in FEP is summarized, leading to specific clinical recommendations for relapse prevention following FEP. We conclude with priorities for further research.

The Recognition and Management of Early Psychosis: A Preventive Approach, ed. Henry J. Jackson and Patrick D. McGorry. Published by Cambridge University Press. © Cambridge University Press 2009.

Defining and assessing psychotic relapse

Prospective naturalistic follow-up studies and follow-up treatment studies have provided a rich source of evidence regarding FEP. Relapse has been one of many critical dependent variables of interest. The total pool of these studies is surprisingly small: a search of PsychLit, Medline, in addition to a hand search of journals, was completed using the search terms 'early psychosis', 'first-episode psychosis/schizophrenia', 'relapse' and 'reoccurrence'. This revealed approximately 30 prospective studies published between 1982 and 2006 that reported relapse rates. The limited number of these studies is a consequence of the enormity of the task; new patients have to be consecutively recruited, often over several years, and considerable resources and doggedness is required to achieve adequate follow-up and retention. Data suggest that relapse is less frequent in the first year after treatment is commenced compared with subsequent years (Gleeson, 2005), so it is necessary to commit resources for the long haul if relapse rates are to be evaluated. The burden on participants is also considerable, especially if follow-up intervals are frequent, so retention is not surprisingly an issue in many of these studies.

One issue of major concern to investigators has been the definition of relapse. In the absence of definitive markers of relapse, researchers have usually relied upon objective ratings of changes in symptom severity. It is generally agreed that readmission or clinical judgement alone, while useful supplementary criteria, are less than ideal (Falloon, 1983). Most definitions of relapse in published studies over the previous 10 years would be consistent with our proposed general definition:

Significant increases in positive psychotic symptoms (using a-priori cutoff scores or change criterion on standardized clinician-rated instruments), which are sustained over at least 1 week and which follow on from a period of absence or only mild severity ratings on positive psychotic symptoms which are sustained for at least 1 month.

In practice, researchers have tended to collapse more mild exacerbations together with full-threshold relapses (Gitlin *et al.*, 2001). Unfortunately, there is enormous variability in the specific operational criteria for relapse.

Most studies did not include a duration criterion in order to discriminate relapses from brief flurries of symptoms, although the four exceptions utilized a 1-week period (Linszen *et al.*, 1996; Linszen *et al.*, 1998; Robinson *et al.*, 1999; Stirling *et al.*, 1991). The degree of change criterion, the range of symptoms required and the method of measurement have varied markedly, with the more objective definitions including a-priori changes on clinician-rated instruments. Seven studies utilized the Brief Psychiatric Rating Scale for this purpose, based on the criteria developed by the group at the University of California at Los Angeles (Gaebel *et al.*, 2002; Gitlin *et al.*, 2001; Gleeson *et al.*, 2005a; Linszen *et al.*, 1994a, 1996, 1998; Nuechterlein *et al.*, 1992a); two used the Present State Examination (Barrelet *et al.*, 1990; Leff *et al.*, 1990; Linszen *et al.*, 1994a) and three studies used the Clinical Global Impression instrument as an additional measure (Gaebel *et al.*, 2002; Robinson *et al.*, 1999; Schooler *et al.*, 2005). The largest study, with 555 participants, utilized the Positive and Negative Syndrome Scale to define relapse (Schooler *et al.*, 2005).

To our knowledge, no study has included negative symptoms in the operationalization of relapse and no specific consideration in the literature has been given to defining criteria for psychotic relapse in the context of schizoaffective disorder or mood disorder with psychotic features. There has also been an unfortunate lack of consensus regarding definitions of relapse or a consensus regarding equivalence of severity ratings across instruments, although considerable efforts have been made to establish consensus definitions and equivalency ratings for remission and recovery in schizophrenia (Andreasen *et al.*, 2005). These inconsistencies remain important to resolve, because it has been demonstrated that the various established relapse criterion sets result in considerable differences in the classification of clinical outcome (i.e. 'relapse' or 'no relapse') at the level of the individual patient (Linszen *et al.*, 1994a). No doubt this will receive further attention.

Surveys regarding the concept of relapse from a clinical perspective warrant mention. For example, one study utilized the Delphi consensus technique with a group of UK-based academic and clinical experts in schizophrenia, who agreed upon three aspects to the definition of relapse: (1) the core of relapse is an increase in positive symptoms, (2) relapse may be occurring despite the absence of elicited positive symptoms, and (3) relapse is not usually determined by either service response or response to service. In terms of clinical practice, it appears that idiographic indicators of relapse are often utilized (e.g. deterioration in an aspect of functioning) to infer that a relapse has occurred in the absence of direct evidence of an increase in positive symptoms (Burns, Fiander & Audini, 2000). Unfortunately, no published studies have examined these constructs from the consumers' perspective.

Relapse rates

These conceptual and methodological challenges notwithstanding, some general conclusions can be gleaned from the FEP studies that have prospectively examined relapse rates. First, it is evident that a relatively small proportion of patients relapse during the first year of treatment: 7 of the 11 studies that have reported a 1-year follow up described rates in the range 20% to 36%. This rate is probably sensitive to variations in recruitment and measurement timing: for example, whether only those who fully remit are included and whether relapses are counted from the commencement of treatment or only after full remission is reached.

This minority of patients relapsing in the first year is unfortunately steadily added to by their peers. Eight studies have reported relapse rates at 2-year follow-up, six studies have described 5-year data, three have reported 10-year outcomes and one study has extended to 15 years. Although rates vary, the findings from the majority of the studies fall in the range 40–50% at 2 years. At 5 years, the rates reported have been in the range 70–90%. Two studies have reported on the occurrence of a second relapse by the 5-year follow-up, with rates of 78% and 53%, respectively (Robinson et al., 1999; Scottish Schizophrenia Research Group, 1992). There is some evidence that by 10 years the relapse curve plateaus, with 15% remaining in remission after 9 years in the only 15-year study available (Wiersma et al., 1998).

Interestingly, relapse rates seem to vary across developing and developed countries, with both Leff et al. (1990) and Sartorius et al. (1986) reporting 2-year relapse rates below 40% in developing nation cohorts. Also, the 10-year rate of 78% in a Madras cohort (Thara et al., 1994) appeared more consistent with the 5-year rates obtained from Western industrialized nations.

The reasons for the shape of the relapse curve are unknown and deserving of further study. It is noteworthy that some estimates of the rate of transition (41%) to FEP amongst the ultra-high-risk group of patients over a 1-year period appear higher or are at least comparable with the rate of relapse over the first year after treatment is commenced (Yung et al., 2003). One might speculate that this first-year relapse rate is related to the availability of intensive treatments and greater initial participation in treatment by patients and families, or other protective steps taken by the patient (e.g. avoidance of substance abuse) to reduce their exposure to stress. Perhaps the degree of exposure to risk and the rate of non-adherence with treatment subsequently increases (Robinson et al., 2002). These are hypotheses worthy of investigation as they may assist with enhancing the resilience of patients over the longer term. Comparisons of relapse rates across cohorts have also suggested that relapse rates have remained stable. For example, the 2-year relapse rate of the 1978–1980 first-episode incidence cohort ($n = 82$) did not differ from that of the 1997–1999 cohort ($n = 42$) in the same catchment area in the Netherlands (48% and 53%, respectively) with comparable background incidence rates (1.1 and 1.9 per 10 000, respectively) (Wiersma, 2004; Wiersma et al., 1998).

Factors associated with the risk for relapse

Factors associated with an increased risk for relapse in FEP have been described in detail elsewhere (Gleeson, 2004) and are reviewed here in brief and summarized in Table 19.1. Overall, these variables, including medication non-adherence, substance abuse, stress and life events, early warning signs and premorbid adjustment, do not appear to be specific to FEP patients, although once again there is a considerably smaller number of studies in this group compared with

Table 19.1. Summary of predictors of psychotic relapse following first-episode psychosis

Area	Predictors
Patient-related factors	• Poorer premorbid adjustment • Antisocial personality (positive); agreeableness (negative) • Use of cannabis • Non-adherence to medication • Cognitive flexibility (negative)
Environment-related factors	• Stressful life events • Expressed emotion
Risk factors requiring further research	• Duration of untreated psychosis • Intensive psychosocial interventions (negative) • Variables that mediate response to environmental factors (e.g. coping style) • Amphetamine use • Early warning signs of relapse
Protective factors requiring further research	• Targeted versus continuous medication • Intensive psychosocial treatments alone • Personal resilience

established schizophrenia, and the gaps in knowledge are noteworthy.

Medication non-adherence

Non-compliance to medication is strongly implicated in risk for relapse. One often-cited study indicated a five-fold relapse risk associated with medication discontinuation over a 5-year follow-up period in FEP patients diagnosed with schizophrenia or schizoaffective disorder (Robinson *et al.*, 1999). The study included a rigorous treatment protocol for medication, involving several steps until an a-priori 'treatment response' was achieved. Thereafter, the dose was lowered by up to 50%, and if patients were clinically stable for 1 year they were given the option of discontinuing use of antipsychotic medication. Preliminary results in a recent Dutch 5-year intervention study with 187 FEP patients that examined continuity of care in a

randomized clinical trial showed an increase in relapse from 24% to 40% from 2- to 3-year follow-up. Medication non-adherence was a predictor of relapse (Linszen *et al.*, 2006).

On further analysis, these findings appear inconsistent with results from some other studies that included non-maintenance medication conditions. For example, Gaebel and colleagues (2002) found that there was no statistically significant difference in relapse rates in 115 FEP patients who were treated with continuous maintenance medication or randomized to targeted regimens with additional monitoring and intervention for relapse prodrome symptoms over a 2-year follow-up period. A completed Dutch randomized controlled trial with a follow-up period of 18 months also compared maintenance and targeted treatment (guided discontinuation) strategies (Wunderink *et al.*, 2007). The study was conducted in seven mental healthcare organizations, covering a catchment area of 3.1 million inhabitants, and recruited a sample of 131 remitted FEP patients aged 18 to 45 years and with a diagnosis of schizophrenia or a related psychotic disorder. After 6 months of remission on positive symptoms, they were randomly and openly assigned to a discontinuation strategy or to a maintenance treatment. Maintenance treatment was carried out according to American Psychiatric Association guidelines – preferably using low-dose atypical antipsychotic drugs. The discontinuation strategy was carried out by gradual symptom-guided tapering of dosage and discontinuation, if feasible. Follow-up was 18 months. Main outcome measures were relapse rates and social and vocational functioning.

Twice as many relapses occurred in the discontinuation strategy than the maintenance treatment (43% and 21%, respectively, $p = 0.007$). Of patients who received the strategy, 20% successfully discontinued. Recurrent symptoms caused another 30% to restart antipsychotic treatment, while in the remaining patients discontinuation was not feasible at all. There were no advantages of the discontinuation strategy regarding functional outcome or quality of life. The conclusion was that only a limited number of patients can successfully discontinue therapy. High relapse rates do not allow discontinuation strategy to be universal practice. However, if the relapse risk can be carefully managed by close monitoring, a guided discontinuation strategy may offer a feasible alternative to maintenance treatment in some remitted FEP patients.

Further studies are clearly needed with FEP patients. However, these mixed findings raise questions as to whether continuous maintenance medication is significantly more protective against relapse for all FEP patients compared with other regimens, and also whether background psychosocial treatments may moderate the effects of medication non-compliance upon relapse risk. Further support for this hypothesis also comes from the retrospective reanalysis of the 2-year outcome data from the Soteria Project, which included 179 young patients who were diagnosed with first- or second-episode psychosis. The reanalysis reported on the outcome of the subgroup of 43% of patients who were randomized to the experimental condition, where they did not receive antipsychotic medication but followed an intensive psychosocial programme, including supportive residential care staffed by non-mental health professionals. In a comparison of the experimental condition with traditional treatment within the state hospital system, the experimental strategy had better outcomes, including rates of readmission to hospital (Bola & Mosher, 2002; Fenton et al., 1998).

An additional study of the 2-year outcome of a group of 106 FEP patients compared the 'needs-adapted treatment model' with usual treatment with neuroleptic drugs (Lehtinen et al., 2000). Although both groups received psychosocial treatments, a greater proportion of the experimental group received psychological and family therapies. In addition, 43% of the experimental group did not receive any medication. At the 2-year follow-up, 51% in the experimental group had less than 2 weeks in hospital during the follow-up period, compared with 26% of the control group. Further studies are needed that involve tighter control of background psychosocial treatments and, ideally, randomization to different conditions and measurement of potentially confounding variables, such as comorbid personality disorders or personality traits (Compton et al., 2005; Gleeson et al., 2005b). More evidence is also required regarding the relative risk of non-adherence at different time points throughout the critical period.

Expressed emotion

We have identified 15 prospective follow-up studies in FEP that have examined expressed emotion (EE). Several issues have been of interest to researchers including the stability of EE over the early course, the predictors of EE and the predictive validity of EE in relation to relapse (Chapter 17). At least three studies have reported that EE is not stable over the early course (Leff et al., 1990; Lenior et al., 2002; Patterson, Birchwood & Cochrane, 2000), and others have reported that EE is predicted by relatives' appraisals of the illness and the patient's behaviour, rather than objectively rated symptom severity measures (Heikkila et al., 2002; Raune, Kuipers & Bebbington, 2004).

Patterson, Birchwood & Cochrane (2005) found some support for the hypothesis that EE can best be understood as a reaction to loss. In relation to predicting relapse, the balance of studies now appears to support a positive association, with five studies showing a positive association (Barrelet et al., 1990; Huguelet et al., 1995; Linszen et al., 1997; Nuechterlein, Snyder & Mintz, 1992b; Pourmand, Kavanagh & Vaughan, 2005) while two studies have not shown an association (Macmillan et al., 1986; Stirling et al., 1991). The study by Leff and colleagues (1990) in India only found an association between hostility and relapse but not other components of EE. Unfortunately, there are significantly fewer studies that have examined burden in families of FEP patients (Tennakoon et al., 2000; Wolthaus et al., 2002).

Although the relationship between EE and relapse in early psychosis was initially viewed with caution (Gleeson et al., 1999), subsequent findings have strengthened the likelihood of a positive association. However, it is clear that research is required that tests the hypotheses regarding potential mediating variables in order to improve understanding of the EE–relapse pathway (Nuechterlein et al., 1992b). This is likely to require experimental paradigms that enable the perceptions and reactions of patients to EE to be examined in controlled conditions.

Substance abuse

In our experience, the link between substance abuse and relapse in early psychosis is taken for granted in clinical practice. The assumption underpins psycho-educational materials and has been the basis for interventions to reduce substance use, especially cannabis (Edwards *et al.*, 2003) and amphetamines (Baker & Dawe, 2005). The link appears to be based largely on clinical observation; for example, in relation to cannabis and relapse in FEP, there are only two published studies with prospective follow-up designs (Linszen, Dingemans & Lenior, 1994b; Sorbara *et al.*, 2003).

Linszen and colleagues (1994b) recruited patients with a DSM-IIIR diagnosis of schizophrenia (APA, 1987) to participate in a 15-month treatment programme, with the cannabis study conducted during the outpatient phase of treatment that followed a 3-month hospital admission. Cannabis use was categorized into mild use (between once per week and once per day) and heavy use (more than one cigarette per day). Of 93 participants, 26% met DSM-IIIR criteria for abuse and 54% of these were heavy users. Relapse was recorded in 42% of those diagnosed with abuse compared with 17% of non-abusers over the 12-month follow-up period of the study. Abusers also had a significantly shorter time to relapse. Furthermore, 61% of heavy users had a relapse compared with 18% of mild users, and there was a greater risk of relapse with longer-term previous use.

Sobara and colleagues (2003) described 2-year outcome data on a sample of 58 patients with a mean age of 31.3 years who presented for treatment for the first time with a DSM-IV psychotic disorder (APA, 1994). Although relapse rates were not described, DSM-IV-defined substance misuse or abuse (predominantly cannabis) was associated with a three-fold risk of readmission to hospital over the 2-year period. Importantly, this study controlled for potential confounding variables including medication adherence, age, sex, diagnosis and duration of untreated psychosis (DUP).

Despite the robust findings from these studies, we believe that more studies are required and that a broader range of illicit substances should be studied, particularly amphetamines. Once again, comorbid personality disorders appear to be a potential uncontrolled confounding variable.

Stress and life events

The link between stress and relapse in FEP has been supported by a small group of early studies that measured prospective life events 'independent' of symptoms and beyond the control of the patient. These studies have shown an association between life events and added risk for relapse in the weeks following life events (Bebbington, Wilkens & Jones, 1993; Birley & Brown, 1970; Chung, Langeluddecke & Tennant, 1986; Ventura *et al.*, 1989).

In the 1960s, Birley and Brown (1970) found a higher frequency of 'independent' life events in the 3 weeks prior to hospital admission that indicated greater vulnerability to stress. Two decades later, Nuechterlein *et al.* (1992a) found that the mean number of independent life events (0.8) prior to relapse was higher for medicated participants than for medication-withdrawal relapsing participants (mean, 0.06), which suggested that medication plays a role in increasing the threshold for relapse.

Unfortunately, the role of mediating psychological variables has been rarely studied. Pallanti, Quercioli & Pazzagli (1997) examined the role of coping in mediating the impact of life events in a group of participants with recent-onset psychosis. Patients who relapsed without severe life events during the month before relapse had more subjective complaints and less coping capacity than did relapsing patients with antecedent life events in the month prior to relapse.

In summary, a small number of studies have indicated a correlation between stressful events and heightened risk for relapse, with one available study of patients with recent-onset psychosis suggesting that patients with lower coping capacity may be more prone to relapse in response to stressful events. Alternative methodologies are required to elucidate the interaction of biological and psychological processes. In relation to relapse, this line of enquiry could usefully be informed by recent research examining interactions between personality variables, stress and biological changes (Pruessner *et al.*, 2005).

Early warning signs

Early warning signs of relapse have been identified from a number of retrospective and prospective follow-up studies in schizophrenia and have been discussed in previous reviews (Fitzgerald, 2001). In brief, these studies indicate that it is possible to achieve moderate levels of predictive validity in relation to relapse with specifically designed early warning signs measures in schizophrenia. Use of the Early Warning Signs Scale (Birchwood et al., 1989) achieved moderate positive predictive validity in a FEP cohort, although problems occurred with the rate of false positives (Gleeson et al., 2005a). Further work is required with larger sample sizes, which would allow use of preferred statistical analysis, such as analysis of receiver operator curve characteristics and more complex regression models, which could combine early warning signs with trait and state risk factors.

Personality and premorbid adjustment

The study of personality in relation to outcome in psychosis has followed two somewhat discrete lines of enquiry: the association between premorbid adjustment and outcome, and the association between prospective measurement of personality traits and outcome.

Kane and colleagues (1982) reported significantly worse premorbid adjustment in the subgroup of patients who relapsed compared with those who remained stable over 1 year in their prospective treatment study of first-episode schizophrenia. Specifically, they found significant differences on items that measured the extent of isolation during preadolescence (6 to 13 years) and adolescence (14 to 20 years). More recently, Robinson et al. (1999) reported that patients with poor premorbid adaptation to school and premorbid social withdrawal, as measured by the Premorbid Adjustment Scale (Cannon-Spoor, Potkin & Wyatt, 1982), relapsed earlier.

The relationship between personality traits and course of psychosis has been a limited field of enquiry. Dingemans, Lenior & Linszen (1998) examined the impact of a personality disorder diagnosis and clinical outcome and reported an increased risk of relapse in a prospective follow-up study of 93 first-episode adolescent patients who scored relatively high on measures of axis II antisocial personality disorder traits (APA, 1994). More recently, a significant association between lower levels of agreeableness and higher neuroticism and risk of relapse has been reported (Gleeson et al., 2005b). When premorbid adjustment was controlled for, the effect of agreeableness, but not neuroticism, remained significant. It is speculated that lower agreeableness may be related to stress-eliciting interpersonal patterns. There is some evidence that personality variables in FEP may be associated with greater frequency of dependent life events (i.e. life events that are influenced by an individual's behaviour, excluding events directly affected by psychotic symptoms) (Horan et al., 2005). This work could be expanded to examine other trait variables related to personality, including schema and cognitive biases such as jumping to conclusions and source monitoring (Garety, Hemsley & Wessely, 1991), which may be associated with the reoccurrence of specific symptoms or symptom combinations. Personal resilience to relapse has not been studied in early psychosis to our knowledge. Perhaps a starting point would be to undertake retrospective research with the minority of those diagnosed with schizophrenia remaining relapse free by 5 and 10 years after their initial treatment response.

Cognitive deficits

There is no doubt that cognitive deficits (e.g. verbal memory, executive functioning) are often found in schizophrenia. The only study that has investigated the predictive value of cognition at onset on relapse rates found no significant effect (Robinson et al., 1999). In a 2-year follow-up of 103 FEP patients (Holthausen et al., 2007), cognitive performance at inclusion did not predict the number of relapses during follow-up. However, selective attention and verbal fluency were significant predictors for time spent in a psychotic phase and verbal fluency was also a significant predictor for time in full remission. Chen and colleagues (2005) reported that perseverative errors on the Wisconsin Card Sorting Test – indicative of reduced cognitive flexibility – were associated with an increased risk (odds ratio, 2.4) of relapse over a 3-year follow-up period amongst a cohort of 93 FEP patients diagnosed with schizophrenia-spectrum psychosis.

Duration of untreated psychosis

The concept of DUP is well known in FEP research and clinical practice because of its positive correlations with the probability of reaching remission and time to remission (Marshall *et al.*, 2005; Perkins *et al.*, 2005).

However, findings regarding DUP and relapse are mixed. Reviewers have often cited a study by May *et al.* (1976), which included 288 participants with schizophrenia recruited between 1959 and 1962 at their first admission. Patients were randomized to five treatment groups including (1) individual psychotherapy, (2) stelazine only, (3) individual psychotherapy plus stelazine, (4) electroconvulsive therapy and (5) a comparison milieu group who received none of the above. Importantly, in terms of the analysis of DUP, the 48 treatment failures from the psychotherapy and comparison group were later given antipsychotic medication and group therapy.

Follow-up-data indicated that the drug therapy group continued to do better on clinical and other outcome measures up to 3 years after the randomization to treatment. The authors concluded that the drug therapy group had a reduced length of stay initially – an advantage that persisted in terms of days in hospital 4 years from the date of first admission, or 3 years after discharge. Patients who initially received drug therapy tended to be admitted less and for shorter periods. Shortcomings of the study included the subjective ratings of clinicians, the exclusion of quick remitters and readmission as an indicator of psychotic relapse. We know of five prospective correlational FEP studies of DUP and relapse that have been published since the May *et al.* (1976) study, with mixed results (e.g. Johnstone *et al.*, 1986; Robinson *et al.*, 1999).

In summary, despite a growing interest in the relationship between DUP and clinical outcome in FEP, its relationship with relapse remains unresolved, and the existing findings are equivocal. Methodological problems abound, particularly problems with distinguishing duration of untreated illness from DUP and lack of objective rating instruments with a-priori definitions for psychotic relapse.

The prevention of relapse in first-episode psychosis

In schizophrenia, both pharmacological (Gilbert *et al.*, 1995) and psychosocial interventions (Pilling *et al.*, 2002) for the prevention of relapse have been supported in published reviews and meta-analyses. Furthermore, health economic analyses have indicated quadrupled costs associated with failure to prevent relapse (Almond *et al.*, 2004). Below, the status of specific evidence for the prevention of relapse following FEP is examined.

Relapse and antipsychotic medication

A number of trials of antipsychotic medication have measured relapse rates as a clinical outcome. This group of studies has been principally concerned with the following questions. Is maintenance antipsychotic medication for early psychosis more efficacious than placebo in the prevention of relapse? Is maintenance medication superior to targeted medication in preventing relapse? What is the effect on relapse rates of medication withdrawal following stabilization after the first episode? What is the relative effectiveness of newer atypical neuroleptic drugs in the prevention of relapse?

It should be emphasized that almost no studies have controlled for background psychosocial interventions and the overall service model, which makes it difficult to generalize across studies. This is particularly salient because the findings from the Lambeth Early Onset Programme suggested superior outcomes in relation to readmission when patients were randomized to a first-episode service compared with service as usual (Power *et al.*, 2004).

The surprisingly small evidence base in FEP has supported the superiority of antipsychotic medication over placebo treatments for the prevention of relapse, particularly during the first year of treatment (Crow *et al.*, 1986; Kane *et al.*, 1982). Discontinuation has been associated with significantly elevated relapse rates (Gitlin *et al.*, 2001; Robinson *et al.*, 1999), although the decision regarding discontinuation is a complex one (Nuechterlein, Gitlin & Subotnik, 1995) and other recent findings have indicated that targeted treatment does not necessarily lead to deterioration in psychopathology, functioning or quality of life – at least for a portion of patients (Wunderink *et al.*, 2007). In brief, more studies are required with randomization to varying durations of maintenance after stabilization together with controls for background psychosocial treatments.

The comparison of newer antipsychotic drugs with typical agents has only been addressed relatively recently. The large multicentre trial of Schooler and colleagues (2005) reported that 42% of patients randomized to a risperidone group experienced a relapse compared with 55% in the haloperidol group, and the median time to relapse was 466 days for risperidone-treated subjects and 205 days for those given haloperidol. However, the overall relapse rates appeared to be at the high end of the expected range, which might be explained by their use of a somewhat inclusive definition of relapse (Csernansky, Mahmoud & Brenner, 2002), which included deliberate self-injury, clinically significant suicidal or homicidal ideation, and violent behaviour.

In conclusion, the current evidence supports the effectiveness of antipsychotic agents in the prevention of relapse in FEP. Open questions include the optimal length of follow-up treatment, whether continual maintenance medication is superior to targeted approaches in FEP in the same way as in schizophrenia and whether equivalent relapse rates can be achieved in the absence of medication in a subgroup of patients by using optimal intensive psychosocial interventions alone.

Individual psychological interventions

Specific individual relapse-prevention therapy for FEP, in the absence of additional family therapy, has not been described in the literature, but relapse has been a dependent variable within the scarce psychosocial and psychotherapeutic trials, discussed above. Nonetheless, individual relapse-prevention therapies have been described for schizophrenia, including monitoring for early warning signs with targeted CBT

interventions (Birchwood & Spencer, 2001; Gumley *et al.*, 2003; Herz *et al.*, 2000; J. Arends, C.J. Slooff, D. Wiersma, M. van den Gaag & R.J. van den Bosch, unpublished data). Specific trials of CBT for relapse prevention in FEP are warranted, bearing in mind that identification of early warning signs may be more problematic because there are fewer retrospective clinical data to guide assessment of idiographic early warning signs. This gap could be filled by prospective investigations of ultra-high-risk patients that extend beyond their transition to psychosis to encompass their first relapse.

Family interventions for relapse prevention

Individual family interventions have been based upon the behavioural family tradition in schizophrenia (Falloon & Lillie, 1988; Mueser & Glynn, 1999), with the aim of modifying the communication patterns of high-EE relatives towards the patient. The typical components of these interventions include comprehensive communication skills training and structured learning in the problem-solving model (Ch. 17).

In short, the limited family-based interventions are varied in composition and in the comparison condition. Zhang *et al.* (1994), for example, compared family-based interventions with standard outpatient follow-up and showed positive outcomes in relation to admission rates over an 18-month follow-up period for the intervention group. However, comparison of an individual-orientated psychosocial programme with the identical programme plus a family intervention did not demonstrate additional benefits in terms of relapse rates over an 18-month period (Linszen *et al.*, 1996). Linszen and colleagues concluded that family therapies may need to be carefully targeted to specific families, and that an initial focus upon psychoeducation and emotional support may be more appropriate.

McFarlane has pioneered the development of multi-family work in schizophrenia, which has been provided as an alternative to both individual family therapy and individual case management. The approach utilizes the collective support and problem-solving resources of the group to address individual family concerns. Recently, the intervention has been modified for prodromal and early psychosis, with lowered relapse rates reported (McFarlane *et al.*, 2003).

We would encourage the development and evaluation of longer-term sustainable approaches for family members, including the use of technology such as the Internet and email support based on a coaching model (Vale *et al.*, 2003). This may be preferable for some family members as they strive to maintain work routines and may be more compatible with their preference for a more self-sufficient coping style.

At the Early Psychosis Prevention and Intervention Centre (EPPIC), a study entitled EPISODE II has been completed. It was funded by an independent research grant from Eli Lilly via the Lilly Melbourne Academic Psychiatry consortium. This study compares combined and parallel family and individual CBT with standard EPPIC follow-up care (Gleeson, 2005; Gleeson *et al.*, 2008a, b). Participants were recruited from November 2003 until May 2005, with a total of 82 providing consent to be randomized into the study. The treatment phase of the study concluded in January 2006. The individual therapy incorporated many of the

components of relapse prevention from schizophrenia trials, including a focus upon identification of early warning signs, but also contained additional interventions for other risk factors, including cannabis abuse and personality factors. The family intervention dovetailed with the individual therapy in joint sessions, usually during the final phase. Initial outcome results are in press (Gleeson *et al.*, 2008b) and the research team is currently analyzing the final outcome data.

Recommendations regarding relapse prevention in first-episode psychosis

Despite the disconcerting gaps in evidence regarding effective interventions for relapse prevention in FEP, research findings and clinical expertise can generate several recommendations for relapse prevention in FEP, which are summarized in Table 19.2. First, it is important to consider the timing of relapse-prevention interventions, with both the patient and their relatives. Response to treatment should be carefully monitored

Table 19.2. Summary of relapse-prevention guidelines in first-episode psychosis

Guidelines	Components
Guiding principles	• Relapse prevention should be a major priority of the treatment team once symptoms have remitted for 1 month or longer
	• The goal of relapse prevention should be integrated with ongoing goals of the recovery phase, including treatment of comorbid conditions and return to work/ school/ recreational pursuits; the young person should be assisted to strike a balance between relapse prevention and quality of life
	• Relapse-prevention interventions should ideally involve both the young person and their family
Specific interventions	
Assessment	• Develop an individualized relapse-risk formulation based on thorough history taking and the known risk factors from research
Medication	• After 6 months to 1 year of uncomplicated remission, consider a trial off antipsychotic medication
	• Consider targeted medication as an alternative strategy where engagement is good and where there is a shared understanding of early warning signs
Individual interventions	• Identify potential early warning signs based on review of prodrome phase
	• Consider motivational interviewing for non-adherence and substance abuse where indicated
	• Cognitive–behavioural interventions for coping with stressful life events
Family interventions	• Allow opportunities for emotional support, with a focus upon grief, loss and burden
	• Psychoeducation regarding risks of relapse
	• Where indicated, include specific sessions for communication skills training and problem-solving training

over the early recovery phase, and if symptoms persist then the focus should remain on acute treatment and then prevention of treatment-resistant psychosis.

Once symptoms have remained at a mild level of severity for 1 month or longer, we would argue that it is appropriate to increase the emphasis in treatment upon secondary prevention, bearing in mind that comorbid syndromes may require ongoing active treatment with both biological and psychosocial interventions. We believe that this is best achieved within specialist FEP services or teams, where the case-management system needs to be flexible in integrating attention to the long-term goal of relapse prevention with shorter-term goals, such as return to study or work. The case vignette of Moira illustrates the kind of flexibility that is required in some cases.

Case vignette: Moira

Moira is a 17-year-old girl. At admission to EPPIC, she lived with her mother, who had a long-standing history of schizophrenia and heroin dependence. Moira developed depressive symptoms at age 14, which subsequently evolved into an episode of psychosis 2 years previously. She has a history of emotional neglect and long-standing behavioural and adjustment problems at school. She commenced using cannabis on a daily basis at age 16. Relapse prevention, one of several treatment priorities, commenced with negotiating alternative supported accommodation arrangements for Moira. Psychoeducation and motivational interviewing, along with basic behavioural strategies regarding cannabis abuse and medication adherence, were also major priorities. Individual work with Moira focused on attempting to increase her awareness of her pattern of placing herself in situations where she was at risk of abuse and exploitation – a risk for relapse and other negative outcomes.

Once remission has been established, we would encourage clinicians to conceptualize an additional assessment phase based upon the risk factors for relapse outlined above. The goal, in our opinion, is to work with the patient and the family in developing an idiographic relapse-risk formulation, considering their level of awareness of psychosis, their attitudes and adherence to treatment, their coping and interpersonal patterns, substance abuse and their exposure to ongoing interpersonal conflict and other stress. Resilience factors, such as social support, can also be incorporated into the formulation. Psychoeducation is critical during this stage to alert the family and the individual to the risks of relapse, as illustrated in the case vignette of Geoff. In our experience this is often dealt with superficially, or is information which is not integrated by the family and the young person. Communicating hope is, of course, critical by emphasizing the preventive benefits of active self-management.

Case vignette: Geoff

Geoff, a 23-year-old brick-layer, presented to EPPIC a year ago with a 6-month history of gradually worsening depressive symptoms and psychotic symptoms, characterized by paranoid beliefs regarding his neighbours and frequent auditory hallucinations. His symptoms remitted over a 4-month period of outpatient treatment, which followed a 2-week admission to hospital after an overdose. He lived at home with his parents, who were actively involved with his treatment. Relapse prevention, undertaken by his case manager and outpatient psychiatrist, initially focused upon increasing the understanding of the risks for relapse. After work-related demands were jointly identified as a potential risk for relapse, individual sessions with Geoff included CBT to encourage a widening of his coping skills at work. Potential early warning signs were assessed and an action plan was jointly devised with his parents' involvement.

In the light of the existing scarce data, we would concur with treatment guidelines stipulating that, if a rapid and uncomplicated remission is achieved early in the course of treatment, as in the example of Geoff, and is maintained after 1 year of maintenance treatment (or at least 6 months), with patients showing (1) insight into their illness, (2) an understanding of likely prodromal signs and (3) abstinence from cannabis and amphetamines, then a period of medication withdrawal should be considered with the patient, balancing the decision against known risk factors for relapse.

We would assert that a balance is needed between vigilance for early signs of relapse and 'space' to recover and resume the challenges of normal development, which, in practice, might mean that some patients who have made a good remission on positive symptoms of psychosis may experiment with earlier periods off medication. In these cases, we would argue for the fall-back option of targeted medication regimens, bearing in mind that this is reliant upon a positive therapeutic alliance in order to enable regular and collaborative monitoring of early warning signs of relapse, and upon an appropriate skill level amongst the treating team in order to institute targeted CBT interventions. We would also encourage further studies to evaluate this option.

In relation to psychosocial interventions, we would emphasize the integration of individual and family-based interventions. Once a shared, written formulation has been developed, potential early warning signs of relapse and an associated relapse-prevention plan can be developed with the additional assistance of the family. Selective attention needs to be given to non-adherence to treatment, substance abuse, stressful life events and comorbid anxiety and depression, as also illustrated in the case vignette of Moira.

Traditional family CBT for schizophrenia can be the basis for family interventions; however, we think more careful tailoring is required, with greater emphasis upon issues of burden and grief, and psychoeducation regarding relapse and its prevention. In our opinion, problem-solving and communication skills should be introduced selectively – where it can be established that families are more consistently stuck within problematic communication patterns.

Further research and conclusions

Psychotic relapse results in an obvious human and economic cost. Unfortunately, significant gaps remain in the knowledge base required to address this impact, which includes a scant understanding of the mechanisms of relapse, and a paucity of data to guide critical clinical decisions, such as the optimal timing of medication discontinuation. This means that the research efforts in relation to relapse prevention in FEP need to be significantly increased, alongside efforts at increasing remission rates and reducing response times.

The evidence highlights that relapse rates are high although a small minority appears not to relapse over the long term. At this stage, long-term follow-up is indicated to prevent relapse, even in those with good prognosis, and an integrated approach to treatment is strongly recommended. Further significant innovations are required before we can confidently claim, for the next generation of FEP patients and their family members, that we can prevent relapse. Ultimately, the most effective interventions are likely to be based on a significantly improved understanding of psychotic relapse. Finally, we would encourage that relapse prevention itself needs to be kept in perspective, as one means to the large end of improving quality of life and independence for patients and families.

REFERENCES

Almond, S., Knapp, M., Francois, C., Toumi, M. & Brugha, T. (2004). Relapse in schizophrenia: costs, clinical outcomes and quality of life. *British Journal of Psychiatry*, **184**, 346–51.

APA (1987). *Diagnostic and Statistical Manual of Mental Disorders*, 3rd edn revised. Washington, DC: American Psychiatric Press.

APA (1994). *Diagnostic and Statistical Manual of Mental Disorders*, 4th edn. Washington, DC: American Psychiatric Press.

Andreasen, N. C., Carpenter, W. T. Jr, Kane, J. M. *et al.* (2005). Remission in schizophrenia: proposed criteria and rationale for consensus. *American Journal of Psychiatry*, **162**, 441–9.

Baker, A. & Dawe, S. (2005). Amphetamine use and co-occurring psychological problems: review of the literature and implications for treatment. *Australian Psychologist*, **40**, 88–95.

Barrelet, L., Ferrero, F., Szigethy, L., Giddey, C. & Pellizzer, G. (1990). Expressed emotion and first-admission schizophrenia: nine month follow-up in a French cultural environment. *British Journal of Psychiatry*, **156**, 357–62.

Bebbington, P., Wilkens, S. & Jones, P. (1993). Life events and psychosis. *British Journal of Psychiatry*, **162**, 72–9.

Birchwood, M. (1999). Early intervention in psychosis: the critical period. In P. D. McGorry & H. J. Jackson (eds.), *The Recognition and Management of Early Psychosis: A Preventive Approach*. New York: Cambridge University Press, pp. 226–64.

Birchwood, M. & Spencer, E. (2001). Early intervention in psychotic relapse. *Clinical Psychology Review Special Issue: Psychosis*, **21**, 1211–26.

Birchwood, M., Smith, J., Macmillan, F. *et al.* (1989). Predicting relapse in schizophrenia: the development of an early signs monitoring system using patients and families as observers, a preliminary investigation. *Psychological Medicine*, **19**, 649–56.

Birley, J. L. T. & Brown, G. W. (1970). Crises and life changes preceding the onset or relapse of acute schizophrenia. *British Journal of Psychiatry*, **116**, 327–33.

Bola, J. R. & Mosher, L. R. (2002). At issue: predicting drug-free treatment response in acute psychosis from the Soteria project. *Schizophrenia Bulletin*, **28**, 559–75.

Burns, T., Fiander, M. & Audini, B. (2000). A Delphi approach to characterising 'relapse' as used in UK clinical practice. *International Journal of Social Psychiatry*, **46**, 220–30.

Cannon-Spoor, H. E., Potkin, S. G. & Wyatt, R. J. (1982). Measurement of premorbid adjustment in chronic schizophrenia. *Schizophrenia Bulletin*, **8**, 470–84.

Chen, E. Y.-H., Hui, C. L.-M., Dunn, E. L.-W. *et al.* (2005). A prospective 3-year longitudinal study of cognitive predictors of relapse in first-episode schizophrenic patients. *Schizophrenia Research*, **77**, 99–104.

Chung, R. K., Langeluddecke, P. & Tennant, C. (1986). Threatening life events in the onset of schizophrenia, schizophreniform psychosis and hypomania. *British Journal of Psychiatry*, **148**, 680–5.

Compton, M. T., Rudisch, B. E., Weiss, P. S., West, J. C. & Kaslow, N. J. (2005). Predictors of psychiatrist-reported treatment-compliance problems among patients in routine US psychiatric care. *Psychiatry Research*, **137**, 29–36.

Crow, T. J., Macmillan, J. F., Johnston, A. L. & Johnstone, E. C. (1986). The Northwick Park study of first episodes of schizophrenia II. A randomized controlled trial of prophylactic neuroleptic treatment. *British Journal of Psychiatry*, **148**, 120–7.

Csernansky, J. G., Mahmoud, R. & Brenner, R. (2002). A comparison of risperidone and haloperidol for the prevention of relapse in patients with schizophrenia. *New England Journal of Medicine*, **346**, 16–22.

Dingemans, P. M. A. J., Lenior, M. E. & Linszen, D. H. (1998). Personality and schizophrenia relapse. *International Clinical Psychopharmacology*, **13**(Suppl 1), S89–95.

Edwards, J. & McGorry, P. D. (2002). *Implementing Early Intervention in Psychosis: A Guide to Establishing Early Psychosis Services*. London: Martin Dunitz.

Edwards, J., Hinton, M., Elkins, K. & Athanasopolous, O. (2003). Cannabis abuse and first-episode psychosis. In H. L. Graham, A. Copello, M. Birchwood & K. T. Mueser (eds.), *Substance Misuse in Psychosis: Approaches to Treatment and Service Delivery*. Chichester, UK: John Wiley, pp. 283–304.

Falloon, I. R. (1983). Relapse in schizophrenia: a review of the concept and its definitions. *Psychological Medicine*, **13**, 469–77.

Falloon, I. R. & Lillie, F. J. (1988). Behavioral family therapy: an overview. In I. R. Falloon (ed.), *Handbook of Behavioral Family Therapy*. New York: Guilford Press, pp. 3–26.

Fenton, W. S., Mosher, L. R., Herrell, J. M. & Blyler, C. R. (1998). Randomized trial of general hospital and residential alternative care for patients with severe and persistent mental illness. *American Journal of Psychiatry*, **155**, 516–22.

Fitzgerald, P. B. (2001). The role of early warning symptoms in the detection and prevention of relapse in schizophrenia. *Australian and New Zealand Journal of Psychiatry*, **35**, 758–64.

Gaebel, W., Jaenner, M., Frommann, N. *et al.* (2002). First vs multiple episode schizophrenia: two-year outcome of intermittent and maintenance medication strategies. *Schizophrenia Research*, **53**, 145–59.

Garety, P. A., Hemsley, D. R. & Wessely, S. (1991). Reasoning in deluded schizophrenic and paranoid patients: biases in performance on a probabilistic inference task. *Journal of Nervous and Mental Disease*, **179**, 194–201.

Gilbert, P. L., Harris, M. J., McAdams, L. & Jeste, D. V. (1995). Neuroleptic withdrawal in schizophrenic patients: a review of the literature. *Archives of General Psychiatry*, **52**, 173–88.

Gitlin, M., Nuechterlein, K., Subotnik, K. L. *et al.* (2001). Clinical outcome following neuroleptic discontinuation in patients with remitted recent-onset schizophrenia. *American Journal of Psychiatry*, **158**, 1835–42.

Gleeson, J. F. (2004). The first psychotic relapse: understanding the risks and the opportunities for prevention. In J. F. Gleeson & P. McGorry (eds.), *Psychological Interventions in Early Psychosis: A Treatment Handbook*. Chichester, UK: John Wiley, pp. 157–74.

Gleeson, J. F. (2005). Preventing EPISODE II: relapse prevention in first-episode psychosis. *Australasian Psychiatry*, **13**, 384–7.

Gleeson, J. F., Jackson, H. J., Stavely, H. & Burnett, P. (1999). Family intervention in early psychosis. In P. D. McGorry & H. J. Jackson (eds.), *The Recognition and Management of Early Psychosis: A Preventive Approach*. New York: Cambridge University Press, pp. 376–406.

Gleeson, J. F., Rawlings, D., Jackson, H. J. & McGorry, P. D. (2005a). Early warning signs of relapse following a first episode of psychosis. *Schizophrenia Research*, **180**, 107–11.

Gleeson, J. F., Rawlings, D., Jackson, H. J. & McGorry, P. D. (2005b). Agreeableness and neuroticism as predictors of relapse after first-episode psychosis: a prospective follow-up study. *Journal of Nervous and Mental Disease*, **193**, 160–9.

Gleeson, J. F., Wade, D., Castle, D. *et al.* (2008a). The Episode II trial of cognitive and family therapy for relapse prevention in early psychosis: rationale and sample characteristics. *Journal of Mental Health*, **17**, 19–32.

Glesson, J. F., Cotton, S., Alvarez-Jimenez, M. *et al.* (2008b). An RCT of relapse prevention therapy for first-episode psychosis patients. *Journal of Clinical Psychiatry*, in press.

Gumley, A., O'Grady, M., McNay, L. *et al.* (2003). Early intervention for relapse in schizophrenia: results of a 12-month randomized controlled trial of cognitive behavioural therapy. *Psychological Medicine*, **33**, 419–31.

Heikkila, J., Karlsson, H., Taiminen, T. *et al.* (2002). Expressed emotion is not associated with disorder severity in first-episode mental disorder. *Psychiatry Research*, **111**, 155–65.

Herz, M. I., Lamberti, J. S., Mintz, J. *et al.* (2000). A program for relapse prevention in schizophrenia: a controlled study. *Archives of General Psychiatry*, **57**, 277–83.

Holthausen, E. A. E., Wiersma, D., Cahn W. *et al.* (2007). Predictive value of cognition for different domains of outcome in recent-onset schizophrenia. *Psychiatry Research*, **149**, 71–80.

Horan, W. P., Subotnik, K. L., Reise, S. P., Ventura, J. & Nuechterlein, K. H. (2005). Stability and clinical correlates of personality characteristics in recent-onset schizophrenia. *Psychological Medicine*, **35**, 995–1005.

Huguelet, P., Favre, S., Binyet, S., Gonzalez, C. & Zabala, I. (1995). The use of the Expressed Emotion Index as a predictor of outcome in first admitted schizophrenic patients in a French speaking area of Switzerland. *Acta Psychiatrica Scandinavica*, **92**, 447–52.

Johnstone, E. C., Crow, T. J., Johnston, A. L. & Macmillan, J. F. (1986). The Northwick Park study of first episodes of schizophrenia I. Presentation of the illness and problems relating to admission. *British Journal of Psychiatry*, **148**, 115–20.

Kane, J. M., Rifkin, A., Quitkin, F., Nayak, D. & Ramos-Lorenzi, J. (1982). Fluphenazine versus placebo in patients with remitted, acute first-episode schizophrenia. *Archives of General Psychiatry*, **39**, 70–3.

Leff, J., Wig, N. N., Bedi, H. *et al.* (1990). Relatives' expressed emotion and the course of schizophrenia in Chandigarh: a 2-year follow-up of a 1st-contact sample. *British Journal of Psychiatry*, **156**, 351–6.

Lehman, A. F., Kreyenbuhl, J., Buchanan, R. W. *et al.* (2004). The Schizophrenia Patient Outcomes Research Team (PORT): updated treatment recommendations 2003. *Schizophrenia Bulletin*, **30**, 193–217.

Lehtinen, V., Aaltonen, J., Koffert, T., Räkköläinen, V. & Syvälahti, E. (2000). Two-year outcome in first-episode psychosis treated according to an integrated model. Is immediate neuroleptisation always needed? *European Psychiatry*, **15**, 312–20.

Lenior, M. E., Dingemans, P. M. A. J., Schene, A. H., Hart, A. A. M. & Linszen, D. H. (2002). The course of parental expressed emotion and psychotic episodes after family intervention in recent-onset schizophrenia. A longitudinal study. *Schizophrenia Research*, **57**, 183–90.

Linszen, D. H., Dingemans, P. M., Lenior, M. E. *et al.* (1994a). Relapse criteria in schizophrenic disorders: different perspectives. *Psychiatry Research*, **54**, 273–81.

Linszen, D. H., Dingemans, P. M. & Lenior, M. E. (1994b). Cannabis abuse and the course of recent-onset schizophrenic disorders. *Archives of General Psychiatry*, **51**, 273–9.

Linszen, D. H., Dingemans, P., van der Does, J. W. *et al.* (1996). Treatment, expressed emotion and relapse in recent onset schizophrenic disorders. *Psychological Medicine*, **26**, 333–42.

Linszen, D. H., Dingemans, P. M., Nugter, M. A. *et al.* (1997). Patient attributes and expressed emotion as risk factors for psychotic relapse. *Schizophrenia Bulletin*, **23**, 119–30.

Linszen, D. H., Lenior, M., de Haan, L., Dingemans, P. & Gersons, B. (1998). Early intervention, untreated psychosis and the course of early schizophrenia. *British Journal of Psychiatry*, **172**(Suppl 33), s84–9.

Linszen, D. H., de Haan, L., Dingemans P. M. & Wouters, L. (2006). Can long-term critical period interventions in the early phase of schizophrenia-like disorders prevent deterioration? *Schizophrenia Research*, **81**(Suppl 6), 8.

Macmillan, J. F., Gold, A., Crow, T. J., Johnson, A. L. & Johnstone, E. C. (1986). The Northwick Park study of 1st episodes of schizophrenia. 4. Expressed emotion and relapse. *British Journal of Psychiatry*, **148**, 133–43.

Marshall, M., Lewis, S., Lockwood, A. *et al.* (2005). Association between duration of untreated psychosis and in cohorts of first-episode outcome patients: a systematic review. *Archives of General Psychiatry*, **62**, 975–83.

May, P., Tuma, A., Yale, C., Potepan, P. & Dixon, W. (1976). Schizophrenia: a follow-up study of the results of five forms of treatment. *Archives of General Psychiatry*, **33**, 776–84.

McFarlane, W. R., Dixon, L., Lukens, E. & Lucksted, A. (2003). Family psychoeducation and schizophrenia: a review of the literature. *Journal of Marital and Family Therapy*, **29**, 223–45.

McGorry, P. (2005). Royal Australian and New Zealand College of Psychiatrists clinical practice guidelines for the treatment of schizophrenia and related disorders. *Australian and New Zealand Journal of Psychiatry*, **39**, 1–30.

Mueser, K. T. & Glynn, S. M. (1999). *Behavioral Family Therapy for Psychiatric Disorders*, 2nd edn. Oakland, CA: New Harbinger.

NICE (2002). *Schizophrenia: Core Interventions in the Treatment and Management of Schizophrenia in Primary and Secondary Care. [Clinical Guideline 1]*. London: National Institute for Health and Clinical Excellence.

Nuechterlein, K. H., Dawson, M. E., Gitlin, M. *et al.* (1992a). Developmental processes in schizophrenic disorders: longitudinal studies of vulnerability and stress. *Schizophrenia Bulletin*, **18**, 387–424.

Nuechterlein, K. H., Snyder, K. S. & Mintz, J. (1992b). Paths to relapse: possible transactional processes connecting patient illness onset, expressed emotion, and psychotic relapse. *British Journal of Psychiatry*, **161**(Suppl 18), s88–96.

Nuechterlein, K. H., Gitlin, M. J. & Subotnik, K. L. (1995). The early course of schizophrenia and long-term maintenance neuroleptic therapy. *Archives of General Psychiatry*, **52**, 203–5.

Pallanti, S., Quercioli, L. & Pazzagli, A. (1997). Relapse in young paranoid schizophrenic patients: a prospective study of stressful life events, P300 measures, and coping. *American Journal of Psychiatry*, **154**, 792–8.

Patterson, P., Birchwood, M. & Cochrane, R. (2000). Preventing the entrenchment of high expressed emotion in first episode psychosis: early developmental attachment pathways. *Australian and New Zealand Journal of Psychiatry*, **34**(Suppl), S191–7.

Patterson, P., Birchwood, M. & Cochrane, R. (2005). Expressed emotion as an adaptation to loss: prospective study in first-episode psychosis. *British Journal of Psychiatry*, **187** (Suppl), s59–64.

Perkins, O. D., Gu, H., Boteva, K. & Lieberman, J. A. (2005). Relationship between duration of untreated psychosis and outcome in first-episode schizophrenia: a critical review and meta-analysis. *American Journal of Psychiatry*, **162**, 1785–804.

Pilling, S., Bebbington, P., Kuipers, E. *et al.* (2002). Psychological treatments in schizophrenia: I. Meta-analysis of family intervention and cognitive behaviour therapy. *Psychological Medicine*, **32**, 763–82.

Pourmand, D., Kavanagh, D. J. & Vaughan, K. (2005). Expressed emotion as predictor of relapse in patients with comorbid psychoses and substance use disorder. *Australian and New Zealand Journal of Psychiatry*, **39**, 473–8.

Power, P., Iacoponi, E., Russell, M. *et al.* (2004). A randomised controlled trial of an early detection team in first-episode psychosis: provisional findings of the LEO CAT study. *Schizophrenia Research*, **70**(Suppl 1), 131.

Pruessner, J. C., Baldwin, M. W., Dedovic, K. *et al.* (2005). Self-esteem, locus of control, hippocampal volume, and cortisol regulation in young and old adulthood. *Neuroimage*, **28**, 815–26.

Raune, D., Kuipers, E. & Bebbington, P. E. (2004). Expressed emotion at first-episode psychosis: investigating a carer appraisal model. *British Journal of Psychiatry*, **184**, 321–6.

Robinson, D. G., Woerner, M. G., Alvir, J. M. J. *et al.* (1999). Predictors of relapse following response from a first episode of schizophrenia or schizoaffective disorder. *Archives of General Psychiatry*, **56**, 241–7.

Robinson, D. G., Woerner, M. G., Alvir, J. M. J. *et al.* (2002). Predictors of medication discontinuation by patients with first-episode schizophrenia and schizoaffective disorder. *Schizophrenia Research*, **57**, 209–19.

Sartorius, N., Jablensky, A., Korten, A. *et al.* (1986). Early manifestations and first-contact incidence of schizophrenia in different cultures: a preliminary report on the initial evaluation phase of the WHO Collaborative Study on Determinants of Outcome of Severe Mental Disorders. *Psychological Medicine*, **16**, 909–28.

Schooler, N., Rabinowitz, J., Davidson, M. *et al.* (2005). Risperidone and haloperidol in first-episode psychosis: a long-term randomized trial. *American Journal of Psychiatry*, **162**, 947–53.

Scottish Schizophrenia Research Group (1992). The Scottish first episode schizophrenia study VIII. Five year follow-up: clinical and psychosocial findings. *British Journal of Psychiatry*, **161**, 496–500.

Sorbara, F., Liraud, F., Assens, F., Abalan, F. & Verdoux, H. (2003). Substance use and the course of early psychosis: a 2-year follow-up of first-admitted subjects. *European Psychiatry*, **18**, 133–6.

Stirling, J., Tantam, D., Thomas, P. *et al.* (1991). Expressed emotion and early onset schizophrenia: a one year follow-up. *Psychological Medicine*, **21**, 675–85.

Tennakoon, L., Fannon, D., Doku, V. *et al.* (2000). Experience of caregiving: relatives of people experiencing a first episode of psychosis. *British Journal of Psychiatry*, **177**, 529–33.

Thara, R., Henrietta, M., Joseph, A., Rajkumar, S. & Eaton, W. W. (1994). Ten-year course of schizophrenia: the Madras longitudinal study. *Acta Psychiatrica Scandinavica*, **90**, 329–36.

Trimbos Institute (2005). *Multidisciplinary Guideline: Schizophrenia. Guidelines for Diagnosis, Organization of Care and Treatment of Adult People with Schizophrenia*. Utrecht: Trimbos Institute.

Vale, M. J., Jelinek, M. V., Best, J. D. *et al.* (2003). Coaching patients on achieving cardiovascular health (COACH): a multicenter randomized trial in patients with coronary heart disease. *Archives of Internal Medicine*, **163**, 2775–83.

Ventura, J., Nuechterlein, K. H., Lukoff, D. & Hardesty, J. (1989). A prospective study of stressful life events and schizophrenic relapse. *Journal of Abnormal Psychology*, **98**, 407–11.

Wiersma, D. (2004). The short and longer term course of psychoses. In *Proceedings of the Geestkracht Symposium on*

Vulnerability and Resilience in First-Episode Psychoses, University Medical Center Utrecht, the Netherlands, June 2004.

Wiersma, D., Nienhuis, F. J., Sloof, C. J. & Giel, R. (1998). Natural course of schizophrenic disorders: a 15-year follow-up of a Dutch incidence cohort. *Schizophrenia Bulletin*, **24**, 75–85.

Wolthaus, J. E. D., Dingemans, P. M. A. J., Schene, A. H. *et al.* (2002). Caregiver burden in recent-onset schizophrenia and spectrum disorders: the influence of symptoms and personality traits. *Journal of Nervous and Mental Disease*, **190**, 241–7.

Wunderink, A., Nienhuis, F. J., Sytema, S. *et al.* (2007). Guided discontinuation versus maintenance treatment in remitted first episode psychosis: Relapse rates and functional outcome. *Journal of Clinical Psychiatry*, **68**, 654–62.

Yung, A. R., Phillips, L. J., Yuen, H. P. *et al.* (2003). Psychosis prediction: 12-month follow up of a high-risk ('prodromal') group. *Schizophrenia Research*, **60**, 21–32.

Zhang, M., Wang, M., Li, J. & Phillips, M. R. (1994). Randomised-control trial of family intervention for 78 first-episode male schizophrenic patients: an 18-month study in Suzhou, Jiangsu. *British Journal of Psychiatry*, **165**(Suppl 24), s96–102.

20

Treatment resistance in first-episode psychosis

Christian G. Huber and Martin Lambert

Introduction

Outcome in first-episode psychosis (FEP) varies on a continuum from complete remission and full recovery to complete failure of response – so-called treatment resistance (TR). Treatment resistance can only be considered when every other possible cause for non-response has been excluded, including an inadequate delivery of first-line pharmacotherapeutic and/or psychotherapeutic treatments, poor tolerability and medication non-adherence (Ch. 12). Currently, a minimum of 10% of first-episode patients experience incomplete recovery owing to TR, and 10–50% of FEP patients show long-term TR (Edwards *et al.*, 1998; Manchanda *et al.*, 2005; Ram *et al.*, 1992; Wiersma *et al.*, 1998). Early identification and management of TR may help to reduce these percentages (Lambert *et al.*, 2008; Robinson *et al.*, 1999).

Traditionally, research into TR has mainly been conducted in schizophrenia and major depressive disorder (MDD). However, since FEP samples include patients who are in the early stages of illness and are, therefore, less chronically affected and also patients with schizoaffective or bipolar I disorder, there needs to be a focus on TR specifically within these samples, with the aim of preventing long-term or chronic disorder. Despite the clinical importance of TR in non-affective *and* affective psychotic disorders, diagnosis-specific definitions of TR do not exist, are not updated or remain controversial. With respect to schizophrenia, positive symptoms were thought for a long time to be the most important outcome measure and were the standard index of TR assessment. This focus on positive symptoms arose because other symptoms were either not clinically well recognized or understood (e.g. cognitive disorganization) or were considered unresponsive to treatment (e.g. negative symptoms). More recently, a wider range of objective and subjective outcome measures have been recognized. These include other symptoms related to schizophrenia itself (e.g. negative symptoms) or to comorbid psychiatric disorders (i.e. affective symptoms and aggressive behaviour), functioning level (i.e. employment, independent living skills and social relationships) and quality of life (i.e. life satisfaction or satisfying subjective well-being; Andreasen, Carpenter & Kane, 2005).

This chapter provides an overview of the definitions and prevalence of TR in FEP (first-episode schizophrenia and schizoaffective disorder, bipolar disorder and MDD). Predictors of TR and strategies for TR prevention and early detection will be outlined. Lastly, diagnosis-specific management of TR in FEP will be discussed, with a major focus on pharmacotherapeutic interventions. A case vignette is presented to illustrate successful management of TR in an individual with FEP.

Definitions of treatment resistance

Schizophrenia and schizoaffective disorder

Definitions of TR differ markedly. For example, treatment response can be considered dichotomously (i.e. response or non-response) or as existing on a continuum of responsiveness. Other definitions consider type and duration of previous pharmacological treatment,

The Recognition and Management of Early Psychosis: A Preventive Approach, ed. Henry J. Jackson and Patrick D. McGorry.
Published by Cambridge University Press. © Cambridge University Press 2009.

as well as type and severity of psychopathological symptoms and concurrent behavioural abnormalities.

The traditional definition by Kane *et al.* (1988) was pharmacologically driven and relatively narrow in scope. The criteria included (1) aspects of the patient's clinical history (level of functioning over the past 5 years and three sufficient previous antipsychotic trials in the preceding 5 years without significant relief), (2) cross-sectional measures (score on Brief Psychiatric Rating Scale (BPRS) or Clinical Global Impression (CGI) scale) and (3) prospective assessments (reduction of BPRS score; post-treatment BPRS score and CGI score). From the present perspective, this definition has several weaknesses: (1) it implies that schizophrenia constitutes a homogeneous group of patients who either respond or do not respond; (2) it does not highlight that schizophrenia has a wide spectrum of symptoms including negative, cognitive and/or affective symptoms as well as functional deficits; (3) the dosage recommended for sufficient trials (60 mg haloperidol per day) is no longer considered adequate (Kapur *et al.*, 1996; Lambert & Naber, 2004a; Robinson *et al.*, 1999); (4) the observation period of 5 years before considering a patient as TR cannot be supported as continuous positive symptoms for the first 3–6 months after the start of initial antipsychotic treatment are highly predictive for non-remission of positive symptoms after 18–24 months, at least for more than 60–70% of patients with FEP (Craig *et al.*, 1999; Lambert *et al.*, 2008); (5) finally, although patients with schizoaffective disorder are often included in TR studies, definitions of TR have not recognized the special clinical issues of these patients, who often experience high rates of incomplete remission of psychotic and/or depressive symptoms (Marneros, 2003).

The contemporary definition of TR includes the criteria of persistent negative, cognitive and depressive-anxiety symptoms, including suicidality, and persistent behavioural disturbances, including aggression and/or hostility (Pantelis & Lambert, 2003; Peuskens, 1999), in addition to the traditional criterion of persistent positive symptoms (cf. Kane *et al.*, 1988). Furthermore, functional criteria included level of functioning in independent living, social relationships and employment/occupation plus criteria related to quality of life,

subjective well-being and life satisfaction. Finally, the definition also includes continuous hospitalization or frequent readmission.

Bipolar disorder

In bipolar disorder, TR is characterized by treatment-refractory manic states, continuous subthreshold hypomanic or depressive symptoms and resistant rapid cycling, but particularly recurrent or resistant depression (Goldberg, Garno & Harrow, 2005; Sachs, 1996; Sackeim, 2001). Although no consensual definition of each of these resistant conditions is available yet, Sachs (1996) provided a set of working definitions. For manic states, TR was defined as a manic episode that had not remitted despite 6 weeks of adequate therapy with at least two antimanic agents in the absence of mood-elevating agents. For mood cycling, TR was defined as continued cycling despite maximally tolerated lithium in combination with valproate or carbamazepine for either three times the average cycle length *or* 6 months in the absence of antidepressants. As the number of pharmacotherapeutic agents has increased over the last several years, these definitions need to be adapted to current pharmacological recommendations (Gitlin, 2001). For bipolar depression, no specific TR definition is available yet. Therefore, it is not known whether the TR definition for MDD (see below) is also applicable to bipolar depression.

Major depressive disorder

Because major depression is common in FEP patients, its importance demands consideration here. Considering the individual and social impact of chronic or treatment-resistant depression (TRD) (Gilmer *et al.*, 2005), it is surprising how poorly TRD is defined. This can be attributed to the lack of a consensus definition of TRD, and to the intrinsic heterogeneity of the depressive disorders (Malhi *et al.*, 2005a). The World Psychiatric Association provided one of the earliest descriptions of resistant depression, defining TRD to have occurred when there was an absence of clinical treatment response after a tricyclic antidepressant (e.g. imipramine or equivalent drug) had been tried for 4–6 weeks at a minimum dose of 150 mg/day (World Health Organization, 1974). In the past decades, despite substantial changes in MDD treatment regimens, little attention has been given to formalizing criteria for evaluating the nature and extent of TRD. Souery and colleagues (1999), for example, proposed an operational definition of TRD that included the failure to respond to at least two adequate trials of different classes of antidepressant. The definition of TRD also includes an adequate dose of antidepressant medication for a sufficient duration of time (at least 4 weeks), and with good adherence. More recently, TRD is considered to be present after inadequate response to at least one antidepressant trial of adequate dose and duration (Fava, 2003).

Prevalence of treatment resistance

Reported prevalence of TR markedly depends on the diagnostic subgroup assessed. As FEP samples are made up of patients with various psychotic disorders other than schizophrenia (e.g. schizoaffective or bipolar I disorder), development of TR in patients with these diagnoses must also be taken into account.

Schizophrenia and schizoaffective disorder

Lambert and colleagues assessed a subsample of an epidemiological cohort of FEP patients over an 18-month follow-up (Lambert *et al.*, 2005a) and found that 33% of patients with schizophrenia had continuous positive symptoms of varying severity and another 22% experienced continuous positive symptoms following relapse (Lambert *et al.*, 2008). Overall, 35% of patients were found to be in symptomatic remission at 18 months, but 20% had persistent psychoses. Other FEP studies, often using informed consent designs with selected samples and not assessing those who are lost to follow-up, have mostly found lower rates of persistent psychoses, varying from 6% to 22% in a 12- to 24-month follow-up period (Edwards *et al.*, 1998; Lieberman *et al.*, 1993; Loebel *et al.*, 1992; Manchanda *et al.*, 2005; Robinson *et al.*, 1999). Nevertheless, in a 15-year follow-up study, Wiersma *et al.* (1998) found

that 63% of patients developed a chronic course of illness after the index first episode, with increased probability of chronicity with each subsequent episode.

The long-term course is also combined with considerable resistance to treatment. Several follow-up studies (5 to 25 years) have shown that response and recovery rates are markedly dependent on the criteria used. Studies using moderately strict criteria found recovery rates of 6% to 17% (Harrison *et al.*, 2001; Robinson *et al.*, 2004). When more narrow recovery criteria were applied (i.e. widely reduced functional and clinical signs of the illness), recovery rates decreased to 0–10% (Lauronen *et al.*, 2005; Leff *et al.*, 1992). As half of the recovered patients relapse in the following 10 years (Torgalsboen & Rund, 1998), recovery is in many cases a time-limited remission (Lauronen *et al.*, 2005). This prognosis was also found in patients with schizoaffective disorder (Tsuang & Coryell, 1993).

Bipolar disorder

One year after the index episode, only 50% of first-episode patients are in syndromal recovery and 35% in functional recovery (Strakowski *et al.*, 2005). In a 2- to 4-year follow-up period, 28% of patients remained symptomatic; only 43% achieved functional recovery and 57% switched or had new illness episodes (Tohen *et al.*, 2003). Observations from Judd *et al.* (2002) on the weekly symptomatic status over a 12- to 20-year follow-up period have indicated that patients experience subthreshold hypomanic and depressive symptoms half of the time, suggesting that one of the major treatment goals – long-term euthymia – is reached less frequently than normally believed.

Major depressive disorder

Unfortunately, many patients with MDD do not achieve durable long-term remission. Approximately 30% to 45% of patients will experience a recurrent or chronic course of illness for which long-term treatment is recommended (Fava, 2003). Moreover, only 25% to 35% of patients treated with traditional antidepressants fully recover from a depressive episode (Kocsis, 2000) and at least 20% of patients do not respond satisfactorily to several antidepressant medication treatment trials (Kennedy *et al.*, 2001). Finally, 80% to 90% of those having experienced two or more episodes will have further recurrences (Crown *et al.*, 2002). Therefore, MDD is often not an episodic or self-limiting disorder but rather a recurrent and chronic illness that can be TR (Crown *et al.*, 2002).

Summary

In summary, high TR prevalence rates are reported for all FEP diagnoses throughout the current literature. However, through early identification and management of TR, the course of illness can be positively influenced and rates of TR can be significantly reduced.

Predictors of treatment resistance

Treatment may be completely or partially unsuccessful for a variety of reasons including illness-, patient- and treatment-related factors (Fig. 20.1). The knowledge of these factors is important for early detection of TR, for the development of an adequate treatment plan, to reduce the appearance of TR and for a fast and appropriate adaptation of interventions.

A series of predictors of poor symptomatic and overall outcome as measured at 1- to 15-year follow-up have been consistently found in adolescents and adults, as well as in dual-diagnosis patients. These predictors include poor premorbid level of functioning and poor functioning in the last year before first treatment (Flyckt *et al.*, 2006; Malla *et al.*, 2006; Meng *et al.*, 2006; Rosen & Garety, 2005), insidious onset and severe negative symptoms (Bromet *et al.*, 2005; Ropcke & Eggers, 2005), (persistent) substance use (Lambert *et al.*, 2005b; Wade *et al.*, 2006), a long duration of prodrome and/or psychosis (Robinson *et al.*, 2004; Rosen & Garety, 2005), male gender (Flyckt *et al.*, 2006; Manchanda *et al.*, 2005; Maziade *et al.*, 1996; Robinson *et al.*, 2004; Rosen & Garety, 2005), (persistent) poor insight (Caton *et al.*, 2006), (persistent) cognitive deficits (Robinson *et al.*, 2004), partial and complete medication non-compliance (Malla *et al.*, 2006; Robinson

et al., 2004) and poor early treatment response within the first 6 to 12 weeks (de Haan *et al.*, 2008; Emsley, Rabinowitz & Medori, 2006; Perkins *et al.*, 2004), especially with regard to subjective well-being (de Haan *et al.*, 2008; Lambert *et al.*, 2007). Despite limited research evidence, repeated service disengagement is also likely to be another important poor prognosis factor (Schimmelmann *et al.*, 2006). These predictors are highly inter-related; this implies that not all are necessarily independently predictive of poor outcome, for example when weighted against one another in multivariate regression analyses.

Management

With respect to management of TR in FEP there are four key aims: (1) optimizing interventions to prevent treatment non-response, (2) early detection of TR and for patients with TR, (3) pharmacologic treatment adaptations and (4) psychosocial treatment adaptations.

Optimizing interventions to prevent treatment resistance

Service prerequisites

A successful acute and long-term needs-adapted integrative treatment of patients with psychotic disorders requires specific service prerequisites. The most important are (1) transfer of inpatient resources to outpatient services with the possibility of long-term treatment; (2) treatment of adolescents and young adults in one single service with continuity of care; (3) cooperation of child, youth and adult psychiatrists in one treatment team; (4) a multidisciplinary treatment team; (5) continuous community awareness and health professional education programmes to improve access and to reduce treatment delay; (6) continuous education of service employees with regard to psychological and pharmacological interventions aimed at enhancing quality of care; (7) implementation of a specialized assertive community treatment team with the tasks of initial and ongoing service engagement, adherence assurance, longitudinal diagnostic assessment and

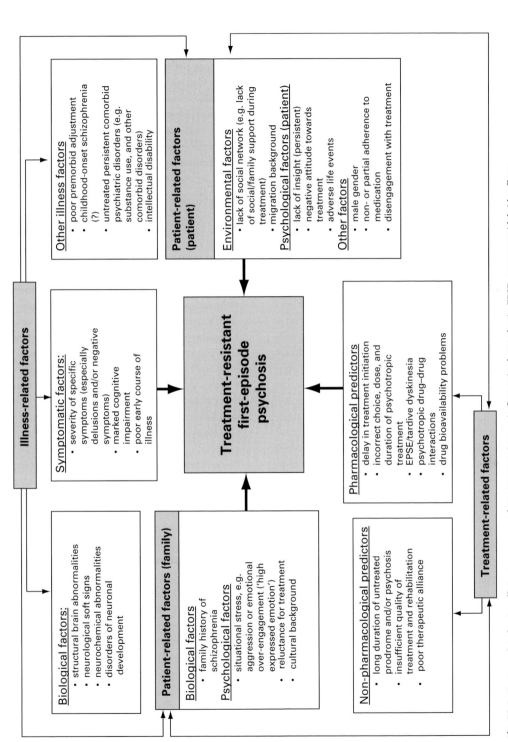

Fig. 20.1. Factors related to insufficient response and treatment resistance in first-episode psychosis. EPSE, extrapyramidal side effects.

crisis intervention; and (8) treatment of each patient and their family by the same team of clinicians throughout the complete treatment period. These demands are of great importance, as many of the previously described predictors are related to poor early detection (giving rise to a long duration of untreated illness) and partly to poor service performance (e.g. lack of specific interventions to reduce substance use, to promote adherence or to reduce service disengagement).

Definition of clinical effectiveness

Defining criteria for 'clinical effectiveness' in psychotic disorders is a necessary prerequisite for assessing whether interventions are successful or not. In schizophrenia, for example, the Remission in Schizophrenia Working Group have published a consensus statement on operational criteria for remission that included sustained symptomatic (i.e. positive, negative, cognitive and affective symptoms, operationalized as BPRS item scores < 3) and functional improvement (i.e. vocational functioning, independent living, regular social contacts) as well as a satisfying quality of life (Andreasen *et al.*, 2005). The working group defined a period of 6 months as a minimum time frame during which these improvements must be maintained in order to achieve remission. Furthermore, Lieberman, Stroup & Schneider (2002) have provided an operational definition of complete recovery from schizophrenia, which included improvement measured by the same criteria for 2 consecutive years. Comparable definitions also exist for MDD, for example (Nierenberg & DeCecco, 2001; Nierenberg & Wright, 1999).

Management strategies to prevent treatment resistance

Prevention is of particular importance, since a psychotic relapse often means a prolonged time to remission, more residual symptoms, increased impairment of psychosocial functioning and decreased quality of life. Therefore, optimizing therapeutic interventions can contribute a great deal to the prevention of poor response to treatment. Most recently, several treatment guidelines for patients with schizophrenia-spectrum

disorders (APA, 2004a; NICE, 2002; Royal Australian and New Zealand College of Psychiatrists, 2005), bipolar disorder (APA, 2004b; Royal Australian and New Zealand College of Psychiatrists, 2004) and MDD (APA, 2004c) have been published. As these guidelines represent a consensus of the best treatment currently available, interventions should be adopted according to the respective recommendations and any updates by these organizations.

Early detection of treatment resistance

While early identification of TR is a high clinical priority, it represents a significant clinical challenge as it is complicated by several factors. These include the multidimensional definition of TR; the absence of distinct categories along the continuous spectrum from treatment response to complete non-response, requiring clinical judgement as to when a patient has crossed the threshold into TR; and the lack of generally valid predictors for TR. Early identification, however, remains a primary objective since pharmacological and psychological interventions for treatment-refractory patients differ from those for non-refractory patients, and early identification and treatment of TR may prevent progression to more chronic stages of psychotic disorder.

The possibility of primary TR should be considered from the initiation of treatment. This recommendation, evident for all psychotic disorders, is based on several research findings. There are two key findings. First, most of the illness- and patient-related factors as well as some treatment-related factors associated with an increased risk of partial or non-response are already evident at initial presentation (e.g. brain structure abnormalities, long duration of untreated psychosis or poor functioning) and may no longer be that malleable. Second, response in the first 6–12 weeks after start of initial antipsychotic treatment is highly predictive of subsequent partial or non-remission. Furthermore, with each relapse, there is a great risk for secondary TR. Therefore, some patients with FEP, especially those with prolonged duration of untreated psychosis or untreated illness, those already diagnosed with schizophrenia or schizoaffective disorder at initial presentation, those with a comorbid persistent substance dependence, those with poor premorbid functioning and/or high severity of negative symptoms at baseline, are at great risk for insufficient response and subsequent TR, regardless of the medication used (Lambert *et al.*, 2005a,b,c). These patients have to be identified early, possibly at initial presentation or during the first 3 months of treatment, and subsequent treatment must be adapted in order to maximize the chances of full recovery.

Pharmacological treatment adaptations for treatment resistance

Schizophrenia and schizoaffective disorder

Patients with schizophrenia and schizoaffective disorder and TR require specific pharmacological interventions, best applied according to a TR management algorithm, as outlined in Fig. 20.2.

Pharmacological management of TR can be conducted in four phases.

Phase 1. At first, the phenomenological domain affected by TR must be identified (Fig. 20.2). There are a variety of confounding factors that have to be explored and excluded before TR is diagnosed (Fig. 20.1). Probably the most common and important are insufficient previous pharmacological interventions, repeated medication non-adherence, a persistent substance-use disorder or lack of or inadequate prior psychosocial treatment. A review of the course of illness and treatment history should concurrently guide the optimization of interventions. This includes the reassessment of diagnosis (especially with respect to schizoaffective or delusional disorder, but also to borderline personality disorder), the administration of antipsychotic medication at sufficient dosage and with sufficient compliance for at least 4–6 weeks, the successful treatment of possible comorbid psychiatric disorders, especially affective and substance-use disorders, and concurrent management of medication side effects, especially those that can affect antipsychotic response (e.g. extrapyramidal motor symptoms) or induce persistent symptoms (e.g. depression or negative

symptoms related to untreated extrapyramidal motor symptoms). In the case of medication non-adherence, intramuscular depot preparations, preferably atypical compounds (currently the only compound available is risperidone), should be used. At this point, if the patient is still not responding to treatment, phase 2 can be entered.

Phase 2. This starts with the implementation of the best treatment available for the combination of affected phenomenological domains, depending on previous treatment success, patient's preference and current pharmacological guidelines. Each of these new treatment steps should always be combined with the corresponding psychological interventions. Many atypical antipsychotic drugs have shown efficacy in each of the possible domains alone and in combination, including negative, cognitive or affective symptoms and quality of life and, so, should be the first-line choice. Therefore, patients previously treated with first-generation antipsychotic drugs should be switched to a second-generation one that has the best evidence for efficacy in treating the respective domain. If the patient had been previously treated with a second-generation antipsychotic drug that was predominantly a dopamine D_2-receptor blocker (e.g. amisulpride), it is recommended that the regimen is switched to another second-generation drug with either higher potency (e.g. risperidone) or with a 'mixed receptor profile' (e.g. olanzapine or quetiapine). If the patient was previously treated with a second-generation drug from the latter group, a switch to a second-generation drug with mainly a D_2-receptor-blocking action is recommended. Another subsequent treatment option is to increase to the highest possible dose, which can be considered, if well tolerated. For patients with resistant positive symptoms, the trial duration should be 6–8 weeks. If the patient exhibits predominantly negative symptoms, and confounders such as depression and extrapyramidal motor symptoms are excluded, a lower antipsychotic dosage should be used (e.g. amisulpride 100–300 mg/day; aripiprazole 5–15 mg/day) and a longer trial should be considered before changes are

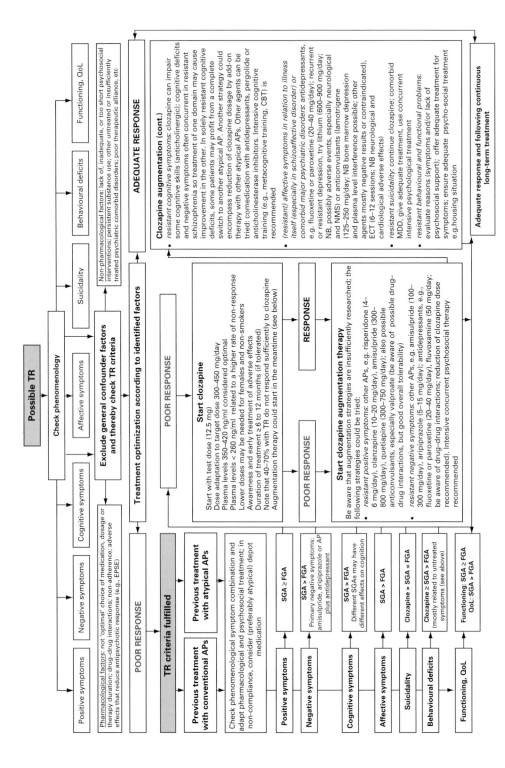

Fig. 20.2. Pharmacotherapy for treatment resistance. These are general guidelines that must be adapted to the individual needs of each patient. AP, antipsychotic drug; CBT, cognitive–behavioural therapy; ECT, electroconvulsive therapy; EPSE, extrapyramidal side effects; FGA, first-generation antipsychotic drug; MDD, Major depressive disorder; NMS, neuroleptic malignant syndrome; QoL, quality of life; SGA, second-generation antipsychotic drug; TR, treatment resistance; ≥, more effective than or equally effective as; >, more effective than.

expected (i.e. 3–6 months). Within these antipsychotic dosages, an improvement of concurrent cognitive deficits is also possible. Affective and anxiety symptoms should be treated concomitantly, as they tend to have a negative effect on response in other domains. Improvement in social and role functioning as well as quality of life are a consequence of the best achievable symptomatic control, including the lowest possible severity of negative and cognitive symptoms as well as depression. As functional outcome depends on additional variables to those intrinsic to schizophrenia itself, the patient needs specific vocational and functional support.

Phase 3. If there is no or insufficient response to the other second-generation antipsychotic drugs, and if no contraindications exist, the next treatment option is a switch to clozapine, regardless of the predominant psychopathology. Clozapine is considered to be the most effective antipsychotic in TR, which holds true when compared with both first and second-generation antipsychotic drugs. However, the drug's benefits must be weighted against its serious adverse effects, including potential risks of neutropenia and agranulocytosis, weight gain, obesity and diabetes, epileptic seizures and cardiomyopathy. There are conflicting findings regarding the necessary duration of treatment before response can be evaluated properly. Treatment-refractory patients in several studies showed strongest improvement within the first 8–12 weeks, while other studies report longer periods of 6–12 months (Pantelis & Lambert, 2003; Remington *et al.*, 2005; Schulte, 2003). However, there is consensus that clinicians should consider a minimum trial duration of 6 months. The decision as to when clozapine should be discontinued is also difficult, mainly because of the lack of alternatives, negative experiences after patients were switched from clozapine back to another antipsychotic drug and the fact that clozapine potentially has additional important benefits (e.g. reduction of aggressive behaviour, reduced suicidality, and a positive influence on tardive dyskinesia and comorbid substance-use disorder). Phase 3 also encompasses optimization of clozapine treatment,

especially with respect to dosage and plasma concentrations. A dose of approximately 300–450 mg/day was considered to be sufficient for many patients who maintained optimal plasma concentrations of 350–420 ng/ml. Nevertheless, even with an optimal treatment regimen, as many as 40% to 70% of patients treated with clozapine do not respond adequately (Buckley *et al.*, 2001; Pantelis & Lambert, 2003).

Phase 4. Remington *et al.* (2005) have reviewed augmentation treatment options in clozapine-resistant schizophrenia patients. In terms of choosing an augmentation strategy, decision making can be guided by several sources, including the problematic symptom domain and the individual preference of the patient. Specific recommendations – depending on symptom domain – are shown in Fig. 20.2. Unfortunately, current evidence for these recommendations is limited; many of these options are in fact poorly researched in randomized controlled trials, but nevertheless, they have been repeatedly replicated in observational studies and case reports.

Bipolar disorder

As discussed above, bipolar disorder can be refractory to treatment. Therefore, pharmacological treatment strategies for bipolar disorder that is TR include agents to improve response in mania and depression as well as drugs to reduce cycling. If partial or non-response is established, further treatment strategies depend on the resistant syndrome (mania or depression including respective subthreshold syndromes or symptoms), or resistant rapid cycling.

Treatment-resistant bipolar mania or mixed episodes

In the case of inadequate symptom control with first-line treatment (APA, 2004b) and after increasing the chosen medication to the highest dose possible/tolerated, there are several additional treatment options for bipolar mania or mixed episodes. (1) The mood stabilizer used can be switched, from lithium to valproate or vice versa or to an alternative mood stabilizer (e.g. oxcarbazepine). (2) Therapy can switch from one atypical antipsychotic drug to another. Currently, there is limited evidence regarding which specific drug should be chosen after failure of another specific atypical antipsychotic drug; therefore, the decision should be based on safety and tolerability aspects. Clozapine should also be considered, especially when concurrent resistant psychotic features are evident. (3) A mood stabilizer combination can be tried (e.g. lithium and valproate or other combinations). (4) Electroconvulsive therapy (ECT), comparable to its applicability in resistant bipolar depression, should be considered as one of the first options in treatment-resistant bipolar mania. Typically 6–12 treatment sessions are recommended.

There is little empirical evidence to guide which of these four strategies is preferred in the individual patient (Bowden, 2005). Because many of these treatment options are combination therapies, selecting a combination with an acceptable tolerability is of particular importance.

Treatment-resistant bipolar depression

In the case of inadequate symptom control with first-line treatment (APA, 2004b; Perlis, 2005) or new episodes that occur despite preventive treatment, there are several options for bipolar depression that is TR. Preference for one of the following treatments should be guided mainly by the severity and chronicity of the depressive state. Depressive episodes that do not respond to the combination therapy mentioned above often warrant ECT (typically 6–12 treatments), which according to the American Psychiatric Association, should be considered as one of the first options in treatment-resistant bipolar depression (APA, 2004b) and should be administered concurrently with pharmacological treatment. Apart from ECT, in most cases further pharmacological treatment options should be explored in a stepwise fashion. These options include the following. (1) The mood stabilizer drug can be switched, from lithium to lamotrigine (first option) or other anticonvulsants (e.g. valproate or topiramate for obese bipolar patients; second option). (2) The antidepressant can be switched from a selective serotonin reuptake inhibitor (SSRI) to another SSRI or to one of the types of antidepressant with broader effects on neuropharmacological systems (e.g. serotonin–noradrenaline reuptake inhibitor, selective serotonin–noradrenaline reuptake inhibitor, or noradrenergic and specific serotonin antidepressant). (3) One atypical antipsychotic drug can be switched to another, possibly to a non-sedative atypical antipsychotic drug with intrinsic activation, such as aripiprazole. Low-dose clozapine also shows efficacy, especially in combination with ECT. (4) Antidepressant combination therapy can be started, for example an SSRI with add-on of bupropion. The latter, a selective norepinephrine and dopamine reuptake inhibitor, has been suggested not only because of its antidepressant effects but also because of a probably lower risk of inducing switches to hypomania or mania. Furthermore, venlafaxine and monoamine oxidase inhibitors, such as tranylcypromine, are found to be effective. As in resistant mania, there is only little evidence regarding which of these strategies should be preferred in the individual patient. Therefore, selecting a combination with an acceptable tolerability is of special importance. In the USA, the combination of olanzapine and fluoxetine (Symbyax) is approved for the treatment of bipolar depression.

Treatment-resistant rapid cycling

Unfortunately, knowledge about the specific pharmacological treatment of rapid cycling bipolar disorder remains limited (Kilzieh & Akiskal, 1999). Although it seems to be more lithium resistant and has less likelihood of being symptom free, the most successful pharmacological strategy is probably discontinuation of antidepressants and use of a combined mood-stabilizer therapy, of which valproate is probably the most useful, plus making additional use of atypical neuroleptic drugs. Furthermore, thyroid and nimodipine augmentation can be considered in those with the most unfavourable course (Kilzieh & Akiskal, 1999).

Major depressive disorder

If partial or non-response is confirmed, treatment strategies for TRD should be applied stepwise, including (1) switching to another antidepressant monotherapy, (2) combination of two or more agents or (3) augmentation therapy. Unfortunately, there is little evidence as to which of these strategies should be applied for the individual patient (Ros *et al.*, 2005). Therefore, the choice of therapy should be guided by efficacy and tolerability of previous pharmacological interventions.

With first-line interventions, the initial symptomatic response may be detected within the first 7–28 days, but sufficient response is often delayed by several weeks. Traditionally, an adequate trial of an antidepressant was thought to take 6–8 weeks, but it is not unusual for the full benefit to be delayed for up to 12 weeks, especially in chronic MDD. Quitkin and colleagues (1996) have suggested that 4 weeks with optimal dosage may be a clinically meaningful time period for re-evaluation of the antidepressant effect. At this point, patients can be separated into responders, partial responders and non-responders. Patients with partial response can be treated for another 2 weeks, while patients with non-response should be switched and subsequently treated with other strategies (see below; Marangell, 2001).

Possible advantages of *switching* to a different monotherapy, compared with combination or augmentation, are reduced medication costs, fewer drug–drug interactions, better adherence and less side effect burden (Marangell, 2001). Response rates for switching (approximately 50%) are comparable to other treatment strategies for TRD. However, in partial response, combining antidepressants is preferable to switching as it avoids the loss of the level of response already obtained. The selection of a specific second antidepressant is hampered by the lack of studies and, therefore, is dependent on the patient's preference, safety and tolerability, drug–drug interactions and the possible effects of the respective agent on any comorbid psychiatric disorders. In most cases, switching should be done using a crossover strategy. Compared with tricyclic antidepressants, switching within one class is possibly more successful in the SSRIs (Kennedy *et al.*, 2001), where 50–60% of first-line non-responders to SSRI monotherapy will respond to another SSRI after switching (Kennedy *et al.*, 2003). Further guidelines for switching strategies can be found in Marangell (2001).

There is currently some evidence to support the combination of two or more antidepressants as a strategy for the management of TRD (Kennedy *et al.*, 2001). From the neuropharmacological perspective, it is important to combine mechanisms of action, rather than simply using one drug with another, and to aim at synergistic effects on the serotonergic, noradrenergic and dopaminergic systems (Fava, 2001; Rojo *et al.*, 2005). Beside switching or combining antidepressants, several augmentation strategies have been studied in TRD (Fava, 2001; Klein *et al.*, 2004; Ros *et al.*, 2005).

In MDD and TRD, there is an increasing interest in the acute and long-term efficacy of atypical antipsychotic drugs as augmentation therapy, mainly in combination with SSRIs. Several studies have documented a robust increased antidepressant effect in such combinations, possibly explained by the enhancement of both serotonin and noradrenaline release (Blier & Szabo, 2005). Most studies are available for risperidone (0.5–2 mg/day) and olanzapine (2.5–10 mg/day); positive results also exist for quetiapine (300–600 mg/day), ziprasidone (40–120 mg/day), amisulpride (50–100 mg/day) and aripiprazole (5–10 mg/day) (Malhi *et al.*, 2005b; Nemeroff, 2005; Simon & Nemeroff, 2005). Less-well-studied substances include anticonvulsants, pindolol, serotonin precursors, dopaminergic agents, psychostimulants, oestrogens, modafinil and antiglucocorticoids (Ros *et al.*, 2005). In most cases, clinical improvement following augmentation therapy tends to occur within 3 to 4 weeks (Fava, 2001). Most augmentation therapies in TRD should be pursued for 6 to 9 months after achieving remission and then should be gradually discontinued.

Non-pharmacological management of treatment resistance

Schizophrenia and schizoaffective disorder

Management of TR should always encompass pharmacological as well as non-pharmacological strategies, including all interventions that are also found to be effective in patients without TR (Lambert & Naber, 2004b). Furthermore, there are some specific interventions for patients with TR, such as specialized cognitive–behavioural therapy (CBT; Sensky *et al.*, 2000; Valmaggia *et al.*, 2005). Chapter 12 describes various psychosocial interventions for incomplete recovery (including TR) in FEP. Beside psychological interventions, repetitive transcranial magnetic stimulation (TMS) was found to influence resistant hallucinations in particular (Fitzgerald *et al.*, 2005). Despite favourable outcomes in some studies, this method needs further exploration in clinical trials.

Treatment-resistant bipolar disorder

High-quality specific psychosocial interventions in bipolar disorder, as in other psychiatric disorders, are a necessary prerequisite to achieve and sustain remission and recovery. Evidence indicates that combining pharmacotherapy with high-quality psychosocial interventions reduces relapse, improves patients' adherence, and decreases the number and length of hospitalizations, all of which are factors that have been associated with the development of TR in bipolar disorder.

Psychosocial interventions that have been specifically recommended in bipolar disorder include psychoeducation (individual and group sessions), CBT, family-focused therapy and interpersonal and social rhythm therapy (Colom & Vieta, 2004). Psychoeducation has been applied in different ways and has been associated with improvement of the course of illness, for example in 7–12 individual sessions with a special focus on recognition of early warning signs and subsequent help-seeking behaviour (Perry *et al.*, 1999), or in 21 weekly group therapy sessions with special attention to causes and triggers of bipolar disorder, medications and coping strategies (Colom *et al.*, 2003). The use of CBT, with the goal of improving the interactions between thinking, mood and behaviour, was found to be effective in individual settings over various time periods (mostly 6–12 months) with improved depressive and manic symptoms, decreased non-compliance rates and reduced relapse rates during follow-up (mostly 12–18 months; Vieta, 2005). Structured family interventions, provided as integrated care, can reduce depression and relapse (Miklowitz *et al.*, 2000). Interpersonal and social rhythm therapy is an individualized

psychotherapy that focuses on improving the patient's psychosocial and interpersonal relationships as well as stabilizing social and biological rhythms (Vieta, 2005).

Major depressive disorder

Non-pharmacological strategies in MDD include psychotherapy, ECT, high-frequency left-sided repetitive TMS as well as low-frequency repetitive TMS for the right prefrontal cortex and vagus nerve stimulation. To maximize prevention of TRD and as a prerequisite for an effective treatment, structured psychotherapeutic interventions should be delivered to as many patients with MDD as possible (McPherson *et al.*, 2005; Thase, 2000). Pharmacological interventions without concomitant psychotherapy increase the risk of developing TRD. Here, CBT or interpersonal therapy particularly have shown efficacy as short-term interventions leading to sustained long-term improvement and increased quality of life (McPherson *et al.*, 2005).

Use of ECT has also been shown to be effective, especially in patients with severe depression and/or TRD (Bauer *et al.*, 2007; Lisanby, 2007). As in bipolar depression, ECT should be considered early in the treatment algorithm, especially in the presence of very severe depression (Bowden, 2005). After ECT, an initial improvement has been reported in vegetative symptoms, such as insomnia and fatigue, and catatonic symptoms. Improvements in affective symptoms, followed by improvements in cognitive (e.g. impaired self-esteem, hopelessness) and behavioural symptoms (e.g. suicidality) are seen later in the course of ECT (Lisanby, 2007). A substantial proportion of non-responders to antidepressants will recover with ECT; patients with melancholic and psychotic presentations respond best. Therapeutic effects of ECT may be evident within three treatments, but treatment may require as many as 12 sessions in some patients. Relapse rate after discontinuation is high (30–70% within 1 year), partly depending on the degree of medication resistance before starting ECT. Prophylactic treatment with an antidepressant should be administered in almost all patients; combination therapy of lithium and an antidepressant has been found to be especially effective (Bauer *et al.*, 2007; Lisanby, 2007).

Repetitive TMS for 10 sessions is a promising novel treatment method that is currently under investigation in several psychiatric disorders and has already shown substantial treatment efficacy in patients with TRD (Avery *et al.*, 2006; Fitzgerald *et al.*, 2005; Rossini *et al.*, 2005). Latest publications on vagal nerve stimulation have also shown sustained efficacy in patients with TRD (Nahas *et al.*, 2005).

Conclusions

In the preceding sections, we have provided an overview on predictors and management of TR in FEP. To enhance this picture, the Case vignette describes a 17-year-old patient with TR first-episode schizophrenia.

Case vignette

Daniel is a school student who presented with a first episode of psychosis at the age of 17. At the time, he was living with his family, who referred him to the service. With respect to his past history, his mother remembered that Daniel was born prematurely and that he had not started talking until 3 years of age. In kindergarten, he had difficulties in making friends and kept to himself most of the time. On referral, his father reported that Daniel was still anxious in many situations, whereas his 19-year-old sister was gregarious, socially adept and connected to others.

At the age of 12, Daniel described his first depressive symptoms, combined with severe difficulties in concentrating at school. Despite his wish to be more connected to other people, he started to isolate himself even more. His parents thought that he was a normal teenager undergoing puberty–being moody, not wanting to go out and not wanting to tidy up his room. At the age of 14, he started to smoke cannabis. Over the next year, he increased his use of cannabis to 2 g per day. At this time, he had several short episodes where he experienced auditory hallucinations. At the age of 16, his parents became worried about his odd behaviour. Daniel started to talk to himself and he became very paranoid and suspicious of people around him. He thought that other students were plotting against him and he stopped leaving his room because he was worried about people reading his thoughts, or people implanting thoughts in his head.

At the time of first treatment contact, Daniel presented with continuous auditory hallucinations experienced since the age of 15 and systematized delusions since the age of 16.

Additionally, he clearly displayed negative symptoms, cognitive deficits and a poor premorbid and current level of functioning. At first presentation, Daniel showed no insight that something was wrong with him. A systematic diagnostic interview revealed a diagnosis of schizophrenia and comorbid cannabis dependency. The duration of untreated psychosis was 118 weeks and the duration of untreated prodrome approximately 5 years. A magnetic resonance scan showed enlarged ventricles, and neuropsychological testing revealed a global reduction in cognitive functioning.

Daniel was first started on an atypical antipsychotic drug and the dosage was slowly increased. He did not respond to low-dose medication; his voices and delusions remained virtually unchanged. Within the next 4 weeks, the dosage was slowly increased to the maximum. At this time, he was still using cannabis from time to time and a one-to-one substance-use treatment approach was commenced. He was able to stop using cannabis and his mental state slowly improved. However, because of insufficient overall response, the medication was changed to a different atypical antipsychotic drug. After another 6 weeks trial, his voices stopped, but his delusions remained widely unchanged. Reviewing his case after 3 months of treatment, the treating team offered him a trial of clozapine in combination with individualized CBT. He was treated with 350 mg/day and the clozapine plasma concentration was kept above 350 ng/ml. Within 4 weeks of starting clozapine, his functional level improved dramatically. During the CBT sessions, he started to talk about his delusional fears and was better able to handle them than before. Three months later, he was in complete symptomatic remission and was able to return to school.

During the following 3 years, he experienced several depressive episodes and so he was started on concurrent mood-stabilizing therapy. Since then he is still experiencing mood swings, but there has been no recurrence of major depression. Today he is working part-time and is actively involved in a peer-support project that involves giving psychoeducation to other FEP patients.

This chapter has summarized recent findings and guidelines with respect to the definition and management of TR in psychotic disorders. The definition of TR should be considered from a multidimensional perspective that includes a broad range of symptoms, functional disabilities and quality of life relevant to patients with psychotic disorders. Additionally, the definition of TR depends on the underlying diagnosis. This aspect is especially important for FEP cohorts, which include patients with various psychotic disorders.

The reported prevalence of TR necessarily depends on the diagnostic subgroup assessed, on the criteria applied and on the follow-up period. Within a first-episode sample, it has been estimated that 5–10% of patients with schizophrenia could be defined as TR in a 2-year follow-up period. However, these rates reflect treatment outcomes in cohorts mostly treated with conventional antipsychotic drugs and not being treated in specialized first-episode centres.

Factors other than choice of medication that may influence a patient's recovery include individual factors relating to the patient, the illness and the treatment. Many of these factors could be seen as confounding factors relevant in establishing and perpetuating TR. The most important factors are non-compliance with medication, ongoing substance use, service disengagement and lack of integrated multidimensional care. After exclusion of these confounders, the chosen intervention largely depends on the underlying diagnosis, as outlined above.

Recent studies of the response to (antipsychotic) treatment have highlighted the importance of early adequate response in a broad range of outcome domains. These findings show the importance of quality of care and the need for early identification of TR.

In summary, TR remains a major treatment challenge in patients with psychotic disorders. However, through early detection of FEP and offering best care by integrating optimal pharmacological and needs-adapted psychosocial interventions from the first day of treatment, prevention of TR is possible. When TR is identified, early and appropriate treatment adaptation(s) are vital for minimizing the chances of more chronic forms of disorder. Enhancement of early detection and treatment strategies for the risk factors for TR, in addition to preventing relapse, are future research and clinical goals for promoting adequate treatment response and full recovery in FEP.

REFERENCES

Andreasen, N. C., Carpenter, W. T., Jr, Kane, J. M. *et al.* (2005). Remission in schizophrenia: proposed criteria and rationale for consensus. *American Journal of Psychiatry*, **162**, 441–9.

APA (2004a). *Practice Guidelines for the Treatment of Psychiatric Disorders, Compendium 2004*, 2nd edn: *Practice Guideline for the Treatment of Patients with Schizophrenia*. Washington, DC: American Psychiatric Press, pp. 249–440.

APA (2004b). *Practice Guidelines for the Treatment of Psychiatric Disorders, Compendium 2004*, 2nd edn: *Practice Guideline for the Treatment of Patients with Bipolar Disorder*. Washington, DC: American Psychiatric Press, pp. 525–612.

APA (2004c). *Practice Guidelines for the Treatment of Psychiatric Disorders, Compendium 2004*, 2nd edn: *Practice Guideline for the Treatment of Patients with Major Depressive Disorder*. Washington, DC: American Psychiatric Press, pp. 440–524.

Avery, D. H., Holtzheimer, P. E., III, Fawaz, W. *et al.* (2006). A controlled study of repetitive transcranial magnetic stimulation in medication-resistant major depression. *Biological Psychiatry*, **59**, 187–94.

Bauer, M., Bschor, T., Pfennig, A. *et al.* (2007). World Federation of Societies of Biological Psychiatry (WFSBP) guidelines for biological treatment of unipolar depressive disorders in primary care. *World Journal of Biological Psychiatry*, **8**, 67–104.

Blier, P. & Szabo, S. T. (2005). Potential mechanisms of action of atypical antipsychotic medications in treatment-resistant depression and anxiety. *Journal of Clinical Psychiatry*, **66** (Suppl 8), 30–40.

Bowden, C. L. (2005). Treatment options for bipolar depression. *Journal of Clinical Psychiatry*, **66**(Suppl 1), 3–6.

Bromet, E. J., Finch, S. J., Carlson, G. A. *et al.* (2005). Time to remission and relapse after the first hospital admission in severe bipolar disorder. *Social Psychiatry and Psychiatric Epidemiology*, **40**, 106–13.

Buckley, P., Miller, A., Olsen, J. *et al.* (2001). When symptoms persist: clozapine augmentation strategies. *Schizophrenia Bulletin*, **27**, 615–28.

Caton, C. L., Hasin, D. S., Shrout, P. E. *et al.* (2006). Predictors of psychosis remission in psychotic disorders that co-occur with substance use. *Schizophrenia Bulletin*, **32**, 618–25.

Colom, F. & Vieta, E. (2004). A perspective on the use of psychoeducation, cognitive-behavioral therapy and interpersonal therapy for bipolar patients. *Bipolar Disorders*, 6, 480–6.

Colom, F., Vieta, E., Martinez-Aran, A. *et al.* (2003). A randomized trial on the efficacy of group psychoeducation in the prophylaxis of recurrences in bipolar patients whose disease is in remission. *Archives of General Psychiatry*, **60**, 402–7.

Craig, T., Fennig, S., Tanenberg-Karant, M. & Bromet, E. J. (1999). Six-month clinical status as a predictor of 24-month clinical outcome in first-admission patients with schizophrenia. *Annals of Clinical Psychiatry*, **11**, 197–203.

Crown, W. H., Finkelstein, S., Berndt, E. R. *et al.* (2002). The impact of treatment-resistant depression on healthcare utilization and costs. *Journal of Clinical Psychiatry*, **63**, 963–71.

de Haan, L., van Nimwegen, L., van Amelsvoort, T., Dingemans, P. & Linszen, D. (2008). Improvement of subjective well-being and enduring symptomatic remission; a 5 year follow up of first episode schizophrenia. *Pharmacopsychiatry*, **41**, 125–8.

Edwards, J., Maude, D., McGorry, P. D., Harrigan, S. M. & Cocks, J. T. (1998). Prolonged recovery in first-episode psychosis. *British Journal of Psychiatry*, **172**(Suppl), s107–16.

Emsley, R., Rabinowitz, J. & Medori, R. (2006). Time course for antipsychotic treatment response in first-episode schizophrenia. *American Journal of Psychiatry*, **163**, 743–5.

Fava, M. (2001). Augmentation and combination strategies in treatment-resistant depression. *Journal of Clinical Psychiatry*, **62**(Suppl 18), 4–11.

Fava, M. (2003). Diagnosis and definition of treatment-resistant depression. *Biological Psychiatry*, **53**, 649–59.

Fitzgerald, P. B., Benitez, J., Daskalakis, J. Z. *et al.* (2005). A double-blind sham-controlled trial of repetitive transcranial magnetic stimulation in the treatment of refractory auditory hallucinations. *Journal of Clinical Psychopharmacology*, **25**, 358–62.

Flyckt, L., Mattsson, M., Edman, G., Carlsson, R. & Cullberg, J. (2006). Predicting 5-year outcome in first-episode psychosis: construction of a prognostic rating scale. *Journal of Clinical Psychiatry*, **67**, 916–24.

Gilmer, W. S., Trivedi, M. H., Rush, A. J. *et al.* (2005). Factors associated with chronic depressive episodes: a preliminary report from the STAR-D project. *Acta Psychiatrica Scandinavica*, **112**, 425–33.

Gitlin, M. J. (2001). Treatment-resistant bipolar disorder. *Bulletin of the Menninger Clinic*, **65**, 26–40.

Goldberg, J. F., Garno, J. L. & Harrow, M. (2005). Long-term remission and recovery in bipolar disorder: a review. *Current Psychiatry Reports*, **7**, 456–61.

Harrison, G., Hopper, K., Craig, T. *et al.* (2001). Recovery from psychotic illness: a 15- and 25-year international follow-up study. *British Journal of Psychiatry*, **178**, 506–17.

Judd, L. L., Akiskal, H. S., Schettler, P. J. *et al.* (2002). The long-term natural history of the weekly symptomatic status of bipolar I disorder. *Archives of General Psychiatry*, **59**, 530–7.

Kane, J., Honigfeld, G., Singer, J. & Meltzer, H. (1988). Clozapine for the treatment-resistant schizophrenic. A double-blind comparison with chlorpromazine. *Archives of General Psychiatry*, **45**, 789–96.

Kapur, S., Remington, G., Jones, C. *et al.* (1996). High levels of dopamine D2 receptor occupancy with low-dose haloperidol treatment: a PET study. *American Journal of Psychiatry*, **153**, 948–50.

Kennedy, J. S., Jeste, D., Kaiser, C. J. *et al.* (2003). Olanzapine vs haloperidol in geriatric schizophrenia: analysis of data from a double-blind controlled trial. *International Journal of Geriatric Psychiatry*, **18**, 1013–20.

Kennedy, S. H., Lam, R. W., Cohen, N. L. & Ravindran, A. V. (2001). Clinical guidelines for the treatment of depressive disorders. IV. Medications and other biological treatments. *Canadian Journal of Psychiatry*, **46**(Suppl 1), 38S–58S.

Kilzieh, N. & Akiskal, H. S. (1999). Rapid-cycling bipolar disorder. An overview of research and clinical experience. *Psychiatric Clinics of North America*, **22**, 585–607.

Klein, N., Sacher, J., Wallner, H., Tauscher, J. & Kasper, S. (2004). Therapy of treatment resistant depression: focus on the management of TRD with atypical antipsychotics. *CNS Spectrums*, **9**, 823–32.

Kocsis, J. H. (2000). New strategies for treating chronic depression. *Journal of Clinical Psychiatry*, **61**(Suppl 11), 42–5.

Lambert, M. & Naber, D. (2004a). Current issues in schizophrenia: overview of patient acceptability, functioning capacity and quality of life. *CNS Drugs*, **18**(Suppl 2), 5–17; discussion 41–3.

Lambert, M. & Naber, D. (2004b). *Current Schizophrenia*. Hamburg: Science Press.

Lambert, M., Conus, P., Schimmelmann, B. G. *et al.* (2005a). Comparison of olanzapine and risperidone in 367 first-episode patients with non-affective or affective psychosis: results of an open retrospective medical record study. *Pharmacopsychiatry*, **38**, 206–13.

Lambert, M., Conus, P., Lubman, D. I. *et al.* (2005b). The impact of substance use disorders on clinical outcome in 643 patients with first-episode psychosis. *Acta Psychiatrica Scandinavica*, **112**, 141–8.

Lambert, M., Conus, P., Naber, D., McGorry, P. D. & Schimmelmann, B. G. (2005c). Olanzapine in subjects with a first-episode psychosis non-responsive, intolerant or non-compliant to a first-line trial of risperidone. *International Journal of Psychiatry in Clinical Practice*, **9**, 244–50.

Lambert, M., Naber, D., Eich, F. X. *et al.* (2007). Remission of severely impaired subjective well-being in 727 patients with schizophrenia treated with amisulpride. *Acta Psychiatrica Scandinavica*, **115**, 106–13.

Lambert, M., Conus, P., Klosterkötter, J. *et al.* (2008). Results of First-Episode Psychosis Outcome Study (FEPOS) and resulting treatment recommendations. *Nervenarzt*, in press.

Lauronen, E., Koskinen, J., Veijola, J. *et al.* (2005). Recovery from schizophrenic psychoses within the northern Finland 1966 birth cohort. *Journal of Clinical Psychiatry*, **66**, 375–83.

Leff, J., Sartorius, N., Jablensky, A., Korten, A. & Ernberg, G. (1992). The International Pilot Study of Schizophrenia: five-year follow-up findings. *Psychological Medicine*, **22**, 131–45.

Lieberman, J., Jody, D., Geisler, S. *et al.* (1993). Time course and biologic correlates of treatment response in first-episode schizophrenia. *Archives of General Psychiatry*, **50**, 369–76.

Lieberman, J., Stroup, S. & Schneider, L. (2002). Prevention of relapse in schizophrenia. *New England Journal of Medicine*, **346**, 1412–13.

Lisanby, S. H. (2007). Electroconvulsive therapy for depression. *New England Journal of Medicine*, **357**, 1939–45.

Loebel, A. D., Lieberman, J. A., Alvir, J. M. *et al.* (1992). Duration of psychosis and outcome in first-episode schizophrenia. *American Journal of Psychiatry*, **149**, 1183–8.

Malhi, G. S., Parker, G. B., Crawford, J., Wilhelm, K. & Mitchell, P. B. (2005a). Treatment-resistant depression: resistant to definition? *Acta Psychiatrica Scandinavica*, **112**, 302–9.

Malhi, G. S., Berk, M., Bourin, M. *et al.* (2005b). Atypical mood stabilizers: a 'typical role' for atypical antipsychotics. *Acta Psychiatrica Scandinavica*, **111**(Suppl), S29–38.

Malla, A., Norman, R., Schmitz, N. *et al.* (2006). Predictors of rate and time to remission in first-episode psychosis: a two-year outcome study. *Psychological Medicine*, **36**, 649–58.

Manchanda, R., Norman, R. M., Malla, A. K., Harricharan, R. & Northcott, S. (2005). Persistent psychoses in first episode patients. *Schizophrenia Research*, **80**, 113–16.

Marangell, L. B. (2001). Switching antidepressants for treatment-resistant major depression. *Journal of Clinical Psychiatry*, **62** (Suppl 18), 12–17.

Marneros, A. (2003). Schizoaffective disorder: clinical aspects, differential diagnosis, and treatment. *Current Psychiatry Reports*, **5**, 202–5.

Maziade, M., Gingras, N., Rodrigue, C. *et al.* (1996). Long-term stability of diagnosis and symptom dimensions in a systematic sample of patients with onset of schizophrenia in childhood and early adolescence. I: nosology, sex and age of onset. *British Journal of Psychiatry*, **169**, 361–70.

McPherson, S., Cairns, P., Carlyle, J. *et al.* (2005). The effectiveness of psychological treatments for treatment-resistant depression: a systematic review. *Acta Psychiatrica Scandinavica*, **111**, 331–40.

Meng, H., Schimmelmann, B. G., Mohler, B. *et al.* (2006). Pretreatment social functioning predicts 1-year outcome in early onset psychosis. *Acta Psychiatrica Scandinavica*, **114**, 249–56.

Miklowitz, D. J., Simoneau, T. L., George, E. L. *et al.* (2000). Family-focused treatment of bipolar disorder: 1-year effects of a psychoeducational programme in conjunction with pharmacotherapy. *Biological Psychiatry*, **48**, 582–92.

Nahas, Z., Marangell, L. B., Husain, M. M. *et al.* (2005). Two-year outcome of vagus nerve stimulation (VNS) for treatment of major depressive episodes. *Journal of Clinical Psychiatry*, **66**, 1097–104.

Nemeroff, C. B. (2005). Use of atypical antipsychotics in refractory depression and anxiety. *Journal of Clinical Psychiatry*, **66**(Suppl 8), 13–21.

NICE (2002). *Clinical Guideline 1. Schizophrenia. Core Interventions in the Treatment and Mangement of Schizophrenia in Primary and Secondary Care*. London: National Institute for Health and Clinical Excellence.

Nierenberg, A. A. & Wright, E. C. (1999). Evolution of remission as the new standard in the treatment of depression. *Journal of Clinical Psychiatry*, **60**(Suppl 22), 7–11.

Nierenberg, A. A. & DeCecco, L. M. (2001). Definitions of antidepressant treatment response, remission, nonresponse, partial response, and other relevant outcomes: a focus on treatment-resistant depression. *Journal of Clinical Psychiatry*, **62**(Suppl 16), 5–9.

Pantelis, C. & Lambert, T. J. (2003). Managing patients with 'treatment-resistant' schizophrenia. *Medical Journal of Australia*, **178**(Suppl), S62–6.

Perkins, D., Lieberman, J., Gu, H. *et al.* (2004). Predictors of antipsychotic treatment response in patients with first-episode schizophrenia, schizoaffective and schizophreniform disorders. *British Journal of Psychiatry*, **185**, 18–24.

Perlis, R. H. (2005). The role of pharmacologic treatment guidelines for bipolar disorder. *Journal of Clinical Psychiatry*, **66**(Suppl 3), 37–47.

Perry, A., Tarrier, N., Morriss, R., McCarthy, E. & Limb, K. (1999). Randomised controlled trial of efficacy of teaching patients with bipolar disorder to identify early symptoms of relapse and obtain treatment. *British Medical Journal*, **318**, 149–53.

Peuskens, J. (1999). The evolving definition of treatment resistance. *Journal of Clinical Psychiatry*, **60**(Suppl 12), 4–8.

Quitkin, F. M., McGrath, P. J., Stewart, J. W., Taylor, B. P. & Klein, D. F. (1996). Can the effects of antidepressants be observed in the first two weeks of treatment? *Neuropsychopharmacology*, **15**, 390–4.

Ram, R., Bromet, E. J., Eaton, W. W., Pato, C. & Schwartz, J. E. (1992). The natural course of schizophrenia: a review of first-admission studies. *Schizophrenia Bulletin*, **18**, 185–207.

Royal Australian and New Zealand College of Psychiatrists. (2004). Australian and New Zealand clinical practice guidelines for the treatment of bipolar disorder. *Australian and New Zealand Journal of Psychiatry*, **38**, 280–305.

Royal Australian and New Zealand College of Psychiatrists. (2005). Royal Australian and New Zealand College of

Psychiatrists clinical practice guidelines for the treatment of schizophrenia and related disorders. *Australian and New Zealand Journal of Psychiatry*, **39**, 1–30.

Remington, G., Saha, A., Chong, S. A. & Shammi, C. (2005). Augmentation strategies in clozapine-resistant schizophrenia. *CNS Drugs*, **19**, 843–72.

Robinson, D. G., Woerner, M. G., Alvir, J. M. *et al.* (1999). Predictors of treatment response from a first episode of schizophrenia or schizoaffective disorder. *American Journal of Psychiatry*, **156**, 544–9.

Robinson, D. G., Woerner, M. G., McMeniman, M., Mendelowitz, A. & Bilder, R. M. (2004). Symptomatic and functional recovery from a first episode of schizophrenia or schizoaffective disorder. *American Journal of Psychiatry*, **161**, 473–9.

Rojo, J. E., Ros, S., Aguera, L., de la Gandara, J. & de Pedro, J. M. (2005). Combined antidepressants: clinical experience. *Acta Psychiatrica Scandinavica*, **112**(Suppl), S25–31.

Ropcke, B. & Eggers, C. (2005). Early-onset schizophrenia: a 15-year follow-up. *European Child and Adolescent Psychiatry*, **14**, 341–50.

Ros, S., Aguera, L., de la Gandara, J., Rojo, J. E. & de Pedro, J. M. (2005). Potentiation strategies for treatment-resistant depression. *Acta Psychiatrica Scandinavica*, **112**(Suppl), S14–24.

Rosen, K. & Garety, P. (2005). Predicting recovery from schizophrenia: a retrospective comparison of characteristics at onset of people with single and multiple episodes. *Schizophrenia Bulletin*, **31**, 735–50.

Rossini, D., Lucca, A., Zanardi, R., Magri, L. & Smeraldi, E. (2005). Transcranial magnetic stimulation in treatment-resistant depressed patients: a double-blind, placebo-controlled trial. *Psychiatry Research*, **137**, 1–10.

Sachs, G. S. (1996). Treatment-resistant bipolar depression. *Psychiatric Clinics of North America*, **19**, 215–36.

Sackeim, H. A. (2001). The definition and meaning of treatment-resistant depression. *Journal of Clinical Psychiatry*, **62**(Suppl 16), 10–17.

Schimmelmann, B. G., Conus, P., Schacht, M., McGorry, P. & Lambert, M. (2006). Predictors of service disengagement in first-admitted adolescents with psychosis. *Journal of the American Academy of Child and Adolescent Psychiatry*, **45**, 990–9.

Schulte, P. (2003). What is an adequate trial with clozapine? Therapeutic drug monitoring and time to response in treatment-refractory schizophrenia. *Clinical Pharmacokinetics*, **42**, 607–18.

Sensky, T., Turkington, D., Kingdon, D. *et al.* (2000). A randomized controlled trial of cognitive-behavioral therapy for persistent symptoms in schizophrenia resistant to medication. *Archives of General Psychiatry*, **57**, 165–72.

Simon, J. S. & Nemeroff, C. B. (2005). Aripiprazole augmentation of antidepressants for the treatment of partially responding and nonresponding patients with major depressive disorder. *Journal of Clinical Psychiatry*, **66**, 1216–20.

Souery, D., Amsterdam, J., de Montigny, C. *et al.* (1999). Treatment resistant depression: methodological overview and operational criteria. *European Neuropsychopharmacology*, **9**, 83–91.

Strakowski, S. M., DelBello, M. P., Fleck, D. E. *et al.* (2005). Effects of co-occurring alcohol abuse on the course of bipolar disorder following a first hospitalization for mania. *Archives of General Psychiatry*, **62**, 851–8.

Thase, M. E. (2000). Treatment of severe depression. *Journal of Clinical Psychiatry*, **61**(Suppl 1), 17–25.

Tohen, M., Zarate, C. A., Jr, Hennen, J. *et al.* (2003). The McLean–Harvard First-Episode Mania Study: prediction of recovery and first recurrence. *American Journal of Psychiatry*, **160**, 2099–107.

Torgalsboen, A. K. & Rund, B. R. (1998). 'Full recovery' from schizophrenia in the long term: a ten-year follow-up of eight former schizophrenic patients. *Psychiatry*, **61**, 20–34.

Tsuang, D. & Coryell, W. (1993). An 8-year follow-up of patients with DSM-IIIR psychotic depression, schizoaffective disorder, and schizophrenia. *American Journal of Psychiatry*, **150**, 1182–8.

Valmaggia, L. R., van der Gaag, M., Tarrier, N., Pijnenborg, M. & Slooff, C. J. (2005). Cognitive-behavioural therapy for refractory psychotic symptoms of schizophrenia resistant to atypical antipsychotic medication. Randomised controlled trial. *British Journal of Psychiatry*, **186**, 324–30.

Vieta, E. (2005). The package of care for patients with bipolar depression. *Journal of Clinical Psychiatry*, **66**(Suppl 5), 34–9.

Wade, D., Harrigan, S., Edwards, J. *et al.* (2006). Substance misuse in first-episode psychosis: 15-month prospective follow-up study. *British Journal of Psychiatry*, **189**, 229–34.

Wiersma, D., Nienhuis, F. J., Slooff, C. J. & Giel, R. (1998). Natural course of schizophrenic disorders: a 15-year followup of a Dutch incidence cohort. *Schizophrenia Bulletin*, **24**, 75–85.

World Health Organization. (1974). Symposium on therapy-resistant depression. *Pharmacopsychiatry*, **7**, 69–224.

SECTION 8

Service models

Using research and evaluation to inform the development of early-psychosis service models: international examples

Meredith Harris, Thomas Craig, Robert B. Zipursky, Donald Addington, Merete Nordentoft and Paddy Power

Introduction

Since the late 1980s, there has been enormous growth and investment in the development of clinical and research initiatives focused on early intervention in psychosis, and in several countries large-scale service reform has been initiated. The underlying evidence base, while far from complete, has expanded rapidly to encompass the basic and clinical research, treatment and intervention research, and health services research domains.

This chapter describes five advanced models of early intervention that couple the provision of optimal treatment with the conduct of substantial programmes of 'real world' clinical research. The services included in this chapter include a range of specified treatment components; they also conduct programmes of research and/ or evaluation that is integral to the ongoing development of the service model and contribute substantially to the advancing literature evaluating early-psychosis treatment services and interventions. The illustrated services do not, however, represent an exhaustive list, and there are several other model programmes around the world that have achieved a similar profile.

The focus of this chapter is limited to services, research and evaluation for the treatment of first-episode psychosis (FEP). Service models and research relating to reduction of the duration of untreated psychosis (DUP) and the prodromal period prior to the onset of FEP are not reviewed here, although the services described may include clinical or research components addressing these issues.

The Early Psychosis Prevention and Intervention Centre, Melbourne

The Early Psychosis Prevention and Intervention Centre (EPPIC) (McGorry *et al.*, 1996) in Melbourne, Australia, is a model of early intervention that provides clinical services focused on early detection and provision of optimal treatment in psychosis and is fully integrated with a large clinical research programme. The centre has undergone significant evolution over a 20-year period, which has been progressively and extensively documented in treatment manuals, clinical guidelines, scientific articles and other documents and resources over that time (see Edwards & McGorry, 2002). Here, the EPPIC service model is summarized with an emphasis on newer clinical service developments. The closely related Personal Assessment and Crisis Evaluation (PACE) clinic in Melbourne provides treatment for young people identified as being at ultra-high risk of developing a psychotic illness; however, discussion of this model is outside the scope of this chapter (see Ch. 7).

Overview

The EPPIC programme is a component of ORYGEN Youth Health (OYH), a clinical service for young people with mental health problems living in the northwestern and western metropolitan region of Melbourne (population nearing 1 million people in 2006). The EPPIC programme provides a comprehensive, community-based, specialized service for individuals living in the catchment

The Recognition and Management of Early Psychosis: A Preventive Approach, ed. Henry J. Jackson and Patrick D. McGorry.
Published by Cambridge University Press. © Cambridge University Press 2009.

area who are experiencing a first treated episode of psychosis (defined as not more than 6 months of previous pharmacological treatment for psychosis) and are aged 15 to 24 years inclusive. The upper age criterion was reduced from 29 years in 2002, in line with broader youth mental health service developments within OYH.

The programme provides care for up to 18 months, or up to the age of 18 years for patients who enter the programme at age 15 or 16. On average, 260 new patients are accepted into EPPIC annually. Epidemiological coverage is considered to be relatively complete, as EPPIC is mandated to treat all eligible individuals who present to public mental health services in the catchment area. Further, there are few private psychiatrists practising in the region, and these routinely refer patients with suspected FEP to EPPIC. Investigation of age-specific treated incidence rates revealed a high incidence of psychosis in the catchment (16.7 per 10 000 person-years in males aged 15 to 29, and 8.1 per 10 000 person-years in females (Amminger *et al.*, 2006)).

Service model components

Youth access team

The youth access team is a multidisciplinary team providing mobile assessment, crisis intervention and community treatment for individuals referred to EPPIC with suspected psychosis. The team operates 24 hours a day, every day of the year. A triage service provides the first point of contact with EPPIC, accepting referrals from any source, primarily by telephone. The access team provides a 'gate-keeper' function for the EPPIC programme, undertaking all new assessments of potentially eligible presentations. The team also provides intensive home-based treatment for patients and families, usually in the period immediately following assessment or during transition into and out of inpatient care, with the aim of providing continuous treatment, maintaining engagement and reducing the number of necessary admissions. Psychoeducation and support for families is provided during the initial engagement period. The youth access team also provides crisis intervention to EPPIC clients who, at any time during their episode of care, are unable to wait for a routine appointment. The

ratio of referrals to accepted clients is approximately 2:1. Referrals most frequently come from mental health services (29%) or family/friends or self (25%), followed by general hospitals (13%), non-mental health and welfare services (19%), primary care physicians (9%), and police in only a small number of cases (2%).

The continuing care team

The EPPIC continuing care team is the linchpin of the EPPIC service model. Upon acceptance into EPPIC, each patient is rapidly allocated an outpatient case manager and doctor. The case manager provides direct clinical intervention and coordinates treatment and involvement of other EPPIC programmes, including acute services, as well as linkage to external programmes. Core goals of case management and details of specific psychological interventions are described in the EPPIC Case Management Manual (EPPIC, 2001). Other key materials for case managers include a range of specialized intervention manuals, plus psychoeducational documents and audiovisual materials (Edwards & McGorry, 2002). Guidance to clinicians regarding the optimal timing and/or intensity of clinical interventions and activities is provided via the EPPIC Clinical Guidelines (Edwards & McGorry, 2002; Harris *et al.*, 2004). The continuing care team is staffed by approximately 13.0 full-time equivalent case managers and 3.9 full-time equivalent medical staff, and it manages a steady caseload of 350–400 patients. The average standing caseload for full-time case managers is approximately 30.

Clinical subprogrammes

A range of internal clinical subprogrammes are available to EPPIC patients, tailored to individual need and phase of illness (Edwards & McGorry, 2002). Group programmes (Albiston, Francey & Harrigan, 1998) target social relationships, health promotion, psychoeducation, personal development and creative expression, and a vocational stream focuses on prevocational skill development and vocation planning. Family work interventions (Gleeson *et al.*, 1999) include multifamily group interventions and individual sessions with family members, supported by specialist family workers, and a series of psychoeducation sessions called 'Family & Friends'. A further multifamily intervention is provided via the Treatment Resistance Early Assessment Team (TREAT) (see below) to provide support and psychoeducation for families of patients experiencing a prolonged recovery. Other subprogrammes include accommodation support and a range of vocational rehabilitation strategies (Edwards & McGorry, 2002).

Several subprogramme developments initiated over the past few years are described below. A major development has been the establishment of the EPPIC intensive case management team (Box 21.1). The TREAT approach (Edwards et al., 2002a) was originally developed with a focus on individuals experiencing persistent positive and/ or negative symptoms following a first or subsequent acute episode. A regular screening system identifies these clients and a clinical consultation 'panel' provides technical assistance to treating clinicians in implementing optimal treatment strategies based on a biopsychosocial model. More recently, TREAT has expanded to include an early detection and monitoring system and a secondary consultation service for clients experiencing suicidal or risk issues, and those with a psychotic diagnosis with comorbid cluster B personality traits, psychosis NOS (not otherwise specified), or brief psychotic disorder. A neuropsychology unit has been established for patients who have preexisting cognitive problems (e.g. attention-deficit hyperactivity disorder, learning or intellectual difficulties) that require ongoing attention, or new difficulties with concentration, memory or learning associated with their mental health problem. The unit conducts a range of cognitive, behavioural and personality tests to assess the nature and severity of problems, and their impact on the young person's school, work or home functioning. Referral is via the case manager. Test results are discussed with the young person and their family, carers or school, with recommendations offered for the management of particular problem areas. The Substance Use Research and Recovery Focused (SURRF) programme supports two dual-diagnosis workers within EPPIC.

Inpatient care

A 16-bed inpatient unit provides acute care for individuals who cannot be managed in the community by

---

Box 21.1. The Early Psychosis Prevention and Intervention Centre intensive case management team, Melbourne

Patients experiencing persistent psychotic symptoms and who are reluctant to engage with the service, who possess few social supports to enable ongoing monitoring of their mental state and level of functioning, or are at unknown or unassessable risk for suicide, have been identified as a high clinical priority. However, the implementation of the assertive outpatient follow-up for these patients has, in the past, been hampered by (1) a lack of dedicated, funded mobile support teams for the 18+ year age group, (2) service developments that have increased demand for assessment and decreased time available for acute-phase home-based treatment, and (3) high caseloads that limit clinicians' ability to provide intensive support for these individuals.

In response, the intensive case management (ICM) team was established in 2002 to provide intensive, multidisciplinary, outreach-based care, focusing on community assessment, treatment and support for the centre's clients aged 18–24 years meeting the above criteria, and their families/carers. The programme has expanded and is now staffed by 3.5 full-time equivalent case managers and 1.0 full-time equivalent medical staff.

An audit of the first 2 years of operation (50 clients) of the pilot ICM team found that, compared with the general client group at the centre, ICM clients were more likely to be male, to have a lower level of education and to have a comorbid substance-abuse diagnosis. Antisocial personality traits and a family history of schizophrenia were each present in approximately half of the ICM group. A comparison of pre-and post-ICM treatment showed significant improvement on indicators of improvement in primary treatment goals recorded in individualized management plans, including positive and negative symptoms, engagement with treatment, critical incidents, unplanned contacts and inpatient readmissions (Brewer et al., 2006).

---

outpatient services, through risk of harm to self or others, refusal or inability to comply with treatment or assessment or lack of adequate support in the community. Brief admissions focus on symptom reduction and containment and prepare the person for community support, provided by the youth access team or the EPPIC continuing care team. While the majority of

EPPIC patients will require an inpatient admission, usually during the initial acute phase, a substantial minority are managed exclusively as outpatients (Power *et al.*, 1998; Wade *et al.*, 2006a). Low doses of antipsychotic medication are standard practice during the acute phase. Restrictive practices such as the use of seclusion and police transport or escort to admission are required for only a small number of patients (Wade *et al.*, 2006b).

Youth participation and family/carer programmes

Although not specific to the EPPIC programme, a number of OYH initiatives have been developed to strengthen youth participation and programmes for families and carers (McGorry, Parker & Purcell, 2007; www.orygen.org.au). In place of more traditional consumer consultation models, OYH has implemented a youth participation model that supports young people who are users of OYH's clinical services to participate in the development of programmes and services, and to advocate for themselves and their peers. Participatory activities include the platform team, a group of OYH clients who meet regularly to discuss possible improvements to the service and also produce a newsletter for clients of OYH. Trained, paid, peer-support workers who are past OYH clients visit the inpatient unit and staff the 'platform' room to provide support to other clients. Young people also participate in educating the wider community about mental health issues by speaking at schools and talking to youth workers and the media. Family/carer programmes include peer family-support workers, who themselves have had experience of OYH services and who provide phone and face-to-face support to new family carers whose relative enters EPPIC. Other services include family-support groups and a family resource room with access to a wide range of information. The Health Arts project is an integrated arts strategy that encompasses therapeutic and non-therapeutic creative projects of benefit to clients, staff and visitors to OYH. The projects use knowledge gained from clinical practice and research activities at OYH to advocate for high-quality mental health services for young people.

Research and evaluation

A comprehensive approach to programme description and evaluation

Programme description and evaluation at EPPIC is guided by a comprehensive, five-phase model focused on maintaining treatment integrity within day-to-day clinical practice (Edwards & McGorry, 2002; Harris *et al.*, 2004). Ongoing process evaluations, involving reviews of aspects of clinical care against existing best practice standards, such as the EPPIC Clinical Guidelines, have been critical in informing improvements in service delivery, including the establishment of the intensive case management team (Box 21.1), and identifying the need for service-based strategies to identify and routinely monitor clients at increased risk of suicide (see TREAT above). Large-scale clinical audits have enabled a broad range of clinical practices, treatment patterns and patient characteristics to be examined in complete and unbiased cohorts of EPPIC service users. Published audits have examined the fidelity of treatment for the initial acute phase of treatment diagnostic stability in FEP over the first 18 months of treatment, the prevalence and impact of substance use, and rates and predictors of service disengagement (e.g. Lambert *et al.*, 2005; Wade *et al.*, 2006b).

An integrated clinical and research programme

The clinical services of EPPIC are fully integrated with the research arm of OYH, the ORYGEN Research Centre, a substantial clinical research initiative in youth mental health established in 2002. One stream of research conducted at this centre encompasses a broad range of biological and psychosocial investigations and interventions in FEP and first-episode mania. This stream builds upon EPPIC's long-standing commitment to developing, evaluating and disseminating the results of innovative, phase-specific treatments for FEP, particularly psychological interventions (e.g. cognitively oriented psychotherapy for early psychosis, cannabis use, suicide prevention and relapse prevention; Edwards *et al.*, 2002a, 2006; Edwards, Harris & Bapat, 2005) as well as optimal pharmacological treatments. Building on prior research at the ORYGEN Research Centre on comorbid cannabis use and psychosis, a substance-use research stream includes neurobiological research into a range of emerging substance-use disorders and, in collaboration with other drug and alcohol services, is supporting the development of early-intervention strategies and integrated models of care. A relatively new research stream focuses on suicide prevention. Current projects specific to, or including, the FEP population include a follow-up study over 5–7 years of young people who were treated at EPPIC between 1998 and 2000 to examine clinical- and treatment-based predictors of suicide risk and a retrospective cohort study comparing EPPIC patients with age-matched contemporaries who received treatment in the generic public mental health system care in Victoria in 1991–1999, to determine the impact of specialist mental healthcare on suicide risk. Other research areas include the phenomenology and clinical and functional outcomes 18 months after an initial manic episode, and a comparison of alternative treatment strategies for first-episode mania; underlying neurobiology of emerging psychotic disorder; evaluation of best-practice models of supported employment and education for clients recovering from an episode of psychosis; and evaluation of a combined individual, group and family-based psychosocial intervention aimed at relapse prevention following remission from the first episode.

The comprehensive EPPIC service model has previously been evaluated through a historical cohort study, which demonstrated superior effectiveness and cost-effectiveness of the EPPIC model compared with the pre-EPPIC model of care (McGorry *et al.*, 1996; Mihalopoulos, McGorry & Carter, 1999). In newer developments, a prospective naturalistic follow-up study, designed to assess whether the demonstrated short-term benefits of early intervention are sustained in the medium-to-long term, has recently been completed. The EPPIC Long Term Follow-up Study involves 765 patients followed for a median of 7.5 years after initial diagnosis and treatment at the EPPIC and pre-EPPIC services. Other service-level evaluation projects include a multisite, prospective study to determine whether adherence to clinical practice guidelines improves the effectiveness of such services providing treatment to young people with FEP (Catts *et al.*, 2005).

The Clinical Practice Improvement Network for Early Psychosis project evaluates the first 6 months of treatment in approximately 450 patients from eight public mental health services, including EPPIC, across three states in Australia.

The Lambeth Early Onset service

The Lambeth Early Onset (LEO) service in south London, UK, was assembled in phases through research grants but has gradually been converted to mainstream funding. Each incremental step of its development has been informed by local evaluations and randomized controlled trials.

Introduction and historical context

The LEO service provides comprehensive care for all patients aged 16 to 35 presenting with a FEP within a defined geographical catchment area in Lambeth, an inner city location in south London. The service currently comprises an early detection and crisis assessment team (LEO CAT), a dedicated 18-bed inpatient unit, and an assertive outreach team (the community team) that case manages all LEO patients during the 2 years after initial presentation. A fourth team (Outreach and Support in South London (OASIS)) for young people at ultra-high risk of psychosis is closely associated with LEO. It covers a larger catchment area (population 1 million) in south London, sees patients aged 14–35 years and operates from the same team base as LEO CAT. The OASIS initiative operates on a service development grant with plans for mainstream funding if successful.

The Borough of Lambeth (population 227 300 aged 16–64 years) is ranked as the seventh most deprived of the 376 local authority boroughs in England and Wales (Department of Health, 2001a,b) and is home to a sizeable ethnic minority population (37% compared with 13% nationally) with unemployment rates twice the national average (Office of National Statistics, 2003). The incidence of psychosis is high in this population; age-adjusted inception rates in LEO for the years 2002–2004 were 40/100 000/year (Kirkebride *et al.*,

2006). Specialist mental health services are provided by a single National Health Service (NHS) trust (the South London and Maudsley NHS Trust) with negligible 'leakage' to other providers (e.g. in the private sector). Prior to LEO, specialist care for FEP patients was delivered through generic adult teams, each providing a range of assessment, treatment and continuing care to a geographically defined sector. Each of these sector teams is associated with inpatient facilities on one of three hospital sites.

One important catalyst for the decision to establish the specialist early-onset service across the borough was local evidence that a significant proportion of patients, particularly those from the black and ethnic minority population, were dissatisfied with standard services. These groups suffer from a higher incidence of psychosis, longer DUP and greater likelihood of service access via 'negative' routes involving crises, contact with the police and compulsory hospitalization (Morgan *et al.*, 2005). They are also more likely to engage poorly with services, dropout of follow-up and discontinue treatment early (Garety & Rigg, 2001).

Service model components

The community team: assertive outreach

The LEO community team was the first component of LEO, established initially as an experimental intervention aimed at improving continuity of care and preventing relapse following FEP. This multidisciplinary team comprises 10 clinicians (including psychiatrist, clinical psychologist, vocational specialist and community psychiatric nurses) and provides an assertive outreach model of case management with a single point of access for all mental health and social welfare needs of its patients. It operates an extended hours service 6 days per week. The first 3 years of operation of the team was evaluated through a randomized controlled trial comparing clinical and social outcomes over 18 months with patients managed by the standard psychiatric service (Craig *et al.*, 2004; Garety *et al.*, 2006). In summary, 144 patients aged between 16 and 40 residing in Lambeth and presenting for the first time with a non-affective psychosis were randomized to follow-up

by either LEO or standard care. The LEO service aimed to maintain contact with patients for 2 years and provide a range of interventions aimed at helping the patient to retain or recover functional capacity to return to study or work, to resume leisure pursuits and retain or reestablish supportive social networks. Interventions included medication management, cognitive–behavioural therapy (CBT), family support and vocational assistance. These followed protocols and manuals developed by EPPIC (EPPIC, 1997; Edwards & McGorry, 2002) and, for CBT, pilot work conducted locally (Jolley *et al.*, 2003). A carers' support group was established, as was a social activity programme open to all patients in the service.

Over an 18-month follow-up, the LEO community team proved superior to standard care. Level of engagement was higher among LEO clients, with no differential dropout across ethnic minority groups. Adherence to prescribed medication was significantly greater, as were the proportions of patients offered, accepting and receiving psychological interventions, including CBT for residual psychotic symptoms, family interventions and vocational support. There were fewer recorded adverse events. The LEO patients maintained vocational engagement for longer and reported significantly improved personal relationships at follow-up. Benefits were also noted in relapse and rehospitalization rates, service satisfaction and quality of life.

During the life of the first LEO randomized controlled trial of the community team, case loads were capped at 15, but this proved difficult to sustain beyond the research period. Numbers have tended to creep upwards (currently 20), largely as the result of delays in meeting discharge deadlines but also reflecting gaps and changes in staffing.

Inpatient care

For much of the research period, inpatient care was provided by general psychiatric wards; however, a shortage of local facilities also resulted in admissions to private hospitals often some distance away from the patient's home and family. An audit of these out-of-area placements showed that significant numbers were for younger patients experiencing either initial hospitalization or readmission within the first few years of a psychotic illness, and this was used to justify a successful bid to fund a specialized early-psychosis inpatient unit, run by LEO, with 18 beds (10 male and 8 female beds with a communal day area). The unit provides a safe and engaging environment for young patients and their families, with collaborative approaches to treatment and a group programme focused on recovery and relapse prevention. The unit opened in 2001, initially occupied almost exclusively by FEP patients, usually admitted within the initial days of contact with services, and a small proportion are readmitted within the 2 years of follow-up by the LEO service.

The experimental service was switched to mainstream funding in early 2002 and from that point LEO was established as the sole specialist service for all FEP patients within Lambeth, broadening to accept all diagnostic groups although reducing the upper age limit from 40 to 35 years of age.

The LEO early detection and crisis assessment team

An important service development has been the establishment of the LEO CAT service (Box 21.2).

Research and evaluation

Specialist services such as LEO provide an excellent basis for ensuring that new initiatives are subject to ongoing process and outcome evaluation. Research has underpinned LEO from its inception through to its current more developed structure, as already described. A research and audit steering committee (the LEO Research Coordination Group) of academics and clinicians meets regularly to review research and research capacity, to discuss and prioritize proposals and to review findings. As far as possible, LEO has attempted to develop services to address problems identified in local research and to test these service models in randomized controlled trials. Nonetheless, there remains a need for studies of the specific interventions that make up the complex LEO service model, such as vocational interventions and treatments targeting substance abuse.

> **Box 21.2.** The Lambeth Early Onset service early detection and crisis assessment team, London
>
> The crisis assessment team (CAT) at the Lambeth Early Onset (LEO) service was established in 2002 with a 2-year service development grant. It is a multidisciplinary team made up of six staff members, with backgrounds in psychiatry, psychology, social work and nursing. The first point of contact for all referrals to LEO is the LEO CAT, which carries out initial assessments and home treatment of the acute phase prior to handing over to the LEO community team for recovery work and follow-up. Although focused on the acute presentation, the full range of pharmacological and psychological interventions is provided as necessary, in partnership with the LEO community service. The team also provides information, advice and training to primary care physicians (GPs) in order to facilitate earlier referral to the specialist service.
>
> The UK Department of Health policy implementation guide for early intervention services has established a target of 'shortening' DUP to 3 months or less. The effectiveness of a GP-based education intervention provided by LEO CAT in shortening DUP is being evaluated through a cluster-randomized controlled trial. However, it is recognized that much more work in the wider population, through media, schools and local authority services, will ultimately be needed.
>
> Both the LEO and the LEO CAT randomized controlled trials have an economic evaluation component. Preliminary findings indicate economic benefits for the two interventions particularly through reduction in hospitalization costs. Since early 2003, the demand on beds for FEP patients has decreased dramatically despite consistent referral rates of 110 new FEP patients per year. Now just over half of the beds at any time are occupied by FEP patients, reflecting the impact of LEO CAT on initial hospitalization rates and the ongoing effect of the LEO community team on readmissions beyond those identified in the original LEO trial. To what degree any savings can be sustained in the long term is yet to be evaluated.

The LEO Research Coordination Group is also concerned with monitoring fidelity to the LEO model and ensuring that this is maintained over the longer term. Key performance indicators such as readmission rates, lengths of stay in the different components of the service and serious incidents are reviewed regularly against benchmark guidelines that, as far as possible, can be determined from available evidence.

A relatively recent aspiration has been to persuade clinicians routinely to collect basic information on their patients including DUP, symptoms, social functioning and quality of life, using standardized measures derived from research. In collaboration with colleagues in the London Early Intervention Research Network, a simple minimum dataset for routine data collection has been developed. It uses a Microsoft Access package with easy-to-use data-entry forms and live feedback of outcomes in the form of graphs. It forms the basis of routine clinical audit for the service and is the platform upon which formal research evaluations can be added. While all agree on the ultimate value of this approach, such routine data collection by clinicians remains patchy and is best achieved where clinical teams have included some dedicated research staff.

The First Episode Psychosis Program, Toronto

The First Episode Psychosis Program (FEPP) in Toronto, Canada, was established as an integrated inpatient/outpatient programme and has evolved organically since the early 1990s. Along with the EPPIC and the LEO programmes, FEPP was one of the first examples of a specialized inpatient service providing care during the acute phase of psychosis that was also integrated with outpatient services.

Service overview

The FEPP was developed at the Clarke Institute of Psychiatry, now the Centre for Addiction and Mental Health, in 1992. Both have been affiliated with the Department of Psychiatry at the University of Toronto, which is the largest such department in Canada and is responsible for training approximately 30% of all psychiatrists graduating annually in Canada. The development of the FEPP reflects the shared priorities of these hospitals and the Department of Psychiatry: research, education and clinical care. The initiation of the FEPP was also underpinned by a desire to advance the understanding of the neurobiology of schizophrenia and to study broadly defined determinants of

clinical outcome, particularly pharmacological treatments. This is achieved optimally by studying patients at the beginning of the illness, independent of the long-term effects of the illness and its treatment.

Service components

The evolution of the service components specific to the treatment of FEP is described below. The service also incorporates the Prevention through Risk Identification Management and Education (PRIME) Clinic, a research-based, outpatient service dedicated to the early identification, treatment and evaluation of individuals aged 12 to 30 considered to be at high-risk for developing psychosis.

Inpatient service

The programme began in 1992 when a 12-bed inpatient unit at the Clark Institute of Psychiatry was transformed to become a specialized inpatient unit for the assessment and treatment of patients experiencing a first episode of non-affective psychosis. This was considered ideal at that time for a number of reasons.

1. It was expected that the majority of FEP patients would require an inpatient stay, primarily for successful initiation of antipsychotic treatment, which at that time was limited to first-generation antipsychotic drugs (which were associated with a high risk of acute extrapyramidal symptoms and akathisia).

2. Inpatient admission allowed the treatment team to carry out necessary evaluations rapidly and for education with the patient and their family to achieve engagement and acceptance of the treatment plan.

3. Young patients would benefit from being in a milieu with other young people facing similar challenges and exposure to individuals who may have experienced a difficult and disabling course of illness would be limited.

4. The availability of inpatient beds facilitated the rapid referral of appropriate patients. This was critical from a research perspective, as research studies required patients to be naive for neuroleptic drugs.

The unit has now expanded to 18 beds and been renamed the Early Psychosis Unit. Beds are used for first admissions as well as for patients who have relapsed and require readmission to hospital. While most patients can now be treated initially as outpatients, the unit is increasingly used to meet the needs of patients who are hospitalized involuntarily.

The first-episode psychosis clinic

In addition to the inpatient unit, the hospital created a new position in 1992 for a full-time outpatient nurse to provide follow-up care in a new outpatient clinic. The outpatient team consisted of one nurse as well as a psychiatrist, inpatient social worker and psychiatric residents shared with the inpatient unit. As clinical demand has grown, the core staffing profile of the clinic now includes two nurses, a social worker, an occupational therapist and a part-time CBT therapist, together with five part-time psychiatrists, psychiatric fellows and residents. The programme has greatly benefited from the availability of a publicly funded high-school programme within the hospital, which over the years has become increasingly focused on providing educational support to younger patients to complete their high-school education.

Patients in the First Episode Psychosis Clinic are offered care for up to 3 years. Each patient is assigned a psychiatrist and a case manager. The case manager is a mental health professional trained as a registered nurse, social worker or occupational therapist. The case manager works with the patient to develop a treatment plan, which includes a range of goals relating to work, schooling, family education, social and recreational activities, housing, income support and medication coverage. Case managers and psychiatrists interact with families for education, support and treatment planning. Additional family support is provided through family education groups and family therapy offered through the Learning, Education, Advocacy and Recreation Network (LEARN) programme (Box 21.3).

Since the early 1990s, the clinical services of the FEPP have grown and new resources have subsequently been added as detailed below.

Box 21.3. The Learning, Education, Advocacy and Recreation Network programme

The LEARN programme was developed following an invitation from benefactors working through the hospital charitable foundation to enhance the care of patients in the First Episode Psychosis Programme. A consultant was hired to work with patients, families, family support organizations, staff, benefactors and the hospital charitable foundation, as well as an architect and planner, to develop a plan for a community-based centre to facilitate the vocational, educational and social recovery of patients. The concept of the LEARN programme was developed as a storefront centre to meet the needs of patients with FEP and their families.

Current staffing includes a full-time general education development teacher, an occupational therapist and a social worker. The teacher has developed a highly successful programme to facilitate completion of a high-school diploma for adult patients (patients under 20 years of age have access to a Toronto Board of Education School programme based in the hospital). Occupational therapists work closely with patients to facilitate rapid return to work or school. A social worker specializes in providing group and individual support to families. A weekly psychiatric clinic is also held where case managers and a psychiatrist see patients in order to facilitate the integration of clinical and rehabilitation services. Experience has indicated that many patients are willing to follow up with their psychiatrists but are reluctant to commit to other components of care (e.g. education, group therapy, supported employment, family education) considered by the treatment team as critical to the recovery process.

The Home Intervention Programme for Psychosis

In 2001, the Government of Ontario provided funding to establish the Home Intervention Programme for Psychosis (HIP) programme, modelled on the youth access team developed by EPPIC (described earlier in this chapter and by Edwards & McGorry (2002)). The team assesses patients in the community and provides community-based care at a higher level of intensity than is available in the outpatient clinic. The team comprises a nurse intake coordinator, a full-time psychiatrist, two psychiatric nurses, two psychiatric social workers and an occupational therapist.

The Learning, Education, Advocacy and Recreation Network

A recent development has been the LEARN programme (Box 21.3), designed to integrate multiple aspects of care in one community-based centre and improve the engagement of patients with the full range of available interventions.

The First Episode Assessment and Care Team Clinic

The Centre for Addiction and Mental Health is mandated to provide inpatient psychiatric services to the region of Peel, located adjacent to the western border of the City of Toronto. However, ongoing meetings with the Ministry of Health and stakeholders in this region led to the request to develop FEP outpatient services for Peel that integrated with the Toronto-based FEPP. The First Episode Assessment and Care Team Clinic (FACT-PEEL) was opened in 2001 and offers services dedicated to the assessment and treatment of individuals from 16 to 45 years living in the region of Peel who are experiencing signs of FEP. Current staffing includes 1.5 psychiatrists, 5 nurses, 2 social workers, an occupational therapist and a psychologist.

Services for first-episode bipolar psychosis

The province of Ontario has introduced a policy framework for early intervention and a funding stream of 28 million dollars of annual funding to support the development of new treatment programmes throughout Ontario (population 12.5 million) (Ministry of Health and Long-Term Care, 2004). This funding has enabled the development of new services to meet the needs of individuals experiencing a first episode of bipolar psychosis. While most of the resources involve outpatient services, a small number of inpatient beds are now dedicated to this group and serviced by this specialty programme. This has been an important addition to local resources, allowing patients with psychotic mood disorders to be transferred to this specialized resource and so allowing the existing services to focus more specifically on the needs of young patients recovering from schizophrenia. It is not currently known whether it is optimal to have different programmes for patients with schizophrenia and bipolar disorder. There are clearly ways in which the needs of these two groups overlap substantially (need for rapid assessment and treatment, education and support for patients and families, etc.); however, the nature of the persisting deficits and disabilities may be quite different and require different longer-term approaches.

Referral criteria and service pathways

Patients enter the programme via referral to the outpatient clinics, the HIP team or the inpatient unit. Referrals by family physician, or psychiatrist either within the hospital or in the community, are preferred, although referrals by family members or self-referrals are accepted to facilitate rapid access to the service. An experienced psychiatric nurse screens all new referrals and distributes them to the most appropriate team. The programme is committed to providing rapid access to new referrals and aims to see all new patients within 2 weeks. Waiting lists for assessment or for ongoing care are avoided.

Programme criteria are generally consistent across the services; however, minor variations have been required as a condition of funding. Referral criteria are age 16 to 45 years of age and experiencing a non-affective FEP, but funding for the HIP team mandates that the service also accepts patients with an affective FEP. Patients with a provisional diagnosis of substance-induced psychosis, psychosis secondary to a general medical condition, a developmental disorder or mental retardation are not accepted. Currently, patients are accepted if they have been in treatment for less than 1 year. The hospital serves as a provincial resource; consequently, the programme does not operate within a defined catchment area (with the exception of the HIP team, which operates within the limits of the City of Toronto). The research mandate has always been a high priority, although willingness to participate in research is not a requirement for receiving services. Over the past 3 years, the programme has accepted approximately 300 new referrals per year (double the number accepted in 2001), but as the population of the City of Toronto is 2.5 million and the metropolitan area is 5.0 million, it is evident that the programme is only seeing a minority of incident cases per year.

Research mandate

The major focus of research efforts have been in the areas of psychopharmacology and neurobiology. Magnetic resonance imaging and positron emission tomography (PET) studies have been a priority for the programme since its inception, and, as a result, it was also critically important to have the opportunity to study patients with little or no exposure to antipsychotic medications. Now only a small minority of patients present untreated and only a small number of these are both capable and willing to participate in research. As a result, a large volume of new referrals are required in order to study even 10–15 neuroleptic-naive patients annually.

Initial studies provided support for the use of low-dose typical antipsychotic drugs in the treatment of patients with FEP (Kapur *et al.*, 1996; Zhang-Wong *et al.*, 1999) at a time when it was standard treatment to be using dosages in the range of, for example, haloperidol 20 mg/day. These observations led to the use of PET to investigate dopamine D_2 receptor binding of both first-generation (e.g. Kapur *et al.*, 1996, 1997) and second-generation (e.g. Remington *et al.*, 2006) antipsychotic drugs and the relationship between this binding and treatment response in patients with FEP (Kapur *et al.*, 2000; Tauscher-Wisniewski *et al.*, 2002). Studies with PET (Lewis *et al.*, 1999), magnetic resonance imaging (e.g. Zipursky et al, 1998) and transcranial magnetic stimulation (Daskalakis *et al.*, 2002) have investigated measures of brain structure and function in young patients with little or no exposure to antipsychotic medication. The PRIME clinic was established to facilitate research into the prodromal phase of schizophrenia and the role of psychosocial and pharmacological interventions (McGlashan *et al.*, 2006).

Research efforts have also focused on broader clinical and functional outcomes. A systematic review using meta-analytic techniques (Menezes, Arenovich & Zipursky, 2006a) was undertaken to examine the outcomes that might be achievable in FEP populations. This review identified major methodological limitations in the literature on outcome from first-episode schizophrenia that greatly limit the conclusions that can be reached. In comparison with meta-analyses involving patients with more chronic disorders, a larger percentage of FEP patients improved over time. However, the study also found that sample design issues may influence outcome findings. For example, non-epidemiologically representative samples were associated with better outcomes, possibly reflecting greater levels of protective factors (e.g. social support, education) in samples recruited from academic settings. In contrast, naturalistic, prospective studies may show poorer outcome, possibly through higher rates of non-compliance and dropout. While existing literature has stressed how such variables as DUP, gender and age of onset may be important determinants of outcome, the review also underscored the importance of the interventions offered. The study found the use of combination psychosocial/pharmacological therapy to be associated with better outcome, whereas use of typical neuroleptic drugs and being treatment naive at study entry were associated with poorer outcome, although it is not clear to what extent these effects may reflect the effects of time, sampling biases or differing outcome definitions between studies.

In order to examine outcomes specifically from the FEPP service model, FEPP has collaborated with three other FEP programmes in Ontario to examine 1-year outcomes from these programmes. Consistent with the findings of the meta-analysis, results to date from this study of 200 patients with FEP indicate the importance of methodological considerations in carrying out multisite evaluation research, particularly issues related to sampling (Menezes *et al.*, 2006b). Research is also investigating specific components of treatment that may be critical in improving outcome. A pilot randomized controlled trial is being undertaken comparing outcomes for patients treated in the outpatient clinic compared with those treated by the newer HIP team.

The Calgary Early Psychosis Treatment Service

The Calgary Early Psychosis Treatment Service (CEPTS) in Canada was designed by the University of Calgary

Psychosis Research Unit and first offered a clinical service in 1996, originally funded by a competitive service grant from the Alberta Provincial Mental Health Advisory Board. It has evolved over to include both health services research and population-based research to the original clinical research base.

Service characteristics

The CEPTS (Addington & Addington, 2001a) was designed to provide optimal, evidence-based, patient- and family-focused early psychosis services to an entire population. The health services are operated by a single organization – the Calgary Health Region – that is responsible for the continuum of healthcare services from acute care to community care and public health. The local economy is strong and the local population highly educated. In the decade that the service has been in operation, the population has grown by about 20 000 per year and the local boundaries of the health region have expanded beyond an urban population to include a rural area. This has meant that the population served has grown from about 750 000 to about 1.2 million. Healthcare services are provided free at the point of delivery and are paid for by a combination of taxes and healthcare premiums.

Service components

The CEPTS provides a comprehensive 3-year service to individuals experiencing non-affective FEP, who have not received more than 3 months of adequate antipsychotic treatment for FEP. Two thirds of patients enter the programme without having experienced an admission to hospital. From the programme's inception, service provision has been informed by well-researched optimal care strategies, including second-generation antipsychotic drugs for all patients (Canadian Psychiatric Association Working Group, 2005), family intervention (Dixon & Lehman, 1995), case management (Ziguras & Stuart, 2000), patient education (Mueser & McGurk, 2004) and integrated addiction therapy with treatment (Drake *et al.*, 1998). Key features of treatment are described elsewhere (Addington & Addington, 2001a) but are summarized below.

Case management and psychiatric management. All patients are assigned a psychiatrist and case manager for the duration of their 3 years in the programme; these undertake assessment, monitoring, pharmacotherapy, supportive therapy and referral to a full range of psychiatric, rehabilitation and community support services.

CBT. Cognitive therapy is offered to help in adaptation to the psychotic illness, to address secondary morbidity and to reduce psychotic symptoms.

Group programmes. A range of groups, such as 'psychosis education', 'recovery group', 'moving on group', 'good health modules' and 'substance use', are offered, each designed for a different phase of recovery following the first episode.

Family interventions. Individual family work, provided over six to eight sessions in the first year, focuses on education about psychosis, recommendations for coping with the disorder, communication skills and problem-solving training. This is followed by a six-session multifamily group.

Continued assessment, case management and family work are provided during inpatient admission to any of three city hospitals.

A number of strategies have helped to ensure a patient and family focus to the service. First, the programme is outpatient based, with all patients allocated a case manager who provides access to a full range of mental health services from acute inpatient care to day hospital care, work rehabilitation, educational accommodation for students and consumer-led support programmes such as a clubhouse or treatment for comorbid addictions. Second, each family is provided with a family worker whose focus is the needs of the family. Third, there is no waiting list and referral can be made by either the patient or a family member.

Approach to programme evaluation

Programme evaluation has progressed in two stages. The first involved reporting on a number of outcomes derived from the routine use of a number of well-established assessment measures (Addington & Addington, 2001a). The second stage is still evolving and involves the use of performance measures specifically developed for evaluating FEP treatment services (Addington *et al.*, 2005a).

Effectiveness research

The structure of the service has allowed the researchers to develop a focus on effectiveness research: that is, collecting evidence that applying evidence-based services can function in the real world. Calgary has some advantages for such an undertaking. It is relatively isolated, with no overlapping or neighbouring population centres or health service jurisdictions. At the same time, it has a population large enough to generate reasonable sample sizes within a few years. The results of the programme evaluation have demonstrated a number of outcomes of interest, briefly summarized below.

There have been few reports of the outcome of early-psychosis treatment services for substance abuse. In Calgary, it was demonstrated that the programme had a positive impact on the use of substances (Addington & Addington, 2001b), with statistically significant reductions in marijuana and alcohol abuse. Improvements in positive symptoms were also observed, with 80% achieving a remission by 1 year. There was little change in negative symptoms over time, while depression initially increased over the first quarter but then declined over the next three quarters (Addington, Leriger & Addington, 2003a). Depression is a predictor of suicide and attempted suicide, but the actual rate of attempted suicide was 15% over the year prior to programme entry; only 2.9% made an attempt during the first year that they were in the programme (Addington *et al.*, 2004).

A study of medication adherence provided results that were initially somewhat disappointing in the light of the use of second-generation antipsychotic drugs, family education and patient education (Coldham, Addington & Addington, 2002). In their first year in the programme, 39% were non-adherent, 20% inadequately adherent and 41% adherent. Non-adherent patients demonstrated more positive symptoms, more relapses, more alcohol and cannabis use, reduced insight and poorer quality of life. They were younger, had an earlier age of onset and were less likely to have a family member involved in treatment. It was concluded

that non-adherence has to be anticipated and relationships maintained with patients and families to allow intervention as soon as possible to minimize the consequence of non-compliance.

The onset of a psychotic illness appears to have a large impact on families. A study examining the impact of an individualized family work intervention (Addington *et al.*, 2003b) found that 24% of families demonstrated severe distress and 23% moderate distress at baseline. No change in proportions was observed at 6 months, but by 12 months the proportion experiencing moderate stress had improved to normal levels, whereas there was no change for those experiencing severe stress. For this group, change was not observed until 2 years. The most significant predictor of poor psychological well-being was the family's appraisal of the impact of the illness on themselves, and not the severity of symptoms or impaired functioning of the patient. This family intervention embedded within a treatment programme proved to be effective and highly acceptable, evidenced by a high participation rate (Addington, McCleary & Addington, 2005b).

Finally, a study of pathways to care found that help-seeking attempts began in the prodromal phase of the illness and continued into the psychotic phase (Addington *et al.*, 2002). A range of contacts were made early but emergency services were most often the contact that helped individuals to obtain appropriate treatment for psychosis. From this study, it was concluded that improved gatekeeper and public education might reduce the time required before individuals developing a psychosis received timely and adequate care. Gatekeeper education was initiated from the start of the programme, with both a programme for family physicians and a programme for school and college counsellors. A more recently delivered multimedia public education programme is currently being evaluated with funding from a competitive research grant. The results to date indicate a positive impact of the education programme, as indicated by increases in the general population's awareness of illness signs and information on how to access treatment services, increased hits on a website and increased numbers of referrals. The impact on DUP and hospital stays is still being assessed.

In conclusion, a decade of studies has demonstrated that an early-psychosis treatment service that operates in a 'real world' environment without extraordinary resources can provide timely and efficient services that deliver good outcomes. These good outcomes are realized not only by the patients but also by the families, who experience reduced distress and a reduction in the negative experience of care giving.

Performance measurement

Recently, the emphasis of evaluation has shifted from one based upon specific outcome measures to one based upon performance measures that fit within a nationally recognized framework (Box 21.4).

OPUS: intensive integrated treatment in the early phase of psychosis in Denmark

The OPUS service evolved in a different way to the services discussed above. It was initiated by the Danish Government as a randomized controlled trial in 1998. The trial was conducted in Copenhagen and Aarhus between January 1998 and December 2000. From January 2002, the experimental treatment was turned into a permanent service in both Copenhagen and Aarhus; the service was expanded and now includes 27 staff members in Copenhagen and 17 in Aarhus. Recently, a similar service was established in Odense, the third largest city in Denmark.

Overview of the service

Patients are accepted into the treatment programme if they fulfil the following criteria:

- diagnosis of schizophrenia, schizotypal disorder, schizoaffective disorder, delusional disorder, acute or transient psychotic disorder, induced delusional disorder or unspecified non-organic psychosis (F20–29 in ICD-10; WHO, 1993) (in Aarhus, only individuals with schizophrenia are included)
- aged between 18 and 35 years with a legal residence in Aarhus County or in the catchment area of

Box 21.4. Performance measures for early-psychosis treatment services, Calgary

The Calgary Early Psychosis Treatment Service has recently completed two studies, the first designed to identify and select appropriate performance measures, and the second designed to apply these measures to a specific programme (Addington *et al.*, 2005a). The first study was conducted in two stages. First, a literature review gathered articles published from 1995 to July 2002, and experts were consulted to determine performance measures. Second, a consensus-building technique, the Delphi process, was used with nominated participants from seven groups of stakeholders. Twenty stakeholders participated in three rounds of questionnaires. Seventy-three performance measures were identified from the literature review and consultation with experts. The Delphi method reduced the list to 24 measures rated as essential. The resulting measures reflected the interests of all stakeholders, across seven domains.

Domain	Performance measures
Accessibility	Median DUP, service availability, education to patients and family, wait time
Appropriateness	Acute phase medication, maintenance phase medication, hospital readmission rate
Continuity	Community follow-up after hospitalization, change in principal mental health provider, dropout rate, documented discharge plan
Effectiveness	Global functioning, symptom remission, relapse, positive symptoms, negative symptoms, depressive symptoms
Competence	Evaluation component in early-psychosis programme
Safety monitoring	Side effects, tardive dyskinesia, suicides, suicide attempt, akathisia
Acceptability	Confidentiality.

The second study examined the feasibility and utility of applying the previously identified set of consensus-derived performance measures to evaluate an early-psychosis treatment service. Operational definitions were developed for the measures and attempts were made to collect all measures from existing sources including corporate databases, clinical databases and chart review. Scoring covered 41 measures, including 12 effectiveness measures. The measures covered seven of eight domains recommended for service-level evaluation by the Canadian Institute for Health Information. The set of measures proved feasible to collect and provides a performance framework that assesses key processes and documents achievement of programme objectives. The next phase of this research includes risk adjustment of the original measures on a new and larger sample of subjects.

Copenhagen Hospital Corporation (the municipalities of Copenhagen and Frederiksberg)

- not more than 6 months prior exposure to continuous antipsychotic medication.

Exclusion criteria are evidence of organic brain disease or a psychotic condition caused by acute poisoning or a withdrawal state. However, individuals are not excluded on the basis of misuse of psychoactive drugs if they most likely suffer from schizophrenia-spectrum disorder.

Patients can be referred to treatment from all inpatient and outpatient mental health services in Copenhagen and Aarhus, the two largest cities in Denmark. The referring units in Copenhagen include six hospitals and all 11 community mental health centres connected to the psychiatric departments of the five inner city hospitals. The referring units in Aarhus include three hospitals and five community mental health centres. Primary care physicians and private psychiatrists also refer patients, and in some cases patients themselves, or their parents, contact the service. In very few cases, assessment is carried out as an assertive outreach meeting in the home of the patient; in even fewer cases, the first contact is established in relation to a compulsory admission. Diagnostic assessments are carried out by a psychiatrist together with another staff member using the Schedule for Clinical Assessment in Neuropsychiatry (SCAN 2.0 in 1998, SCAN 2.1 since 1999; WHO, 1998).

Service model

The integrated psychiatric treatment has four elements, all provided by a multidisciplinary team: (1) assertive community treatment, (2) medication, (3) psychoeducational family treatment and (4) social skills training.

Assertive community treatment

The integrated treatment can be defined as an enriched assertive community treatment model (Stein & Santos, 1998; Stein & Test, 1980) that includes protocols for family involvement and social skills training. Three multidisciplinary teams, two in Copenhagen and one in Aarhus, were established and intensively trained by external experts to provide the integrated treatment. Each team includes the following disciplines: psychiatrist, psychologist, psychiatric nurse, occupational therapist and social worker. All team members receive group supervision continuously. Caseload is approximately 10 and never exceeds 12 for each professional team member. Each patient is offered integrated treatment for 2 years. A primary team member is designated to each patient and is then responsible for maintaining contact and cocoordinating treatment within the team and across different treatment and support facilities, and across the social and health sectors. Patients are visited in their homes, at their workplace, in other places in their community or are seen at the office, according to a patient's preference. The offices are based in facilities outside the hospital. The team practises case sharing, which means that any team member may become involved in the treatment of a patient, as necessary. Hours of operation are Monday to Friday from 8 a.m. to 6 p.m.

All team workers have a mobile telephone with an answering function. Patients are encouraged to call at any time if they need help or advice. After hours, they can leave a message, knowing that the team will respond the next morning. In a crisis, patients are instructed to get help from significant others and to use the local psychiatric emergency room. A specific crisis plan is developed for each patient in collaboration between the patient and the clinician with primary responsibility for the patient. The team attempts to avoid developing dependency by reducing the intensity of help offered to patients with a high level of functioning. The patient is encouraged to take responsibility for his or her own affairs as soon as possible during the process of recovery. During hospitalization, treatment responsibility is transferred to the hospital, but a team member visits the patient once a week and takes part in treatment-planning conferences.

In instances where the patient wishes to discontinue psychiatric treatment before the 2 years of treatment have elapsed, the team practises assertive outreach to maintain contact and tries to motivate the patient to continue treatment and to find a common focus for therapy. Psychoeducation is provided along with antipsychotic medication, and team members pay close attention to adverse events. Very good fidelity (70%) to the programme model, measured with the Index of Fidelity of Assertive Community Treatment (McGrew *et al.*, 1994), has been achieved in both Copenhagen and Aarhus. Factors responsible for reduced fidelity are time-limited treatment, 24-hour coverage in other settings and about two contacts weekly with each patient, patient's family and collaborating partners. Patients requiring continued treatment beyond the 2 years of integrated treatment are transferred to other treatment facilities, most often community mental health centres.

Psychopharmacological treatment

Psychopharmacological treatment follows the guidelines issued by the Danish Psychiatric Society (1998), which recommends use of the newer atypical antipsychotic medications and lower dosages for recent-onset psychosis. The same guidelines were applied to patients treated by the standard mental health services throughout the study period.

Psychoeducational family intervention

Within the first month after inclusion, patients are encouraged to allow the primary team member to invite relatives into collaboration. Psychoeducational family treatment is offered to patients in contact with at least one significant other. Most often parents are involved in treatment, but any significant relative, friend or other non-professional caregiver may be invited to participate. Family treatment has three components modelled on Psycho-educational Multiple Family Group Treatment (McFarlane *et al.*, 1995): (1) at least three individual family meetings without the patient, with the aim of creating an alliance with the family and reviewing the present crisis; (2) survival skills workshop (Anderson, Reiss & Hogarty, 1986) where four to six families are given formal education about psychosis and its management, aetiology and prognosis through lectures and discussions; and (3) the family group treatment with four to six families plus the patients and two family therapists; the group meets for 1½ hours every other week for 18 months. The focus is on problem solving and development of coping skills.

Social skills training

Patients who lack basic skills for independent living or are unable to work in a group are offered individual training and practical help in their homes. Patients with an intermediate level of impaired social skills are offered social skills training in a group with a maximum of six patients and two therapists, one being a psychologist. The training programme is organized in modules to overcome the patient's symptomatic and cognitive barriers to learning (Liberman *et al.*, 1986). The five selected modules are medication self-management, coping with symptoms, conversation, problem-solving and conflict-solving skills. Some patients do not need social skills training. Patients receive individual psychoeducation during meetings with their primary team worker.

Evaluation of integrated treatment

The OPUS randomized controlled trial has examined whether the provision of integrated treatment leads to better course and outcome in young patients with schizophrenia-spectrum disorders compared with patients treated with standard care. Key findings to date are summarized in Box 21.5.

Conclusions

This chapter has presented an overview of the service models and research and evaluation programmes of five well-established early-psychosis programmes. Each service conducts an ongoing programme of research and/or evaluation that is integral to the continued development of the service model. One major difficulty in defining the parameters of early-psychosis services has been identified by the services reviewed here, that is, for how long should patients with FEP be followed up by early intervention services and, in particular, for how long should fully recovered patients continue treatment. As yet, the evidence base to support an optimal duration of treatment has not been firmly established. Hence, services face difficulty in establishing best-practice protocols around this issue, and in negotiating for funding to extend early-psychosis care significantly into, and beyond, the critical period. Where demand exceeds preferred caseload levels, the services reviewed here have had to develop strategies to manage demand, or revise the duration of their episode of care.

Because of funding constraints, the maximum episode of care offered by EPPIC is 18 months for most clients. The 18-month time frame is short, allowing only a 'front-end' approach. At the conclusion of the maximum period of EPPIC treatment, almost one-third of patients (32%) required transfer to office-based

follow-up with psychiatrists or primary care physicians; 38% were referred to non-specialist mental health services in the same catchment area; 11% did not require a referral for follow-up care; and around 20% had already disengaged from the service because they moved to another area or were no longer in contact with the service (Edwards, Harris & Herman, 2002b). In the LEO service, it was originally envisaged that continuing care and supervision would be provided over the first 3 years following onset, with a gradual and closely managed transfer of care to generic services where this was needed at the end of that time. In practice, however, funding and service pressures have constrained follow-up with the LEO service to 2 years. At this point, around half of the patients continue to require the level of supervision and support provided by a specialist FEP service but have to be handed on to overstretched generic community teams.

Similarly, the FEPP programme in Toronto has experienced pressure to reduce the episode of care or, alternatively, to increase caseloads in order to meet the ongoing demand for new referrals. A flexible approach has had to be developed. The programme is committed to accept new referrals even when full clinical capacity has been reached, reflecting its clinical and research priorities. Where it is clear, before the 3-year point, when a patient's needs could be met in a clinic with a less-intensive model of care, efforts are made to transfer the care of such patients. Similarly, it is sometimes clear within the first year or two that patients require more intensive services, such as those of an assertive community treatment team, at which point efforts are made to facilitate the transfer. In situations where patients have been stabilized, have returned to work or school and have minimal ongoing needs, it is often possible for psychiatrists to provide the ongoing infrequent follow-up without the involvement of a case manager, whose time can then be devoted to the more intensive needs of new referrals.

Recent studies provide some evidence that, for most patients, treatment intensity should not be reduced within the first 5 years (e.g. Linszen, Dingemans & Lenoir, 2001). Patients 'graduating' from specialized early-psychosis programmes may experience negative consequences arising from disruptions to continuity of care and reduced levels of support or treatment available from subsequent treatment services; however, this needs to be monitored through careful long-term follow-up. More research is needed to establish the optimal duration of specialized treatment and to determine whether it is possible to reduce the intensity of specialized treatment over a longer time frame, at least in certain subgroups of patients. This information is critically needed to guide appropriate service development.

REFERENCES

Addington, D., McKenzie, E., Addington, J. *et al.* (2005a). Performance measures for early psychosis treatment services. *Psychiatric Services*, **56**, 1570–82.

Addington, J. & Addington, D. (2001a). Early intervention for psychosis: the Calgary Early Psychosis Treatment and Prevention Program. *Canadian Psychiatric Association Bulletin*, **33**, 11–13.

Addington, J. & Addington, D. (2001b). Impact of an early psychosis program on substance abuse. *Psychiatric Rehabilitation Journal*, **25**, 60–7.

Addington, J., van Mastrigt, S., Hutchinson, J. & Addington, D. (2002). Pathways to care: help seeking behaviour in first episode psychosis. *Acta Psychiatrica Scandinavica*, **106**, 358–64.

Addington, J., Leriger, E. & Addington, D. (2003a). Symptom outcome 1 year after admission to an early psychosis program. *Canadian Journal of Psychiatry*, **48**, 204–7.

Addington, J., Coldham, E. L., Jones, B., Ko, T. & Addington, D. (2003b). The first episode of psychosis: the experience of relatives. *Acta Psychiatrica Scandinavica*, **108**, 285–9.

Addington, J., Williams, J., Young, J. & Addington, D. (2004). Suicidal behaviour in early psychosis. *Acta Psychiatrica Scandinavica*, **109**, 116–20.

Addington, J., McCleery, A. & Addington, D. (2005b). Three-year outcome of family work in an early psychosis program. *Schizophrenia Research*, **79**, 77–83.

Albiston, D., Francey, S. M. & Harrigan, S. M. (1998). Group programs for recovery from early psychosis. *British Journal of Psychiatry*, **172**(Suppl 33), s117–21.

Amminger, G. P., Harris, M. G., Conus, P. *et al.* (2006). Treated incidence of first-episode psychosis in the catchment area of EPPIC between 1997 and 2000. *Acta Psychiatrica Scandinavica*, **114**, 337–45.

Anderson, C. M., Reiss, D. J. & Hogarty, G. E. (1986). *Schizophrenia in the Family. A Practitioner's Guide to Psycho-education and Management.* New York: Guilford Press.

Brewer, W. J., Murphy, B., Lambert, T. *et al.* (2006). Intensive case management (ICM) for high suicide risk: evaluating a unique model of care for poorly engaged clients with first episode psychosis. *Schizophrenia Research*, **81**(Suppl 1), 229.

Canadian Psychiatric Association Working Group (2005). Clinical practice guidelines for treatment of schizophrenia. *Canadian Journal of Psychiatry*, **50**(Suppl 1), 1s–56s.

Catts, S. V., O'Toole, B., Carr, V. *et al.* (2005). The feasibility of routine effectiveness evaluation in public mental health services: what does it take? *Australian and New Zealand Journal of Psychiatry*, **39**(Suppl 2), A85.

Coldham, E. L., Addington, J. & Addington, D. (2002). Medication adherence of individuals with a first episode of psychosis. *Acta Psychiatrica Scandinavica*, **106**, 286–90.

Craig, T. K. J., Garety, P., Power, P. *et al.* (2004). The Lambeth Early Onset (LEO) team: randomised controlled trial of the effectiveness of specialised care for early psychosis. *British Medical Journal*, **329**, 1067–8.

Danish Psychiatric Society (1998). Behandlung med antipsy-kotika: vejledende ratningslinier. [Guidelines for treatment with antipsychotic drugs]. *Ugeskrift for Laeger*, **160**(Suppl 5).

Daskalakis, Z. J., Christensen, B. K., Chen, R. *et al.* (2002). Evidence for impaired cortical inhibition in schizophrenia using transcranial magnetic stimulation. *Archives of General Psychiatry*, **59**, 347–54.

Department of Health (2001a). *Compendium of Clinical and Social Indicators.* London: The Stationery Office.

Department of Health (2001b). *The Mental Health Policy Implementation Guide.* London: The Stationery Office.

Dixon, L. B. & Lehman, A. F. (1995). Family interventions for schizophrenia. *Schizophrenia Bulletin*, **21**, 631–43.

Drake, R. E., Mercer-McFadden, C., Mueser, K. T., McHugo, G. J. & Bond, G. R. (1998). Review of integrated mental health and substance-abuse treatment for patients with dual disorders. *Schizophrenia Bulletin*, **24**, 589–608.

Edwards, E., Elkins, K., Hinton, M. *et al.* (2006). Randomized controlled trial of a cannabis-focused intervention for young people with first-episode psychosis. *Acta Psychiatrica Scandinavica*, **114**, 109–17.

Edwards, J. & McGorry, P. D. (2002). *Implementing Early Intervention in Psychosis: A Guide to Establishing Early Psychosis Services.* London: Martin Dunitz.

Edwards, J., Maude, D., Herrmann-Doig, T. *et al.* (2002a). A service response to prolonged recovery in early psychosis. *Psychiatric Services*, **53**, 1067–9.

Edwards, J., Harris, M. & Herman, A. (2002b). The Early Psychosis Prevention and Intervention Centre, Melbourne, Australia: an overview, November 2001. In C. Ogura (ed.),

Recent Advances in Early Intervention and Prevention in Psychiatric Disorders. Tokyo: Seiwa Shoten, pp. 26–33.

Edwards, J., Harris, M. G. & Bapat, S. (2005). Developing services for first episode psychosis and the critical period. *British Journal of Psychiatry*, **187**(Suppl 48), s91–7.

EPPIC (1997). *Early Psychosis Training Pack*. Melbourne: Early Psychosis Prevention and Intervention Centre.

EPPIC (2001). *Case Management in Early Psychosis: A Handbook*. Melbourne: Early Psychosis Prevention and Intervention Centre.

Garety, P. A. & Rigg, A. (2001). Early psychosis in the inner city: a survey to inform service planning. *Social Psychiatry and Psychiatric Epidemiology*, **36**, 1–8.

Garety, P. A., Craig, T. K. J., Dunn, G. *et al.* (2006). Specialised care for early psychosis: symptoms, social functioning and patient satisfaction. *British Journal of Psychiatry*, **188**, 37–45.

Gleeson, J., Jackson, H. J., Stavely, H. & Burnett, P. (1999). Family intervention in early psychosis. In P. D. McGorry & H. J. Jackson (eds.), *Recognition and Management of Early Psychosis: A Preventive Approach* New York: Cambridge University Press, pp. 376–406.

Harris, M., Edwards, J., Ratnaike, D. *et al.* (2004). Evaluating treatment integrity in early psychosis programs: comparing what is promised with what is delivered. In T. Ehman, G. W. MacEwan & W. G. Honer (eds.), *Best Care in Early Psychosis: Global Perspectives*. London: Taylor & Francis, pp. 167–74.

Jeppesen, P., Petersen, L., Thorup, A. *et al.* (2005). Integrated treatment of first-episode psychosis: effect of treatment on family burden: OPUS trial. *British Journal of Psychiatry*, **187** (Suppl 48), s85–90.

Jolley, S., Garety, P., Craig, T. *et al.* (2003). Cognitive therapy in early psychosis: a pilot randomized controlled trial. *Behavioral and Cognitive Psychotherapy*, **31**, 473–8.

Kapur, S., Remington, G., Jones, C. *et al.* (1996). High levels of dopamine D2 receptor occupancy with low-dose haloperidol treatment: a PET study. *American Journal of Psychiatry*, **153**, 948–50.

Kapur, S., Zipursky, R., Roy, P. *et al.* (1997). The relationship between D_2 receptor occupancy and plasma levels on low dose oral haloperidol: a PET study. *Psychopharmacology*, **131**, 148–52.

Kapur, S., Zipursky, R., Jones, C., Remington, G. & Houle, S. (2000). Relationship between dopamine D(2) occupancy, clinical response, and side effects: a double-blind PET study of first-episode schizophrenia. *American Journal of Psychiatry*, **157**, 514–20.

Kirkbride, J., Fearon, P., Morgan, C. *et al.* (2006). Heterogeneity in incidence rates of schizophrenia and other psychotic syndromes: findings from the 3-centre ÆSOP study. *Archives of General Psychiatry*, **63**, 250–8.

Lambert, M., Conus, P., Lubman, D. I. *et al.* (2005). The impact of substance use disorders on clinical outcome in 643 patients with first-episode psychosis. *Acta Psychiatrica Scandinavica*, **112**, 141–8.

Lewis, R., Kapur, S., Jones, C. *et al.* (1999). Serotonin 5-HT$_2$ receptors in schizophrenia: a PET study using [18F] setoperone in neuroleptic-naive patients and normal subjects. *American Journal of Psychiatry*, **156**, 72–8.

Liberman, R. P., Mueser, K. T., Wallace, C. J. *et al.* (1986). Training skills in the psychiatrically disabled: learning coping and competence. *Schizophrenia Bulletin*, **12**, 631–47.

Linszen, D., Dingemans, P. & Lenior, M. (2001). Early intervention and a five year follow up in young adults with a short duration of untreated psychosis: ethical implications. *Schizophrenia Research*, **51**, 55–61.

McFarlane, W. R., Lukens, E., Link, B. *et al.* (1995). Multiple-family groups and psychoeducation in the treatment of schizophrenia. *Archives of General Psychiatry*, **52**, 679–87.

McGlashan, T. H., Zipursky, R. B., Perkins, D. *et al.* (2006). Randomized, double-blind trial of olanzapine versus placebo in patients prodromally symptomatic for psychosis. *American Journal of Psychiatry*, **163**, 790–9.

McGorry, P. D., Edwards, J., Mihalopoulos, C., Harrigan, S. M. & Jackson, H. J. (1996). EPPIC: an evolving system of early detection and optimal management. *Schizophrenia Bulletin*, **22**, 305–26.

McGorry, P. D., Parker, A. & Purcell, R. (2007). Youth mental health: a new stream of mental healthcare for adolescents and young adults. In G. Meadows, B. Singh & M. Griggs (eds.), *Mental Health in Australia*, 2nd edn. Cambridge, UK: Cambridge University Press, pp. 438–49.

McGrew, J. H., Bond, G. R., Dietzen, L. & Salyers, M. (1994). Measuring the fidelity of implementation of a mental health program model. *Journal of Consulting and Clinical Psycholology*, **62**, 670–8.

Menezes, N. M., Arenovich, T. & Zipursky, R. B. (2006a). A systematic review of longitudinal outcome studies of first episode psychosis. *Psychological Medicine*, **36**, 1349–62.

Menezes, N. M., Malla, A., Norman, R. *et al.* (2006b). Predictors of outcome from first episode psychosis programs in Ontario, Canada. *Schizophrenia Research*, **81** (Suppl 1), 246.

Mihalopoulos, C., McGorry, P. & Carter, R. (1999). Is phase-specific, community-oriented treatment of early psychosis an economically viable method of improving outcome? *Acta Psychiatrica Scandinavica*, **54**, 1–9.

Ministry of Health and Long-term Care (2004). *Program Policy Framework for Early Intervention in Psychosis*. Ontario: Government of Ontario, pp. 1–29.

Morgan, C., Mallett, R., Hutchinson, G. *et al.* for the ÆSOP Study Group (2005). Pathways to care and ethnicity. 2: Source of referral and help-seeking. *British Journal of Psychiatry*, **186**, 290–6.

Mueser, K. T. & McGurk, S. R. (2004). Schizophrenia. *Lancet*, **363**, 2063–72.

Nordentoft, M., Thorup, A., Petersen, L. *et al.* (2006). Transition rates from schizotypal disorder to psychotic disorder for first-contact patients included in the OPUS trial. A randomized clinical trial of integrated treatment and standard treatment. *Schizophrenia Research*, **83**, 29–40.

Office of National Statistics (2003). *Census 2001*. London: Office of National Statistics.

Petersen, L., Jeppesen, P., Thorup, A. *et al.* (2005a). A randomised multicentre trial of integrated versus standard treatment for patients with a first episode of psychotic illness. *British Medical Journal*, **331**, 602–5.

Petersen, L., Nordentoft, M., Jeppesen, P. *et al.* (2005b). Improving 1-year outcome in first-episode psychosis: OPUS trial. *British Journal of Psychiatry*, **187**(Suppl 48), s98–103.

Power, P., Elkins, K., Adlard, S. *et al.* (1998). Analysis of the initial treatment phase in first-episode psychosis. *British Journal of Psychiatry*, **172**(Suppl 33), s71–6.

Remington, G., Mamo, D., Labelle, A. *et al.* (2006). A PET study evaluating dopamine D_2 receptor occupancy for long-acting injectable risperidone. *American Journal of Psychiatry*, **163**, 396–401.

Stein, L. I. & Santos, A. B. (1998). *Assertive Community Treatment of Persons with Severe Mental Illness*. New York: W.W. Norton.

Stein, L. I. & Test, M. A. (1980). Alternative to mental hospital treatment. I. Conceptual model, treatment program, and clinical evaluation, *Archives of General Psychiatry*, **37**, 392–7.

Tauscher-Wisniewski, S., Kapur, S., Tauscher, J. *et al.* (2002). Quetiapine: an effective antipsychotic in first-episode schizophrenia despite only transiently high dopamine-2 receptor blockade. *Journal of Clinical Psychiatry*, **63**, 992–7.

Thorup, A., Petersen, L., Jeppesen, P. *et al.* (2005). Integrated treatment ameliorates negative symptoms in first episode psychosis-results from the Danish OPUS trial. *Schizophrenia Research*, **79**, 95–105.

Wade, D., Harrigan, S., Harris, M. G., Edwards, J. & McGorry, P. D. (2006a). Pattern and correlates of inpatient admission for patients with first-episode psychosis. *Australian and New Zealand Journal of Psychiatry*, **40**, 429–36.

Wade, D., Harrigan, S., Harris, M. G., Edwards, J. & McGorry, P. D. (2006b). Treatment for the initial acute phase of first-episode psychosis in a real-world setting. *Psychiatric Bulletin*, **30**, 127–31.

WHO. (1993). *The ICD-10 Classification of Mental and Behavioural Disorders. Diagnostic Criteria for Research.* Geneva: World Health Organization.

WHO. (1998). *Schedules for Clinical Assessment in Neuropsychiatry*, version 2.1. *Present State Examination*. Geneva: World Health Organization.

Zhang-Wong, J., Zipursky, R. B., Beiser, M. & Bean, G. (1999). Optimal haloperidol dosage in first-episode psychosis. *Canadian Journal of Psychiatry*, **44**, 164–7.

Ziguras, S. J. & Stuart, G. W. (2000). A meta-analysis of the effectiveness of mental health case management over 20 years. *Psychiatric Services*, **51**, 1410–21.

Zipursky, R. B., Lambe, E. K., Kapur, S. & Mikulis, D. J. (1998). Cerebral gray-matter volume deficits in first episode psychosis. *Archives of General Psychiatry*, **55**, 540–6.

Index

ABC study, emotional and personality dysfunctions, 284

abstract language disturbance, prodrome basic symptoms, 99

abuse, depression, 288

access problems, treatment delays, 165–6

acoustic perception disturbances, prodrome basic symptoms, 100

Active Cognitive Therapy for Early Psychosis (ACE) study, 205

acute psychotic phase, emotional and personality dysfunctions, 285–6

acute risk containment, suicide prevention, 272–3

adherence
  bipolar disorder treatment, 228–9, 235
  see also medication adherence/non-adherence

admission *see* inpatient admission

adolescence
  CNS changes, 61
  emotional and personality dysfunctions, 284

adoption studies, environmental risk factors, 49

affective-dynamic disturbances, SPI-A, 91

affective psychosis
  atypical antipsychotic 191
  pharmacotherapy, 186, 191, 192

age, FEP, substance misuse, 244

age of onset, bipolar disorders, 233

AKT1 gene/protein, 32

Alcohol, Smoking and Substance Involvement Screening Test (ASSIST), 250

alcohol use
  bipolar disorder, 234
  suicide risk, 266

Alcohol Use Disorders Identification Test (AUDIT), 250

allele association studies, 34
  single nucleotide polymorphisms, 34

ambiguity, in diagnosis, 19

ambiguous loss, 315

Amish study, bipolar disorder prodrome identification, 232

amisulpride, 194
  incomplete recovery therapy, 215
  treatment-resistant major depressive disorder, 375
amphetamine use, psychosis relapse, 354
amygdala, structural neuroimaging, 69
anger/irritability, at-risk mental state, 114
anterior cingulate cortex, structural neuroimaging, 70
antidepressant medication
  bipolar disorders, 225
  suicidal behaviour treatment, 273
  treatment-resistant bipolar depression, 374
antipsychotic medication
  adverse effects, 110, 187, 193–6
    diabetes, 188–9, 195
    endocrine effects, 189, 195–6
    extrapyramidal motor symptoms, 188, 194–5, 228
    metabolic effects, 193
    metabolic syndrome, 188–9, 195
    obesity, 188, 195
    sexual side effects, 189, 195–6
    tardive dyskinesia, 188, 194–5, 228
    weight gain, 188, 195
  atypical 194
    affective psychosis, 191
    maintenance therapy, 352
    non-affective psychosis, 189
    suicidal behaviour treatment, 273
    treatment-resistant bipolar depression, 374
    treatment-resistant bipolar mania, 374
  bipolar disorder, 227, 228, 233
  borderline personality disorder, 294
  combination therapy, 375
  DUP offset, 126
  first-generation, 213
  low-dose, FEP, 187, 193
  monotherapy, 375
  professionals, beliefs about, 151
  public, beliefs about, 150, 151
  relapse prevention, 356–7
  response studies, 378
  second-generation, 214
    incomplete recovery therapy, 215
    treatment-resistant schizophrenia, 371
  treatment-resistant major depressive disorder, 375
  treatment-resistant schizophrenia, 371
  unacceptability to service users, 111
anxiety
  at-risk mental state, 94, 114
  incomplete recovery, FEP, 208

persecutory delusions, 287
aripiprazole, 194
  treatment-resistant major depressive disorder, 375
assertive community treatment team, FEPP, 401
assessment phases, relapse prevention, 359
Association of Cognitive Analytic Therapy, 297
at-risk mental state, 7, 83–105
  common problems, 114
  hypothalamic–pituitary–adrenal axis, 96–7
    cortisol, 96
  identification, 85–93
    basic symptoms criteria, 88–92
    false positives, 85
    rationale, 84–5
    referral source effects, 88
    see also specific methods
  'madness' concerns, 111
  management see at-risk mental state management
  neurobiological variables, 96–7
    gyrification index, 97
    hippocampus, 96
    pituitary gland, 97
    reduced grey matter, 97
  neurocognitive changes, 84
  neurocognitive variables, 95–6
  predictors, 93–7
  psychopathological variables, 93–5
    anxiety, 94
    basic symptoms, 94
    depression, 94
    distress, 94
    negative symptoms, 93–4
    poor functioning, 94–5
    positive psychotic phenomena, 93
    schizotypal personality features, 93
    stress, 95
    substance use, 95
  signs and symptoms, 107
  see also prodrome, UHR
at-risk mental state management, 114, 165
  antipsychotic medication, 108–11
    evidence against, 110–11
    support of, 108–10
    see also specific studies
  criteria, 107
  ethics, 108
  interventions, 108–15
    see also specific interventions
  monitoring, 113

no interventions, 113
psychoeducation, 118
psychological interventions, 111–13
evidence against, 112–13
support of, 111–12
see also specific studies
retrospective studies, 107
social interventions, 113
attentional defects, neuropsychological studies, 65
attention captivation, prodrome basic symptoms, 99
attention division inability, prodrome basic symptoms, 99
Attenuated Psychotic Symptoms (APS) Group, UHR criteria, 86
attenuated symptoms, prodrome, 83
attributions, family interventions, 322
atypical antipsychotic drugs, *see* antipsychotic medication, atypical
auditory P50 inhibition deficits, psychophysiological studies, 66

basic symptoms
at-risk mental state, 88–92, 94
prodrome, 83, 98–100
behavioural disturbances, FEP, 178–9
benzodiazepines, psychiatric emergencies, 193
bilateral cingulate grey matter, neuroimaging, 70
biological markers, 62–3
diagnosis (of early psychosis), 19
family history *see* family history of psychosis
see also endophenotypes
bipolar affective disorder, neuroimaging, 68
bipolar depression, 230
identification, 232, 233
pharmacotherapy, 191
treatment resistance, 374–5
bipolar disorders, 10–11, 223–39
case studies, 226–7, 229
Clinical Global Impressions (CGI) score, 234
comorbidities, 234
depression *see* bipolar depression
early intervention, 223–5
outcome, 224
psychotic disorders vs., 225
targets, 229–30
first-episode mania, 230
comorbidities, 230
identification of, 231–2, 233
non-recognition of, 230
functional recovery, 225
identification

age of onset, 233
earlier identification, 231–2
initial prodrome, 232–3
manic episodes, 232
problems, 231, 233
initial prodrome, 230–1
psychological interventions, 234–5
CBT, 234
developmental issues, 234
family input, 235
psychoeducation, 234
rapid cycling *see* rapid cycling bipolar disorders
recovery rates, 229
relapse prevention, 235
substance use, 225
symptomatic remission, 225
syndromal remission, 224
treatment, 227–9, 233–4
adherence, 228–9, 235
antidepressants, 225
antipsychotic medication, 227, 228, 233
current guidelines, 227–8
current practice, 228
delay 226
delay, consequences of 226
delay, factors 226
treatment resistance
definition, 366
non-pharmacological management, 376
pharmacological treatment, 373
prevalence, 367
see also specific disorders
birth cohort studies, neuropsychological studies, 63
body perception disturbance, SPI-A, 91
borderline personality disorder, 12, 293–4
antipsychotic medication, 294
cognitive analytic therapy, 296
co-occurring psychosis, 294
therapeutic interventions, 295–7
Helping Young People Early Clinic, 297
psychotic symptoms, 294
brain-derived neurotrophic factor (neurotropin 3), 37–8
C-270T polymorphism, 37
functional neuroimaging, 40
G196A polymorphism, 37
linkage studies, 41
brief limited intermittent psychotic symptoms group, 86
Brief Psychiatric Rating Scale (BPRS), 86
relapse definitions, 350

C270T polymorphism, brain-derived neurotrophic factor, 37

Calgary Early Psychosis Treatment Service *see* CEPTS

cannabis use
  COMT gene, 54–5, 246
  FEP, 243, 246, 247
  psychosis relapse, 354

cardiovascular disease, FEP, 184

care pathways, 397

care provision, EPPIC, 386

carer–patient contact, expressed emotion, 306

case examples
  emotional and personality dysfunctions, 295
  relapse prevention, 359

case management, 396

Case Management Manual, EPPIC, 386

case studies
  at-risk mental state management, 116–17
  bipolar disorders, 226–7, 229
  treatment resistance, 377–7

catechol-*O*-methyltransferase *see COMT*

CBT (cognitive–behavioural therapy)
  Active Cognitive Therapy for Early Psychosis study, 205
  at-risk mental state management, 112
  bipolar disorders, 234
  CEPTS, 396
  definition, 292
  early-recovery phase, 205–6, 212
  emotional/personality dysfunction, 291–3
  FEP, substance misuse, 248, 252–3
  LEO Service, 390
  Norfolk Early Intervention Service programme, 344
  PRIME study, 115
  relapse prevention, 357, 360
  staging model, 24
  treatment-resistance schizophrenia, 375

central nervous system (CNS), adolescence, changes in, 61

CEPTS (Calgary Early Psychosis Treatment Service) 207, 395–8
  care pathways, 397
  case management, 396
  CBT, 396
  characteristics, 396
  components, 396
  effectiveness research, 397–8
  family, impact on, 397
  family interventions, 396
  group programme, 396
  medication adherence, 397
  performance measurement, 398
  programme evaluation, 396–8

psychiatric management, 396
  substance abuse, 397

children
  emotional and personality dysfunctions, 284
  see also adolescence

CHRNA7 (nicotinic acid receptor) gene/protein, 32, 38

chromosomal translocations, schizophrenia, 36

chronic illness *see* illnesses, chronic

Clinical Global Impression Severity (CGI-S) Score, 189
  relapse definitions, 350

clinical judgement, diagnosis (of early psychosis), 19

Clinical Practice Improvement Network for Early Psychosis, EPPIC, 389

clinical studies, psychological variables in relapse, 354

clinician errors, treatment delays, 171

clozapine, 194
  FEP, 214
  incomplete recovery therapy, 215
  suicidal behaviour, 273
  treatment-resistant bipolar mania, 374
  treatment-resistant schizophrenia, 373

clubhouse model, 335–8
  Program of Assertive Community Treatment vs., 336
  studies in, 336–8
  supported employment vs., 338
  transitional employment, 335

cognition, endophenotypes, 64

cognition activation tasks, functional neuroimaging, 67

cognitive analytic therapy, 295–7
  borderline personality disorder, 296
  Helping Young People Early Clinic, 297
  psychosis, 296–7

cognitive assessment, FEP, 184

Cognitive Assessment and Risk Evaluation (CARE) Clinic, 87

cognitive–attentional impediments, SPI-A, 91

cognitive–behavioural therapy, *see* CBT

cognitive impairment, 94
  at-risk mental state, 95
  COMT gene, 36
  FEP, 182
    incomplete recovery, 209
  relapse, 355–6
  SPI-A, 91

cognitively oriented psychotherapy for early psychosis, 205

cognitive models, social anxiety, 290–1

cognitive therapy
  Early Detection and Intervention Evaluation, 111
  EPPIC, 340–1
  UHR, 97

cohort characteristics, DUP follow-up studies, 133–6

Cologne Early Recognition and Intervention Centre for Medical Crisis *see* FETZ (Früh-Erkennungs and Therapie-Zentrum für psychische Krisen)

Cologne Early Recognition Study, 88–9

community campaigns, mental health literacy, 153–5

community efforts, treatment delay reduction, 168

community mental health literacy, 8

Community Treatment Orders, 276

comorbid disorders, *see* FEP assessment

comorbid psychiatric disorders, FEP, 188, 194–5

The Compass Strategy (Australia), 154–5, 156, 158

Comprehensive Assessment of At Risk Mental State (CAARMS)
   Early Detection and Intervention Evaluation, 116
   PACE UHR criteria, 86, 87

comprehensive treatment services, FEP, substance misuse, 249

COMT (catechol-*O*-methyltransferase) gene, 32, 36
   associated behaviour, 31
   cannabis use, 54–5, 246
   cognitive impairment, 36
   as endophenotype, 38
   functional neuroimaging, 67
   manic-depressive illness, 36
   Val158Met genotype, 36, 55

concentration/attention problems, at-risk mental state, 114

coping strategies, family interventions, 322–3

cortical folding patterns, structural neuroimaging studies, 68

cortisol, hypothalamic–pituitary–adrenal axis, 96

counselling, public, beliefs about, 150

counsellors, public, beliefs about, 149

crisis assessment team, LEO, 389, 391

Criteria for Prodromal Symptoms (COPS), PRIME study, 109

cultural factors, suicide risk factors, 267–8

cultures, expressed emotion, 306, 311

cytoskeleton, DISC1, 37

DAAO gene/protein, 32

DAOA gene/protein, 32, 35
   NMDA receptor, 35
   single nucleotide polymorphisms, 35

Dartmouth Assessment of Lifestyle Instrument (DALI), 250

data extraction, DUP follow-up studies, 132–3

debriefing, suicide prevention, 275

Delphi consensus technique
   CEPTS, 398
   relapse definitions, 350

delusions
   at-risk mental state, 114

emotional and personality dysfunctions, 286–7
   FEP, 182
   persecutory
     anxiety, 287
     emotional and personality dysfunctions, 287

demography, treatment delay, 166–7

depression, 285–6
   abuse, 288
   at-risk mental state, 94, 114
   bipolar disorders *see* bipolar depression
   incomplete recovery, FEP, 208
   postpsychotic, 286
   public recognition of, 148
   suicidal behaviours, 261

derealization, prodrome basic symptoms, 99

Developmental Processes in Schizophrenic Disorders Project, UCLA Aftercare Research Program, 342

diabetes, antipsychotic medication, 188–9, 195

diagnosis (of early psychosis), 17–27
   aims of, 18
   ambiguity, 19
   biological markers, 19
   clinical judgement, 19
   crystallized disorders vs., 18–19, 134–5
   non-specific symptoms, 19
   timing difficulties, 19
   validity, 18–20

DISC1 gene/protein, 32, 36–7, 72
   cytoskeleton, 37
   functional neuroimaging, 67
   linkage studies, 41

discrimination decrease, prodrome basic symptoms, 99

disrupted in schizophrenia-1 gene/protein *see* DISC1 gene/protein

distress, at-risk mental state, 94

distress level studies, family caregiving, 313, 314

DNA methylation, 50
   epigenetics, 39

dorsolateral hyperfrontality, functional neuroimaging, 67

DRD3 gene/protein, 38

DTNBP1, 32
   linkage studies, 41

DUP (duration of untreated psychosis), 7–8, 125–45, 147
   estimates, 161
   follow-up studies, 129, 130–3
     cohort characteristics, 133–6
     data extraction, 132–3
     measurement methods, 130–2
     outcome types, 132

DUP (duration of untreated psychosis) (cont.)
  premorbid adjustments, 136-8, 139
  quantitative data analysis, 133
  results, 133-9
  see also specific results
  search strategies, 130
  sensitivity analysis, 138-9, 140-1
  study characteristics, 18-19, 133, 134-5
  study selection, 130
  validity assessment, 132
  Hillside study, 142
  initial assessment, 180
  lack of correlation, 142
  minimization aims, 24
  'neurotoxic' effects, 161
  offset definition, 125-7
  onset definition, 125-7
    consistency lack, 125
    illness status, 127
    retrospective data, 127
    symptom inconsistency, 126
  outcome effects, 129-30, 131, 136, 213
    heterogeneity effects, 136
    long-duration vs. short-duration groups, 136, 137, 138
    participant numbers, 136
  P300 abnormality, 66
  patient vs. carer accounts, 127-8
  professional contact to treatment delay, 161, 164-5
  relapse effect, 356
  retrospective assessment, 127
  sample bias, 128
  standardized assessment instruments, 128-9
  Suffolk County study, 142
  symptom to professional contact delay, 161
  see also treatment delay reduction
duration of active psychosis, 213
duration of treated psychosis
  definition, 127
  negative outcomes, 127
duration of untreated illness, 180
duration of untreated prodromal psychosis, 180
duration of untreated psychosis *see* DUP
duration of untreated psychosis in treatment, 213
dysbindin, 34
  functional neuroimaging, 67
dystrophin-associated protein complex (DPC), 34

Early Case Identification Program (Canada), 155
Early Detection and Intervention Evaluation, 111-12, 115-16

cognitive therapy, 111
Comprehensive Assessment of At Risk Mental State, 116
transition rates, 87
early detection effects
  bipolar disorders, 231-2
  DUP outcome effects, 129
early initial prodrome state
  FETZ, 89, 90, 116
  German Research Network on Schizophrenia, 89, 90
early intervention
early intervention targets, bipolar disorders, 229-30
  suicidal behaviour treatment, 275
Early Psychosis Intervention Program, 155, 169
  family intervention stage models, 320
  success of, 170
Early Psychosis Prevention and Intervention Centre *see* EPPIC
early psychosis service models, 14, 385-404
  see also specific models
early recovery phase, 10, 201-14
  pharmacology, 202-4
    long-acting novel antipsychotic drugs, 203-4
    poor efficacy, 203
    poor tolerability, 203
    relapse, 204
    reviews, 203
    switching treatment, 203
  psychosocial treatments, 204-7
    CBT, 205-6, 212
    family therapy, 207
    phase-specific group treatment, 206
    psychoeducation, 204
    recovery stage model, 207
    vocational interventions, 206-7
    see also specific clinical trials
early warning signs, relapse, 355
Early Warning Signs Scale, 355
ECT *see* electroconvulsive therapy
Edinburgh High-Risk Study (EHRS), 64
  emotional and personality dysfunctions, 284
  symptom severity, 64
education level, treatment delays, 166
electroconvulsive therapy
  suicidal behaviour treatment, 273
  treatment-resistant bipolar depression, 374
  treatment-resistant bipolar mania, 374
  treatment-resistant major depressive disorder, 376
emergency departments, inpatient admission, 165
emotional and personality dysfunctions, 12, 283-302
  acute psychotic phase, 285-6

case example, 295
CBT, 291–3
historical aspects, 283–4
persecutory delusions, 287
prior to onset, 284
prodromal phase, 284–5
psychosis interactions, 286–8
   adolescents vs. adults, 289
   delusions/hallucinations, 286–7
   diagnostic implications, 289
   maintenance processes, 287–8
   psychological reaction, 289–91
   shame/stigma, 289–90
   shared developmental pathways, 288–9, 290
   social anxiety, 289–90
   traumatic reactions, 289
psychosis link, 286–91
safety behaviours, 287
see also borderline personality disorder; *specific dysfunctions*
emotions, suicidal behaviours, 259
employment
   barriers to *see* work functioning
   rates, 333
   specialists, UCLA Aftercare Research Program, 342
Employment Intervention Demonstration Project, 336
endocrine effects, antipsychotic medication, 189, 195–6
endophenotypes, 6–7, 38–9, 61–80
   characteristics, 61
   chronic illness effects, 62
   cognition, 64
   deficits, 62
   definition, 38
   established disease effects, 61
   event-related brain potentials, 62
   executive functions, 71
   family history *see* family history of psychosis
   frontal lobe integrity, 71
   functional neuroimaging *see* neuroimaging functional
   general cognition, 63
   GRM3 gene/protein, 39
   markers of inhibitory control, 71
   neuroanatomy, 61
   neuropsychological studies *see* neuropsychological studies
   neuropsychological test performance, 38
   psychophysiological studies *see* psychophysiological studies
   structural neuroimaging *see* neuroimaging, structural
   study selection, 56
   temporal effects, 62
   working memory, 72

environmental risk factors, 5, 47–59
   adoption studies, 49
   epidemiology, 49
   family studies, 49
   gene relations, 47–8
   see also gene–environment correlation, gene–environment
      interactions
   measurement of, 56
   paternal age, 50, 53
   psychometric psychosis liability, 49–50
   schizophrenia, 40
   twin studies, 49
epigenetics, 39
   DNA methylation, 39
EPIP *see* Early Psychosis Intervention Program
EPPIC, 169, 385–9
   bipolar disorders, 225, 234
   care provision, 386
   Case Management Manual, 386
   clinical guidelines, 386
   Clinical Practice Improvement Network for Early
      Psychosis, 389
   clinical subprogrammes, 386–7
   cognitive therapy studies, 340–1
   comprehensive service model, 389
   continuing care team, 386
   early recovery phase, 208
   emotional and personality dysfunctions, 295
   family/carer programmes, 388
   family interventions, 358
   family work interventions, 386
   funding constraints, 401
   incomplete recovery treatment, 214
   inpatient care, 387–8
   intensive care management team, 387, 388
   Long Term Follow-Up Study 389
   ORYGEN research centre, 388
   preexisting cognitive problems, 387
   psychosis incidence, 386
   relapse prevention, 358
   research and evaluation, 388–9
   service model components, 386–8
   suicidal behaviour, 261
   suicide risk monitoring, 271
   TREAT programme 387
   vocational interventions, 340–1
   Youth Access Team, 386
   youth participation, 388
ERBB4 gene/protein, 32

ethics, at-risk mental state management, 108
ethnicity
    LEO, 390
    suicide prevalence, 267
    treatment delays, 166
European Prediction of Psychosis Study, 91
event-related brain potentials, 62
executive functions, 71
expressed emotion (EE), 306–12
    detection problems, 308–12
    emotional overinvolvement vs., 311
    in FEP, 307–8, 309–10
        level monitoring, 315
        outcome effects, 308
    loss reaction, 353
    patient conflicts, 311
    predictive validity, 306–7
    relapse mechanisms, 307
    relapse predictors/risk factors, 353
    social context, 311
    in UHR, 307–8, 309–10
expressive speech disturbance, prodrome basic
        symptoms, 99
extrapyramidal motor symptoms, antipsychotic medication,
        188, 194–5, 228

false positives
    at-risk mental state identification, 85
    prodrome, 92
families
    bipolar disorders, 235
    caregiving, 312–15
        distress level studies, 313, 314
        EPPIC, 388
        experiences of, 312–15
        illness duration effects, 313
        individual differences, 315
        loss and grief issues, 315
        specific issues, 313
    during course of psychosis, 305–12
    emotion see expressed emotion
    history of psychosis, 62
        first-generation studies, 51, 52
        follow-up periods, 62
        gene–environment interactions, 48, 51–3
        twin studies, 49, 51
        studies, 63
        treatment delays, 168
    LEO, 390

as psychotic cause, 305
    recovery model, 316–20
    segregation studies, 33
    studies, environmental risk factors, 49
    suicide risk factors, 267–8
    therapy
        early recovery phase, 207
        incomplete recovery therapy, 216
    treatment, seeking of, 163, 170
family interventions, 13, 305–29
    CEPTS, 396
    components and guidelines, 320–1
    coping strategies, 322–3
    FEP, 315–21
        substance misuse, 248
    future work, 323–4
    implementation, 323
    psychoeducation, 322
        attributions, 322
        OPUS, 400
    relapse prevention, 357–8
    stage models, 316–20
    supportive interventions, 321–2
    treatment aims, 321
    work interventions, EPPIC, 386
fear of psychosis, 112
FEP (first-episode psychosis) 9, 21, 23, 24
    assessment see FEP assessment
    cognitive dysfunction, 184
    early recovery phase see early recovery phase
    emotional/personality dysfunctions, 294
        prevalence, 294–5
    expressed emotion see expressed emotion
    family interventions, 315–21
    incomplete recovery from see incomplete recovery, FEP
    recovery from, 201
    remission, 201
    substance abuse see FEP substance abuse
    suicide, 260
        acute phase, 260–2
    treatment see FEP treatment
    vocational interventions, 339–45
FEP assessment, 9–10, 177–200
    aims, 177–80
    see also specific aims
    behavioural disturbances, 178–9
    biomedical evaluation, 184
    clinical history, 180–2
    comorbid disorders, 181, 182–3

diagnostic evaluation, 185
differential diagnosis, 186, 191
initial contact planning, 178
integrated treatment plan, 179–80
mental state examination, 181, 182
neuropsychological assessment, 184–5
personal context recognition, 178
personal history, 180–2
problems with, 177
psychobiological assessments, 180–5
psychosis recognition, 178
recommendations, 184, 189–91
remission, 179
risk assessment, 181, 183–4
social assessment, 181
therapeutic alliance, 177–8
FEP substance abuse, 243–5
assessment feedback, 251
cannabis, 243, 246, 247
psychological interventions, 247
correlates/consequences, 244–5
engagement, 249
information sources, 251
initial assessment, 249–50
motivation to cease, 250–1
persistence, 244
prevalence, 243
psychological interventions, 247–53
CBT, 248, 252–3
comprehensive treatment services, 249
established psychotic disorders, 247
family interventions, 248
harm minimization, 252
motivational interviewing, 248, 252
psychoeducation, 251–2
randomized controlled trials, 247
stepped care, 249
types, 247
rate and patterns, 243–4
reasons for, 245–7
common factors, 246–7
personality traits, 246
psychosis causes substance abuse, 245
self-medication hypothesis, 245
substance abuse causes
psychosis, 245–6
temporal order, 244
tobacco, 243, 244
psychological interventions, 248

FEP treatment, 9–10, 177–200
adherence to, 212–13
impaired adherence therapy, 213–14
outcome definitions, 201
pharmacology, 185–9, 191
changes in, 188–9, 195
comorbid psychiatric disorders, 188, 194–5
integrated treatment, 187
low-dose antipsychotic drugs, 187, 193
non-affective vs. affective psychosis, 184, 186, 187, 189–91, 192
patient/relation input, 187
principles, 185
response, timing of, 181, 189
treatment adherence, 188, 195
treatment delay reduction, 185
unfavourable outcome identification, 189, 195–6
see also antipsychotic medication
treatment resistance, 202, 214
FETZ (Früh-Erkennungs and Therapie-Zentrum für psychische
Krisen), 89, 90, 116
early initial prodrome state, 89, 90, 116
Early Recognition Study 88–9
late initial prodrome state, 89, 90, 116
FEZ1 gene/protein, 32
first aid skills, pubic knowledge/beliefs, 148–9
first-episode bipolar psychosis services, FEPP, 394
first-episode mania *see* bipolar disorders
first-episode psychosis *see* FEP
First Episode Psychosis Program, *see* FEPP
FEEP (First Episode Psychosis Program), 207, 392–5
Assertive Community Treatment Team, 401
First Episode Assessment and Care Team Clinic 387
FACT-PEEL 394
components, 392–5
see also specific components
early psychosis unit, 393
family intervention stage models, 316–20
FEP bipolar services, 394
First Episode Psychosis Clinic, 387
funding constraints, 401
Home Intervention Program for Psychosis, 393
inpatient service, 392–3
Learning, Education, Advocacy and Recreation Network
(LEARN) programme, 393, 394
PRIME clinic, 392, 395
referral criteria, 394–5
research mandate, 395
service pathways, 394–5
services, 392

first-generation antipsychotic drugs *see* antipsychotic
    medication, first-generation
forensic history, FEP, 180
formal caregivers, expressed emotion, 307
frontal lobe integrity, endophenotypes, 71
fronto-striatal function, functional neuroimaging, 68
functional magnetic resonance imaging functional
    neuroimaging *see* neuroimaging; functional 67
functional recovery, bipolar disorders, 225
functioning levels, treatment delays, 167
funding constraints
    EPPIC, 401
    FEPP, 401
    LEO Service, 401

GAD1 (glutamic acid decarboxylase 1), 32
gender
    expressed emotion, 306
    FEP, substance misuse, 244
    treatment delays, 166
    gene–environment links 47–8
        correlation (rGE), 47, 48
        confounding, 56
        evocative, 56
        passive, 56
    interactions, 40, 47, 48, 50
        first-generation studies, 48, 51–3
        migration designs, 49
        rearing environment measures, 49
        sample size, 56
        second-generation studies, 54–5
        see also endophenotypes
general cognition, endophenotypes, 63
general education development, Learning, Education,
    Advocacy and Recreation Network programme, 393
general population screening, prodrome, 92
general practitioners
    inpatient admission, 165
    primary help seeking, 163
    public, beliefs about, 149
genetics, 4–5, 31–46
    allele association studies, 34
    environment relations *see* gene–environment link
    linkage studies, 33, 41
    multiple tests, 57
    structural neuroimaging, 70
    suicide risk, 266
    susceptibility genes, 31, 32
    see also specific genes

genome-wide linkage studies, 33
    early initial prodrome state, 89, 90
    late initial prodrome state, 89, 90
    needs-focused intervention, 91
Global Assessment of Functioning (GAF) scale,
    PRIME study, 109
glutamic acid decarboxylase 1 *see* GAD1 (glutamic acid
    decarboxylase 1)
    functional neuroimaging, 67
grey matter
    density, structural neuroimaging studies, 68
    reduced in at-risk mental state, 97
GRM3 gene/protein, 32
    as endophenotype, 39
group programme, CEPTS, 396
group therapy, incomplete recovery
    therapy, 216
gyrification index, at-risk mental state, 97

hallucinations, triggering, emotional and personality
    dysfunctions, 288
haloperidol, maintenance medication, 357
harm minimization, FEP, substance misuse, 252
health belief model, FEP treatment, 212
health professionals
    knowledge/beliefs of, 151–3
    pubic knowledge/beliefs, 149, 150
Helping Young People Early Clinic
    borderline personality disorder, 297
    cognitive analytic therapy, 297
heterogeneity effects, DUP outcome effects, 136
Hillside Recognition and Prevention Program
    Criteria, 92
    Clinical high-risk patients, 92
    duration of untreated psychosis, 142
hippocampus
    at-risk mental state, 96
    structural neuroimaging, 69
Home Intervention Program for Psychosis,
    FEPP, 393
$5HT_{2a}$ gene/protein, 38
hyperprolactinaemia, antipsychotic drugs, 196
hypothalamic–pituitary–adrenal axis
    structural neuroimaging studies, 69
    see at-risk mental state

ICD-10 schizophrenia diagnosis, OPUS, 398
identification (of psychosis), 7–8
    see also diagnosis (of early psychosis)

illicit drug use *see* substance abuse/misuse

illness duration effects, family caregiving, 313

illnesses, chronic
  endophenotypes, 62
  suicide risk, 266

illness status, onset, 127

impaired adherence therapy, FEP treatment, 213–14

imprinting, 50

incidence (of psychosis) *see* psychosis

incomplete recovery, FEP, 10, 201–14
  anxiety, 208
  cognitive defects, 209
  comorbidities, 211
  depression, 208
  negative symptoms, 208
  ongoing positive symptoms, 208
  outcome confounders, 209–13
  pharmacotherapy, 215
    positive symptoms, 215
  psychological adjustments, 212
  psychosocial therapy, 215–16
  social deficits, 208–9
  treatment approaches, 214–16

individual placement, vocational interventions, 338–9

individual placement and support approach, 338–9, 340, 342–3
  assessment of, 338–9
  FEP, 340

individual psychotherapy
  FEP, incomplete recovery, 215–16
  incomplete recovery therapy, 215–16

individual training programmes, mental health literacy, 157

industrial therapy, 334

information sources, FEP, substance misuse, 251

inhibitory control, endophenotypes, 71

initial contact planning, FEP, 178

initial prodrome, bipolar disorders *see* bipolar disorders

initial risk assessment, suicide prevention *see* suicide
    prevention

inpatient admission
  emergency departments, 165
  general practitioners, 165
  professionals, beliefs about, 151
  public, beliefs about, 150, 151

inpatient care
  EPPIC, 387–8
  FEPP, 392–3
  LEO Service, 389, 390–1

intensive care area, psychiatric emergencies, 193

intensive care management team, EPPIC, 387, 388

intermediate phenotypes *see* endophenotypes

International Center for Clubhouse Development, 335

International Early Psychosis Association
  relapse prevention, 349
  treatment guidelines, 117

interpersonal and social rhythm therapy,
    treatment-resistant bipolar disorder, 376

interpersonal difficulties, at-risk mental state, 114

Interview for the Retrospective Assessment of the Onset of
    Schizophrenia (IRAOS), DUP measurement, 130

Italy, social firms, 335

job agencies, vocational interventions, 341

Lambeth Early Onset Service *see* LEO Service

late initial prodrome state
  FETZ, 89, 90, 116
  German Research Network on Schizophrenia (GRNS), 89, 90

Learning, Education, Advocacy and Recreation Network
    (LEARN) programme *see* FEPP

LEO (Lambeth Early Onset Service), 389–92
  CBT, 390
  crisis assessment team (LEO CAT), 389, 391
  ethnic populations, 390
  funding constraints, 401
  historical context, 389–90
  inpatient care, 389, 390–1
  LEO Research and Coordination group, 391
  Outreach and Support in South London (OASIS), 389
  outreach team, 389, 390
  psychosis incidence, 389
  Research and Coordination Group 391
  research and evaluation, 391–2
  service model components, 390–1
  see also specific components

life events, relapse predictors/risk factors, 354

LifeSPAN therapy, suicidal behaviour treatment, 274

linkage studies, 33, 41
  brain-derived neurotrophic factor, 41
  DISC1 gene/protein, 41
  DTNBP1, 41
  NRG1 gene/protein, 41

lithium, suicidal behaviour treatment, 273

Liverpool University Neuroleptic Side-Effect Rating Scale, 203

long-acting novel antipsychotics drugs, 203–4

longitudinal studies
  neuropsychological studies, 65
  psychophysiological studies, 66
  structural neuroimaging studies, 69

long-term studies, neuropsychological studies, 63
loss and grief issues, family caregiving, 315

'madness' concerns, at-risk mental state, 111
magnetic resonance spectroscopy, 69
maintenance therapy, 353
   atypical antipsychotic drugs, 352
   emotional and personality dysfunctions, 287–8
   needs-adapted treatment model, 353
   relapse prevention, 356
major depression, selective serotonin-reuptake inhibitors, 191
major depressive disorder, treatment resistance
   definition, 366–7
   non-pharmacological management, 376–7
   pharmacological therapy, 374–5
   prevalence, 367–8
maladaptive beliefs, emotional and personality
     dysfunctions, 287
manic-depressive illness, *COMT* gene, 36
manic episodes, bipolar disorders, 232
markers of inhibitory control, endophenotypes, 71
medial temporal structures, structural neuroimaging, 69
medical disorders, FEP, 183
medication
   LEO Service, 390
   suicide prevention, 273
   suicide risk, 267, 269
   see also specific diseases/disorders; specific medications
medication adherence/non-adherence
   CEPTS, 397
   relapse predictors/risk factors, 352–3
medication discontinuance
   OPUS, 399
   relapse predictors/risk factors, 352, 356
Mental Health First Aid Course, 157
mental health literacy, 147–60
   definition, 147
   historical improvements, 153
   interventions, 153–8
     community campaigns, 153–5
     individual training programmes, 157
     school-based programmes, 155–7
     see also pubic knowledge/beliefs
mental health service provision models, suicide prevention,
     275–6
Mental Illness Aware Week (USA), 155
Mental Illness Education (Australia), 114
mental state examination, *see* FEP assessment
metabolic syndrome, antipsychotic medication, 188–9, 195

migration designs, gene–environment interactions, 49
mismatch negativity, psychophysiological studies, 66
monitoring
   at-risk mental state management, 113
   psychiatric emergencies, 193
mood cycling, treatment resistance, 366
mood stabilizers
   affective psychosis, 191
   bipolar disorder, 227, 228
   treatment-resistant bipolar depression, 374
   treatment-resistant bipolar mania, 373
motivational interviewing, FEP, substance misuse, 248, 252
motivation problems, at-risk mental state, 114
MRDS1 gene/protein, 32
multifamily work, relapse prevention, 357
multiple family group treatment, OPUS, 400
mutations, 50
MUTED gene/protein, 32

N-acetylaspartate (NAA), 69
National Institute for Health and Clinical Excellence (NICE),
     relapse-prevention treatment guidelines, 349
needs-adapted treatment model, maintenance medication, 353
negative symptoms, at-risk mental state, 93–4, 114
neocortical surface, structural neuroimaging, 71
Netherlands Mental Health Survey and Incidence Study, bipolar
     disorder, 226
networks, suicide prevention, 268
neuregulin (NRG1), 32, 35
   functional neuroimaging, 67
   linkage studies, 41
neuroanatomy, endophenotypes, 61
neurobiology, 5–6
   prodrome, 84
   see at-risk mental state
neurocognitive variables
   at-risk mental state, 84
   prodrome, 84
neurodevelopment
   schizophrenia, 39
   staging model, 20
neuroimaging
   functional neuroimaging, 67–8
     brain-derived neurotrophic factor, 40
     cognition activation tasks, 67
     COMT gene/protein, 67
     DISC1, 67
     dorsolateral hyperfrontality, 67
     dysbindin, 67

fronto-striatal function, 68
GAD1, 67
neuregulin, 67
normal developmental changes, 71
parietal regions, 67
prefrontal cortex, 67
schizophrenia, 40
working memory, 67
schizophrenia, 33, 40
structural neuroimaging, 68–71
amygdala, 69
anterior cingulate cortex, 70
bilateral cingulate grey matter, 70
bipolar affective disorder, 68
cortical folding patterns, 68
disease areas of overlap, 69
genetic associations, 70
grey matter density, 68
hippocampus, 69
hypothalamic–pituitary–adrenal axis, 69
longitudinal studies, 69
medial temporal structures, 69
neocortical surface, 71
paracingulate sulcus, 70
pituitary size, 69
prefrontal cortex, 71
regions of interest, 68
schizophrenia, 68
twin studies, 68
UHR, 69
voxel-based morphometry, 68
neuroleptic treatment, DUP outcome effects
use, 129
withheld, 129
neuropathology, schizophrenia, 39
neuropsychological assessment, *see* FEP assessment
neuropsychological studies, 63–5
attentional defects, 65
birth cohort studies, 63
as endophenotype, 38
longitudinal studies, 65
long-term studies, 63
olfactory identification, 65
performance IQ, 64
progressive deficits, 65
spatial working memory, 64
story recall tasks, 65
tests, 64
verbal memory deficits, 65

visual reproduction, 65
working memory, 65
see also specific studies
'neurotoxic' effects, DUP, 161
neurotropin 3 4–5 *see* brain-derived neurotrophic factor
(neurotropin 3)
New York High-Risk Study, 63
NMDA receptor, 35
non-affective psychosis
atypical antipsychotic drugs, 189
pharmacotherapy, 189, 190
non-genetic insults, 70
non-psychotic disorders, PACE UHR criteria, 87
non-psychotic state, suicidal behaviours, 258–9
Norfolk early intervention service programme
(UK), 343–5
CBT, 344
social recovery aims, 344
Nottingham Onset Schedule, DUP measurement, 130
NRG1 gene/protein *see* neuregulin

obesity, antipsychotic medication, 188, 195
offset definition, 127
olanzepine, 194
clinical trial, 98
treatment-resistant major depressive
disorder, 375
olfactory identification
at-risk mental state, 95
neuropsychological studies, 65
onset definition, 127
OPUS, 398–400, 401
assertive community treatment, 399–400
ICD-10 schizophrenia diagnosis, 398
psychoeducational family interventions, 400
psychopharmacological therapy, 400
referral to, 399
service model, 399–400
social skills training, 400
treatment evaluation, 400
ORYGEN Research Centre, EPPIC, 388
ORYGEN Youth Health, PACE UHR criteria, 87
Outreach and Support in South London (OASIS), LEO
Service, 389
outreach team LEO Service, 389, 390

P300 abnormality, DUP, 66
P300 event-related potential, psychophysiological
studies, 66

PACE (Personal Assessment and Crisis Evaluation Clinic), 115, 385
  at-risk mental state criteria, 107
  UHR criteria, 85–8
    attenuated psychotic symptoms group, 86
    brief limited intermittent psychotic symptoms group, 86
    non-psychotic disorders, 87
    operation, 86
    primary symptom-based, 86
    sequential screening, 86
    trait and state risk factor group, 86
PACT (Program of Assertive Community Treatment)
  Clubhouse model vs., 336
PANSS (Positive and Negative Syndrome Scale for Schizophrenia), 189, 212
  relapse definitions, 350
paracingulate sulcus, structural neuroimaging studies, 70
paranoia, at-risk mental state, 114
parietal regions, functional neuroimaging, 67
participant numbers, DUP outcome effects, 136
paternal age, environmental risk factors, 50, 53
patient conflicts, expressed emotion, 311
patient stressors, expressed emotion, 307
perception disturbance, SPI-A, 91
perceptual abnormalities, at-risk mental state, 114
performance IQ, neuropsychological studies, 64
performance measurement, CEPTS, 398
persecutory delusions see delusions
Personal Assessment and Crisis Evaluation Clinic see PACE
personal circumstances, treatment delay, 166–7
personal context recognition, FEP, 178
personal history see FEP assessment
personality traits
  FEP, substance misuse, 246
  psychosis, course of, 355
  relapse, 355
pharmacology
  early recovery phase see early recovery phase; medication; specific disorders
phase-specific group treatment, early recovery phase, 206
phenotypes, intermediate see endophenotypes
physical treatments, suicide prevention, 273
pituitary gland
  at-risk mental state, 97
  structural neuroimaging, 69
placement, individual, vocational interventions, 338–9
pleasurable experiences, psychosis, 111
poor functioning, at-risk mental state, 94–5

population-based association studies, 34
population screening, prodrome, 92
Positive and Negative Syndrome Scale for Schizophrenia see PANSS (Positive and Negative Syndrome Scale for Schizophrenia)
positive psychotic phenomena, at-risk mental state, 93
positron emission tomography, FEPP, 395
postpsychotic depression, 286
PPP3CC gene/protein, 32, 38
predictive validity, expressed emotion see expressed emotion
preexisting cognitive problems, EPPIC, 387
prefrontal cortex
  functional neuroimaging, 67
  structural neuroimaging, 71
premorbid adjustments
  DUP follow-up studies, 136–8, 139
  relapse, 355
premorbid functioning
  FEP, 180
  FEP, substance misuse, 244
pre-psychosis onset, treatment, seeking of, 162
prevalence (of psychosis), 3
preventative intervention, 17
Prevention and Early Intervention Program Canada, treatment delay, 164, 165
Prevention and Early Intervention Program for Psychoses (PEPP), 164, 169
Prevention through Risk Identification, Management and Education see PRIME (Prevention through Risk Identification Management and Education) study
primary care physicians see general practitioners
primary health care
  treatment, seeking of, 163–4
  treatment delay reduction, 169, 171
primary help seeking, general practitioners, 163
PRIME (Prevention through Risk Identification Management and Education) study, 109–10, 115
  CBT, 115
  Criteria for Prodromal Symptoms, 109
  FEPP, 392, 395
  Global Assessment of Functioning scale, 109
  PACE UHR criteria, 87
  SOPS scores, 109
  SIPS, 87, 109
  supportive therapy, 115
PRODH2 gene/protein, 32, 38
prodrome phase, 83–4
  attenuated symptoms, 83
  'basic symptoms,' 83, 98–100

bipolar disorders, 230–1
common symptoms, 84
emotional and personality dysfunctions 284–5
identification drawbacks, 92–3
neurobiological changes, 84
neurocognitive abnormalities, 84
non-specific features, 85
suicide, 260, 261
symptoms and signs, 83
  FEP, 180
thoughts, 98, 99
visual perception disturbance, 99
professional contact to treatment delay, DUP, 161, 164–5
professional help, public encouragement of, 149
Program of Assertive Community Treatment see PACT
progressive deficits, neuropsychological studies, 65
protective factors, suicide risk factors, 269
protocols, suicide prevention, 275
psychiatric emergencies, pharmacotherapy, 188, 191
psychiatric management, CEPTS, 396
psychiatrists, public, beliefs about, 149
psychobiological assessments, FEP, 180–5
psychoeducation
  at-risk mental state management, 118
  bipolar disorders, 234
  early recovery phase, 204
  family interventions see family interventions
  FEP, substance misuse, 251–2
  relapse prevention, 359
  treatment-resistant bipolar disorder, 376
  see also public knowledge/beliefs
psychological adjustments, incomplete recovery,
      FEP, 212
Psychological Assistance Service (PAS) (Newcastle), transition
      rates, 87
psychological interventions
  management at-risk mental state, 111–13
    evidence 111–13
  bipolar disorders see bipolar disorders
  public, beliefs about, 150, 151
  relapse prevention, 357
  suicide prevention, 273–4
psychological reactions, emotional and personality
      dysfunctions, 289–91
psychometric psychosis liability, environmental risk factors,
      49–50
psychopathological variables, see at-risk mental state
psychopharmacological therapy, OPUS, 400
psychophysiological studies, 65–6

auditoryP50 inhibition deficits, 66
  longitudinal studies, 66
  mismatch negativity, 66
  P300 event-related potential, 66
psychosis
  affective see affective psychosis
  bipolar disorders, 225
  cognitive analytic therapy, 296–7
  emotional and personality dysfunction interactions see
        emotional and personality dysfunctions
  expense of, 333
  fear of, 112
  first episode see FEP
  incidence
    EPPIC, 386
    LEO Service, 389
  non-affective see non-affective psychosis
  pleasurable experiences, 111
  recognition, 178
  stage definitions, 20
  stigma of, 112
  symptoms, borderline personality disorder, 294
psychosocial therapy
  early recovery phase see early recovery phase
  FEP, incomplete recovery, 215–16
  suicide prevention, 274
  treatment-resistant bipolar disorder, 376
psychotherapy, individual see individual
      psychotherapy
pubic knowledge/beliefs, 147–50
  first aid skills, 148–9
  of professionals, 149, 150
  professionals vs., 151–3
  recognition of psychosis, 147–8
  schizophrenia/split personality association, 149
  treatments, 150
  see also psychoeducation
public education
  treatment delay reduction, 168, 170
  see also psychoeducation
publicly funded health care loss, employment
      barriers, 332

qualifications/experience, employment barriers, 332
quality of life, early recovery phase, 208
quality of life scale, early recovery phase, 208
quantitative data analysis, DUP follow-up studies, 133
quetiapine, 194
    treatment-resistant major depressive disorder, 375

randomized controlled trials
  CBT, 205
  FEP, substance misuse, 247
  see also specific trials
RAP *see* Hillside Recognition and Prevention Program
rapid cycling bipolar disorders, 374
  treatment resistance, 374, 375–7
rate of transition, relapse rates, 351
realization of illness, suicidal behaviours, 262
rearing environment measures, gene–environment
      interactions, 49
receptive language disturbance, prodrome basic symptoms, 99
recovery phase, suicide *see* suicide
recovery rates, bipolar disorders, 229
recovery stage model, early recovery phase, 207
reduced grey matter, at-risk mental state, 97
referral criteria
  FEPP, 394–5
  OPUS, 399
relapse
  cognitive deficits, 355–6
  definition/assessment, 350–1
  expressed emotion, 306
  personality adjustment, 355
  prediction *see below*
  premorbid adjustment, 355
  prevention *see below*
  rates of, 351
  suicide, 261, 263
relapse prediction/prevention, 14, 349–64
  antipsychotic medication, 356–7
  bipolar disorders, 235
  CBT 360
  early warning signs, 355
  family interventions, 357–8
  International Early Psychosis Association, 349
  psychological interventions, 357
  recommendations, 358–9
    targeted medication regimens, 360
  risk factors, 351–6
    environment-related, 352
    expressed emotion, 353
    life events, 354
    medication discontinuance, 352, 356
    medication non-adherence, 352–3
    patient-related, 352
    stress, 354
    substance abuse, 354
  treatment guidelines, 349

Remission in Schizophrenia Working Group, 370
repetitive transcranial magnetic stimulation
  treatment-resistant major depressive disorder, 376, 377
  treatment-resistant schizophrenia, 376
resistance to treatment *see* treatment resistance
retrospective data, DUP onset, 127
reviews, suicide risk monitoring, 269
RGS4 (regulator of G-protein signalling-4), 32, 35–6
risk assessments
  FEP, 179, 181, 183–4
  suicide prevention *see* suicide prevention
risperidone, 194
  adverse effects, 110
  at-risk mental state management, 108
  clinical trial, 97
  maintenance medication, relapse, 357
  treatment-resistant major depressive disorder, 375
routine risk monitoring, suicide prevention, 269–72
Royal Park Multidiagnostic Instrument for Psychosis
      (RP-MIP), DUP measurement, 128, 132

safety behaviours, emotional and personality dysfunctions, 287
sample bias, DUP, 128
sample size, gene–environment interactions, 56
Scale of Prodromal Symptoms *see* SOPS
schizoaffective disorder, treatment resistance
  definition, 365–6
  non-pharmacological management, 375–6
  pharmacological management, 371–3
  prevalence, 367
schizophrenia
  chromosomal translocations, 36
  environmental effects, 40
  functional neuroimaging, 40
  illicit drug use, 40
  neurodevelopmental hypothesis, 39
  neuroimaging, 33, 40
  neuropathology, 39
  phenotype, 32–3
  split personality association, 149
  structural neuroimaging, 68
  suicide risk factors, 263
  treatment resistance, 365
    definition, 365–6
    non-pharmacological management, 375–6
    pharmacological management, 371–3
    prevalence, 367
Schizophrenia Patient Outcomes Research Team (PORT),
      relapse-prevention treatment guidelines, 349

Schizophrenia Proneness Instrument, Adult Version *see* SPI-A
schizotypal personality features, at-risk mental state, 93
school-based programmes, mental health literacy, 155–7
SocRATES trial, CBT, 205
screening, sequential, PACE UHR criteria, 86
search strategies, DUP follow-up studies, 130
secondary prevention, relapse prevention, 359
second-generation antipsychotic *see* antipsychotic medication drugs
second generation studies, gene–environment interactions, 54–5
selective serotonin-reuptake inhibitors (SSRIs), suicidal behaviour treatment, 273
self-experiencing disturbances, SPI-A, 91
self-focus attention, 290
self-harm, 260
self-help, suicide prevention, 274–5
self-medication hypothesis, FEP, substance misuse, 245
self-preservation, suicidal behaviours, 260
sensitivity analysis, DUP follow-up studies, 138–9, 140–1
sensory gating, at-risk mental state, 96
sequential screening, PACE UHR criteria, 86
serotonin
   breakdown product and suicide risk, 266
   selective serotonin-reuptake inhibitors, suicidal behaviour treatment, 273
services
   Factors
      FEP, 216
      incomplete recovery, 216
      suicide risk, 268–9
   reviews, suicide prevention, 275
   social services
      suicide prevention, 276
      treatment delay reduction, 169
   see also specific service models
sexual side effects, antipsychotic medication, 189, 195–6
shame, emotional and personality dysfunctions, 289–90
shared developmental pathways, emotional and personality dysfunctions, 288–9, 290
single nucleotide polymorphisms
   allele association studies, 34
   DAOA, 35
SIPS (Structured Interview for Prodromal Symptoms), PRIME study, 87, 109
sleep disturbances, at-risk mental state, 114
smoking, FEP, 243, 244, 245, 248
social anxiety, 286
   cognitive models, 290–1
   emotional and personality dysfunctions, 289–90

social assessment, FEP, 181
social contexts, expressed emotion, 311
social deficits, incomplete recovery, 208–9
social factors, suicide risk factors, 267–8
social firms, 334–5
   disadvantages, 335
   Italy, 335
   supported employment vs., 338
   UK, 335
Social Functioning Scale, treatment delays, 168
social groups, suicide prevalence, 267
social interventions, at-risk mental state management, 113
social networks, treatment delays, 166
Social Phobia and Anxiety Inventory, 208
social policies, suicide prevention, 276
social problems
   at-risk mental state, 125–45
   withdrawal, 114
social recovery aims, Norfolk Early Intervention Service, 344
social services *see* services; social services
social skills training, OPUS, 400
socioeconomic status, treatment delays, 166
SOPS (Scale of Prodromal Symptoms) scores
   scores in PRIME study, 109
Soteria Project, maintenance medication, 353
spatial working memory, neuropsychological studies, 64
SPI-A (Schizophrenia Proneness Instrument, Adult Version), 91–2
   affective–dynamic disturbances, 91
   body perception disturbance, 91
   cognitive–attentional impediments, 91
   cognitive disturbances, 91
   perception disturbance, 91
   self-experiencing disturbances, 91
staff awareness, suicide prevention, 275
staging models, 3–4, 17–27, 31
   family interventions, 316–20
   as heuristic model, 22
   neurodevelopmental framework, 20
   progress in, 18
   stage 0, 21
   stage 1a, 21, 23–4
   stage 1b, 21, 23–4
   stage 2 *see* FEP
   stage 3a, 21, 23, 24
   stage 3b, 21, 23
   stage 3c, 22, 23
   stage 4, 22, 23
standardized assessment instruments, DUP, 128–9

stepped-care, FEP, substance misuse, 249

stigma

emotional and personality dysfunctions, 289–90

psychosis, 112

story recall tasks, neuropsychological studies, 65

stress

at-risk mental state, 95

and coping paradigms, family caregiving, 315

relapse predictors/risk factors, 354

stressful life events, suicide risk factors, 267

'Stress Management' module, at-risk mental state management, 108

structural neuroimaging *see* neuroimaging, structural

Structured Interview for Prodromal Symptoms *see* SIPS

studies

DUP follow-up studies, 18–19, 130, 133, 134–5

longitudinal *see* longitudinal studies

long-term, 63

substance abuse/misuse, 11, 243–56

at-risk mental state, 95

bipolar disorder, 225, 234

CEPTS, 397

EPPIC, 389

FEP, 183

prevalence, 11

relapse predictors/risk factors, 354

schizophrenia, 40

suicide risk, 266

treatment delays, 168

see also specific drugs/substances

substance use disorder, incomplete recovery, FEP, 211

Suffolk County study, DUP, 142

suicidal behaviours, 258–60, 270

depression, 261

FEP, substance misuse, 245

fluctuating course of, 261, 262, 268

non-psychotic state, 258–9

during psychotic state, 259–60, 261

realization of illness, 262

suicide prevention, 272

suicide

EPPIC, 388

factors, 258

FEP, 183, 260

first-episode acute phase, 260–2

incidence, 257

methods chosen, 260

pre-illness, 261

prevalence

between countries, 267, 268

ethnicity, 267

social groups, 267

prevention *see* suicide prevention

prodrome phase, 260, 261

recovery phase, 261, 262

support withdrawal, 262

relapse phase, 261, 263

risk-assessment schedules, 265

risk factors

cultural factors, 267–8

family factors, 267–8

family history of, 267

protective factors, 269

schizophrenia, 263

service factors, 268–9

social factors, 267–8

stressful life events, 267

treatment factors, 268–9

wider effects of, 258

Suicide Intervention Project, 157

suicide prevention, 11–12, 257–81

biological risk markers, 266–7

early intervention effects, 258

future work, 276–7

indicated interventions, 272–5

acute risk containment, 272–3

pharmacological interventions, 273

physical treatments, 273

psychological interventions, 273–4

psychosocial interventions, 274

self-help, 274–5

suicidal factors, 272

Initial Suicide Risk Assessment and Formulation, 265–6

networks, 268

risk assessments, 263–9

critical questions, 264

previous attempts, 264

triggering events, 264

see also specific types

risk management, 269–76

selective interventions, 258–60, 269–72

routine risk monitoring, 269–72

suicide risk assessment schedules, 265

universal interventions, 269, 275–6

debriefing, 275

mental health service provision models, 275–6

protocols, 275

service reviews, 275
social policies, 276
social services, 276
staff awareness, 275
training provision, 275
supported employment, 338
clubhouse model vs., 338
social firms vs., 338
see also individual placement and support approach
supportive interventions
family interventions, 321–2
PRIME study, 115
Survival Skills Workshop, OPUS, 400
susceptibility genes, 31, 32
suspiciousness, at-risk mental state, 114
symptomatic remission, bipolar disorders, 225
Symptom Onset in Schizophrenia Inventory (SOS), DUP
measurement, 130
symptoms
FEP, substance misuse, 244
inconsistency, DUP onset, 126
symptom to professional contact delay, DUP, 161
syndromal remission, bipolar disorders, 224
Systematic Treatment of Persistent Psychosis (STOPP),
incomplete recovery therapy, 216

tardive dyskinesia
antipsychotic medication, 188, 194–5, 228
bipolar disorder, 228
targeted medication regimens, relapse prevention, 360
Texas Medication Algorithm Program, 215
thoughts in prodromal basic symptoms
blockage, 99
interference, 98
perseveration, 98
pressure, 98
timing
relapse prediction/prevention, 358
relapse prevention, 358
tobacco use, FEP, 243, 244, 245, 248
TOPP Clinic (Norway), transition rates, 87
training programmes, mental health literacy, 157
training provision, suicide prevention, 275
tranquilization, psychiatric emergencies, 193
transitional employment, clubhouse model, 335
traumatic reactions, emotional and personality dysfunctions, 289
TREAT (Treatment Resistance Early Assessment Team)
programme
EPPIC, 387

incomplete recovery, 214
suicide risk, 271
treatment, seeking of, 162–6, 170
barriers to, 164
facilitation variation, 165, 170
family actions, 163, 170
non-psychosis symptoms, 162
pre-psychosis onset, 162
primary health care advisors, 163–4
treatment adherence, FEP treatment, 184, 188, 195
Treatment and Intervention in Psychosis (TIPS) study,
153, 169
DUP, 125
success of, 170
treatment delay
access problems, 165–6
aspects of illness onset, 167–8
family history of psychosis, 168
functioning levels, 167
suddenness effects, 167
bipolar disorders *see* bipolar disorders
clinician errors, 171
demography/personal circumstances, 166–7
prediction of, 166–8
substance abuse, 168
treatment delay reduction, 8–9, 161–74
antipsychotic drug response, 185
community efforts, 168
FEP treatment, 185
primary health care, 169, 171
public education, 168, 170
social service providers, 169
treatment evaluation, OPUS, 400
treatment resistance, 14, 365–81
definitions, 365
early detection, 370–1
from treatment initiation, 370
factors, 378
FEP treatment, 202, 214
incidence, 365
major depressive disorder *see* major depressive disorder,
treatment resistance
management, 368–77
clinical effectiveness definitions, 370
intervention optimization, 368–70
non-pharmacological, 374, 375–7
pharmacological adaptations, 371–5
prevention strategies, 370
service prerequisites, 368–70

treatment resistance (cont.)
mood cycling, 366
predictors, 368, 369
prevalence, 367–8, 378
schizoaffective disorder *see* schizoaffective disorder,
treatment resistance
symptoms, 366
Treatment Resistance Early Assessment Team *see* TREAT
treatment-resistant depression, 366
triggering hallucinations, emotional and personality
dysfunctions, 288
twin studies
environmental risk factors, 49
first-generation studies, 51, 52
structural neuroimaging, 68

UCLA (University of California at Los Angeles) Aftercare
Research Program, 342–3
brokered model vs., 343
comparison group, 343
Developmental Processes in Schizophrenic Disorders
Project, 342
employment specialists, 342
full implementation, 342
Workplace Fundamentals Module, 342
UHR (ultra-high risk), 63
expressed emotion, 307–8, 309–10
intervention, 97–8
cognitive therapy, 97
supportive therapy vs., 97, 98
structural neuroimaging, 69
supportive therapy, intervention vs., 97, 98
see also at-risk mental state
ultra-high risk, *see* UHR
unemployment, effects of, 332–4
unfavourable outcome identification, FEP treatment, 189,
195–6
United Kingdom (UK)
school-based mental health literacy, 156
social firms, 335
see also specific schemes
universal interventions, suicide prevention *see* suicide
prevention
unstable ideas of reference, prodrome basic
symptoms, 99

vagus nerve stimulation, treatment-resistant major depressive
disorder, 376

Val158Met genotype, *COMT* gene, 36, 55
validity assessment, DUP follow-up studies, 132
velo-cardial facial syndrome, 36
verbal memory deficits, neuropsychological studies, 65
victimization, FEP, 183
violence, FEP, 183
visual perception disturbances, prodrome basic
symptoms, 99
visual reproduction, neuropsychological studies, 65
vocational functioning *see* work functioning
vocational interventions, 334–9
case study, 341
EPPIC, 340–1
FEP, 339–45
incomplete recovery, 212, 216
individual placement, 338–9
industrial therapy, 334
job agencies, 341
LEO Service, 390
see also clubhouse model, Norfolk Early Intervention Service,
social firms, UCLA Aftercare Research Program
voxel-based morphometry, structural neuroimaging, 68
vulnerability–stress–coping model, FEP, 179

weight gain, antipsychotic medication, 188, 195
work functioning, 13–14, 335
early recovery phase, 206–7
employment barriers, 332
employment rates, 333
historical aspects, 331
incomplete recovery therapy, 212, 216
interventions *see* vocational interventions
positive benefits, 334
type of work, 332
working memory
at-risk mental state, 95
endophenotypes, 72
functional neuroimaging, 67
neuropsychological studies, 65
Workplace Fundamentals Module, UCLA Aftercare Research
Program, 342

youth participation, EPPIC, 388

ziprasidone, 194
treatment-resistant major depressive disorder, 375
zoning system, suicide risk monitoring, 270, 271
zotepine, 194